Postgra

The Candi

Postgraduate Surgery
The candidate's guide

M. A. R. AL-FALLOUJI
LRCP & S(Ed & Glas), FRCS(Ed), FRCS(Glas), FRCSI, FICA
Research Fellow, Royal Postgraduate Medical School,
Hammersmith Hospital, London

and

M. P. McBRIEN
MS (Lond), FRCS (Eng)
Consultant Surgeon, West Suffolk and Newmarket Hospitals; Hunterian Professor,
Royal College of Surgeons of England; Lecturer and Demonstrator, St. Thomas'
Hospital and Cambridge Final FRCS Course; Clinical Teacher and Examiner in
Surgery, Cambridge School of Clinical Medicine

Foreword by L. H. Blumgart
Director, University Clinic for
Visceral and Transplantation
Surgery, Bern, Switzerland;
Formerly Professor and Director of Surgery
Royal Postgraduate Medical School

BUTTERWORTH
HEINEMANN

Butterworth-Heinemann Ltd
Linacre House, Jordan Hill, Oxford OX2 8DP

A member of the Reed Elsevier plc group

OXFORD   LONDON   BOSTON
MUNICH   NEW DELHI   SINGAPORE   SYDNEY
TOKYO   TORONTO   WELLINGTON

First published 1986
Reprinted 1988, 1989, 1990, 1992, 1993, 1994

ISBN 0 7506 0836 6

Printed and bound in Great Britain by
The Headway Press Ltd

Contents

Foreword

This volume is not intended to replace or to be a substitute for a surgical textbook. Its aim is essentially two-fold. First, to allow proper orientation of candidates towards the Fellowship examination of the Colleges of the United Kingdom and Ireland and, second, to afford guidance to candidates regarding examination skills and approaches which might lead to success in the examinations of the Colleges. The book is meant to be complementary to a surgical textbook and, more importantly, to serve as a guide for the written part of the Fellowship exam.

While there is no substitute in the Fellowship examination for knowledge gained by hard work, and for evidence of having actually been involved in relevant clinical work, this volume will help candidates, including those from abroad, who may be unfamiliar with the approach necessary to confront the examiners and defeat them on occasion.

There is nothing so distressing as to see a good candidate with adequate knowledge repeatedly fail an examination for lack of sound examination technique. This book should prove to be a valuable source of guidance for those who need it.

L. H. Blumgart
London, 1986

Preface

The FRCS has a reputation for being a difficult examination. Sound basic and updated knowledge coupled with good surgical practice and experience are essential in approaching this examination. Flexibility in substantiating your reasoning for choosing one operation rather than another and familiarity with the examination techniques (practised instinctively according to a well-planned methodical approach) are paramount.

The final FRCS is basically designed to test clinical wisdom, judgement, insight and practicality rather than an encyclopaedic knowledge. This book therefore, is not intended to replace or to be a substitute for a surgical reference textbook. It has two aims:

Part I: Surgery
Proper orientation of the candidate towards:
- Selective surgical topics (theoretical).
- Commonly presented cases (clinical).
- Popular surgical specimens (pathological).
- Commonly examined instruments, X-rays and bones (principles).
- Commonly discussed surgical procedures (operative).

Practical examples, succinct comments, reviews and discussion with the pros and cons of each approach are included (these aspects are common to all Colleges in the United Kingdom and Ireland). We present a well-balanced selection of material, with detailed discussion only when deemed essential.

Part II: Background
Familiarisation of candidates with the type of conduct, skills, techniques and approaches that have proved highly successful in the Colleges' examinations (stemming from our own experience as a candidate and an examiner). Historical background is also provided.

While we are aware of the increasing complexities of surgical approaches (e.g. there are six approaches to femoral hernia repair and many approaches to breast carcinoma management) we stress the importance of one approach (especially the one commonly used) with its substantiation. In the written part you can write about various approaches freely within the limits of the question asked but in the clinical part when you are face to face with the examiner you are very limited in your answer. You therefore have to talk from the most common to the rare and from the general to the specific and to adopt your personal surgical approach to a problem (one operation). Your presentation of the case history, methodical examination and personality all play a definite role in passing the FRCS.

This book is intended to serve not only as an essential theoretical and clinical review but also as a practical guide to the various examination parts in the Colleges. We believe that our combined effort, as an examiner (M. P. McBrien) and as a candidate and organiser of the clinical part of the final FRCS Edinburgh (M. Al-Fallouji) has enabled us to produce a comprehensive and unique guide.

In order to make the volume as compact as possible and to avoid distracting the reader from essential points, we have kept textual references to a minimum. Where important relevant statistics (e.g. 5 year survival rates in treated cancer cases) have been included in studies referred to, the source for these can be found in the appropriate section of the References and Further Reading. Where names and dates are mentioned (e.g. Cuschieri, 1984), these are not usually listed individually in the References and Further Reading, but can be found in one of the main sources listed in the appropriate section.

The book is written primarily for doctors preparing for their final FRCS. However, since the FRCS is historically reputed to be the first examination for surgical qualification and is therefore the prototype for most subsequent examinations, it should also be of benefit to all surgeons sitting similar high postgraduate surgical diplomas such as the Australian, Canadian and South African Fellowships as well as the American and Arabian Boards in Surgery. We feel that there is a great need for such a book not only because it will provide a pan British-Irish comprehensive course condensed in one volume but also because all written books in this field (however excellent they are) represent only one fraction of the final FRCS (written part only) which is probably suitable to one College but not another.

We also believe that examples and illustrated discussions, together with our evaluation of the 'causes of failure' and comments on 'what to read' and 'what to do', based on our experience and the experience of our colleagues, are more important than mere listing or enumeration of topics.

It is common sense, selective reading, proper orientation and clinical approaches together with

the digestion and crystallisation of essential facts
that really prove to be the safe ship in the sea of
examination bewilderment in which the drowning
rate is 80%.

M. A. R. Al-Fallouji
M. P. McBrien
London, 1986

Acknowledgements

We wish to thank the Presidents of the Royal Colleges of Surgeons of England, Edinburgh, Glasgow and Ireland for their kind cooperation in providing the historical data of the Royal Colleges. We are especially grateful to Sir James Fraser (President, Royal College of Surgeons, Edinburgh) and Sir Geoffrey Slaney (President, Royal College of Surgeons, England) for their kind permission to publish samples of the written examination papers. We acknowledge the technical skill and expertise of the Medical Illustration Department of Ipswich Hospital (East Anglia) and Bridge of Earn Hospital (Tayside, Scotland).

We should like to thank all those who helped us with producing this book whether candidates or consultants and in particular Mr C. B. Wood (Consultant Surgeon, Hammersmith Hospital), Mr R. E. C. Collins, (Consultant Surgeon, Kent and Canterbury Hospital), Dr C. Swan (Consultant Physician, Stoke-on-Trent), the British Society of Gastroenterology, Mr S. Meehan, Mr A. Irving (Senior Registrars, University of Dundee, now Consultant Surgeons), Dr S. Field, (Consultant Radiologist, Canterbury and Thanet District) and Mr K. N. Khalid (Registrar in Plastic Surgery, Wexham Park Hospital), who have kindly allowed us to benefit from their extensive experience both in surgery and the examination techniques.

We are indebted to Dr Richard Barling (Editorial Director, Heinemann Medical) for his continuous encouragement during the preparation of this book. Our special thanks go to Mrs Valerie Pringle for enduring the tedious job of typing the manuscript.

Contributors

Although the authors took the responsibility of writing most of the book, many topics were kindly contributed (written and/or reviewed) by our colleagues as indicated below.

N. K. Al-Quisi DA, FFARCS(Eng) Senior Registrar, Clinical Anaesthesia, Royal Victoria Hospital, Belfast (Postoperative analgesia).

S. J. Becker FRCS(Ed) Surgical Registrar, Wakefield Hospitals, W. Yorkshire (Critical review of abdominal stoma, common surgical conditions affecting the hip joint, Medical imaging and interventional radiology).

J. S. G. Blair OBE, ChM, FRCS(Ed) Senior Consultant Surgeon, Examiner in Final FRCS(Ed) and Senior Lecturer in Surgery (University of Dundee), Perth Royal Infirmary, Scotland (Urinary diversion procedures and part of Clinical radiology).

M. F. Butler FRCS(Eng) Senior Consultant Surgeon, Thanet General Hospital, Margate, Kent (Peripheral vascular disease, aortic aneurysm surgery, aortic bypass and arterial embolectomy).

P. W. Davis FRCS(Eng) Consultant Surgeon, Barnet General Hospital, Herts (Solitary thyroid nodule and Cervical swellings examination).

J. A. K. Meikle FRCP, FRCR Consultant Radiologist and Postgraduate Clinical Tutor, Perth Royal Infirmary, Scotland (part of Clinical radiology).

K. Sikora PhD, MRCP, FRCR Director of Ludwig Institute for Cancer Research MRC, Addenbrooke's Hospital, Cambridge (Introduction to clinical oncology, Radiotherapy, Chemotherapy, Tumour markers and cancer screening in surgery).

R. E. B. Tagart ChM, FRCS(Eng) Senior Consultant Surgeon to Newmarket and West Suffolk Hospitals (East Anglia), Hunterian Professor (Principles in colonic surgery).

PART I

Surgery

SECTION 1
The Written Examination

Introduction

The written papers are an essential part of the examination. *You have to pass* the written and the clinical parts *individually* in order to pass the final FRCS. (Borderline marking in some parts could be compensated for by others.) Some people know enough about the subject but are unable to organise their thoughts and write clearly within the time available. Others can write fluently but often do not answer the question asked, through misinterpretation. The following points and hints provide a useful guide on writing answers.

Planning

1. Read the instructions at the top of the paper carefully, and divide the time equally between the questions, allowing 10 minutes for revision. Candidates often answer too many or too few questions, or leave no time for the last one. *The marking system makes it impossible to recover from an unanswered question or even to compensate for a half answered question.*
2. Read the question through several times slowly, noting exactly what is asked for and underline the key words. *The examiners take great care in phrasing each question, but candidates often answer them entirely differently.*
3. Spend about 5 minutes (for planning), jotting down all your relevant thoughts and notes on the scrap paper provided and referring back to the question from time to time.
4. Rearrange and refine your ideas in a logical sequential practical order (for clarity) with common things first, resisting the temptation to dwell on rarities, and avoid repetition. All clinical answers are best considered under the headings:

History   *Examination*   *Special tests*

(History and physical examination are clinical investigation; special tests are mainly laboratory, radiological and other investigations.)

Layout (introduction and body)

The capacity to earn marks is highest at the start of an answer and you should therefore impress the examiner by your introduction. It is easy to get bogged down here, and if you are not sure where to start always revert to the basic principles.

The following hints are helpful.
1. Imagine that you are writing for a tired, bored examiner, who only wants to see if you are fit to become a safe surgeon.
2. Examiners get their first impression of an answer from its physical appearance and the opening of your introduction, so make your answer *legible and concise* (legibility pleases the examiner and conciseness saves your time in writing).
3. Use well-spaced, underlined, and numbered headings and subheadings and start a new paragraph for each new idea you wish to record. (Leave the page margin free and avoid crowding.)
4. Illustrate your answer wherever necessary. Good figures and simple line diagrams are an extra bonus and facilitate interpretation of the answer.
5. Avoid jargon (i.e. unintelligible words and debased language) and unfamiliar incorrect abused terms. Short and common phrases with basic simple English are best.
6. Avoid lists (without further explanation and elaboration).

Revision

Spend about 10 minutes on reading over what has been written for punctuation, correct spelling, sequence of phrases and checking the illustrations.

Special terms

The use of some of the terms used in examination questions needs to be explained.

Describe   Write in details. Usually forms an introduction to a question involving a pathological process and commonly leads to a second part about management (each part of the question should be allotted equal time).

Give an account of Give a comprehensive account of that particular condition including: incidence; pathology; aetiology; symptoms and signs; and treatment.

Discuss Select the most important and controversial aspects of the subject (compare and contrast) and discuss pros and cons; if you are in favour of a particular feature you must give the reasons clearly.

Symptomatology
Clinical findings } Symptoms and signs.

Diagnosis How would you prove what it is? Anatomically—what structure is involved? Pathologically—what is wrong with it? The answer is considered under the headings: *History Examination Special tests.* Differential diagnosis is only referred to incidentally.

Differential diagnosis What else could it be and how would you exclude the other possibilities? This usually calls for a list of the various alternatives that might cause the disease or symptom, with notes on the means of excluding them, by: *History Examination Special tests.* The various possibilities may be thought of in the following way.
● Anatomical structures
● The pathological conditions (e.g. swelling): congenital or acquired
— Congenital (since birth ± family history)
— Traumatic (history)
— Inflammatory
  Acute (days): infective (bacterial, viral, parasitic)
  Subacute (weeks)
  Chronic (months): non-specific or specific (leprosy, tuberculosis, syphilis, actinomycosis)
— Neoplastic (months): benign or malignant
— Allergic (minutes)
— Miscellaneous (metabolic, vascular, rheumatic)

Pathology One's first thought is 'What on earth can I write about for 55 minutes?' but this topic includes:
  Incidence (age, sex, race, geography)
  All relevant *investigations* that can be done by the department of clinical pathology
  Natural history of the disease (including aetiology, pathogenesis, course, spread and final outcome)

Pathological physiology (complications and prognosis).
Morbid anatomy (macroscopy)
Histology (microscopy)

Pathogenesis Underlying mechanisms (of causation and clinical presentation), including predisposing factors (and in cancers, the precancerous conditions).

Aetiology Causes

Treatment This calls for a technical account of the various methods of treatment of the condition and the indications for each:
  Prophylaxis
  Non-operative conservative measures
  Operative measures
  Rehabilitation

Operation In describing an operation, it is convenient to use the headings:
  Preoperative preparation
  Anaesthetic
  Position
  Skin preparation, draping (special draping, e.g. thyroid surgery should be mentioned)
  Access (including incision)
  Procedure
  Postoperative instruction (if any)

Management This describes the handling of the patient from the first presentation in casualty or Outpatients to his return to normal health (i.e. diagnosis and treatment), including rehabilitation and follow-up. Thus the field is large and *the review correspondingly superficial.* If the question concerns a symptom (e.g. diarrhoea) the diagnostic procedures must be described, but if it concerns a diagnosis (e.g. carcinoma of the rectum) this may be assumed to have been established already.

Final points

Write clearly and tidily (erase or delete your mistakes unambiguously) and do not abbreviate.

If your handwriting is poor, print your answers (preferably in capital letters) and save your time by writing the basic principles in a concise, summarised manner. Use a good quality biro (fine point) or fountain pen (with a good nib such as an italic nib). Black ink is preferable. It is also useful to have various coloured pens for illustration purposes whenever necessary. Pack everything in a small case—you may also place your admission card in the case so that you will not forget it.

1.1. Shock

Shock is a clinical syndrome manifested by (in addition to apprehension and irritability) changes in: blood pressure and pulse rate—indicative of cardiac output; skin temperature and colour—indicative of peripheral resistance; state of venous filling and colour of nail beds—indicative of blood flow; and urinary output—indicative of tissue perfusion. The feature that appears to be common to all types of shock is inadequate tissue perfusion. The cardiac output may be inadequate because the heart is damaged or the volume of circulating blood may be less than the capacity of the circulation either because the blood volume is reduced or the capacity is increased.

On this basis, three general types of shock can be delineated (Table 1).

HYPOVOLAEMIC SHOCK

Hypovolaemic shock is also called 'cold shock' and is manifested typically by hypotension, rapid thready pulse, cold, pale, clammy skin, intense thirst, rapid respiration, restlessness and reduced CVP. This type includes traumatic shock, crush syndrome, surgical shock, wound shock and burn shock. The fluid lost in hypovolaemic shock is one of the following.

Blood

- Externally—haemorrhage and gastrointestinal bleeding.
- Internally into the tissues—fractures; pancreatitis; haemothorax; haemoperitoneum; ruptured spleen; ectopic gestation.

Table 1. Differentiation of major shock states

	Hypovolaemic	Septic	Cardiogenic
Place of shock	Street (rarely hospital)	Hospital	Home
Triggering factor	RTA (or cold operation)	Peritonitis or emergency operation	Exercise
Presentation	Bleeding	Fever and rigor	Chest pain
History	? Alcoholic intake (in RTA)	Steroid or insulin (diabetes)	Glyceryl trinitrate (Angised; no external trauma)
Appearance of limbs	Cold/pale	Warm → Pink / Cyanosis	Cold/cyanosis
Other remarks	Rarely pure. Usually with element of septicaemia	Jaundice and splenomegaly Element of hypovolaemia	Basal crepitation (bilateral); 3rd heart sound ± arrhythmia
CVP	Decreased	Increased or decreased	Increased
Special investigation	PCV, Hb, Blood Group and crossmatch	Peripheral smear (toxic granulation in WBC and Dohle bodies in RBC), Blood culture, gas chromatography, limulus test	ECG may show myocardial infarction
Basic treatment	Fluid replacement Arrest bleeding	Antibiotics Blood Steroid Surgical drainage	Intropic drug, e.g. dopamine ? Intra-aortic balloon

RTA = road traffic accident; CVP = central venous pressure; PCV = packed cell volume (haematocrit); Hb = haemoglobin; WBC = white blood cells; RBC = red blood cells

Plasma

- Burns—major problem.
- Inflammation—minor problem, i.e. the exudate.

Extracellular fluid

Loss of extracellular fluid occurs as a consequence of:

- Deviation of normal exchange mechanisms at transcellular level. These losses include: gastrointestinal losses via vomiting (as in pyloric stenosis and intestinal obstruction) and fistulae; and renal losses via urine (as in diabetes mellitus, diabetes insipidus and excessive use of diuretics).
- Increased extracellular fluid loss along a normal pathway as in excessive sweating—insensible water loss without replacement.
- The 'third space phenomenon':
  —Increased capillary permeability as in an inflamed area.
  —Loss of biochemical integrity of cell membrane (due to hypoxia) which increases the level of cellular sodium and decreases the level of cellular potassium. This is presumably related to increased permeability of cell membrane or damage to the sodium/potassium pump mechanism. The effective extracellular fluid volume is thus reduced.

CARDIOGENIC SHOCK

This type of shock is caused by failure of the heart pump action, which takes two forms.

Pump failure proper The commonest cause is sudden myocardial infarction; other less common causes are arrhythmia (as in electrocution), severe congestive heart failure with low cardiac output, following open heart surgery, and acute septal perforation.

Mechanical vascular obstruction as in massive pulmonary embolus, tension pneumothorax, cardiac tamponade, dissecting aortic aneurysm, intracardiac lesions (e.g. ball valve thrombus, atrial myxoma), regurgitation caused by a ruptured cusp, papillary muscle dysfunction and valve damage. The picture of pulmonary embolism is well known. Effects vary from immediate death to the almost symptomless and late development of cor pulmonale.

The symptoms of cardiogenic shock are those of shock plus congestion of the lungs and viscera due to failure of the heart to pump out all the venous blood returned to it and is therefore called 'congestive shock'. It occurs in 10% of myocardial infarction patients (when at least 45% of the left ventricular myocardium has been damaged).

Cardiogenic shock is differentiated from hypovolaemic shock by:

- No history and no signs of blood loss.
- Raised rather than lowered CVP.
- ECG evidence.

LOW RESISTANCE SHOCK

Includes a number of entities in which the circulatory volume is normal while the capacity of the circulation is increased by massive vasodilation; it is therefore called 'warm shock'.

Vasovagal syncope or fainting (neurogenic shock)

Occurs in response to strong emotion, such as overwhelming fear and grief. Also seen in spinal cord injury, in drug-induced shock (anaesthesia, ganglion-blockers and other antihypertensive drugs, overdose of barbiturates, glutethimide, phenothiazines) and in orthostatic hypotension (primary autonomic insufficiency and peripheral neuropathies). Valsalva's manoeuvre occurring during defaecation, vomiting or labour may reduce the venous return to the heart and produce fainting. Micturition syncope due to the reflex bradycardia induced by voiding, carotid sinus syncope due to tight collars, cough syncope and effort syncope are all types of fainting. Severe pain (e.g. a blow on the testes can also cause fainting). The physiological chain of events in neurogenic shock is: adrenaline secretion—muscular vasodilation—bradycardia—cerebral hypoxia—fainting.

Septic shock

Due to endotoxaemia (endotoxin is a complex lipopolysaccharide bound to cell wall protein of dead microorganisms) rather than bacteraemia (transient bacteraemia, invariably of no consequence, is a common event in minor surgical procedures such as urinary catheterisation, sigmoidoscopy and biopsy, percutaneous liver biopsy and even barium enema).

Exposure of mammalian cells to endotoxin results in cell injury by several mechanisms:

- Direct cell membrane damage by endotoxin.

- Extracellular release of lysosomal enzymes from leucocytes.
- Activation of the complement cascade.
- Metabolic injury due to tissue anoxia.

The majority of patients with septic shock become infected while in hospital.

Surgical causes

Septic shock occurs in strangulated intestine (strangulated hernia, mesenteric thrombosis) or peritonitis, after gas gangrene and often following operations on the gastrointestinal tract especially the large bowel and rectum or genitourinary tract, particularly when surgery is performed under emergency or semi-elective conditions. Patients with major trauma, burns and transplantations are more susceptible.

Septic shock may also result from manipulation or instrumentation in the presence of obstruction of the urinary tract (e.g. cystoscopy and catheterisation), gastrointestinal tract (e.g. oesophagogastroduodenoscopy and ERCP) or genital tract (e.g. septic abortion after retained placenta; and following the birth of premature and full-term infants).

Parenteral feeding and blood transfusion are sometimes complicated by septic shock.

Non-surgical causes

These causes include pneumonia, endocarditis, meningitis and dermatological infections as well as hospital infection due to misuse and overuse of antibiotics. Advanced age, diabetes, malnutrition, uraemia, malignancy, immunological defects or treatment with chemotherapeutic and corticosteroid drugs (immunosuppression) are risk factors and common associated findings.

The responsible bacteria in order of frequency are: *Escherichia coli*, Proteus species, *Pseudomonas aeroginosa*, Klebsiella, *Bacteroides fragilis*, *Clostridium perfringens*.

The clinical features of infection, e.g. fever, tachycardia, hyperventilation (respiratory alkalosis) and warm extremities (dry, pink or suffused), together with a degree of hypotension, low peripheral resistance, and increased CVP, cardiac index and pulse rate predominate in the early stages (the hyperdynamic phase). Later features are cyanosis, vasoconstriction and increased peripheral resistance, oliguria and confusion with more marked degrees of hypotension as well as decreased CVP and cardiac index. This hypodynamic phase is more common than the hyperdynamic phase.

In the hyperdynamic phase cardiac output is usually high but nevertheless still inadequate to satisfy the metabolic requirements. Also, maldistribution of blood alone (due to constriction, dilatation, shunting) can be sufficient to produce shock even in the presence of high cardiac output and arterial blood pressure.

Jaundice, minor splenic enlargement, septicaemic rash or splinter haemorrhages under the nails are valuable confirmatory signs of toxaemia but their absence does not exclude septicaemia.

Hypovolaemia is almost invariably present in septic shock because of:
- Inadequate fluid intake postoperatively.
- Pyrexia.
- Hyperventilation.
- Gastrointestinal bleeding due to stress ulceration occurring in up to 15% of cases.
- Bleeding diathesis due to thrombocytopenia resulting from:
    - Disseminated intravascular coagulation.
    - Haemodilution.
    - Direct action of endotoxin on platelets.
    - Indirect action via immune complexes.

The treatment of a patient suffering from shock associated with sepsis can be summarised as follows. (*see also* Table 1).

1. Assess adequacy of ventilation. Give oxygen and, if necessary, use mechanical ventilation (monitor blood gases).
2. Assess electrolyte and acid-base status. Insert a CVP line. Restore circulating blood volume and, if possible, correct metabolic imbalance.
3. Insert urinary catheter and assess renal function. Be prepared to treat acute renal failure.
4. Take blood and other cultures. Start appropriate antibiotic therapy. Give antibiotics intravenously. Consider hyperbaric oxygen therapy.
5. Assess haematological status. Should there be evidence of disseminated intravascular coagulation treat accordingly. Use fresh frozen plasma, check fibrinogen level—if this falls or there is bleeding from multiple sites then give heparin 100 units/kg immediately followed by 10 units/kg hourly. If bleeding does not stop use platelets especially when platelet count is less than 40 000/mm^3.
6. Should there be a poor response to (2) and (4), give massive doses of methylprednisolone sodium succinate intravenously.
7. Consider digitalis.
8. Should the condition remain critical consider monitoring cardiac output and the use of drugs affecting the haemodynamic state.
9. Consider surgery.

Anaphylactic shock

This is a rapidly developing, severe allergic reaction that sometimes occurs when a sensitised individual is exposed to antigen, e.g. from injection of anti-tetanus serum or penicillin i.m., injection of iodine contrast medium i.v., or ruptured hydatid cyst fluid intraperitoneally.

The resultant Ag-Ab reaction releases large amounts of histamine leading to increased capillary permeability and widespread dilatation of arterioles and capillaries (splanchnic pooling) with a consequent fall in venous return and cardiac output. It is also associated with bronchospasm. It is treated with 0.5 ml of 1:10 000 adrenaline subcutaneously, i.v. steroids and antihistamine.

Endocrine failure (including Addison's disease and myxoedema)

Adrenocortical shock is mixed septic and haemorrhagic shock following the Waterhouse–Friderichsen syndrome (named after Danish and British physicians) in which intramedullary adrenal haemorrhage increases shock in children suffering from overwhelming infection. Adrenals treated with steroid drugs may be inhibited for up to 2 years after stopping treatment and then may become shocked following minor trauma or operations. The longer the duration of therapy the slower must be the withdrawal. Adrenocortical shock may occur following steroid withdrawal even without sepsis or bleeding. It is treated by prevention through adequate steroid administration i.m. or i.v. in the perioperative period then tailing it down.

1.2. Pain in Surgery

INTRODUCTION

Pain is a subjective experience usually due to an underlying organic lesion. It varies from person to person and within any given individual as a result of the interplay of biological, psychological and environmental factors. There are three basic theories about pain mechanisms.

Specificity theory Maintains that pain is a specific stimulus received by special receptors (free nerve endings discovered by Von Frey, different from touch discovered by Meissner, pressure by Pacini, heat by Ruffini and cold by Krause) that make special connections in the CNS. Pain travels along thick, myelinated, fast-conducting A fibres and along thin, unmyelinated, slow-conducting C fibres, producing respectively immediate short and delayed persistent responses. These fibres synapse with the neurons of the substantia gelatinosa in the dorsal horn of the spinal cord. The second-order neurons cross the midline in the white commissure and ascend in the lateral spinothalamic tract to reach the posterolateral ventral nucleus of the thalamus, whence they are relayed via third-order neurons to the postcentral gyrus of the cerebral cortex.

Pattern theory Suggests that afferent nerves carry all kinds of impulses impartially and that the patterns of impulses are programmed in the spinal cord and interpreted by the brain. Certain spatiotemporal patterns are perceived as pain after intense stimulation of non-specific receptors.

Modulation (gate) theory Melzack Wall (1965) proposed the existence of input control in the substantia gelatinosa, which operates as a gate (Fig. 1). Persistent intense high threshold impulses carried by the C fibres (perceived as severe pain) can be blocked if a 'gate mechanism' in the dorsal horn is first closed by faster low-threshold pain impulses carried by A fibres or by modifying impulses descending from the brain, e.g. initiated by stress or emotion. This theory explained 'combat analgesia': a soldier in the heat of battle can be oblivious to the pain from a serious wound. It also explains intractable post-herpetic neuralgia where selective degeneration of the peripheral thick A fibres is said to leave the gate open to the more persistent C fibre impulses. The gate theory can also explain why pain is relieved (after a painful blow) by rubbing the skin, topical application of counter-irritants (such as liniments), transcutaneous nerve stimulation with an electrode applied to the trigger zone (dermatome), or needles inserted into the meridians in acupuncture. In all these situations peripheral A fibres are stimulated, thus closing the gate against the C fibres.

Enkephalins and endorphins

These represent the brain's own opiates (or endogenous naturally occurring morphines) and were discovered in the 1970s. Enkephalins are penta-peptides and it was found that methionine, or met-

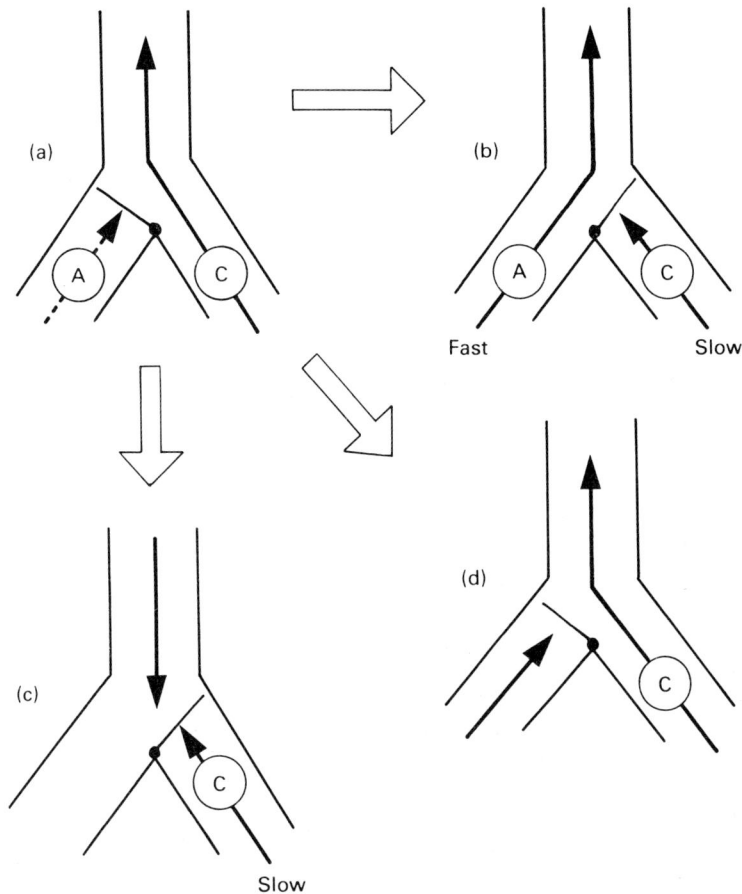

Fig. 1 Gate theory of pain. (a) Persistent severe pain via C fibres after cessation of A fibre impulses. (b) Acupuncture and transcutaneous nerve stimulation. (c) Stress, emotion and stored experience (combat analgesia). (d) Postherpetic neuralgia (degeneration of A fibres)

enkephalin, consisted of the same amino acid sequence as the terminal five amino acids of a much larger peptide, β-lipotrophin. Furthermore, the terminal 31 amino acids of β-lipotrophin are called β-endorphin. It is now certain that the lipotrophin-related peptides and ACTH have a common precursor, 'pro-opiocortin', which codes for the formation of β-endorphin, met- and leu-enkephalins via a special messenger RNA. These opiate peptides are hydrolysed by enkephalinase enzyme, and like morphine their effects are antagonised by naloxone. Enkephalins are distributed in the limbic system, thalamus and substantia gelatinosa as well as in the gastrointestinal tract and adrenal medulla. Endorphin distribution is more restricted, being found abundantly in the pituitary which is devoid of enkephalin. These natural peptides together with their synthetic analogues as well as most narcotic analgesics (notably opiate alkaloids) occupy special receptors (opioid receptors) in the CNS of which μ, κ, σ, δ, and ε were found, the last being specific for β-endorphin only. These endogenous opiates act as neurotransmitters. Morphine and enkephalins inhibit noradrenergic firing of locus ceruleus. Withdrawal of opiates leads to massive neuronal discharges which are associated with the 'opiate abstinence syndrome'. Clonidine acting as an α_2 agonist at these neurons slows the discharge and reverses or prevents the withdrawal syndrome. It was also found that acupuncture-induced analgesia is reversed by naloxone (narcotic antagonist) and conversely, the analgesia is potentiated by giving the enkephalinase-inhibitor D-phenylalanine with electroacupuncture; this suggests that acupuncture is associated with the release of enkephalins and endorphins into CSF. These opiates act only intrathecally or intraventricularly since they cannot cross the blood–brain barrier by parenteral administration. Disappointingly all these opiate peptides produce tolerance and dependence. Their role in psychiatric disorders is not proven yet and it is uncertain whether they have any endocrine function. Therefore, their actual therapeutic use is still not fully explored.

Types of pain

Pain itself can be acute or chronic. *Acute pain* (e.g. postoperative pain, myocardial infarction and colics, whether intestinal, ureteric or biliary) is commonly of less than 1 month's duration and is due to a known and treatable cause. The pain may cause anxiety but treatment is logical and effective with good results and normal life expectancy. *Chronic pain*, on the other hand, is comparatively uncommon (often neglected), of several months' duration and due to an uncertain cause that is difficult to treat, leading to depression. Treatment is empirical, often only partly effective with sometimes disappointing results and possibly short life expectancy (as in malignancy). The causes of chronic pain include:

Traumatic
- Neuromuscular injuries (e.g. neuroma and tendon injuries).
- Fractures.
- Painful scars.
- Amputation stump and phantom pain.

Degenerative
- Disc protrusion, sciatica and low back pain.
- Osteoarthritis.
- Ankylosing spondylitis and Paget's disease.

Inflammatory
- Post-herpetic neuralgia.
- Chronic peptic ulcer.
- Chronic pancreatitis.

Neoplastic

Vascular
- Lower limb ischaemia.
- Sympathetic dystrophy syndrome (Sudeck's atrophy and shoulder—hand syndrome).
- Raynaud's disease.

Neurological
- Nerve lesions, entrapment and neuralgias.

- Trigeminal (facial) neuralgia.
- Headache (migraine).
- Causalgia.

GENERAL PRINCIPLES OF MANAGEMENT

The management of pain involves three aspects: physical, emotional and rational.

The physical aspect

Removal of noxious stimuli

For example, partial gastrectomy to remove hydrochloric acid content in cases of chronic peptic ulcer, or removal of mechanical obstruction in nerve entrapment.

Prevention of neural integration of pain

Natural mechanisms

By counterstimulation which includes rubbing, manipulation, percussion, heating, cooling, acupuncture, electrical stimulation and application of counter-irritants.

Analgesic drugs

The mild non-narcotic analgesics act peripherally by inhibiting prostaglandin synthesis while the narcotics exert their effect on opiate receptors in the CNS. For mild pain—aspirin (may cause gastrointestinal bleeding) or paracetamol. For moderate pain—codeine, dihydrocodeine (may cause constipation), pentazocine (causes dysphoria) and dextropropoxyphene in combination with paracetamol (Distalgesic) is preferred (banned in USA). Pyrazole and indole derivatives have strong anti-inflammatory action and are indicated in chronic painful inflammatory conditions of the joints. As gastric ulcers and serious blood disorders are side-effects, their use is monitored with laboratory tests. Mefenamic acid causes less gastrointestinal bleeding but can cause diarrhoea. For severe and intractable pain, potent analgesics (narcotics) should be considered. Narcotic analgesics fall within the spectrum between pure agonists such as fentanyl and pure antagonists such as naloxone. The following are clinical remarks about some of them.

Morphine Is the most commonly used—sets the standard by which all the others are judged. It produces CNS depression (which promotes analgesia, tranquillisation, sleep, respiratory depression and suppression of cough) as well as excitation (vomiting, anxiety and restlessness). It acts directly on smooth muscles, increasing sphincteric tone and decreasing peristalsis (hence constipation, increase in intrabiliary and pancreatic pressure) and is therefore contraindicated in colonic diverticular disease, irritable colon, pancreatitis and biliary colic (unless preceded by an antispasmodic such as atropine and anticholinergic drugs). It may cause euphoria and addiction. Dose 10–20 mg i.m., i.v. or orally.

Diamorphine (heroin) More powerful analgesic than morphine with more euphoria and less sedation; thus associated with considerable risk of addiction. Its duration of action is half that of morphine, i.e. 2 h, but is otherwise similar to morphine. Dose 5–10 mg i.m. or i.v. on regular basis in terminal care cases.

Methadone Is effective orally with fewer side-effects; thus used in ambulant patients with intractable pain. It does not cause euphoria and is less addictive. Indeed, morphine addiction is treated by gradual replacement with high doses of methadone which can be terminated eventually without causing morphine withdrawal symptoms. Dose 5–10 mg orally or i.m. *Dextromoramide* and *dipipanone* are similarly used orally for ambulant patients with severe chronic pain.

Pethidine Is not well absorbed from the gastrointestinal tract. It has short action, causes dry mouth, tachycardia (atropine-like action), hypotension and dysphoria, and it is painful on injection. Phenoperidine and fentanyl similarly have no place in the treatment of chronic pain but are used in general anaesthesia and intensive postoperative cases. Dose 50–100 mg i.m. or i.v.

Pentazocine (Fortral) Shorter in duration, it causes slight respiratory depression but recently it was found that the CO_2 response curve can be depressed as much by pentazocine 60 mg/70 kg as by morphine 10 mg/70 kg. There appears to be a ceiling effect in the anaesthetic action so that increasing the dose produces no further increase in analgesia. Gastric absorption is good but slow. It causes dysphoria and hallucination with less sedation. Pentazocine is less addictive and has minimal effects on smooth muscle (can therefore be given in irritable colon, diverticular disease, biliary and pancreatic disease). It is a narcotic antagonist and 1 mg/kg has been used to reverse respiratory depression produced by fentanyl leaving adequate analgesia for a prolonged period. Dose 30–60 mg orally, i.m. or i.v.

Buprenorphine (Temgesic) Has powerful agonist and partial antagonist actions with low addiction. There is a ceiling effect for its respiratory depression which could well be the case for its analgesic action. Vomiting is troublesome especially with ambulant patients. The prolonged action (twice that of morphine), availability of the sublingual route and absence of serious side-effects (except for vomiting) makes this drug a considerable advance in the treatment of postoperative pain. Dose 0.3–0.4 mg sublingually.

Butorphanol Is a narcotic antagonist analgesic. It is seven times as potent as morphine and 40–50 times as potent as pethidine and has a similar duration of action. Ceiling effect in its respiratory depression has been reported. Successfully used postoperatively but drowsiness is a common side-effect.

Meptazinol Narcotic antagonist analgesic with potency equal to pethidine in postoperative patients. It produces minimal respiratory depression and sedation.

Nefopam Antihistamine derivative with less anticholinergic and antihistaminic activity. Its nonnarcotic analgesic potency in postoperative pain is in the region of 20 mg nefopam equivalent to 7.5 mg morphine (i.m.) Intravenous injection has ceiling analgesic effect at about 60 mg so that increasing the dose will only increase its side-effects (tachycardia, nausea, sweating and restlessness).

Nerve blocks

Using local anaesthetics can be diagnostic (pain relief confirms the selected responsible nerve pathway), prognostic (if no pain relief, no need for neurolytic block as the case is difficult to treat), palliative, and even curative. This can be performed either directly via a needle or for prolonged use via a catheter. Because local anaesthetics selectively affect amyelinated and thin myelinated fibres, motor function is spared. Blocking sites are:

Local infiltration to: tender spots
trigger areas.

Regional blocks to: brachial plexus
                       cranial nerves
                       peripheral nerves
                       (i.v. and tourniquet—
                       Bier's block).
Sympathetic blocks to: stellate ganglion
                       lumbar ganglion
                       coeliac plexus.
Axial blocks to: paravertebral somatic
                       nerves (epidural or
                       intrathecal).

Note: epidural and intrathecal routes can be used for narcotic injection to block pain receptors only (pure analgesia) and for local anaesthetics to block sensory (anaesthesia) and/or motor fibres depending on injected dose.

Destructive blocks

Chemical blocks

Using intrathecal injection of alcohol or phenol (in glycerine) as neurolytic agents (extrathecal injection should not be used). Intrathecal injection of hypertonic or iced saline is also used. They take effect in 2–5 days and pain relief lasts for 1–3 months. These blocks should bathe only the required dorsal roots with the agent and must be kept away from ventral roots to avoid motor loss (chemical posterior rhizotomy). Sympathetic ganglia blocks using alcohol or phenol can also be used (chemical sympathectomy).

Physical means

Barbotage is repeated (15 ×) aspiration and replacement of CSF via a wide-bore needle. It damages the dorsal root and offers pain relief for up to 3 months in cancer cases. Cooling CSF before replacement may be painful and requires general anaesthesia.

Neurosurgery

Usually needs general anaesthesia. Possible procedures are the following.
- Nerve section or surgical posterior rhizotomy.
- Anterolateral cordotomy on the side opposite the pain. If it is done bilaterally bladder and bowel problems occur and if done bilaterally at the cervical level then the patient may die of sleep apnoea (Ondine's curse).
- Radiofrequency percutaneous cervical cordotomy selectively destroys the lateral spinothalamic tract. It should be done unilaterally.
- Dorsal column stimulation with an electrode implanted intrathecally at laminectomy.
- Stereotactic thalamotomy.
- Cingulotomy.
- Prefrontal leucotomy.
- Pituitary ablation (under image intensifier taking 30 min) by transethmoidal surgery or transnasal radioactive pellets, implantation or alcohol injection or cryoprobe ablation can relieve pain of advanced cancer with secondary deposits (whether hormone-dependent, like breast and prostatic carcinomas, or not).

Other modalities

- Specific treatment of underlying disease, e.g. local resection of tumour.
- Endocrine therapy, e.g. calcitonin in Paget's disease, hormones in breast and prostatic carcinomas.
- Radiotherapy, e.g. for bony deposits.
- Chemotherapy, e.g. for Hodgkin's lymphoma.
- Cryosurgery, e.g. in palliation of residual or recurrent malignancy of the oral cavity.
- In trigeminal neuralgia, where the pain is a specific entity rather than a symptom of underlying lesion (as in malignancy), carbamazepine (Tegretol) should be tried first before destructive means.
- Rarely superadded infection (e.g. in malignancy) can be painful and can be treated symptomatically with antibiotics.
- Steroids although not analgesic can lessen the inflammation, improve appetite and elevate mood.

The emotional aspect

Depends on severity, duration and significance of the pain. Its control involves:
- Psychological support: by good doctor–patient relationship and explanation.
- Drug therapy: since morphine suppresses the limbic system it has an adverse emotional effect. Diazepam (anxiolytic) or even chlorpromazine can be used. For depression, imipramine may be used. Psychotropic drugs are being used more and more for analgesia in chronic pain, apart from their psychological effect.
- Psychosurgery: selective operation on the limbic system (emotion centre) such as cingulotomy, is preferred to extensive prefrontal leucotomy.

The rational aspect

The patient can be helped to learn to live with the pain by:
- Good doctor–patient relationship.
- Occupational therapy (a form of distraction).
- Group therapy (to counteract the psychological and social isolation).
- Mental relaxation: by autohypnosis.

1.3. Nutrition in Surgery

As a general rule, the gastrointestinal tract should be used as frequently and as completely as possible. However, repeated attempts to feed enterally patients who have intermittent episodes of ileus or intolerance to the feedings are ill-advised and parenteral nutrition is a better choice. It may be necessary to use more than one type of enteral nutrition or a combination of enteral and parenteral feedings.

Enteral nutrition is used in patients with a normally functioning gastrointestinal tract who cannot eat enough. It may be given:
- Orally
- Via nasoenteric soft Silastic fine-bore tube (e.g. 8 Fr), cooled in the refrigerator before use (to harden it and facilitate its passage), with continuous slow infusion. Such tubes are tolerated well even for 2 months with few complications. The large-bore nasogastric tube should be avoided since it is badly tolerated and associated with aspiration pneumonia (residual gastric volume should be checked frequently and if it is 150 ml or over the feeding should be stopped) and other complications, e.g. oesophageal erosion with subsequent reflux oesophagitis, haemorrhage, perforation or tracheo-oesophageal fistulation.
- Via tube enterostomies, e.g. pharyngostomy, cervical oesophagostomy, gastrostomy, jejunostomy to bypass a proximal lesion.
- Via continuous rectal infusion (proctoclysis)—rarely done.

Enteral diets are relatively inexpensive. There are three types: blenderised diets, partially hydrolysed and elemental diets. Complications are related to diet hyperosmolarity, e.g. diarrhoea and hyperosmolar hyperglycaemic non-ketotic coma.

Parenteral nutrition is the treatment of choice in the absence of a normally functioning gastrointestinal tract and in rapidly progressive catabolic states.

In addition to standard central i.v. hyperalimentation (total parenteral nutrition) there are other easier to administer and safer forms of parenteral nutrition which can be used for patients with lesser nutritional needs. These include the infusion of amino acids alone or in combination with fat emulsions by either the peripheral (e.g. Perifusin — isotonic amino acid solution) or central venous route.

TOTAL PARENTERAL NUTRITION

Indications

Total parental nutrition (TPN) is indicated for:
- Patients who cannot ingest food as a result of anorexia, neurological disorders, intracranial surgery, central nervous system trauma and coma, multiple injuries especially maxillofacial, head and neck fractures.
- Patients with malfunctioning gastrointestinal tract due to:
  - Short-bowel syndrome secondary to massive small bowel resection.
  - Enteroenteric, enterocolic, enterovesical or enterocutaneous fistulae.
  - Obstruction, e.g. oesophageal neoplasm, stricture or achalasia, gastric carcinoma and pyloric obstruction.
  - Paralytic ileus due to whatever cause.
  - Crohn's disease and ulcerative colitis.
- Hypercatabolic patients with major disease, fever of more than 38°C, tachycardia and increased respiratory rate and urea production rate of more than 20 g/24 h. Seen in:
  - Severe trauma and major fractures.
  - Extensive burns.
  - Selected patients with chemotherapy or radiotherapy particularly for gastrointestinal tumours.
- Infants with major gastrointestinal anomalies (e.g. tracheo-oesophageal fistula, gastroschisis, omphalocele or massive intestinal atresia) or who fail to thrive because of gastrointestinal insufficiency from short-bowel syndrome, malabsorption, enzyme deficiency, meconium ileus or idiopathic diarrhoea.

Administration Route

Directly into the superior vena cava via a subclavian (rarely internal jugular) vein. The occlusive dressing can be placed below the clavicle, allowing optimal catheter care, patient comfort and mobility. The route is safe since solutions of 1500 mol/l, infused at a rate of 2–3 ml/min, are immediately diluted a thousand-fold by a blood flow of 2–3 l/min. Such a large vein also decreases the likelihood of thrombophlebitis. The central venous catheter is 16 Fr and preferably made of silicone as this material is inert, soft, flexible and radiopaque. Under aseptic conditions and using local anaesthesia the catheter is introduced through the subclavicular midclavicular point horizontally towards the suprasternal notch. The needle is attached to a heparinised syringe to ensure intrasubclavian vein location. The catheter is then threaded down and further confirmation is obtained by lowering the bottle below the patient's heart position (blood comes back via the catheter). The catheter is then secured to the skin with sutures and dressing, and subcutaneous tunnelling may be performed. A chest X-ray is obtained immediately thereafter to confirm the position of the radiopaque catheter in the superior vena cava and to check for induced pneumo- or haemothorax.

Complications

- Pneumo-, haemo- or hydrothorax.
- Subclavian artery or vein injury and possible cardiac arrhythmias if the catheter is placed into the ventricle.
- Air embolism (potentially fatal if 40 ml or more of air is introduced)—rare.
- Thrombosis of subclavian vein due to catheter infection. If suspected the catheter should be removed and the tip cultured and venogram done. Heparin and antibiotics are required.
- Catheter-related sepsis is the commonest complication. Any evidence of local infection around the catheter site is an indication for its removal and culture and reinsertion into another location.
- Hyperglycaemia and glycosuria.
- Hyperosmolar, non-ketotic, hyperglycaemic coma.
- Hyperchloraemic metabolic acidosis (amino acids related).
- Mild prerenal azotaemia even in patients with normal renal function, fluid volume depletion as well as fluid overload and possibly pulmonary oedema.
- Hypokalaemia and metabolic alkalosis, hypomagnesaemia and hypophosphataemia, jaundice and essential fatty acid deficiency.

Calculation of Requirements

There is a close relationship between energy and nitrogen requirements and the two must be considered jointly. The calorie: nitrogen ratio is 200:1 and daily nutritional requirements are therefore:

Patient	Nitrogen (g/kg)	Energy (per kg/24 h)
Normal (resting)	0.15	126 kJ (30 kcal)
Surgical (postop)	0.2	167 kJ (40 kcal)
Hypercatabolic	0.3	209–251 kJ (50–60 kcal)
Neonate	0.5	419 kJ (100 kcal)

The sources of energy requirements are approximately: carbohydrate 50%, fat 35%, protein 15%. The patient should never receive less than 12.5% of the total energy from protein. Energy values are:

1 g carbohydrate delivers 17 kJ (4 kcal)
1 g protein delivers 17 kJ (4 kcal)
1 g fat delivers 38 kJ (9 kcal)

Roughly 8.4–16.8 MJ (2000–4000 kcal) in 2–4 litres of fluid can be given daily. Concentrated dextrose solutions are hyperosmolar and may require the concomitant use of soluble insulins; however, they have several advantages over the use of fat as an energy source:

- Carbohydrate appears to have a greater protein sparing action than fat.
- Insulin is a potent anabolic hormone.
- Large quantities of fat may not be metabolised well in certain circumstances, leading to fatty liver, haemorrhagic problems and even fat embolism.

In long-term feeding it is important to provide some fat in order to avoid essential fatty acid deficiency and 1 litre of 10% intralipid/week is considered adequate for this purpose.

The recommended amino acid solution for nitrogen source is Aminoplex 12 which provides 12.44 g of nitrogen per litre.

There are two approaches to the administration of total parenteral nutrition solutions.

- Solutions may be infused directly using a two- or three-way giving set. It is essential that energy and nitrogen sources are administered simultaneously. If insulin is being given, the rate of carbohydrate infusion should remain constant over 24 h.

- The patient's total 24 h requirements of amino acids, non-protein energy, electrolytes, vitamins and trace elements may be aseptically mixed in the pharmacy and supplied to the ward in a 3 litre container. The use of a 3 litre bag provides steady infusion rates for all constituents, removes the infection risks associated with making additives on the ward, avoids the need for airways and results in considerable saving in medical and nursing time.

Central venous administration lines used for total parenteral nutrition should never be used for any secondary purpose, e.g. blood sampling or antibiotic infusion. The rate of administration should not normally exceed 655 kJ (156 kcal) or 0.9 g nitrogen per hour. If for any reason administration falls behind schedule, never attempt to 'catch up', but rather review the administration schedule.

Recommended regimens

Simple basic regimen (for stable patient)

Aminoplex 12	1 litre
Dextrose 50%	1 litre
Dextrose 20%	500 ml

This regimen provides:

Fluid	2.5 litres
Energy	10 MJ (2400 kcal) (non-protein)
Nitrogen	12.44 g
Sodium	35 mmol Na$^+$
Potassium	30 mmol K$^+$
Magnesium	2.5 mmol Mg^{2+}
Chloride	67.2 mmol Cl$^-$
Acetate	5 mmol Ac$^-$

High nitrogen regimen (for severely catabolic patients with no fluid problems)

Aminoplex 12	1.5 litres
Dextrose 50%	1.5 litres

This regimen provides:

Fluid	3 litres
Energy	12.6 MJ (3000 kcal) (non-protein)

Nitrogen	18.66 g
Sodium	52.5 mmol Na$^+$
Potassium	45 mmol K$^+$
Magnesium	3.75 mmol Mg^{2+}
Chloride	100.8 mmol Cl$^-$
Acetate	7.5 mmol Ac$^-$

Each regimen requires the following additions:

Multibionta	1 ampoule
Solivito (water-soluble vitamins)	1 ampoule
Addamel (trace elements)	1 ampoule daily
Addiphos (phosphate and K with Na)	30 mmol daily
Intralipid 10%	500 ml twice weekly
Folic acid	1.5 mg i.m. weekly
Vitamin K	10 mg i.m. weekly

Vitlipid adult (fat soluble vitamins) may be added to the intralipid.

Monitoring and laboratory investigations

Monitoring of blood and urine constituents has an essential role in the management of total parenteral nutrition. However, too frequent estimations waste laboratory resources and the results may be difficult to interpret. The following are suggested as adequate for routine management of most patients receiving total parenteral nutrition.

Daily: Plasma urea, electrolytes and glucose. (When estimations of urea and electrolytes are also required in 24 h collections of urine or other fluids, these will only be available on a daily basis on weekdays unless special arrangements are made with the laboratory.)

Twice Weekly: Plasma calcium, phosphate, albumin, full blood count.

Weekly: Liver function tests. Plasma lipids and magnesium.

Monthly: B$_{12}$ and folate, iron, zinc and prothrombin time.

Collect blood samples from veins remote from i.v. sites. Remember that lipaemia will falsely lower estimated concentrations of water-soluble plasma constituents, so avoid collecting any specimens during or immediately after giving i.v. lipid. Twenty-four hours should elapse between giving i.v. lipid and taking samples for lipid estimations. Samples for microbiological examination should be collected whenever indicated.

In most district hospitals, TPN is supervised by a physician with a special interest or by an anaesthetist who can set up the central line.

1.4. Deep Venous Thrombosis and Pulmonary Embolism

Deep venous thrombosis of a length of the femoral vein causes a painful swollen leg. With lymphangitis the deep venous thrombosis will be protracted (phlegmasia alba dolens or white leg) and lead to varicose veins later on. Massive pulmonary embolism may occur. Such deep venous thrombosis occurs in late pregnancy and the puerperium. On the other hand, extensive deep venous thrombosis of iliofemoral and pelvic deep veins (phlegmasia caerulea dolens or blue leg) may lead to infarction and even sudden venous gangrene of the lower limb. Virchow's triad is still the pathological basis for deep venous thrombosis (i.e. changes in the vessel wall, changes in the blood flow and changes in the composition of the blood). Special risk groups include those with a past history of deep venous thrombosis or pulmonary embolism, malignant disease, polycythaemia, abdominal or pelvic surgery, extensive trauma, congestive heart failure or myocardial infarction, obese and dehydrated patients, the elderly, and those taking the oral contraceptive pill (females) or stilboestrol (males with prostatic cancer).

Deep venous thrombosis

Prophylaxis

Preoperative
  Weight reduction.
  Stoppage of contraceptive pill 1 month prior to surgery.
  Identification of high risk groups.
Peroperative
● Physical means
  Electrical stimulation of calf.
  External intermittent pneumatic compression of calf.
  Passive leg exercise (foot pedalling machine).
● Chemical means (to commence with premedication and to continue postoperatively until the patient is mobile)
  Aspirin (decreases platelet adhesiveness).
  Oral anticoagulants.
  Low-dose subcutaneous heparin.
  Dextran 70.

Postoperative
  Pressure-graduated elastic stockings.
  Early mobilisation, massage and leg movements.
  Adequate hydration.

Diagnosis

● Clinical examination (avoid Homans' sign as it may cause thrombus dislodgment): slight fever and tender swollen calf.
● Ascending deep functioning venography: essential to confirm diagnosis, delineate extent of deep venous thrombosis and detect silent deep venous thrombosis in postoperative pyrexia (after exclusion of all other causes).
● Ultrasound flow detector (Doppler principle): inexpensive, harmless in pregnancy and practical—may give false negative results.
● Radioactive labelled fibrinogen ^{125}I: unreliable above mid-thigh and in the presence of haematoma or healing wound. It carries the risk of serum hepatitis.
● Impedance plethysmography.

Treatment

● Anticoagulant, stocking and rest. Heparin 25 000–40 000 units per day continuous i.v. infusion with warfarin to be continued for 6 months (heparin is stopped after 2 days) and controlled by prothrombin time (should be twice or three times the control) or prothrombin index (should be 10–15 %).
● Surgical thrombectomy (Fogarty balloon catheter).
● Fibrinolysis (streptokinase).
● Vein ligation, plication or filter introduction (e.g. Mobin-Uddin umbrella in a capsule via internal jugular vein under X-ray control).

Pulmonary embolism

About 3 % of all hospital deaths are due to pulmonary embolism.

Small emboli: lead to pulmonary hypertension which requires permanent anticoagulants.

Medium emboli: lodge in branches of the pulmonary artery resulting in a pulmonary infarction. Clinically, sudden chest pain, dyspnoea and haemoptysis occur. Radiologically, an infarcted triangular (wedge) segment is seen. Lung scan reveals the perfusion defect and pulmonary angiography is seldom required. ECG may reveal $S_1 Q_3 T_3$

pattern. Recurrent emboli are frequent. Heparin should be given i.v. and clot removed by Fogarty catheter. Warfarin is administered for six weeks.

Large emboli: lodge in the main pulmonary artery with serious haemodynamic and ECG changes (right ventricular strain). Immediate death may occur in massive pulmonary embolism. Shock is profound with high CVP, low blood pressure, feeble pulse, and severe hypoxaemia in blood gases. Such cases need emergency pulmonary embolectomy with or without cardiopulmonary bypass as well as immediate heparin and streptokinase i.v. administration. Unfortunately the majority die in spite of cardiac resuscitation.

Practical points

All female patients on the contraceptive pill and patients over the age of 40 years undergoing hernia surgery (or anything comparable or of greater severity) must be given deep venous thrombosis prophylaxis. In general, low-dose heparin (Calciparin), 5000 units 8-hourly subcutaneously, is started with the premedication and continued until the patient is fully ambulant. Heparin is given into a fold of abdominal skin and not into the arms or buttocks.

500 ml of Dextran 70, given at induction of anaesthesia and 500 ml immediately postoperatively is another alternative to prevent pulmonary embolism.

There are two groups unsuitable for deep venous thrombosis and pulmonary embolism prophylaxis using the low-dose heparin regimen:
- Those in whom the tiny risk of haemorrhage will be dangerous, e.g. those with recent gastrointestinal tract bleeding, recent cerebrovascular accident, diastolic blood pressure greater than 120 mmHg or known bleeding diathesis such as haemophilia or Christmas disease. Also patients with toxic goitre (very vascular) and head injuries and those patients undergoing open as well as endoscopic urological surgery (to avoid haematuria). This group needs intermittent pneumatic compression boots during operation.
- Those in whom low-dose heparin appears to be an inadequate form of prophylaxis, including those with a history of deep venous thrombosis or pulmonary embolism, and those with hip fractures or those who have had surgery (immobility). They require full anticoagulation therapy.

1.5. Pulmonary Complications After Major Abdominal Operation

More surgical patients probably die of postoperative chest problems than anything else. Such morbidity and mortality can be largely prevented by adequate pre- and postoperative care.

Predisposing factors include the site of operation, sex (males more than females), age (the two extremes of life), chronic bronchitis, smoking, anaesthesia itself (bronchial trauma, prolonged recovery), pain (restricts coughing and deep breathing), patient immobility, dehydration, abdominal distension (leads to paralytic ileus with consequent hypokalaemia which precipitates respiratory failure—vicious circle) and obesity.

After upper abdominal surgery, the vital capacity of the patient's lungs often drops to as low as 25% of its preoperative value. The normal requirement for adequate oxygenation is 10 ml of vital capacity for every kilogram of body weight; if the ratio drops below this, respiratory failure ensues.

This is important in obese patients. For example, if a 120 kg female is undergoing an incisional hernia repair and she is a smoker with a preoperative vital capacity of 4 litres, postoperatively she requires

$$\frac{10}{1000} \times 120 = 1.2 \text{ litres}$$

of vital capacity to avoid respiratory failure. However, with the postoperative reduction, she will have a vital capacity of only 1 litre. She will almost certainly be in respiratory failure and will need mechanical ventilation. The situation is also exacerbated by the reduction in intra-abdominal space, causing competition among the contents, which push up the diaphragm and further reduce the vital capacity. The fact that the patient is a smoker means that the lungs will be even less able to cope with the reduction in vital capacity.

Complications

One complication may lead to another.
- Bronchitis: may arise *de novo* or as an exacerbation of pre-existing bronchitis.
- Bronchopneumonia (aspiration pneumonia): commonly by *Haemophilus influenzae* and pneumococci, rarely by drug-resistant staphylococci and *Pseudomonas pyocyanea*. Here the

radiological patchy consolidation is associated clinically with systemic manifestations.

- Atelectasis (*see below*).
- Lung abscess.
- Empyema.
- Subphrenic abscess: with the three salient radiological features of basal lung consolidation or collapse, hemidiaphragmatic tenting and sub-diaphragmatic pus collection as indicated by fluid level.
- Mendelson's syndrome (*see below*).
- Adult respiratory distress syndrome (*see below*).

ATELECTASIS

Due to bronchial obstruction by viscid secretions of mucus or pus leading to absorption collapse of the involved lobe. Depression of the cough reflex by pain and/or sedation and/or poor ventilation are predisposing factors. Auscultation for good air entry and chest X-rays are important diagnostic means. It is important to remember that the most likely cause of a high fever within 36 h of surgery is pulmonary atelectasis.

Treatment

The best treatment lies in prophylaxis through endotracheal aspiration at the end of surgery, pain control (not to the extent of respiratory depression, e.g. small repeated doses of pethidine 50 mg), preoperative breathing exercises, no smoking, treatment of pre-existing chest infection prior to surgery and reduction of obesity.

Once diagnosed the treatment must be immediate physiotherapy. Antibiotics do not play any part in the initial management of atelectasis. Bronchoscopic removal of secretions may be required. In extreme cases tracheostomy is needed to reduce the 'dead space'.

MENDELSON'S SYNDROME
(Mendelson, USA, 1946)

Caused by aspiration of vomitus or gastric contents with its irritant hydrochloric acid. Occurs *during induction* of anaesthesia in any patient with a full stomach or intestinal obstruction, or in pregnancy. The condition can occur in *coma*, e.g. after head injury, and *preoperatively* in haematemesis, intestinal obstruction and alcoholic or drug poisoning. *Postoperatively* it may occur after premature

removal of the endotracheal tube. The condition can be fatal and is clinically manifested by wheezes, cyanosis, tachycardia, tachypnoea and hypotension. Radiologically widespread lung infiltration occurs more on the right than on the left and more in the lower lobes. Blood gas analysis reveals severe hypoxaemia. Treatment is by prevention, endotracheal aspiration, steroids and bronchodilators.

ADULT RESPIRATORY DISTRESS SYNDROME (shock lung)

Leads to pulmonary insufficiency which is a major cause of death in injured patients and patients receiving intensive care. This syndrome takes many forms:

- Damage to the pulmonary capillary bed by endotoxin action on vascular epithelium with its swelling, microemboli and intravascular coagulation leading to a rise in pulmonary vascular resistance at precapillary and small vein level. Both neurogenic and humoral factors may be involved and the intravascular aggregation of platelets and white blood cells occurs, with local release of vasoactive substances (e.g. prostaglandin $F_{2\alpha}$, 5-hydroxytryptamine, histamine) and lysosomal enzymes.
- Damage to pneumocytes, manifested by interstitial and intra-alveolar oedema (and occasionally haemorrhage) with impairment of gaseous transport.
- Damage to surfactant layer manifested by diffuse patchy atelectasis due to diminished secretion of surfactant (surface-tension reducing substance which normally holds open the smaller air alveoli). The lung compliance is markedly decreased and so it is called stiff lung.
- Pulmonary shunting (bypassing the pulmonary circulation) through dilatation of the arteriovenous communications (which normally exist between the pulmonary and bronchial vasculatures) will further impair gaseous transport. Pulmonary shunting is an excellent guide to the adequacy of pulmonary ventilation and is measured from the oxygen content in arterial and mixed venous blood after the patient breathes 100% O_2 for at least 15 min. The normal physiological shunting should be less than 5%. Acute respiratory failure is defined as an intrapulmonary shunt of 15% or more. A shunt of 40% or more, particularly if it is increasing, is an indication for ventilatory assistance.

- These pulmonary disturbances, although primarily vascular in origin, often tend to be complicated by pneumonitis due to infection by organisms derived from the upper air passages such as those in the klebsiella group and antibiotic-resistant staphylococci (the most lethal).

These are the five elements of shock lung producing a pulmonary vicious circle which can only be broken by achieving improved tissue oxygenation following restoration of blood volume together with intermittent positive pressure ventilation; this is preferably carried out by the technique of positive expiratory end pressure (PEEP) where positive pressure within the lung is maintained throughout the whole respiratory cycle, so that the collapsed alveoli are inflated and the fluid exudation is reversed. Large doses of steroid and antibiotics may also be required. Although the need for oxygen is great and the arteriovenous difference is wide hyperbaric oxygen is useless owing to the failure of oxygen transport in the lungs. Failure of oxygen release from haemoglobin is due to decreased 2,3-DPG concentration, the oxygen dissociation curve swinging to the left.

Clinically shock lung is manifested by tachypnoea and hypoxicaemia in spite of a high inspired oxygen concentration. Radiologically it is seen as diffuse, fluffy infiltrates. The radiological deterioration usually lags behind the clinical and gas exchange disturbances.

Shock lung is a dangerous pathological entity because death is likely to result largely from the additional burdens of respiratory failure; it is not only encountered in septicaemia but also follows extensive intravascular coagulation produced by trauma, after massive transfusion and following heart-lung bypass (pump lung), fat embolism, cardiac failure and oxygen toxicity.

1.6. Antimicrobials in Surgery

Antimicrobials are drugs that damage microorganisms without harming the host tissue cells; they are either -cidal or -static. This is in contrast to antineoplastic drugs which harm both tumour and host cells and are always -cidal.

Antimicrobials fall into two groups:

Synthetic   Includes sulphonamide, nitrofurantoin, nalidixic acid, para-aminosalicylic acid (PASA), isonicotinic acid hydrazide (INH) and co-trimoxazole (Septrin). Most are bacteriostatic (and work by inhibition of folate metabolism). However, INH and co-trimoxazole are bactericidal.

Antibiotics   (natural products of one microorganism affecting another microorganism)
- Bactericidal, including mainly the three major groups: penicillin, aminoglycosides and cephalosporins; or
- Bacteriostatic, e.g. chloramphenicol and tetracycline.

Antibiotic combinations

A combination of bacteriostatic and bactericidal drugs is pharmacologically poor: the bactericidal drug is effective only in killing growing bacteria and once growth is arrested by the bacteriostatic drug, the bactericidal agent is useless. A combination of two bacteriostatic agents yields a bacteriostatic agent except for trimethoprim and sulphamethoxazole (both are folate metabolism inhibitors) which yield a synergistic bactericidal drug, co-trimoxazole. A combination of two bactericidal agents always yields a bactericidal agent. The combination effect may be antagonistic (less than each drug used alone), agonistic (more than each drug used alone), additive (equal to the algebraic sum of the effects of both drugs) or synergistic (more than the algebraic sum of the effects).

Indications for antibiotic combinations

Mixed bacterial infections in which the organisms are not susceptible to a common agent

- Intra-abdominal sepsis secondary to intestinal perforation and postoperative sepsis secondary to gastrointestinal operation. Here the anaerobes (particularly *Bacteroides fragilis*) and the aerobic Gram-negative bacilli, the Enterobacteriaceae (particularly *Escherichia coli*), predominate. The combination of aerobes and anaerobes is synergistic. Elimination of one or other of the organisms reduces the overall infectivity of the inoculum. Antibiotics with anaerobic coverage are metronidazole, clindamycin, lincomycin, chloramphenicol, or semisynthetic penicillins (carbenicillin or ticarcillin). Antibiotics with aerobic coverage are aminoglycoside (with ampicillin to cover the anaerobic

Streptococcus faecalis) or cephalosporins such as cefuroxime. Triple chemotherapy of metronidazole/gentamicin/ampicillin was originally used. This was largely replaced with double chemotherapy of metronidazole/cefuroxime and now a single agent is used—mezlocillin (semisynthetic penicillin) or latamoxef (third-generation cephalosporins). Any of the above regimens, however, may be used prophylactically or therapeutically.

- Polymicrobial bacteraemia in a febrile, neutropenic patient. A bactericidal combination should be used such as semisynthetic penicillin (carbenicillin or ticarcillin) with aminoglycoside *or* cephalosporin with aminoglycoside *or* semisynthetic penicillin with a cephalosporin. These regimens have been shown to decrease the mortality of these infections.
- Endometritis and post-hysterectomy infections caused by aerobic and anaerobic vaginocervical flora.

To achieve synergistic antimicrobial activity against a single organism

Synergism occurs when a combination of drugs produces at least a fourfold decrease in the minimal inhibitory concentration of *each* drug, e.g.

- Penicillin and aminoglycoside (streptomycin) in enterococcal endocarditis are replaced by penicillin and gentamicin to cover possible *Pseudomonas aeruginosa*.
- Trimethoprim and sulphamethoxazole (cotrimoxazole, Septrin, Bactrim). Each drug has only bacteriostatic activity when used alone while their combination is bactericidal.

To overcome bacterial tolerance

Tolerance (*in vitro* phenomenon) is the resistance of an organism to the lethal action of an otherwise bactericidal agent. Tolerance to penicillins, cephalosporins and vancomycin have been described in *Staphylococcus aureus*, *Staphylococcus pneumoniae*, *Streptococcus viridans* and Group G streptococci infections. The goal of *in vitro* tests is to obtain the best single or combined regimen that will assure bactericidal activity against the causative organism.

To prevent the development of bacterial antibiotic resistance

Bacteria can become resistant to drugs by chromosomal mutation, recombination and acquisition of plasmids, e.g.

- Treatment of active tuberculosis particularly with cavitary pulmonary disease. To treat an intrinsically drug-resistant subpopulation as well as to prevent the development of a totally drug-resistant subpopulation of *Mycobacterium tuberculosis*, more than one effective antituberculosis agent must be used.
- Aminoglycoside with semisynthetic penicillins (carbenicillin or ticarcillin) to treat infections due to *Pseudomonas aeruginosa*. These β-lactam antibiotics are excellent antipseudomonal drugs. Rapid development of bacterial resistance to the β-lactam drug caused by β-lactamase inactivating enzymes can be suppressed by the drug synergistic combination and by β-lactamase inhibitors (the prototype of this class of drugs is clavulanic acid).
- Rifampicin incorporation with antistaphylococcal regimen. Rifampicin is the most effective antimicrobial agent against both *S. aureus* and *Staphylococcus epidermidis* (on the basis of minimal inhibitory concentration). However, studies reveal that if staphylococci are exposed to rifampicin alone, they develop total resistance to this drug within 24 h but if a good second antistaphylococcal agent is combined with rifampicin, e.g. aminoglycoside or vancomycin, the totally rifampicin-resistant population is aborted. *S. epidermidis* is the most common organism responsible for endocarditis associated with prosthetic valves and infections associated with ventricular shunt devices and prosthetic joints, and since such regimens have been effective in eradicating this organism the prosthesis does not have to be removed.

To decrease the toxicity of the most effective agent

For example, by treating meningitis due to *Cryptococcus neoformans* with amphotericin B (effective and toxic) and 5-fluorocytocine the duration of the drug administration can be shortened.

Principles of chemoprophylaxis in surgery

- Not a substitute or alternative to aseptic practice and good surgical technique.
- Necessary only in high-risk cases of bacterial contamination.
- Timing is vital. It should start with premedication, aiming at a saturated tissue concentration at the time of surgical manipulation and throughout the operation. Thus administration for 24–48 h is as effective as administration for 7 postoperative days.

- Route of administration should be intravenous since the oral route is not suitable in all patients and may have undesirable side-effects, e.g. pseudomembranous enterocolitis. The topical route is limited although tetracycline lavage has been shown to reduce mortality in faecal peritonitis; kanamycin lavage proved to be toxic and lavage with normal saline alone actually increased the risk of sepsis (by spreading infection). Topical ampicillin is known to reduce wound sepsis but does not provide protection against intra-abdominal abscesses and septicaemia. The intramuscular preoperative route leads to a delayed peak level.
- Chemoprophylaxis should be employed only when scientific evidence shows that it has advantages. However it is logical to adopt a policy of selective use of antibiotics in general surgery in the knowledge that infection is more likely to occur in some situations than others (Fig. 2). It must be remembered, nevertheless, that since *in vitro* sensitivity may be different from *in vivo* sensitivity, culture is far more informative (e.g. biliary and urinary organisms require not only an effective drug but an effective drug that can concentrate in the biliary tree or urinary system in adequate therapeutic concentrations).
- Choice of agent (preferably bactericidal) should be made on the basis of activity against the *pathogens* most commonly encountered. Most of these are endogenous (exogenous *S. aureus* is responsible for only 5% of postoperative sepsis). In the healthy person only a few body fluids, such as cerebrospinal fluid, seem to be permanently sterile, while all other fluids and cavities contain at least a few organisms per millilitre from time to time. The distribution of pathogens does not, however, always mirror their prevalence in infections. There are more Bifidobacteria than Bacteroides in faeces and of the latter, *Bacteroides fragilis* accounts for less than 5%, but in clinical sepsis *B. fragilis* is the dominant pathogen.

Indications for antibacterial prophylaxis

Endogenous contamination

Endogenous bacteria are important in the pathogenesis of infections after gastrointestinal tract surgery.

- Surgery for oesophagogastric carcinoma or gastric ulcer, patients on cimetidine and those undergoing revisional gastric surgery and in emergency surgery. Bacteria are normally destroyed rapidly by gastric acid and when intragastric pH is > 4, microorganisms are almost invariably present. Cephalosporins (cefuroxime) with or without metronidazole are effective in such conditions.
- Biliary tract surgery, especially with high-risk factors: emergency surgery, age over 70 years, jaundice, obesity, exploration of common bile duct, concomitant alimentary procedures. Biliary instrumentation without surgery such as percutaneous transhepatic cholangiography and endoscopic retrograde cholangiopancreatography also requires prophylaxis. Cephalosporins (ceftriaxone or cefazolin), mezlocillin or aminoglycoside (gentamicin) are all effective in reducing the infection from 20% to 2–4%.
- Colorectal surgery is associated with a high rate of sepsis which may be primary (initiated at the time of surgery) or secondary (occurring postoperatively as a result of anastomotic dehiscence). Prophylaxis is mainly effective in preventing primary sepsis (secondary sepsis due to anastomotic leak is affected by other factors). Without prophylaxis, the incidence of wound sepsis has been 35–50%, that of abscesses 4–11% and that of septicaemia 4–35%. Metronidazole/cefuroxime is an appropriate prophylactic regimen, reducing the sepsis rate to less than 10%. For emergency operations (when infection is established), a stoma should be raised and contaminated wounds left open (closing the abdominal wall only, leaving skin and subcutaneous tissues to heal by second intention). For these patients antibiotic therapy should be prolonged (therapeutic not prophylactic).
- In appendicectomy the presence of perforation or local peritonitis justifies prophylaxis but because these complications cannot be identified preoperatively, it is reasonable to give metronidazole to all patients preoperatively and to continue it for 2 days only in those with obvious sepsis.
- Vaginal or abdominal hysterectomy is associated with infection in 25–35%. Metronidazole is very effective.
- Sepsis is rarely a serious problem in urinary tract procedures and inappropriate prophylaxis can produce a population of drug-resistant bacteria which pose a potentially serious threat. There is no evidence that chemoprophylaxis prevents postoperative chest infections or that it is effect-

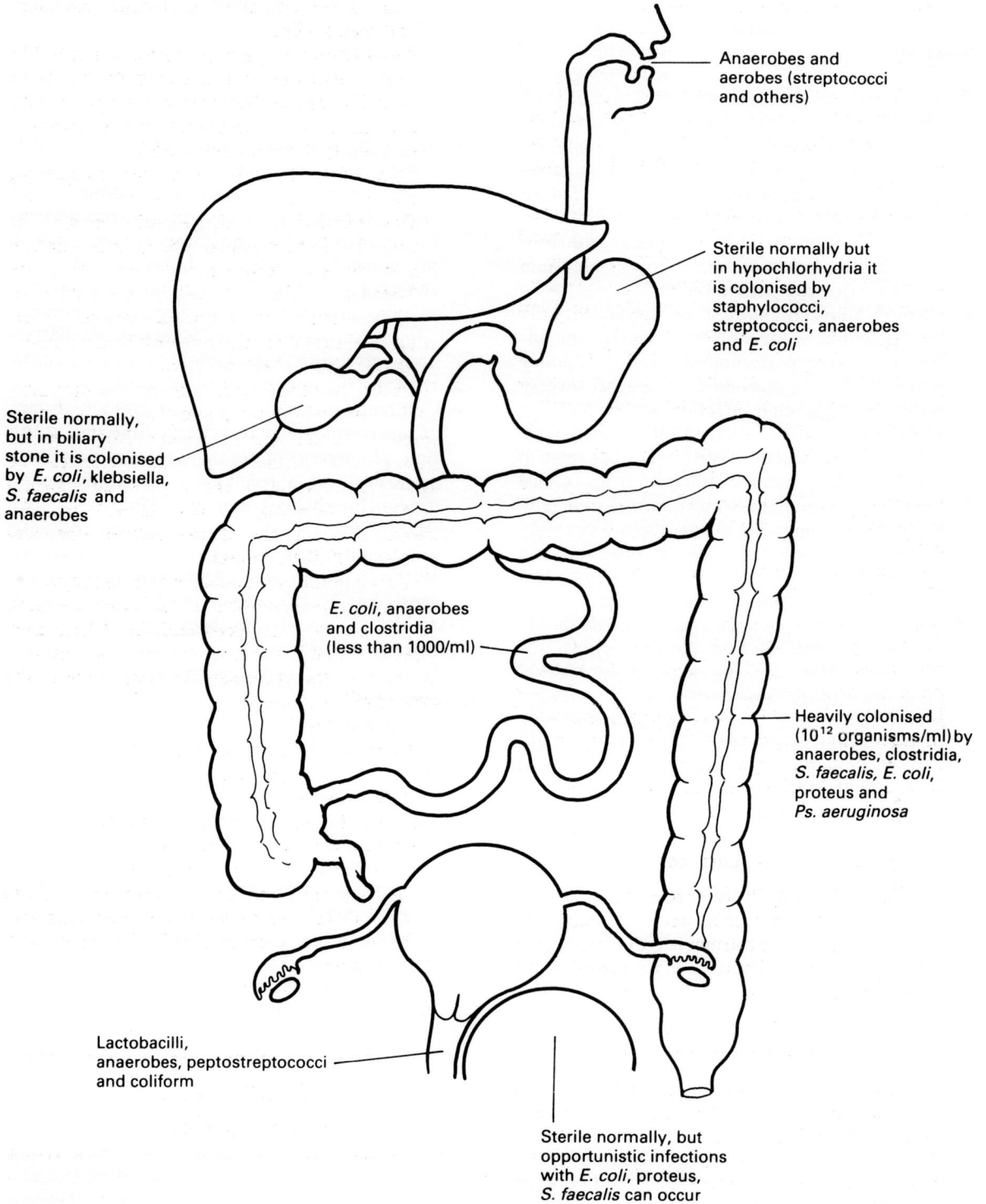

Anaerobes and aerobes (streptococci and others)

Sterile normally but in hypochlorhydria it is colonised by staphylococci, streptococci, anaerobes and *E. coli*

Sterile normally, but in biliary stone it is colonised by *E. coli*, klebsiella, *S. faecalis* and anaerobes

E. coli, anaerobes and clostridia (less than 1000/ml)

Heavily colonised (10^{12} organisms/ml) by anaerobes, clostridia, *S. faecalis*, *E. coli*, proteus and *Ps. aeruginosa*

Lactobacilli, anaerobes, peptostreptococci and coliform

Sterile normally, but opportunistic infections with *E. coli*, proteus, *S. faecalis* can occur

Fig. 2   Bacterial flora

ive in preventing chest infections in tracheos-
tomies or endotracheal intubation.

Exogenous contamination

- Lower limb surgery in the presence of peripheral
  vascular disease carries a small, but important,
  risk of gas gangrene (e.g. above-knee amputation stump) which is eliminated by perioperative benzylpenicillin.
- Prosthetic joint replacement, e.g. hip and knee:
  introduction of any prosthesis may be followed
  by infection (in less than 5% of cases). Because
  of the potentially disastrous consequences antibiotic prophylaxis is justified and effective. Joint
  replacements develop sepsis in 3.4% of untreated cases compared to 0.8% of those with
  prophylaxis. The antibiotic of choice is a β-
  lactamase-stable penicillin such as flucloxacillin.
  In all cases of prosthesis, staphylococci are the
  major pathogens (in heart surgery as well as
  neurosurgery).
- Prosthetic heart valves, e.g. Starr–Edward,
  Björk–Shilly and Porcine valves, and aortic
  grafts.
- Neurological shunts, e.g. Pudenz–Heyer and
  Hirtz–Holter valves.
- Extensive trauma and burns.
- Surgical procedures and instrumentations in
  rheumatic and valvular heart diseases and
  patients with pacemakers to avoid subacute
  bacterial endocarditis. The prophylactic antibiotic of choice depends on the site of operation
  and its prevalent organisms (*see* Fig. 2).
- Insertion of Marlex mesh in hernia repair and
  pacemakers in heart blocks.

Host immune system suppression

Such as in diabetes mellitus, chronic renal failure,
leukaemia, aplastic anaemia, severe malnourish-
ment, carcinomatosis, obstructive jaundice, steroid
therapy and chemotherapy, e.g. azothioprine
(Imuran) and cytotoxics.

Practical points

- *Ps. aeruginosa* infection is difficult to eradicate
  because of three defence mechanisms—a barrier
  preventing antibiotic access, plasmid-mediated
  β-lactamases and inducible β-lactamases. Its
  main habitat is the large bowel and it likes moist
  surfaces, e.g. burns, urinary tract and tracheostomy wounds (intensive care organism). The
  main antimicrobials are:

  —Semisynthetic penicillins (e.g. carbenicillin in
  large doses, ticarcillin, carfecillin, azlocillin
  and mezlocillin).
  —Aminoglycosides, e.g. gentamicin, netilmicin
  (less otonephrotoxic) and tobramycin. Both
  ticarcillin and carbenicillin can be given with
  gentamicin as the combination is synergistic.
  —Colistin (polymyxin antibiotic).
  Some of the third generation cephalosporins,
  e.g. cefsulodin.
  —Povidone-iodine (Betidine) solution with its
  remarkable bactericidal effect. This solution
  can be used freely since it does not cause
  burning or allergy. It can be used for skin
  preparation, intraperitoneal lavage, interparietal spray, intracolonic washout and even
  as an intraurethral ointment.
- In gastrointestinal tract surgery the currently
  used common double prophylactic is cefurox-
  ime/metronidazole combination. Single chemotherapy with mezlocillin or moxalactam can be
  used. However, the latter may produce clinically
  important bleedings in vitamin K store deficiency, e.g. in the elderly and in chemical
  sterilisation of the bowel.
- Avoid clindamycin and lincomycin as they cause
  pseudomembranous colitis which may be fatal.
  It is due to toxin produced by *Clostridium
  difficile* which is sensitive to oral vancomycin.
- Remember the anaerobes for proper antibiotic
  coverage. They are:
  —Bacteroides.
  —Clostridia (gas gangrene and tetanus).
  —*Streptococcus faecalis.*
  —Actinomyces.
- Sources of hospital infection are from:
  —Same patient (autoinfection).
  —Other patients (cross-infection).
  —Hospital staff (cross-infection) whether from
  ward or theatre nurses, surgeon or assistant.
  These three sources should be dealt with
  accordingly.

1.7. Postoperative Analgesia

Over half of patients have severe pain in the
immediate postoperative period. Since pain is a

subjective feeling, measurement is difficult. However, thoracotomy and laparotomy associated with painful breathing do permit direct measurement of FEV_1 and PFR and their improvement with analgesia; otherwise, a (rough) linear analogue is used in which the patient makes a mark on a 10 cm line, one end of which is marked as 'no pain' and the other as 'the worst pain you can imagine'. The position of the mark on the line measures how much pain the patient is experiencing. This technique is better than analgesimetry. With the Cardiff Palliator or Newcastle Interactive Demand apparatuses, operated by the patient himself by pressing a button to add a small increment of i.v. narcotic, pain can be analysed quantitatively by the rate of administration of narcotic analgesic.

The incidence of pain was found to be determined by a single factor: the site of operation (which also accounts for its severity), e.g. thoracic (pain incidence is about 70%), upper abdominal (60%) and lower abdominal (50%). Intermittent i.m. injections of narcotics, even when carried out at regular intervals, can produce fluctuating and unpredictable blood levels of the drug. Therefore continuous i.m. (rare) or i.v. (commonly used) infusion of narcotics via mechanically driven syringes is preferable. This means giving more than the conventional i.m. dose, and continuous respiratory monitoring is necessary. However, the respiratory stimulant doxapram can be given continuously for long periods with no effect on the analgesic action of narcotics. It improves pulmonary function and reduces the incidence of postoperative pulmonary complications. It is probably superior to naloxone (a pure narcotic antagonist).

Narcotics

Mild non-narcotic analgesics have no place in the treatment of immediate postoperative pain for four reasons:
1. Rather large doses are needed to produce the maximum effect (equivalent to 6–10 mg morphine).
2. They are given orally at a time when absorption is uncertain after major operation.
3. Immediately after surgery, the inflammatory response, against which aspirin is effective, has not developed so less analgesia will be expected.
4. Increased side-effects such as bleeding may result, e.g. with indomethacin. Postoperative pain should therefore be treated initially with a narcotic (see Section 1.2, 'General principles') and later with an analgesic and anti-inflammatory agent such as indomethacin.

Inhalational analgesia

Nitrous oxide (e.g. Entonox: $N_2O/O_2 = 50/50$) is a powerful analgesic used with or without mechanical ventilation for not more than 48 h since it depresses the bone marrow and blocks B_{12} activity.

Local analgesic agents

Exert their effect by blocking Na^+ and K^+ channels in nerve membranes. Some have a reliable duration of 3 h especially if combined with 1:200 000 adrenaline, e.g. 1% lignocaine 3 mg/kg (maximum dose) or preferably long-acting 0.5% bupivacaine 2 mg/kg (maximum dose). Used in, for example, ingrowing toenail operations, circumcision and inguinal hernia. The dose can be doubled if mixed with adrenaline (since their absorption will be slowed down) but adrenaline is contraindicated in digital, penile, nasal and ear infiltration.

Intercostal block

Used in thoracotomy, chest trauma with rib fractures, and upper abdominal operations with analgesia duration of 3–18 h. Involves injection of 0.5% bupivacaine and 1:200 000 adrenaline via a needle or indwelling plastic catheter. For upper abdominal incisions seven nerves need to be blocked (T5–T11). Bilateral intercostal block is needed in median and paramedian incisions with the possible risk of bilateral pneumothorax and reduced respiratory function (due to bilateral intercostal muscle paralysis in the presence of impaired diaphragmatic movement). The block is performed posteriorly 7 cm from the midline near rib angles. It is contraindicated in chronic obstructive airway disease. It is superior to the thoracic epidural approach since it is easier to perform and carries no risk of hypotension, leg weakness, urinary retention or early respiratory depression.

Thoracic paravertebral block

Superior to multiple intercostal block. Four nerves can be blocked by one injection. Catheters can be left in for 5 days.

Caudal (sacral epidural) block

Easier in children and used in circumcision, inguinal herniotomy and orchidopexy. Lignocaine + 1:200 000 adrenaline can block up to T12. Lignocaine 1% is used for children under 5 years

(0.5 ml/kg) and lignocaine 1.5% for those over 5 years (0.3 ml/kg). Haemorrhage into the sacral canal is a complication.

Continuous caudal block in adults

Continuous brachial plexus block

Carried out by means of catheters inserted via the supraclavicular, axillary and interscalene approaches.

Abdominal wound continuous infusion of local analgesic solutions

Fine catheters are used (sited between posterior rectus sheath and rectus muscle) sometimes attached to a bacterial filter. Excellent analgesia is produced but visceral pain remains, and if the patient is unable to sleep, additional sedation may be necessary. Wound healing may be impaired and infection introduced.

Epidural (extradural or peridural) analgesia

For reliable analgesia, the catheter must be placed in the mid-thoracic region in thoracic and upper abdominal surgery but such positioning involves risks (see 'Intercostal block'). Owing to narcotic absorption the side-effects are similar to those occurring when the parenteral route is used.

Transcutaneous electrical nerve stimulation

Indicated in soft tissue pain (e.g. myalgia), postherpetic neuralgia, cervical and spine metastases, pudendal pain and root pain as an adjunct to steroids and regional blocks.

Cryoanalgesia

Similar to intercostal block but cryoprobe is applied to the nerve. Rapid N_2O expansion causes extreme cold ($-60°C$) producing local degeneration and interruption of nerve conduction (regeneration of nerves can take place later). This can be done by the surgeon at the conclusion of thoracotomy.

Intrathecal morphine (1–2 mg)

Produces prolonged analgesia of up to 18 h via a needle or catheter. May cause late respiratory depression (after 4 h), itching of unknown mechanism, urinary retention with possible neurotoxicity and arachnoiditis. However, no addiction or classical opiate withdrawal syndrome has been found. Spinal headache is masked by morphine analgesic effect.

1.8. Sutures and Implants in Surgery

A suture is a strand of material used to tie (ligate) blood vessels and/or to sew (approximate) tissues together.
- Suture material should have and maintain adequate tensile strength until its purpose is served. It should not shrink in the tissues.
- It should stimulate minimal tissue reaction and should not create a situation favourable to bacterial growth.
- It should be non-electrolytic, non-capillary, non-allergenic, non-carcinogenic (and non-thrombogenic in vascular surgery).
- The material should handle comfortably and naturally by the surgeon and a knot should hold securely without fraying or cutting.
- It should be inexpensive and easily sterilised.

The histological reactions to *all* sutures are essentially the same for the first 7 days as these changes are secondary to trauma of passage of the needle and suture.

Sutures are classified as absorbable and non-absorbable.

Absorbable surgical sutures

A sterile strand prepared from collagen derived from healthy mammals or a synthetic polymer. It is capable of being absorbed by living mammalian tissue but may be treated to modify its resistance to absorption. It may be impregnated or coated with a suitable antimicrobial agent. It may be coloured by a colour additive approved by the Federal Food and Drug Administration (FDA).

Natural collagens (monofilament in behaviour and classification although made originally from two or more ribbons).

Surgical gut Plain or chromic (treated with chromium salt solution before or after spinning into strands in order to resist body enzymes and prolong absorption time); derived from submucosa of sheep intestine or serosa of beef intestine. After 4 weeks, chromic catgut size 0 loses 60% of its initial tensile strength; plain catgut loses strength more rapidly since it is digested relatively quickly by body enzymes. The rate of absorption differs according to the site sutured, e.g. slower in subcutaneous tissues and extremely rapid if exposed to gastric juice.

Collagen sutures Extruded from a homogeneous dispersion of pure collagen fibres from flexor tendons of beef (plain or chromic).

Biological absorbable sutures Of historical interest, e.g. preserved skin, fascia lata strips (also live autogenous), cadaveric dura mater and kangaroo tendon (strong but scarce and expensive).

Synthetic absorbables (multifilament except PDS)

Polyglycolic (Dexon) and polyglactic acid Are homopolymers of glycolide and copolymer lactide respectively. Absorption is complete within 4 months.

Polyglactin 910 (Vicryl) Copolymer of lactide and glycolide absorbed within 90 days (it is braided). Dexon loses tensile strength more rapidly and is absorbed significantly more slowly than Vicryl. Their handling property is similar to silk—they knot easily and the knot holds well.

Poly Dioxanone Synthetic smooth suture (PDS) The only monofilament synthetic absorbable suture with total absorption at 180 days, thus providing longer wound support. It retains its strength in tissue twice as long as any other synthetic absorbable suture.

Non-absorbable sutures

These are strands of material that effectively resist enzymatic digestion in living tissue. A suture may be mono- or multifilament, of metal or organic fibres, rendered into a strand by spinning, twisting or braiding. Each strand is substantially uniform in diameter throughout its length. The material may be uncoloured, naturally coloured or dyed with an FDA approved dyestuff. It may be coated or uncoated, treated or untreated for capillarity (designated as Type B or A respectively). Capillarity refers to the characteristic that allows the passage of tissue fluids along the strand, permitting infection to be drawn into the wound. Type B is resistant to wicking transfer of body fluids.

Natural non-absorbable materials

Surgical silk Derived from raw silk spun by silkworm larva in construction of its cocoon. Each fibre is processed to remove the natural waxes and gums. Fibres are twisted or braided together to form the suture strand. *In vivo* studies show that it loses all or most of its tensile strength in 1 year and usually cannot be found after 2 years. Thus it behaves as a very slow absorbable suture. Silk is treated to remove its capillary action and to render it serum-proof. It is dyed black for easy visibility in tissues and is used dry because it loses tensile strength when exposed to moisture (the opposite to cotton).

Dermal suture Twisted silk fibres encased in a non-absorbable coating of tanned gelatin or other protein substance.

Virgin silk Consists of several natural silk filaments drawn together and twisted to form a fragile strand of very small diameter.

Surgical cotton Made from individual long staple vegetable cotton fibres combed, aligned and twisted into a strand. It gains tensile strength when wet.

Linen Cellulose material made from twisted long staple flax fibres.

Horsehair and human hair Have been used for plastic and nerve repair.

Surgical stainless steel wire Made of soft annealed iron alloy formula (with nickel, chromium and molybdenum) presenting optimum metal purity, strength, flexibility, uniformity and compatibility with stainless steel implants and prostheses. Both monofilament and twisted multifilament sutures have high tensile strength and low tissue reactivity owing to extreme inertness. Its disadvantages are difficult handling, late fragmentation and the possibility of cutting tissue.

Synthetic non-absorbables

Nylon (Ethilon) Polyamide polymer derived by chemical synthesis. It has high tensile strength and tissue reaction is very moderate. It degrades *in vivo* at a rate of 15% per year (monofilament).

Black braided nylon (Nurolon) Multifilament braided.

Polyester fibre (Mersilene; Ethiflex) Polymer of terephthalic acid and glycolethylene (multifilament braided).

Polyester (Ethibond) Braided polyester fibres coated with polybutilate as a surgical lubricant.

Polypropylene (Prolene) polymer of propylene extruded into a monofilament suture. Extremely inert (minimal tissue reaction) with high tensile strength.

The non-absorbable sutures are all multifilament except monofilament nylon, steel and polypropylene. Multifilament sutures are easier to handle and tie than monofilaments. Synthetic polymeric materials possess the property of 'memory', i.e. the suture 'remembers' that it was originally a straight fibre and as the knots are subjected to movement and various stresses, the suture tends to straighten and the knot slips and unties. The coefficient of friction in monofilament sutures is relatively low and it therefore needs many knots (i.e. at least six).

Metallic clips Dependable stapling instruments are widely used for clipping blood vessels and for skin closures and gastrointestinal anastomoses.

Non-biological implants

Used for repair, reconstruction and replacement.

Metals

- Stainless steels—bone plates, screws and arthroplasties.
- Tantalum titanium—coarse mesh for acetabular floor and fine mesh for hernial repair. Also for bone plates and screws and mandible.
- Chrome-cobalt alloys—bone plates, screws and arthroplasties.

Textiles (used mainly in vascular surgery and hernia repair)

Dacron (Terylene)
- Woven tubes—small interstices with small blood loss, poor penetration by fibrous tissue and poor fixation of pseudointima. Used for large blood vessel replacement.
- Knitted tubes—large interstices so preclotting is necessary, good fibrous tissue penetration and good pseudointima formation; suitable for smaller vessel replacements.
- Sheets and felts for attachment of heart valves and breast prostheses.
- Spun sutures (vascular).

Polyethylene sheets (Marlex) For hernial repair.

Teflon (Fluon) Similar uses to Dacron. Gortex grafts are made from expanded Teflon (polytetrafluoroethilene) and are relatively non-porous. Velour prostheses are modified knitted grafts of Dacron or Teflon.

Biological implants

Biografts (in contrast to manufactured grafts) remain the first choice for aortocoronary bypass and vascular bypass below the groin. Biografts include autografts (autogenous reversed saphenous vein), homografts (umbilical vein prostheses treated with glutaraldehyde-tan) and heterografts (modified bovine arteries).

1.9. Reflux Oesophagitis

Oesophagitis is usually due to gastro-oesophageal reflux (acid-peptic oesophagitis) and rarely to entero-oesophageal reflux (alkaline oesophagitis). In man, the oesophagogastric junction marks the transition from negative intrathoracic pressure to positive intra-abdominal pressure and is normally 3–5 cm in length. This tonically high pressure zone, called the 'lower oesophageal sphincter' (LOS), maintains a resting pressure of approximately 15–30 mmHg. The LOS relaxes with swallowing, allowing food to pass freely into the stomach. Normally, the diaphragmatic crura, the phreno-oesophageal ligaments, the acute angulation of the oesophageal entry into the stomach, the intra-abdominal segment of the oesophagus and the mucosal rosette all contribute to functioning of the LOS as a mechanical flutter valve (mechanical theory of LOS). However, the LOS is also a specialised tonic muscle which acts as a normal protective barrier to reflux via the excitatory and inhibitory effects of many neurotropic, hormonal and pharmacological agents, e.g. vagotomy leads to reflux while metoclopramide and domperidone antagonise the inhibitory dopaminergic receptors of LOS leading to a pressure rise and prevention of reflux. Gastrointestinal hormones exert excitatory and inhibitory effects (sphincter theory).

Pathogenesis

Gastro-oesophageal reflux has been associated with sliding hiatus hernia and a causal relationship has been established. However, the relationship between hiatus hernia *per se* and reflux is probably of no significance since:

- A substantial number of patients with hiatus hernia fail to demonstrate evidence of reflux.
- 20% of patients with reflux have no demonstrable hiatus hernia.
- Reflux may occur without oesophagitis whether or not a hiatus hernia is present.
- Displacement of the sphincter into the thorax, as seen in hiatus hernia, does not diminish its pressure or competence.

Hiatus hernia, gastro- or entero-oesophageal reflux and oesophagitis are therefore three separate and distinct conditions.

The reflux is due to some abnormality in LOS function which causes the sphincter to become weaker and subsequently incompetent, leading to a retrograde flow across the sphincter into the oesophagus. At least three major abnormalities in LOS function have been described in man:

- Decrease in basal LOS pressure, usually to below 10 mmHg or even as low as 2 mmHg, allowing free reflux of gastric content while the patient is asleep in the recumbent position and in the fasting state.
- Reduction in the adaptive response of the LOS to increase in intra-abdominal pressure. Normally there is an adaptive mechanism that allows the LOS pressure to increase to a greater degree than the intra-abdominal pressure during exercise, Valsalva's manoeuvre or the wearing of tight garments. Patients with reflux disease do not demonstrate this physiological response.
- A defect in the release of the hormone, gastrin, during the ingestion of a meal leading to postprandial complaints. Normally, ingestion of a protein meal leads to the antral and duodenal release of gastrin, which in addition to stimulating acid secretion, is the most potent stimulus for increasing LOS pressure in man. Patients with reflux have less gastrin released during a meal and subsequently show a diminished LOS pressure response to a meal. Other hormones such as glucagon, secretin and cholecystokinin and certain prostaglandins reduce LOS pressure. Foods rich in fat may greatly reduce sphincter competence by the release of cholecystokinin.

The causes of LOS incompetence are:
- Idiopathic (the majority of cases).
- Congenital short oesophagus (brachyoesophagus).
- Chalasia of infancy.
- Pregnancy and obesity.
- Prolonged nasogastric intubation.
- Iatrogenic—after operations that disturb the function of the cardia, including oesophagogastric anastomosis and Heller's oesophagocardiomyotomy (acid and pepsin gastro-oesophageal reflux); or after oesophagoduodenostomy, oesophagojejunostomy, distal gastrectomy with Billroth II (gastrojejunostomy); and occasionally after vagotomy and pyloroplasty (alkaline entero-oesophageal reflux).
- Chronic pyloric or duodenal obstruction, sometimes.

Diagnosis and assessment

It is the reflux disease rather than sliding hiatus hernia that should be called the 'masquerader of the upper abdomen'.

Clinical history

Essential. Suggestive symptoms of reflux are burning epigastric or retrosternal pain during or after food ingestion (heartburn), and gastric content regurgitation with effortless vomiting. The aggravation or precipitation of these symptoms by stooping or lying (postural aggravation) is diagnostic for reflux. There is no correlation between the severity and duration of symptoms and the presence or absence of oesophagitis as determined by endoscopy. Some patients complain bitterly of symptoms but with no visible endoscopic evidence of oesophagitis, whereas others present with peptic stricture and dysphagia but with no other symptoms. Inflammation, ulceration and bleeding (melaena or haematemesis) with anaemia occur. Dysphagia is usually a late symptom due to peptic stricture; however, if it occurs earlier it is due to oesophageal spasm triggered by reflux. Other complications of reflux include aspiration pneumonia, abscesses and bronchiectasis. Prolonged reflux can lead to metaplastic mucosal changes with replacement of squamous epithelium by columnar epithelium (Barrett's epithelium); this is rare but considered to be a premalignant condition leading to adenocarcinoma of the oesophagus.

There are no physical signs to be looked for during physical examination.

Investigations

The primary and routine investigations are *radiology* (*barium swallow, especially in the Trendelenburg position, and fluoroscopic study*) *and oesophagoscopy with biopsy*. These are the most informative for diagnosing reflux oesophagitis with or without stricture. Histologically reflux oesophagitis is either: acute, when changes are visible microscopically and not macroscopically; chronic, with visible changes and microscopic fibrosis identical to chronic gastric peptic ulcer; or a combination of acute and chronic, i.e. a subacute ulceration of aberrant gastric mucosa.

Other selective tests are the following.

Intraoesophageal manometry Quantifies the gastro-oesophageal pressure barrier, locates the gastro-oesophageal junction physiologically as a guide to placement of the pH electrode and catheters for other tests, and determines whether other conditions such as scleroderma, spasm or achalasia are present.

pH reflux test (Using a nasogastric pH electrode after introduction of 300 ml of 0.1 N HCl into an empty stomach) The most accurate method for detecting reflux and judging the competence of the cardia.

The acid perfusion test (Bernstein) Perfuse saline at a rate of 6 ml/min for 10 min in a sitting position and switch to 0.1 N HCl (unknown to the patient) at the same rate for 20 min or until the patient spontaneously complains of reflux symptoms or pain. The perfusion is switched back to normal saline. The test is positive when symptoms occur during acid perfusion and not saline perfusion. This test determines whether acid in contact with the oesophagus causes symptoms, and as with the pH reflux test, it may identify the reflux as the cause of the symptoms.

Acid clearing test Measures the motor ability of the oesophagus to empty itself of acid and thus protect itself from damage as a result of prolonged contact with refluxed gastric secretions. It correlates well with the presence of reflux oesophagitis.

Potential difference test Detects whether oesophageal mucosa is squamous or abnormal (non-specific).

The specificity of these tests is shown in Table 2.

Table 2. Specificity of tests for reflux

Test	Specificity
LOS pressure (manometry)	+ + +
Radiology	
Barium swallow	+
Cine barium swallow	+ +
pH acid reflux	+ + +
Mucosal integrity	
Endoscopy	+ +
Biopsy	+ + +
Acid perfusion	+ + +
Acid clearing	+ +

+ + + = excellent; + + = good; + = fair

Treatment

Normal people can have occasional reflux. If gastroduodenal reflux alone without symptoms or complications is demonstrated, no treatment is required. The primary treatment of reflux oesophagitis is medical. The plan of treatment consists of three stages.

Stage I

- Simple therapeutic postural manoeuvres, e.g. patient should sleep with the bed head elevated, avoid reclining immediately after eating and diminish activities that decrease the gravitational advantage of the oesophagus.
- Obesity should be reduced and patients should not wear tight garments or take vigorous exercise after eating. Dietary advice: avoid coffee, smoking, alcohol, chocolate and fatty food (these lower the LOS pressure either through release of Cholecystokinin, directly or through an unknown indirect mechanism).
- Gaviscon and antacids neutralise gastric acidity and directly increase LOS pressure and prevent reflux through their alkalinisation effect. Non-calcium-containing antacids are preferred, e.g. Maalox, to avoid hypercalcaemia from prolonged use.
- Stop contraindicated drugs that reduce LOS pressure, e.g. anticholinergic and β-adrenergic drugs.

About 75 % of patients with uncomplicated reflux will respond to Stage I medical treatment.

Stage II

Those who have failed to improve with traditional Stage I therapy require specific pharmacotherapy.

- Give drugs that increase LOS pressure and are relatively free of side-effects, e.g. bethanecol chloride and metoclopramide hydrochloride (Maxolon).
- Give drugs that inhibit acid secretion by H_2 receptor antagonism, i.e. cimetidine and ranitidine.

A further 20% of patients respond to this therapy, so that only 5–10% of all patients with reflux disease will require surgical intervention (Stage III).

Stage III

Includes antireflux procedures. In the past, the aim of surgery was to repair the hiatus hernia. This approach, as represented by Allison surgical repair, had limited success and many failures since reflux is unrelated to the presence of a hiatus hernia.

Surgical reconstruction or restoration of the competent LOS mechanism leads to functional improvement and clinical cure and should be the aim of any antireflux operation.

Surgical treatment

Indications

- Failure of medical therapy (Stages I and II) and/or severe initial symptoms interfering with patient's occupation.
- Local complications, e.g. oesophagitis (with ulceration visible on barium swallow), haemorrhage (with anaemia), peptic oesophageal stricture.
- Respiratory complications from reflux, e.g. aspiration pneumonia, abscesses, empyema and bronchiectasis.
- Paraoesophageal (rolling) hiatus hernia (10% of cases; the sliding type represents 85% and the mixed type 5% of cases) with postprandial cardiorespiratory distress and dysphagia.
- Associated lesions, e.g. pyloric or duodenal (peptic) ulcers and gall stones.

Surgical approaches

Either the laparotomy or the thoracotomy approach is used.

The advantages of the laparotomy approach are:
- Less painful (no intercostal neuralgia).

- Safer in middle-aged obese patients.
- Able to provide satisfactory examination and surgical treatment for intra-abdominal associated diseases, e.g. duodenal or pyloric petic ulcer and gall stones.

Thoracotomy has the advantages of:
- Better access for severe oesophagitis and shortening of oesophagus.
- Being the best approach for para-oesophageal hiatus hernia repair.
- Definite place in peptic stricture treatment, e.g. Thal's patch.

Types of antireflux operation

Mark IV–Belsy Repair (Belsy—Bristol, 1966) (Fig. 3).

A transthoracic approach through the eighth rib bed. After careful and complete mobilisation of the oesophagogastric junction or cardia and intra-abdominal reduction of the peritoneal hernial sac, the repair is performed in three stages:
(a) Reapproximation of the two halves of the right crus of the diaphragm with stout sutures (snug closure of the oesophageal hiatus behind the oesophagus).
(b) Restoration of an acute oesophagogastric angle by plication of the stomach fundus onto the distal oesophagus via the initial row of mattress sutures.
(c) Restoration of an abdominal segment of the oesophagus via the second row of three mattress sutures.

Fundoplication (Nissen II–Basel, Switzerland 1964)

A transabdominal approach. The right crus margins are identified and approximated. Mobilisation of stomach fundus by dividing the gastrosplenic omentum is followed by wrapping the mobilised fundus around and suturing in front of the abdominal oesophagus to produce an 'unspillable inkwell' effect. In the presence of pyloric or duodenal peptic ulcer, vagotomy and pyloroplasty could be added.

Gastropexy

Simple anterior fixation of anterior surface of stomach (near the lesser curve) to the linea alba (described separately by Boerema of Amsterdam, 1955 and Nissen (I), 1960).

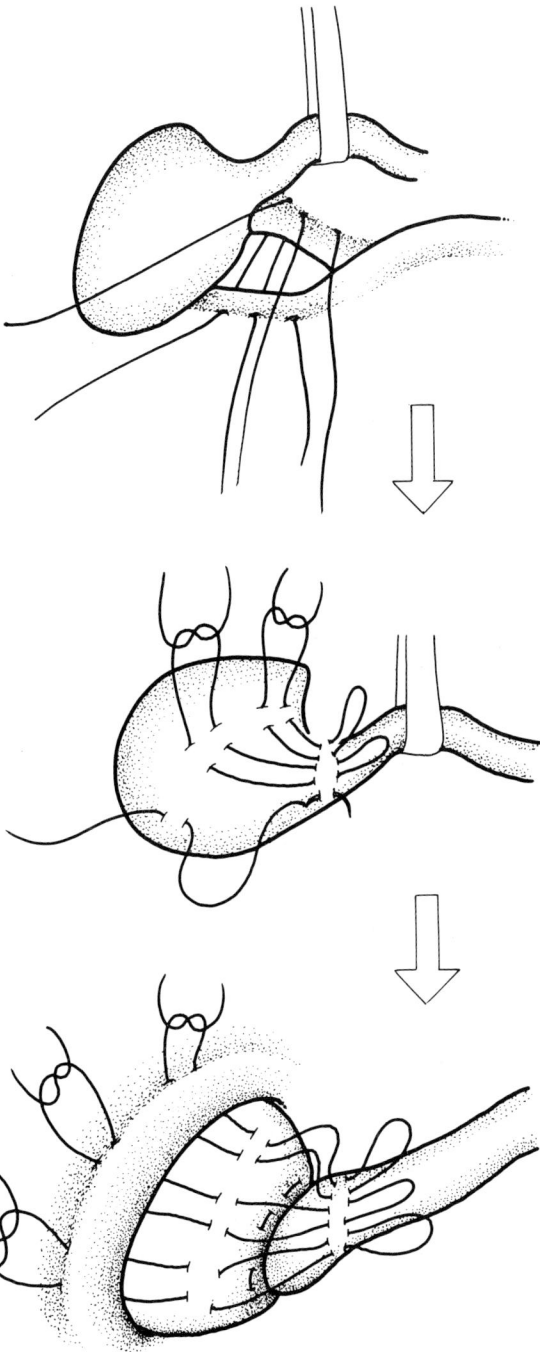

Fig. 3 Mark IV – Belsey repair of hiatus hernia

Posterior fixation by anchoring the gastro-oesophageal junction to the pre-aortic fascia and median arcuate ligament after transabdominal reduction of the hernia and closure of the hiatus posterior to the oesophagus (Hill, 1967).

Others

Collis thoracoabdominal approach with approximation of the right crus in front of the oesophagus and fixation of stomach fundus to the undersurface of the left dome of the diaphragm to maintain an acute angle.

Balanced composite operation (Berman and Berman, 1959): consists of reduction of the hernia, bilateral vagotomy, repair of hiatus, oesophagogastropexy and pyloroplasty.

Silastic ring Angelchick prosthesis placed around oesophagogastric junction—a procedure still undergoing evaluation. So far, the results of randomised trials are promising.

Alkaline reflux oesophagitis (Fig. 4)

Treated in the following ways.
(a) Oesophagoduodenostomy—convert to Roux-en-Y oesophagojejunostomy.
(b) End-to-side oesophagojejunostomy—(i) add enteroenterostomy; or (ii) convert to Roux-en-Y; or (iii) convert to Tanner-19 modification.
(c) Billroth II—convert to (i) Roux-en-Y or (ii) Tanner-19 Alternatively add an enteroenterostomy.
(d) Billroth I—convert to Roux-en-Y (not illustrated).

1.10. Abdominal Wound Dehiscence

Burst abdomen occurs in 1 % of all abdominal operations with 10 % mortality. The peak incidence is between the 6th and 8th postoperative day.

Predisposing factors

Preoperative   Chest infection, systemic sepsis, persistent cough, jaundice, malignancy, anaemia, hypoproteinaemia, diabetes mellitus, steroid therapy, immune deficiency diseases, immune suppression therapy and obesity (general causes—patient's fault).

Operative   Aseptic surgery or operations for peritonitis, poor surgical technique (too tight or too loose suturing, nerve injury and haematoma formation due to vascular injury) (Local causes—surgeon's fault).

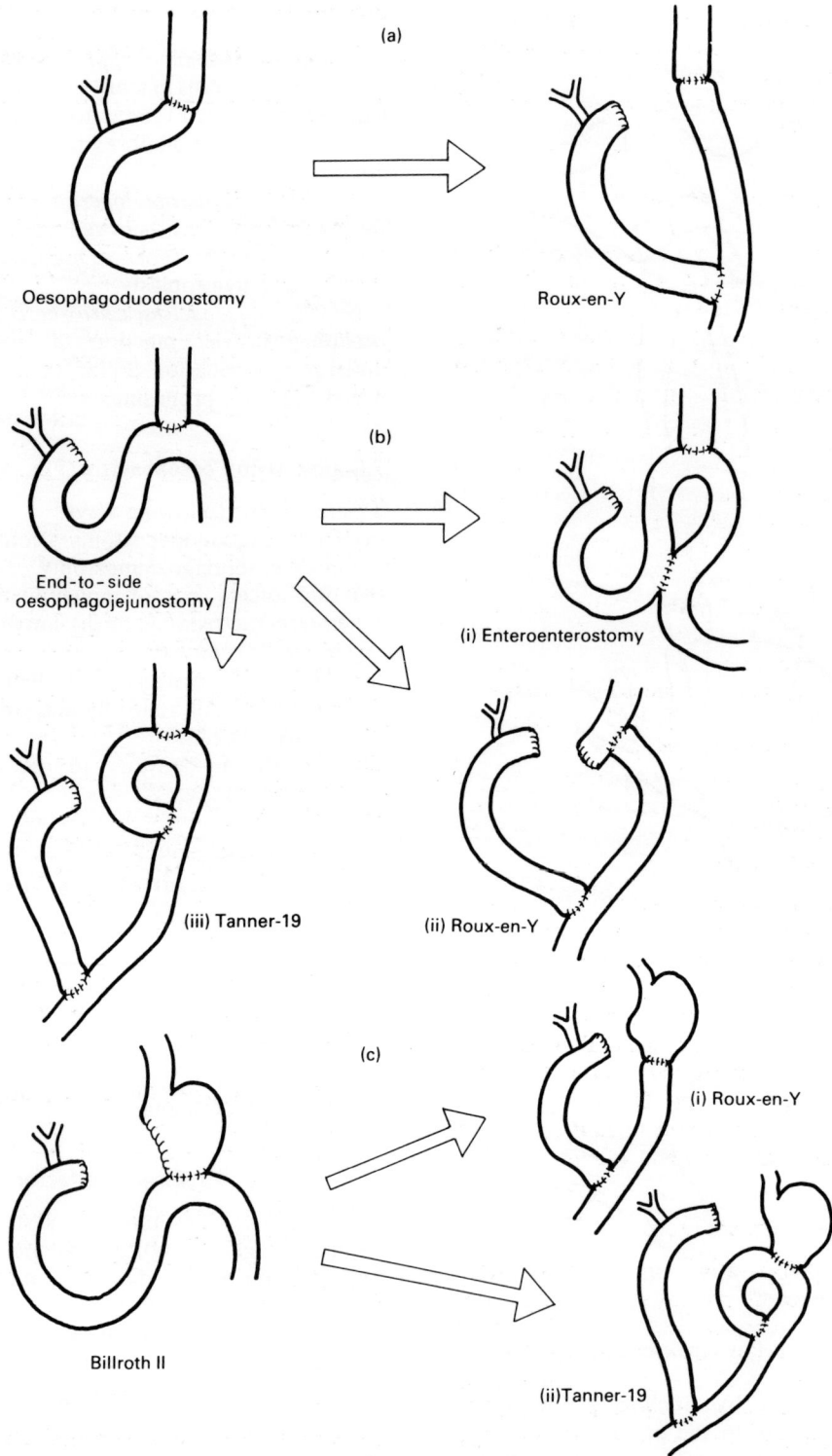

Fig. 4   Choice of treatments for alkaline reflux oesophagitis

Postoperative Persistence of the preoperative problem, postoperative distension (gastric or paralytic ileus), premature removal of deep tension sutures, wound infection and haematoma (nurses' and surgeon's fault).

Types and treatment

Revealed (superficial) Gaping of skin and subcutaneous tissues (only) after removal of stitches 2 weeks postoperatively. Due to wound infection or haematoma. The treatment is to evacuate blood clots, treat the wound infection and let the wound heal by secondary intention (granulation).

Concealed (deep) Separation of all layers of the anterior abdominal wall except the skin. Incisional hernia develops eventually. If the condition is recognised in hospital, delay stitch removal, apply abdominal corset and treat incisional hernia on its merit using non-absorbable nylon size 1 or 0 for the repair either in pleating layers pushing the hernial sac into the abdomen without opening (keel operation—Maingot) or opening the sac and repairing the layers from the inside margins of the sac upwards (Cattell's operation). In huge incisional hernia, a preoperative repeated induced pneumoperitoneum may be required to increase the peritoneal reservoir to cope with subsequent reduction of the intestinal contents and to avoid possible respiratory embarrassment.

Complete (burst abdomen) Occurs either gradually with a 'tell-tale' serosanguinous discharge or suddenly with protrusion of a knuckle of bowel or omentum through the wound on the 10th day. Apply *sterile warm* packs (never dry) and do an urgent repair in theatre under general anaesthesia. Resuture with interrupted non-absorbable through-and-through sutures. Do not try to separate the tissues; skin can be included in suturing or left open to heal with secondary intention.

Prophylaxis

In all cases, preoperative predisposing factors should be corrected before any surgery, e.g. reduction of obesity, treatment of chest infection or sepsis, stoppage of smoking and control of diabetes. Attention must be paid to proper aseptic conditions and meticulous surgical technique minimising bowel manipulation to avoid paralytic ileus. Postoperative nasogastric suction (and i.v. drip) to avoid postoperative distension and timely removal of stitches are essential.

1.11. Early Gastric Carcinoma

Early gastric carcinoma (EGC) is the term adopted by the Japanese Society of Digestive Endoscopy in 1962 and defined as 'Carcinoma limited to the mucosa and submucosa, with or without lymph node metastases'. Surgical treatment usually leads to cure. The Japanese 5 year survival is 92% and becomes 57% and 29% respectively when muscles and serosa are invaded in contrast to 20% or less in the usual gastric carcinoma which has the distinction of being the commonest fatal cancer in the world. Morphologically EGC is classified into three types (Fig. 5).

The diagnosis is reached by the use of a double-contrast barium meal (DCBM) as a screening test coupled with endoscopy and biopsy in suspected cases. The DCBM was used widely for stomach examination in Japan in 1966. It is a six-film technique without fluoroscopy using a medium-density, low-viscosity barium suspension with air introduced originally via a nasogastric tube which is then replaced by a 'bubbly barium', effervescent drinks and effervescent tablets. Results are enhanced by using smooth muscle relaxants (glucagon 0.25 mg i.v. or hyoscine butylbromine (Buscopan) 20 mg i.v.) to induce gastric and duodenal hypotonia. The latter drugs are contraindicated in heart failure, angina, prostatism and glaucoma. In this manner it is possible:

- To detect slight mucosal irregularities, e.g. small cancers, ulcers and ulcer scars.
- To see lesions *en face* and assess the size, shape and margins.

In 1971, a total of 1 886 062 Japanese people were screened (as above) in a mass gastric survey. EGC was detected in 0.15% and the 5 year survival proved to be 63%.

Many British surgeons, however, believe that EGC described in Japan is probably a different disease from gastric carcinoma diagnosed in the UK.

Treatment

Surgery is the only form of curative treatment and is also the main means of palliation in advanced cancer. Preoperative preparation aimed at correction of electrolyte disturbances, dehydration and

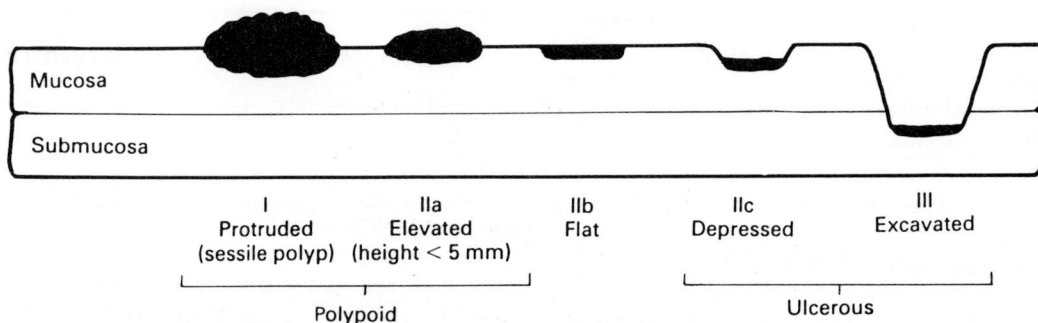

Fig. 5 EGC classification according to the Japanese Society of Digestive Endoscopy, 1962 (uppermost) and Hermanek and Rosch, 1973 (lowermost)

anaemia is essential. Parenteral nutrition and prophylactic antibiotics may be required.

The choice of operation depends on the site, the extent of the growth and the state of the patient. Curative resection should include the entire tumour and a 7–8 cm margin proximally and distally to ensure adequate macroscopic excision with removal of greater and lesser omentum and lymph nodes *en bloc*. A Polya technique utilising a wide stoma should be used. The transverse colon is usually left *in situ*, but can be included if necessary. For antral tumours, distal gastrectomy should include 4 cm beyond the pylorus via the abdominal approach (Fig. 6a). For cardia or fundus tumours, proximal gastrectomy should include the spleen, pancreatic tail and lower part of the oesophagus via a thoracoabdominal approach (Fig. 6b). For extensive or multiple tumours in the body of the stomach, total gastrectomy should include removal of the whole of the stomach, again via the thoracoabdominal approach (Fig. 7). If the lower part of the oesophagus is resected, both vagal trunks are divided and pyloromyotomy or pyloroplasty is needed to prevent pyloric obstruction. However, the Japanese believe that a conservative gastrectomy is satisfactory for EGC.

The postoperative prognosis depends on age, length of history, operation type, tumour site and size, depth of invasion, lymph node metastases, tumour-free margin, tumour macroscopy and microscopy and immune response (represented by infiltration of the tumour by lymphocytes and plasma cells and follicular response in adjacent lymph nodes).

1.12. Critical Review of Peptic Ulcer Management

The operative methods of treating duodenal ulcer are compared in Table 3. These are: partial gastrectomy (PG), vagotomy and antrectomy (V + A), total vagotomy and drainage (TV + D), (whether drainage is in the form of gastrojejunostomy (GJ) or pyloroplasty (P)), and highly selective vagotomy (HSV).

GASTRIC ULCER

Presents in one of two ways.

Combined gastric ulcer + duodenal ulcer (25%)

The duodenal ulcer is the primary and gastric ulcer is secondary. If both are active then gastric ulcer is benign but if duodenal ulcer is scarred then gastric ulcer is probably malignant. Treat medically (while duodenal ulcer is treated as above). If unsuccessful then total vagotomy + hemigastrectomy resecting both ulcers. Alternatively HSV + dilatation with gastric ulcer excisional biopsy.

Gastric ulcer alone (75%)

Ulcer cancer (15% of gastric ulcers) Clinical, radiological, endoscopical (five biopsies) and his-

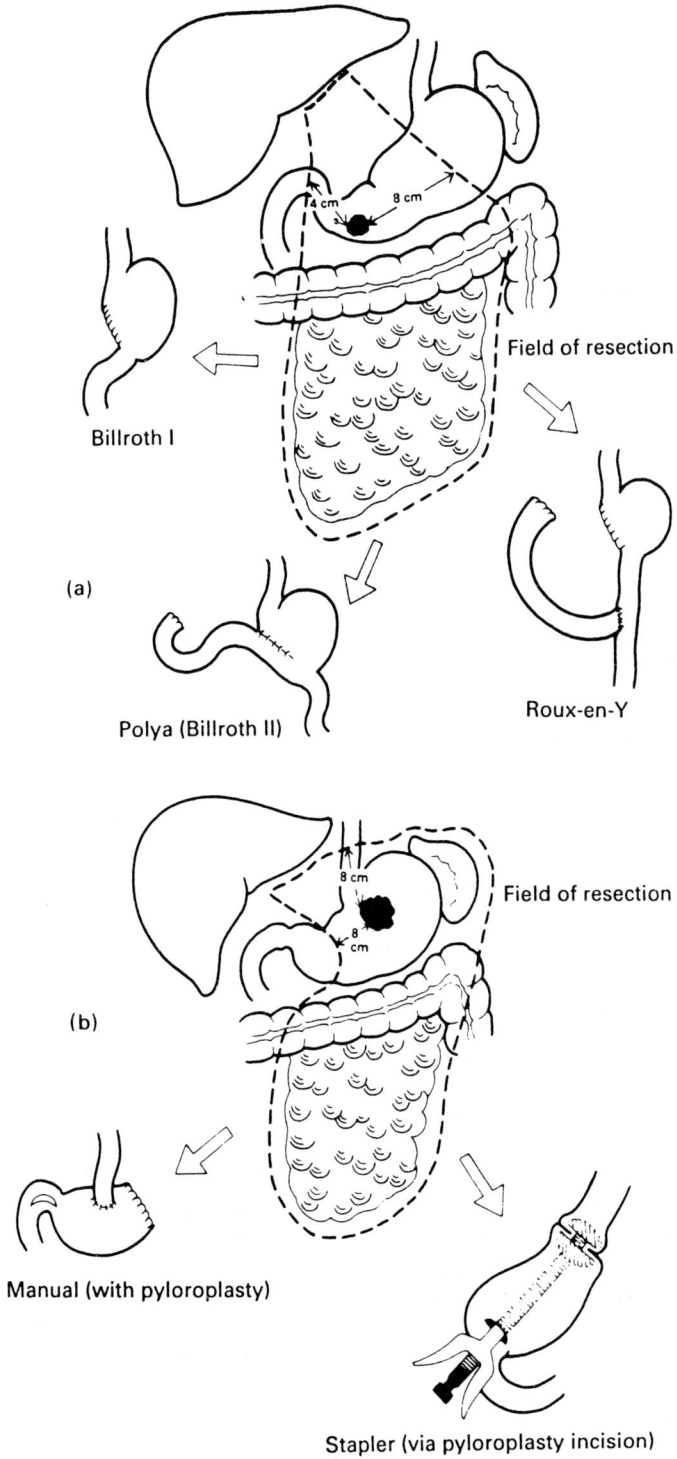

dietary fibre has a protective value in appendicitis, colonic cancer, coronary heart disease, colonic diverticulosis, constipation, haemorrhoids, varicose veins, obesity, gall stones and diabetes which are very common in urban areas and developed countries and by contrast rare in rural areas and developing countries.

Familial Polyposis coli is regarded as a precancerous condition (being an autosomal dominant, the family should be screened with barium enemas). Gardner's syndrome (polyposis coli with osteomas) may be associated with gastroduodenal tumours, e.g. periampullary tumour. Sebaceous cysts in children should always give rise to the suspicion of Gardner's syndrome.

Ulcerative colitis Especially in the presence of pseudopolyps which increase the risk of malignancy by 15%. Generally the risk of cancer is in the region of 3.5% which increases to 12% after 20 years.

Crohn's disease Rarely predisposes to colonic cancer.

Adenoma of rectum (villous, tubular or tubulovillous) A definite premalignant condition.

Carcinogenic metabolites of excessive bile salts Hydrolysed by bacterial flora—mainly nuclear dehydrogenating Clostridia—they may lead to cancer. The relationship between cholecystectomy and colonic cancer is debatable.

Bilharzioma (*Schistosoma mansoni*).

Ureterosigmoidostomy May be complicated by colonic cancer.

Anal canal

Radiotherapy (squamous cell carcinoma)

Leucoplakia

Usual skin premalignant conditions Note that basal cell carcinoma and melanoma can develop in the anus (very rarely).

1.16. Endoscopy and Clinical Surgery

While flexible fibreoptic endoscopy is better tolerated by the patient and provides a diagnostic,

therapeutic, research and screening service, there are also some disadvantages:
- Expensive—£7000 per instrument.
- Fragile instruments—a careless bite could cost £2000.
- Cannot readily be sterilised.
- More dangerous than radiology.

However, endoscopy has the advantage of greater accuracy. The conventional barium meal gives about 67% accuracy, while accuracy with endoscopy is about 95%. Endoscopy also has therapeutic uses, e.g. oesophageal dilatation and colonic polypectomy, which are cost-effective.

INDICATIONS FOR OESOPHAGOGASTRODUODENOSCOPY

Diagnostic

The advantages of fibreoptic endoscopy include: direct visualisation of the lesion and organ in question, making possible an assessment of appearance, movement and contents; biopsy specimens for histopathological study and cytological smears can easily be taken, and permanent records of appearance obtained (still photographs, cine-film and video-tape recordings). Thus, endoscopy complements radiology and may be used to confirm or clarify radiological findings, but is also used diagnostically instead of radiology.

Indications in oesophageal disorders include the investigation of dysphagia and the diagnosis and assessment of varices and oesophagitis, as well as the confirmation and clarification of radiological findings. In the stomach, one of the most important indications is the assessment of gastric ulcers, i.e. their possible malignancy. The duodenum is a common seat of disease and radiology often gives equivocal results: endoscopy is extensively used in the diagnosis of duodenal ulcer and of duodenitis. It is also of particular value in assessing the symptomatic patient who has undergone gastric or gastroduodenal surgery (e.g. recurrent peptic ulcer).

Oesophagogastroduodenoscopy (OGD) is more accurate than radiology in diagnosing the cause of *acute upper gastrointestinal bleeding*, partly as lesions difficult to find radiologically can readily be seen (e.g. Mallory–Weiss tears, acute gastric or duodenal erosions and varices) and partly because the site of recent bleeding can usually be identified when two or more abnormalities are present. Mortality is about 10% and emergency OGD should be done after 4–12 h to allow for gastric

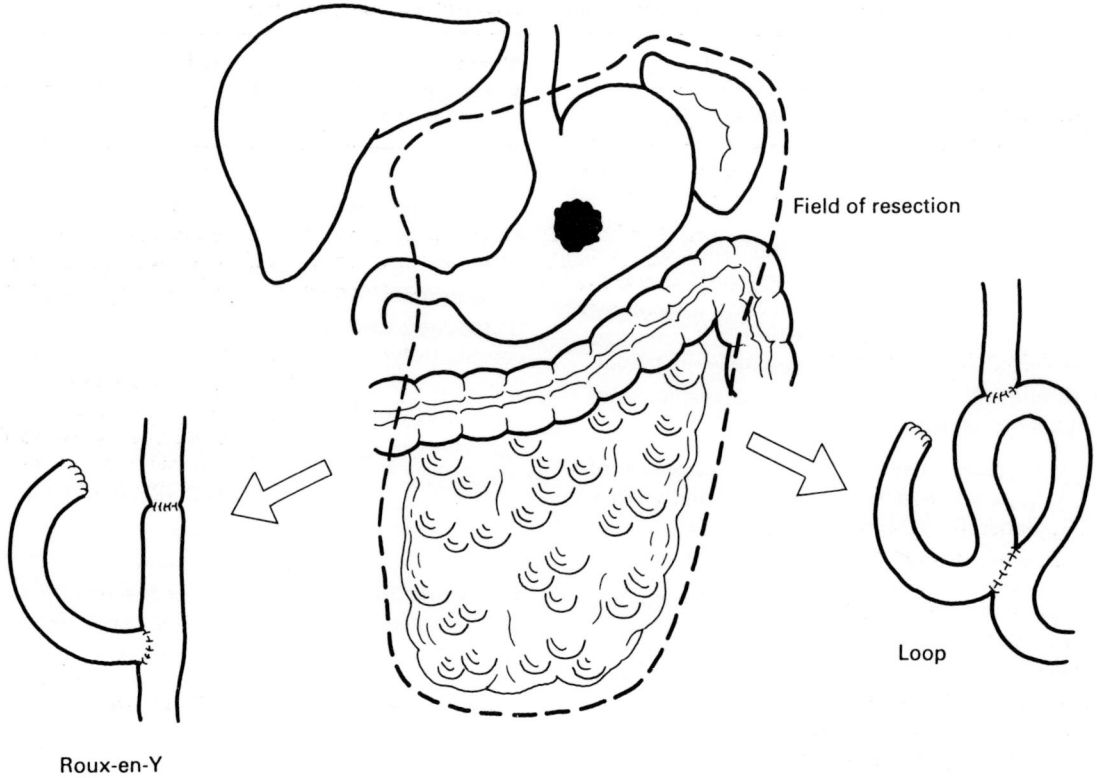

Fig. 7 Total gastrectomy and oesophagojejunostomy showing alternative methods of repair (oesophagoduodenostomy should not be done because of risk of alkaline oesophagitis)

tological confirmation before operation are needed. Treated by gastrectomy (usually Billroth I—PG).

Prepyloric gastric ulcer (behaves like duodenal ulcer)
- Ulcer cancer: treat as above.
- Benign gastric ulcer with MAO more than 40 mEq HCl/h: treat as duodenal ulcer.
- Benign gastric ulcer with normal MAO: treat as gastric ulcer at incisura or lesser curve (Billroth I—PG; *see below*).

Benign gastric ulcer The acid output level is normal. Serum gastrin level is high. Minority have gastric stasis (with coexisting pyloric channel disease or duodenal ulcer). Pressure within pylorus is abnormally low and reflux of duodenal content into stomach is greater than normal.

The reflux of bile salts and lysolecithin breaks the gastric mucosal barrier, leading to gastritis, and release gastrin, rendering gastric mucosa more vulnerable to the action of irritant drugs, acid and pepsin.

Ulcers occur in the junctional zone between the parietal cell mass and alkaline mucosa of the pyloric gland area. The operative principles therefore should be to:
- Reduce the output of acid and pepsin.
- Reduce reflux of bile into stomach.
- Ensure that gastric stasis does not occur.

Treatment

Conservative

Treat with H_2-antagonist (e.g. ranitidine, cimetidine), carbenoxolone (Biogastrone), antacids, rest, regular meals, no smoking. If these measures do not lead to healing of the ulcer in 6 weeks, surgery is indicated (in duodenal ulcer 6 months' medical treatment is required before operative intervention is deemed necessary after failure).

Table 3. Assessment of operative treatment for duodenal ulcer

	PG	*V + A*	*TV + D*	*HSV*
Operative mortality	1.5 %	1.2 %	0.6 %	0.3 %
Postoperative morbidity	Gastric stasis, loop syndrome, ruptured duodenal stump		Anastomotic leak	Lesser curve necrosis 0.1 %
Side-effects	Dumping, diarrhoea, dysphagia (heartburn and reflux oesophagitis), bilious vomiting, postprandial distension. Visick clinical grading: Perfect (1), Good (2), Fair (3) and Poor (4). In HSV (1 + 2) represents 96 % while in V + A or TV + D (1 + 2) represents 76 %.			
Recurrent ulcer after 5–10 years	3 %	1 %	9 % (V + GJ = 7 %) (V + P = 11 %)	8 % Surgeon should clean distal 5 cm of oesophagus downward, leaving only 5–7 cm from pylorus
Long-term metabolic sequelae after 5–30 years (gastric cripple), e.g. weight loss, anaemia (iron and B_{12} deficiency), tuberculosis and bone disease (osteoporosis and osteomalacia)	+ + +	+ +	+	None
Carcinoma of gastric remnant after 15–30 years (due to bile reflux and gastritis). Vagotomy also produces chronic gastric mucosal changes of unknown significance	+ +	+ +	+	? (unknown)
Relative ease or difficulty of salvage operation if first operation fails	Worst ⟶ Best			

Operative

- PG (Billroth I). Recurrent ulcer in 2 % and operative mortality of 2 %.
- TV + D with ulcer excision (indicated in elderly and frail patients and in cases of bleeding gastric ulcer or high gastric ulcer on the lesser curve). Recurrent ulcer on 10 % and operative mortality of 1.5 %.
- HSV + ulcer excision is a good alternative as it reduces hydrochloric acid and pepsin output and increases intragastric pressure, thus preventing bile reflux.

TV + P versus TV + G (merits and demerits)

In *total vagotomy and pyloroplasty* the long-term metabolic sequelae are less severe. The operation:
- Is simpler and quicker.
- Maintains the normal pathway.
- Has a definite place in bleeding peptic ulcer and pyloric stenosis.
- Is safer in elderly and high risk patients (with cardiac and/or respiratory and/or renal problems).
- Diarrhoea is a rare problem.

Total vagotomy + gastrojejunostomy deals with healthier tissue:
- It can be undone easily when a salvage operation is needed.

Invasive
- Endoscopic retrograde cholangiography (ERC) and endoscopic retrograde pancreatography (ERP).
- Chiba needle PTC.

Efficiency of showing the biliary tree (depends upon experience)

ERC is successful in 70–90% of patients regardless of the size of the ducts. However, PTC is successful in 95% of dilated ducts but in only about 50% of non-dilated ducts.

Special considerations

- ERC may be the procedure of choice for:
  —Pancreatitis causing cholestasis.
  —Tumours of the ampulla, duodenum, etc.
  —Endoscopic sphincterotomy.
  —Sclerosing cholangitis.
- ERC and PTC may be complementary in defining the extent of bile duct strictures and tumours.
- Choice is also dependent upon the therapeutic component (drainage, prosthesis, sphincterotomy).

N.B. In a jaundiced patient, the size of the ducts should first be assessed by a non-invasive method (grey scale ultrasonography). If they are dilated, PTC is the procedure most likely to succeed. If the ducts are not dilated, ERC is most successful. After both procedures, if dilated bile ducts are shown, early surgery or non-operative drainage is advised.

ERCP Interpretation

Biliary System (ERC)

ERCP provides information on the *lower duct* but may fail to fill the upper ducts if a block or stenosis is present. Therefore, PTC may provide more useful information on the *upper duct system* where ultrasonography has shown dilated 'intrahepatic' ducts.

The success rate of ERC depends on operator experience but in average hands is about 70%.

Remember the value of *late films* (45 min or later) in demonstrating gall stones not shown on routine cholecystography.

Pancreatic duct (ERP)

ERP is the most accurate technique available for assessing the presence and extent of pancreatic disease. Unfortunately it can be very difficult to distinguish between *benign* or *malignant* disease, and other methods such as *cytology*, *ultrasonography* and *CT* may be required to assist in this differentiation.

Radiological signs of value are:
- *Block* or *stricture* of duct system.
- *Leakage* from duct system.
- *Irregularity* and *beading* of side radical.
- *Cysts*.
- *Delayed emptying* of main duct (more than 10 min) in part or all of the duct system.
- *Calcification* in pancreas and relationship to duct.

N.B. If a *cyst is filled* or there is *leakage from the duct system* at ERP there is a serious risk of secondary complications (e.g. acute pancreatitis or abscess formation) and *surgical treatment* may be required *urgently*.

Duodenoscopic sphincterotomy and gall stone extraction

Allowing spontaneous passage   This is the easiest and least traumatic method of eliminating stones; over 70% will pass spontaneously within 4 weeks. However, ascending cholangitis may still occur, and repeat ERCP is necessary to check. A transnasal biliary catheter facilitates repeat cholangiography and allows flushing of stones.

Extraction of stones   May be done at the time of sphincterotomy or subsequently using 'baskets' or 'balloon catheters'. Balloon catheters are rather fragile. It is possible for the basket to become impacted if the orifice is inadequate.

Selection of patients

Common bile duct stones
- After previous cholecystectomy when risk of surgery is high.
- After previous cholecystectomy if the patient does not want a further operation.
- After 'recent' cholecystectomy if other methods have failed.
- Patients with stones in *both* the gall bladder and common bile duct where surgery is contraindicated on medical grounds and common bile duct stone is causing problems.

Papillary stenosis   If this is a cause of the problem.

Papillary tumour   For palliation or preoperative drainage.

Results

An experienced surgeon should be able successfully to treat over 90 % of common bile duct stones with endoscopic sphincterotomy. Complication rates depend on experience and type of patient treated. A mortality of around 1 % is anticipated on present evidence.

CHOLEDOCHOSCOPY (RIGID AND FLEXIBLE)

Choledochoscopy is the visual examination of the interior of the bile ducts with a choledochoscope. In *operative choledochoscopy* the instrument is placed directly into the common bile duct during the course of a surgical procedure for gall stones. In *postoperative choledochoscopy* the instrument is passed via a T-tube track into the common bile duct and hepatic ducts during the postoperative period as a means of retrieving retained bile duct stones. This is widely used in Japan, but not in the UK.

Operative choledochoscopy

Postexploratory choledochoscopy

The common bile duct is explored by conventional methods and any stones removed. The choledochoscope is then used to provide a postexploratory visual check that the common bile duct and hepatic ducts are clear and no stones or debris have been overlooked. This method of direct visual check is more reliable and quicker than a postexploratory intraoperative cholangiogram which may be difficult to interpret.

Exploratory choledochoscopy

The choledochoscope is placed into the common bile duct as soon as it is opened and used as the exploring instrument. Exploration of the bile ducts for stones is thus carried out by direct vision. This is much less traumatic and more reliable for finding the stones than conventional blind techniques with forceps or bougies.

Stone retrieval

Using exploratory choledochoscopy it is only a short step to stone retrieval under direct vision. Devices which pass along the irrigation channel of the choledochoscope for this purpose include a Fogarty-type balloon catheter, a wire basket, wire stone forceps, a catheter with reversed water jet, and a controllable right-angled curette for dislodging impacted stones and detaching stones from the duct walls. Smaller loose stones are easily flushed out of the ducts by the high-pressure fluid irrigation through the channel of the choledochoscope. These techniques are much less traumatic than blind stone retrieval.

COLONOSCOPY

Indications

Colonoscopy is usually performed after the patient has had a high-quality double-contrast barium enema, although some centres prefer to do colonoscopy or sigmoidoscopy before barium enema. Colonoscopy is indicated for:
- Evaluation of an abnormal barium enema: a suspect area may be inspected and biopsied or cytological brushings taken.
- Persistent symptoms, especially rectal bleeding, with normal barium enema.
- Selected cases of inflammatory bowel disease where it may be helpful in the differential diagnosis to assess the extent of disease or to examine strictures and to search for synchronous or metachronous lesions.
- Assessment of postoperative colonic anastomosis or inspection of bowel segment prior to reconnection.
- Therapeutic polypectomy.

Contraindications

Contraindications to the procedure are those related to the general medical condition of the patient such as recent myocardial infarction, and those directly related to colonic disease such as acute severe colitis of any kind. It is wise to think carefully before performing colonoscopy in those patients who are elderly and frail; those with severe diverticular disease; those who have had extensive previous pelvic or abdominal surgery; and, in particular, after pelvic irradiation and in those with an excessively redundant colon. Newer techniques of intubation and improvements in the instruments, however, make these considerations less important than previously.

Limitations

It may not be possible to pass the instrument and complete the examination because of poor prepar-

skull X-ray showing ballooned sella turcica in multiple adenoma syndrome.

Treatment

Conservative

Give cimetidine and antacids and withdraw alcohol, smoking and ulcerogenic drugs.

Operative

- Revagotomy with or without antrectomy (Billroth I) after TV + D or HSV. Sometimes, Polya PG may be needed.
- Exclude ZES if there is recurrence after PG.
- If gastric ulcer recurs after an operation for duodenal ulcer, it is due to gastric stasis. However, ischaemic gastric ulcer may follow HSV. Do antrectomy including the gastric ulcer.

Prevention

Avoid Albatross syndrome (failures in gastric surgery due to wrongly selected patient developing side-effects; called albatross syndrome due to patient 'hanging about the surgeon's neck'). Such cases include patients with atypical pain and young patients with short peptic ulcer history who smoke and drink, are absent from work and on anti-depressant drugs.

Remember that recurrence after complete vagotomy is usually gastric while after incomplete vagotomy it is usually duodenal.

How to test for complete vagotomy

Intraoperative tests (Fig. 8)

Burge test (UK, 1964).   A manometer is applied via an oesophagogastric balloon, the pylorus is occluded with a clamp, and then the vagotomised area is stimulated. Any detected increase in pressure indicates incomplete vagotomy.

Grassi test (Rome, 1971)   A glass electrode inserted through a small gastrostomy is used to measure pH after vagotomy and MAO stimulation. A pH of 1.2–2 surrounded by a pH of 5.5–7 indicates the presence and actual location of incomplete vagotomy.

Postoperative tests

Peak acid output after pentagastrin   A 50% or more reduction compared to the preoperative value indicates complete vagotomy.

Insulin test   Performed 1 week after vagotomy an insulin test has a prognostic value. If it is positive within such a short time, the chance of recurrence is high; if it is negative, the chance of recurrence is low. The insulin test is contraindicated in epileptics, patients over 65 years of age, those with a history of ischaemic heart disease and diabetics.

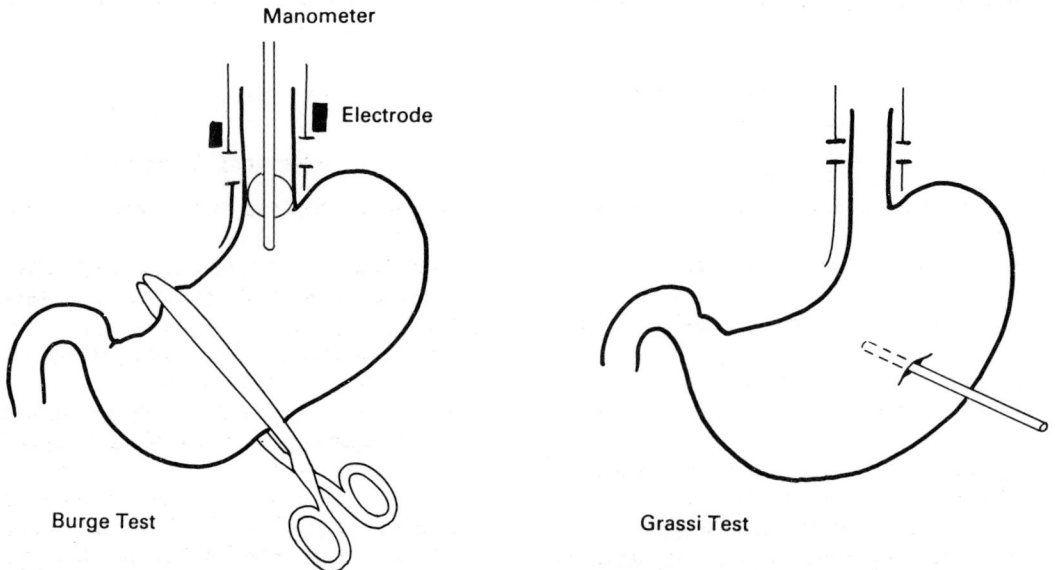

Fig. 8   Intraoperative tests for incomplete vagotomy

1.13. Surgery for Chronic Inflammatory Bowel Disease

ULCERATIVE COLITIS

Indications for surgery:
- Chronic: stricture and carcinoma.
- Acute: bleeding, perforation, toxic megacolon and obstruction.
- Extraintestinal manifestations, e.g. eye, joints and skin: ameliorated by surgery.
- Intractability: in spite of medical treatment in chronic recurrent cases (salazopyrine, bland diet, diarrhoea control and steroid retention enema) and in acute cases (i.v. fluid replacement, parenteral feeding, i.v. prednisolone 60 mg/24 h, blood transfusion and twice daily steroid retention enema).

Surgical options (Fig. 9)

Proctocolectomy and ileostomy
- Most widely used.
- Complete excision of entire colonic mucosa.
- No risk of recurrence or stump carcinoma.
- Impaired sexual function in some patients.
- Ileostomy for life but it is well managed by young patients and the adherent stoma bag is followed up by a stoma therapist.

Subtotal colectomy and ileorectal anastomosis
- Increasingly used operation particularly in the UK.
- Incomplete excision of colonic mucosa.
- Risk of recurrence and carcinoma in rectal mucosa.
- Life-long sigmoidoscopic and rectal biopsy follow-up.
- No ileostomy and no sexual function impairment.
- Loose stools in some patients (mean frequency of 3.5/24 h, range of 1–6/24 h).

Colectomy, ileostomy and rectal mucous fistula
- Performed in emergency situations.
- Incomplete excision of colonic mucosa.
- Safe emergency operation as it is less extensive and can achieve remission via diversion of faecal stream.

- Retains the option of a subsequent restorative procedure such as subtotal colectomy and ileorectal anastomosis.

Proctocolectomy and Kock's continet ileostomy
- Similar to proctocolectomy and ileostomy with complete excision of entire colonic mucosa.
- 'Mini' stoma requiring regular catheterisation.
- Such a reservoir stoma with an intussuscepted nippled valve could become dilated with contents, or could malfunction and produce incontinence (leakage).

Colectomy, rectal mucosectomy, ileoanal anastomosis and pelvic ileal pouch
- Complete excision of entire colonic mucosa.
- No risk of recurrence or cancer.
- Temporary loop ileostomy for 6–8 weeks (to protect the ileoanal anastomosis), but no permanent stoma and no psychological trauma (in young man concerned about sex and marriage).
- Continence is maintained by anal sphincters.
- Sexual function is intact.
- Probably the most promising operation of the future.

The pelvic ileal pouch is constructed either by a J-shaped anastomosis using a stapler or by a triple S-shaped sutured anastomosis. Removal of the rectal mucosal cuff down to the dentate line followed by anastomosis may lead to infection and anastomotic dehiscence—therefore routine ileostomy protection is needed. Postoperative diarrhoea may be troublesome and anastomotic stricture may be marked requiring dilatation.

CROHN'S DISEASE

Indications for surgery

- Anal manifestations, i.e. abscesses, fistulae and strictures.
- Intestinal obstruction, haemorrhage and perforation (perforation is rare because of transmural thickening).
- Extraintestinal manifestations, i.e. uveitis, recurrent polyarthritis and pyoderma gangrenosa.
- Failure of medical measures to suppress the active disease or to aid healing of anal lesions (i.e. salazopyrine, steroids, azothioprine, correction of anaemia and hypoproteinaemia; control of diarrhoea by low-fibre bland diet and administration of codeine, lomotil and cholestyramine to overcome the cathartic action of non-absorbed bile salts on the colon).

the vessels or platelets. If both prothrombin time and partial thromboplastin time are prolonged, the defect is probably in the common pathway. If partial thromboplastin time is prolonged and prothrombin time is normal, the defect is in the intrinsic system. A prolonged prothrombin time and a normal partial thromboplastin time is rare and indicates deficiency of factor VII.

Local vascular disease

The commonest cause of regional bleeding is local vascular disease, e.g. as a result of badly ligated blood vessels or secondary infection, rather than a generalised bleeding disorder. Epistaxis is usually due to a vascular abnormality in the nose and haematuria is usually due to a urinary tract lesion, e.g. bladder tumour or prostatic enlargement. Severe postoperative regional bleeding may be due to platelet deficiency (either quantitative or qualitative) or to an impairment of the clotting mechanism but is rarely caused by generalised vascular damage acting on its own.

Principles of therapy

1. Blood volume maintenance.
2. Treatment of the underlying disorder (as in disseminated intravascular coagulation).
3. Replacement therapy. Platelet transfusions should be given if the count is less than 50 000/ml in a bleeding patient (given in the form of platelet concentrates or fresh blood. ABO compatibility is essential since platelets carry ABO antigens). Clotting factors are replaced, e.g. factor VIII in haemophilia given in the form of cryoprecipitate bags or fresh frozen plasma (contains all factors) (20 ml/kg). Fresh frozen plasma (20 ml/kg) is also given in:
- Liver disease (with vitamin K).
- Disseminated intravascular coagulation (with platelets with or without fibrinogen—the latter carries a significant risk of hepatitis).
- Massive transfusion.
- Anticoagulant therapy bleeding (with i.m. vitamin K 10 mg). With heparin, neutralisation by protamine is necessary. With streptokinase, EACA is a specific antidote—100 mg/kg i.v. over 30 min.

Risk of AIDS

Blood transfusion carries a low but definite risk of transferring AIDS (acquired cellular immunodeficiency syndrome). The risk is high in Factor VIII, IX concentrates and fibrinogen transfusion. AIDS was first recognised as an epidemic in Spring 1981 in the USA and affects 4 Hs, i.e. Homosexuals, Haemophiliacs, Heroin and intravenous drug addicts and Haitian immigrants. AIDS can occur also in women after artificial insemination by donor. (AIDS has been found in normal heterosexuals in some parts of Africa). AIDS is associated with a decrease in helper T-lymphocytes and a high incidence of cytomegalovirus (CMV) infection. It is thought that CMV or another virus (homosexuals usually harbour many viruses, e.g. hepatitis B virus, Epstein–Barr virus and CMV) may possibly cause the cellular immunodeficiency. However a human retrovirus which was isolated and called human T-cell leukaemia-lymphoma virus (HTLV-3) is thought to be the causative agent in AIDS. This virus infection has a mean incubation period of 2 years and is thought to be responsible for persistent generalised lymphadenopathy (PGL) and Kaposi's sarcoma (a multifocal malignancy composed of new blood vessels and large spindle cells; it presents as firm, bluish-brown nodules in the skin usually on the limbs). However not everyone who becomes infected with HTLV-3 will develop AIDS. HTLV-3 is detected by antibody test, using immunofluorescence, radioimmunoassay and enzyme-linked immunoassay.

Clinically there is often a prodromal illness characterised by fever, weight loss, oral thrush (due to candidiasis and possible oesophageal extension and dysphagia), diarrhoea and PGL. The syndrome is frequently complicated by opportunistic infections mainly *Pneumocystis carinii* and CMV pneumonia, bowel infestations with *Giardia lamblia*, *Entamoeba histolytica*, *shigella*, *salmonella* and *campylobacter*, CMV chorioretinitis and *Toxoplasma gondii* encephalopathy. AIDS is also often complicated by malignancies, e.g. Kaposi's sarcoma. The treatment is that of opportunistic infections. Radiotherapy and chemotherapy may be needed for skin malignancies. Neutralising antibodies, interferons, interleukin, thymic hormone, suramin and phosphonoformate drugs have all been tried with no dramatic improvement. The mortality is 40% but rises even higher in the presence of Kaposi's sarcoma of the skin.

General principles in the management of gastrointestinal bleeding

Haematemesis

The sources of upper gastrointestinal bleeding are confined to oesophagogastroduodenal areas (*see*

Section 1.16). All patients should be hospitalised and managed under shared consultation between physicians and surgeons.

Management plan (resuscitate—review—repair)

1. Resuscitation (see Sections 1.12 and 1.18).
2. Establishment of a diagnosis—history/physical examination/endoscopy confirm diagnosis (in 90%); barium meal is less reliable (60%) and rarely visceral angiography may be needed to identify the site of bleeding.
3. Specific management of the cause.
(a) Bleeding peptic ulcer. Operation is indicated in the presence of:
   - Massive and continuous bleeding.
   - Rebleeding.
   - Coexistent systemic condition, e.g. cardiorespiratory incipient failure.
   - Associated pyloric stenosis.
   - Endoscopic evidence of a visible vessel in the ulcer base (bleeding or not) and/or stigmata of recent haemorrhage (signs of recurrent bleeding).

   The type of operation depends on whether the ulcer is duodenal or gastric (see Section 1.12).
(b) Acute gastric erosions, stress ulcer and Mallory—Weiss syndrome are treated surgically (see Section 1.12).
(c) Bleeding oesophageal varices (see Section 1.18 and Section 4.1, Question 4).

Bleeding per rectum

The source of lower gastrointestinal bleeding extends from the duodenojejunal junction downwards to the anus. Haemorrhoids is the commonest cause of bright red bleeding, although massive higher bleeding can be bright. Proximal lesions lead to dark-coloured stool or melaena and are associated with anaemia and a change in bowel habits. The common causes of bleeding per rectum are internal haemorrhoids, anal fissure and large bowel carcinoma (in order of frequency). The common causes of massive bleeding per rectum are diverticular disease, angiodysplasia (congenital vascular malformation), upper gastrointestinal bleeding and aortoenteric fistula. Less common causes are Meckel's diverticulum, intussusception, mesenteric infarction and tumours (small intestine), ulcerative colitis, Crohn's disease and ischaemic colitis (large intestine).

Management plan

1. Resuscitation especially in massive bleeding.
2. Diagnosis: history of bleeding (colour, clots, relation to defaecation, mixed with stool or not, smear on paper or not and amount), perineal and abdominal pain, prolapse, change of bowel habits and diarrhoea, abdominal distension, anaemia, weight loss, pneumaturia, rectal bleeding with menstruation (in endometriosis).
3. Physical examination and treatment. *General examination*—for anaemia, weight loss and lymph nodes; *abdominal examination*—for masses, distension; and *rectal examination* are carried out. Proctoscopy, sigmoidoscopy and biopsy are done if necessary. Then double-contrast barium enema is carried out if necessary as a screening test prior to colonoscopy which is performed selectively in suspicious cases (to reveal high colonic carcinoma or angiodysplasia and possibly for treatment).

If the bleeding source is still unknown then visceral angiography is performed to identify the site and possibly the cause of bleeding, e.g. angiodysplasia, to be followed by elective surgery. However, if there is still continuous bleeding of unknown origin, emergency surgery should be performed with or without repeated angiography preoperatively and with or without on-table colonoscopy.

In bleeding of unknown origin, a blind subtotal colectomy is performed, bringing up the proximal end as an ileostomy and the distal end as a separate colostomy. Postoperative monitoring is carried out. If there is no bleeding then bowel continuity is restored once the patient has recovered. If the distal end starts bleeding through the colostomy then excision of the rectum, completed as for abdominoperineal resection, is recommended, keeping the ileostomy as a permanent stoma. However, if the ileostomy starts bleeding then the patient should be reinvestigated, as initial misdiagnosis is possible. The underlying cause may be in the upper gastrointestinal tract and one should proceed with upper gastrointestinal tract endoscopy with barium meal and repeated angiography.

1.18. Portal Hypertension

Normal portal venous pressure is 80–120 mmH$_2$O and depends on splanchnic blood flow, resistance to

Construction of stoma

In the construction of an ileostomy it is necessary to evert 6 cm of ileum to produce a 3 cm spout. The deeper layer of the ileum needs to be anchored to the abdominal wall either from within or at the level of the external oblique aponeurosis. Whichever technique is chosen care should be exercised in the placement of the sutures. The bite into the bowel should go only through serosa.

The formation of a pericolostomy fistula or a pericolostomy abscess which bursts onto the skin with the subsequent formation of a fistulous track requires surgery. The track should be laid open and left to granulate. In the case of an ileostomy the whole stoma may have to be revised.

Stoma appliances

There are two basic designs of stoma appliance. The one-piece unit consists of a bag which is attached to the skin directly either by adhesive, Stomahesive or karaya gum. The bag itself may be drainable or closed. The two-piece unit consists of a plastic flange which is either attached directly to the skin or bonded to a karaya gum or Stomahesive square. The collecting bag can be detached from the plastic flange and disposed of separately. The two-piece system makes stoma management easier and minimises skin irritation due to constant removal and reapplication of the bag, but it is bulkier than a one-piece bag.

Skin problems

Skin problems associated with an ileostomy are more common since its efflux is liquid and contains proteolytic enzymes. The contact of the efflux with skin rapidly causes irritation, maceration, excoriation and digestion. For this reason an ileostomy is constructed as a spout protruding 2–4 cm beyond the skin of the abdominal wall so that the motions pass directly into the collecting appliance.

Leakage of the stoma efflux may be due to faulty site selection, failure of adherence of the appliance or to complications in the stoma itself which allow escape of the efflux directly onto the skin. Adhesive sensitivity is another cause of skin problems.

Skin problems in relation to a colostomy are seldom so severe since the motions are semisolid and are non-irritant. Leakage of the faeces from a colostomy may be due to faulty site selection; problems of the stoma itself (rendering adherence of the bag difficult) or a loose colostomy appliance which causes skin maceration.

Too frequent change of the one-piece appliance

The use of a one-piece system may result in skin soreness due to the constant minor trauma of removing the bag. If this is the cause of the skin irritation, then the patient should be advised to use a two-piece system. A Stomahesive or karaya square is cut to cover the injured skin and a hole made in it to accommodate the stoma. The square should be left on the skin for as long as possible. A plastic flange is mounted onto the square or may be integral with it. The bag is merely unclipped from the flange at the appropriate time and replaced with a new one. Once the skin has had time to heal the patient can go back to the old appliance or may continue with the new method.

Problems with the two-piece appliance

In applying the plastic flange of a two-piece ileostomy set, care should be taken to ensure that it does not chafe the spout; otherwise it may cause bleeding or pressure necrosis of the stoma and a fistula may develop at skin level. Should this occur the efflux will discharge directly onto the skin, causing excoriation, and the stoma will have to be revised.

Sensitivity to adhesive

Sensitivity to the adhesive can be tested by placing a similar appliance on another part of the patient's body. If a skin reaction occurs, the patient should avoid appliances using adhesive and be advised to use those utilising either a Stomahesive or karaya washer since sensitivity to these materials is virtually unknown.

Established skin excoriation

Established ulceration or weeping macerated skin can be dressed with Stomahesive squares upon which a flange and clip-on bag can be mounted. Healing of the skin below the Stomahesive takes place.

Control of the stoma efflux

Most ileostomies settle to a discharge of 500 ml/24 h and the stool becomes sloppy rather than liquid in its consistency. For those patients with a persistently loose ileostomy which drains large volumes (up to 1500 ml/24 h), leakage and the development of skin irritation can be a major problem. Attempts to improve the consistency of the efflux should be made by the administration of hydrophilic agents such as ispaghula, sterculia or methylcellulose. Kaolin may sometimes help and certain drugs such as codeine phosphate, loperamide and diphenoxylate which reduce intestinal motility can be tried. Should these manipulations prove unsuccessful and the patient cannot manage, then, as a last resort the revision of the ileostomy is contemplated. A reversed interposed loop of ileum proximal to the stoma has been tried and the conversion of the ileostomy into a continent reservoir has also been advocated.

Control of the colostomy is usually much more straightforward. It responds well to dietary and pharmacological agents. A loop colostomy fashioned in the right upper quadrant can be loose and fixture of the bag a problem, but by the measures outlined above the stool can be rendered firmer and the colostomy controlled better.

Stoma complications

Necrosis

Following the fashioning of an end colostomy, necrosis of the bowel adjacent to the mucocutaneous suture line may occur as a result of inadequate intraoperative assessment of the viability of the blood supply of the terminal portion of the bowel, or as a result of thrombosis in the vessels constricted by a tight external oblique aponeurosis.

This complication can be avoided by paying attention to the placement of ligatures on the mesentery when mobilising the sigmoid colon, ensuring that the opening in the abdominal wall is adequate and that there is no tension on the suture line.

Slight separation of the mucosa from the skin merely requires observation since the mucosa will rapidly re-epithelialise the defect. If the colostomy necroses for more than 1.5 cm, the stoma should be revised since the granulating area will fibrose and a stenosis of the stoma will result.

Stenosis (more dangerous than prolapse)

When stomas were not immediately completed by direct mucocutaneous suture stenosis was commonplace. Direct mucocutaneous suture has made this complication rare. It may occur if the distal bowel becomes gangrenous and circumferential granulations undergo fibrosis. It can be remedied by excising the stenotic rim, mobilising the stoma so that viable bowel can be brought to the skin surface without tension and performing direct mucocutaneous suture.

Obstruction

Faecal impaction

Large bowel obstruction may be due to faecal impaction with or without spurious diarrhoea. A glycerine suppository, a colostomy washout or digital evacuation may remedy the situation.

A search should be made for an underlying stenosis of the stoma. This may be at skin level or at the level of the external oblique aponeurosis as revealed by digital examination.

If the stoma is of normal calibre the patient is advised to keep the stool soft by taking a high fibre diet or a faecal softener can be prescribed. If a stenosis is the underlying cause of the faecal impaction then the stoma may have to be revised.

Prolapse of the small bowel through pelvic peritoneum

Following the excision of the rectum and repair of the pelvic floor, if the suture line in the pelvic peritoneum gives way a knuckle of small bowel may herniate into the pelvic space. This may give rise to an obstruction. If at laparotomy the defect cannot be resutured easily, the pelvic peritoneum is opened in its entirety so that the complication cannot recur.

Lateral space obstruction

This complication has been eliminated by the extraperitoneal technique of stoma fashioning. If a direct colostomy or ileostomy is fashioned care should be taken to close the lateral space by suturing the mesentery of the bowel to the lateral wall of the abdominal cavity or, alternatively, a flap of mobilised peritoneum is sutured to the bowel in order to prevent the prolapse of small bowel around the lateral side of the emergent limb of the stoma.

Fistula

The placement of sutures through the serosa of the colon to anchor it to the deeper layers of the abdominal wall should be avoided. It is unnecessary and a misplaced suture which passes through the whole thickness of the bowel is an invitation to a fistula.

Emergency treatment of bleeding varices

Conservative approach

Blood replacement, i.v. vasopressin 20 units in 200 ml of 5% dextrose (or somatostatin given as i.v. bolus injection of 250 μg to be followed by continuous i.v. infusion of 7.5 μg/min or preferably Terlipressin given in initial 2 mg i.v. bolus dose and repeated 4–6 hourly up to a maximum of 24 h) and Sengstaken–Blakemore balloon tamponade for 24–48 h with vitamin K and prehepatic coma prevention (oral non-absorbable antibiotic, colonic washout, lactulose and restriction of proteins) remain the mainstay of the medical therapy.

Bleeding varices can be injected with 5 ml of 5% ethanolamine oleate using a rigid oesophagoscope and a long Macbeth needle followed by tamponade.

Direct surgery to varices

- Transthoracic, transoesophageal ligation of varices (Boerema–Crile operation).
- Transthoracic, oesophageal transection (mucosal or complete) (Milnes–Walker operation) with variceal ligation or reanastomosis by hand or stapler.
- Subcardiac porta-azygous disconnection (Tanner operation)—gastric transection.

Emergency or urgent shunt surgery

- Emergency Portacaval shunt has an overall operative mortality of 57%, which is directly related to the degree of hepatic dysfunction.
- Mesocaval shunt (jump graft) side-to-side Dacron graft between the superior mesenteric vein and inferior vena cava—claimed to have acceptable mortality.

Encephalopathy is caused by:

- Diversion of portal blood from the liver.
- Deteriorating liver cell function.
- Haemodynamic changes precipitated by shunt operation.

The encephalopathy ranges between 12% and 45% but it is around 10% if intestinal antibiotic, lactulose and protein restriction are used for control. Surgical procedures such as subtotal colectomy or colonic exclusion are also claimed to be helpful in reducing this risk.

In general, portacaval shunt carries a 20% risk of encephalopathy (better shunt patency). Lienorenal shunt carries a 10% risk of encephalopathy (but higher risk of shunt thrombosis—20% versus 3% in portacaval shunt). Operative mortality is 10% in both shunts. The jump graft has good patency and less encephalopathy risk. Warren's operation is the least likely to produce encephalopathy (liver function is undisturbed); it has 9% operative mortality, 90% patency with good bleeding control, and 50–60% 5 year survival.

1.19. Acute Pancreatitis

Acute pancreatitis is basically an autodigestion of the pancreas by its own proteolytic and lipolytic enzymes. There are four formulated theoretical mechanisms of pathogenesis:

Obstructive hypersecretion, e.g. acute pancreatitis occurs in pancreatic carcinoma, although rarely.

Duodenal reflux, e.g. acute pancreatitis after Polya gastrectomy and gall stone impaction at ampulla (the majority of small gall stones could be recovered from the faeces of patients with acute pancreatitis) indicating that a transient obstruction with stones passing into the duodenum is more likely.

Bile reflux (common channel theory). Operative cholangiograms frequently outline the pancreatic duct confirming that bile reflux can occur under physiologically abnormal pressures. Gall stone impaction at the ampulla of Vater was found in 5% of fatal cases of acute pancreatitis.

Acinar cell derangement: due to metabolic disturbances induced by hyperlipaemia, anoxia, traumatic vascular damage, hypothermia with venous thrombosis.

Classification

Acute and acute relapsing pancreatitis, chronic and chronic relapsing pancreatitis. Pathologically, oedematous acute pancreatitis and haemorrhagic necrotising acute pancreatitis are merely stages of progression and not distinctive diseases.

CAUSES

- Gall stones (biliary diseases) 60%.
- Alcoholism varies from 20 to 50%.

- Trauma—a rare cause.
  —Direct blunt abdominal trauma.
  —Instrumental trauma due to ERCP.
  —Postoperative in common bile duct exploration, pancreatic biopsy, gastric resection and splenectomy.
- Metabolic: hyperparathyroidism, hyperlipaemia, hypothermia.
- Drugs: opiates, steroids, contraceptive pill, phenformin, chlorothiazides, chlorthalidone, frusemide and azathioprine (Imuran).
- Miscellaneous: liver disease with fulminating liver failure, pancreatic carcinoma, Trinidad scorpion bite (causing selective spasm of sphincter of Oddi), *Ascaris lumbricoides* (wandering worm enters duodenal papilla and obstructs it), mumps in children, blood dyscrasia.
- Idiopathic.

PRIORITIES IN MANAGEMENT

I Confirmation of diagnosis

- High index of suspicion in any acute abdomen especially in patients with known history of gall stones or alcoholism.
- Clinical features: especially upper abdominal severe pain with radiation by penetration associated with vomiting. Fever, tachycardia, jaundice, rigidity, distension and hypotension also may be present.
- Serum amylase of more than 1000 i.u./l. However, acute cholecystitis, biliary peritonitis, perforated peptic ulcer, intestinal obstruction with strangulation, afferent loop obstruction after partial gastrectomy, mesenteric arterial thrombosis, ruptured aortic aneurysm, acute parotitis, post-ERCP and the administration of codeine and other opiates in sensitive people may all be associated with hyperamylasaemia even reaching 1000 i.u./l or more in rare cases.
- Urinary amylase remains elevated for up to 10 days whereas serum amylase subsides within 2–4 days. Thus Rapignost Amylase Teststrip offers a rapid reliable bedside estimation of urinary amylase.
- Diagnostic peritoneal lavage and estimation of peritoneal amylase level (via a dialysis catheter using 1 litre normal saline) in a red or rusty, yellow or turbid peritoneal aspirate fluid.
- P_3 index less than 80% (*see* Comment on P_3 index).
- Laparotomy.

II Assessment of severity

Patients (once diagnosed) should be categorised within 48 h after admission into *mild* or *severe* cases. Clinical assessment is less reliable than objective laboratory results.

The following criteria (from Ranson *et al.*, 1976; Imrie *et al.*, 1978) indicate severe acute pancreatitis:

Clinical (one or more)
- Generalised abdominal signs with rigidity and hypotension or cyanosis
- Grey Turner's sign (loin skin bruising)
- Cullen's sign (discoloured umbilicus or Owl's eye sign)
- Pre-existing diabetes mellitus
- Postoperative acute pancreatitis
- Age more than 55 years

Laboratory (three or more)
- WBC more than $15 \times 10^9/l$
- Serum Ca^{2+} less than 2 mmol/l
- Arterial Po_2 less than 7.5 kPa
- Blood glucose more than 11 mmol/l
- Serum albumin less than 32 g/l
- Blood urea more than 16 mmol/l
- Raised serum bilirubin and/or liver enzymes
- Methaemalbuminaemia
- P_3 index less than 50%

Peritoneal lavage revealing (one or more)
- Volume of more than 10 ml of free peritoneal fluid irrespective of its colour (prior to running in the saline)
- Free fluid of a dark colour (prune juice)
- A mid-straw or darker colour lavage fluid

Comment on P_3 index Electrophoresis of normal human serum shows two main iso-enzyme bands of serum amylase, the salivary S_1 and the main pancreatic iso-enzyme P_2. In acute pancreatitis P_3 iso-enzyme appears and together with S_1 is termed P^1. The distance between P_2 and P^1 in acute pancreatitis represents 60% of the distance between peaks on the standard strip. As the patient recovers clinically the distance between peaks P_2 and P^1 increases towards the control distance owing to the disappearance of P_3 until P^1 is represented entirely by S_1.

$$P_3 \text{ index } = \frac{\text{Distance between } P_2 \text{ and } P^1}{\text{Distance between } P_2 \text{ and } S_1} \times 100$$

P_3 is a reliable indicator in the monitoring of the progress of an attack of acute pancreatitis and in subsequent identification of those who may be at risk from the development of complications.

Large bowel fistulae

These fistulae are not as problematical as small bowel fistulae. However, they may discharge at 'inconvenient' points on the abdominal wall—through an abdominal incision or near to bony points. Since the stools are not corrosive to the skin, excoriation is not a problem. Ingenuity is required to keep a suitable collecting appliance on the skin according to the above principles, in the expectation of final healing.

PROBLEMS ASSOCIATED WITH AN ILEAL CONDUIT

The ileal conduit is a more complicated construction than an ileostomy or a colostomy and the complications that may arise are more numerous.

The surgical construction of an ileal conduit consists of three stages, if a total cystectomy is omitted. (1) A 15 cm piece of ileum is isolated on a vascular pedicle and the continuity of the intestine re-established. (2) The two ureters must be anastomosed to the proximal end of the ileal segment. (3) The urostomy must be constructed as a 2 cm spout through the abdominal wall.

Dehiscence of the intestinal anastomosis

This may present as peritonitis or as a small bowel fistula. This must be treated on its own merits.

Postoperative urinary fistula

Leakage of urine from the site of anastomosis of the ureters to the ileum usually presents as a urine leak from the drain site. Contrast medium can be introduced into the spout of the urostomy to confirm the site of leakage. If the ureters can be visualised and are in continuity with the ileal segment then the fistula can be expected to close spontaneously. If the ureters are not visualised an intravenous urogram is indicated. Complete lack of continuity with the ileal segment will demand reconstruction.

Vascular problems of the ileal segment

The stoma may appear dark red immediately after operation but as oedema of the operation subsides it should regain a healthy pink colour. A persistent dusky stoma or one that turns black indicates that the blood supply to the ileal loop is imperilled and this demands reconstruction.

Control of the urostomy efflux

Unlike for an ileostomy or a colostomy a large volume output from the urostomy is desirable. No efforts should be made to diminish output since large volume flows of urine discourage ascending infections.

Ascending infection and renal failure

Ascending infections are common, and can lead to calculus formation and destruction of renal parenchyma.

1.15. Gastrointestinal Cancer: Precancerous and Predisposing Conditions

Oral cavity

Lips   Exposure to sunlight (countryman lips) with actinic cheilitis; skin precancerous conditions (*see* Section 5: Surgical pathology).

Tongue   Leucoplakia due to 7 S's (smoking, syphilis, sepsis, sharp tooth, spirits, spices and susceptibility). Some benign tumours and lingual thyroid can undergo malignant mitotic changes.

Salivary glands   Benign tumours such as pleomorphic adenoma may develop malignancy.

Oesophagus

Plummer–Vinson (USA) syndrome (or Paterson–Kelly syndrome—two British ENT surgeons). A premalignant condition which leads to postcricoid and cervical oesophageal carcinomas. It affects middle-aged women and is manifested by dysphagia due to high oesophageal web, iron deficiency anaemia with koilonychia, smooth tongue, stomatitis and achlorhydria.

Achalasia of cardia   Auerbach's plexus Absence leads to diverticulA, carcinomA, Aspiration pneumonia, <u>A</u>rthritis (toxic rheumatoid) and <u>A</u>naemia.

Lower oesophageal carcinoma Develops in 0–20% of achalasia cases after a duration of about 17 years.

Ectopic gastric mucosa Associated with hiatus hernia and reflux oesophagitis may lead to a primary adenocarcinoma.

Leucoplakia In a longstanding area of reflux oesophagitis due to any cause.

Benign strictures From various causes, e.g. lye and peptic strictures. Carcinoma may develop in an oesophageal diverticula (probably insignificant association).

Benign tumours (papillomas and adenomatous polyps) Can undergo malignant changes.

Tylosis (with palmar and solar desquamation).

Reverse smoking (smoking with the ignited end in the mouth—common habit in South America).

Stomach

Diet Carcinoma is uncommon in areas where maize is the staple food. Meat, and green and yellow vegetables also lower the risk. Carcinoma is common in areas where potatoes form a major part of diet. Consumption of pickled vegetables and dried/salted fish, ingestion of secondary amines (fish), less milk, and smoking increase the risk. The preparation of food is also important, e.g. talc-treated rice in Japan was found to have an inverse relationship to gastric carcinoma and atherosclerosis.

N-nitrosamines Produced by bacteria and other nitroso compounds, they are precancerous and seen in chronic gastritis, extensive intestinal metaplasia and following Billroth II gastrectomy and gastroenterostomy. The risk of developing carcinoma in partial gastrectomy stump after 25 years is six times the risk after 15 years (the breaking period is 10–15 years after which regular gastroscopy check-up is necessary).

Gastric ulcers Develop malignancy in 3–5% of cases.

Pernicious anaemia Increases the risk four times and gastric carcinoma develops characteristically in the gastric body and/or fundus.

Familial predisposition Relatives of gastric carcinoma patients are four times more at risk than those with unaffected relatives.

Polyp A descriptive term which means a projection into a lumen or cavity. Gastric polyps are classified into:
- Hamartomatous polyps which include:
  —Juvenile polyps.
  —Peutz–Jeghers syndrome (gastrointestinal hamartomatous polyposis with ano-oral melanosis—usually benign).
  —Cronkhite–Canada syndrome (alopecia, nail atrophy and gastric polyposis).
  —Heterotopias: as aberrant pancreatic tissue located submucosally.
- Hyperplastic—regenerative polyps.
- Neoplastic adenomas present in 40% of gastric polyps and are either tubular, villous or tubulovillous.

Giant rugal hypertrophy of the stomach (Ménétrier's disease) is a benign disease with ancedotal evidence of ?malignant changes.

Others Gastric carcinoma develops in patients with blood group A (Japanese however claim blood group B). Asbestosis and immunodeficiencies may be associated with gastric carcinoma.

Hepatobiliary system

Gall stones May be complicated by gall bladder adenocarcinoma.

Clonorchiasis Has a particular role in the pathogenesis of primary cholangiocarcinoma (intrahepatic bile duct carcinoma) in Hong Kong.

Cirrhosis A definite precancerous condition, predisposing to primary hepatocellular carcinoma. Cirrhosis is mainly idiopathic or alcohol-induced rather than malnutrition-induced.

Genetic α_1-antitrypsin deficiency may be an enhancing factor for cirrhosis and even carcinoma.

Natural carcinogens
- Pyrrolizidine alkaloids found in 'bush teas', consumption of which may cause veno-occlusive disease common in the West Indies.
- Cycasin found in camphor oil, cinnamon and bay leaf.
- Ethiopian herbal mixtures and taenicides.
- Nitrosamines found in smoked fish, bacon and mushrooms.

Table 4.   Investigation plan of jaundiced patient

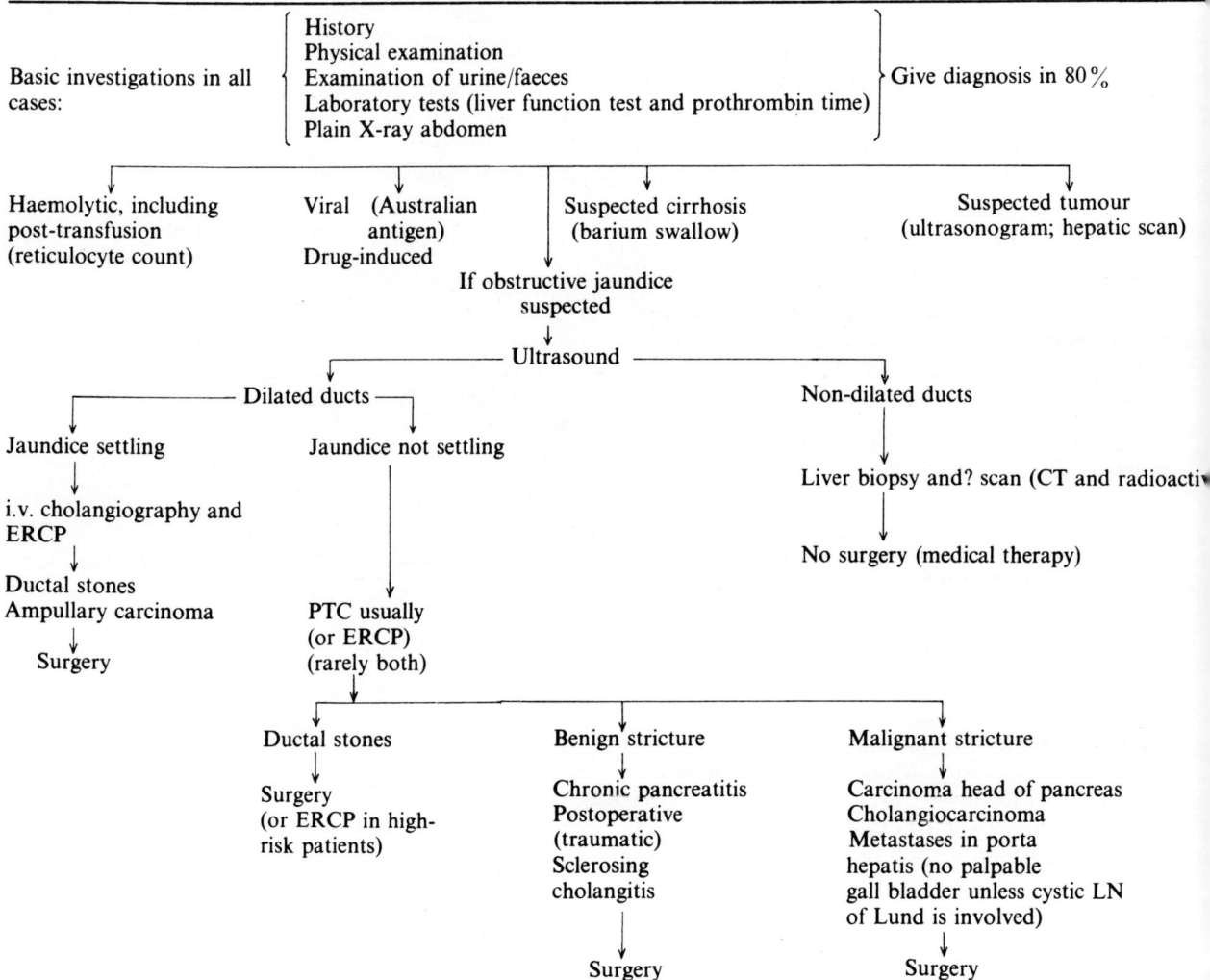

Basic investigations in all cases:

{
History
Physical examination
Examination of urine/faeces
Laboratory tests (liver function test and prothrombin time)
Plain X-ray abdomen
} Give diagnosis in 80%

Haemolytic, including post-transfusion (reticulocyte count)

Viral (Australian antigen)
Drug-induced

Suspected cirrhosis (barium swallow)

Suspected tumour (ultrasonogram; hepatic scan)

If obstructive jaundice suspected

— Ultrasound —

— Dilated ducts —

Non-dilated ducts

Jaundice settling

Jaundice not settling

Liver biopsy and? scan (CT and radioacti▼

i.v. cholangiography and ERCP

No surgery (medical therapy)

Ductal stones
Ampullary carcinoma

PTC usually (or ERCP) (rarely both)

Surgery

Ductal stones

Benign stricture

Malignant stricture

Surgery (or ERCP in high-risk patients)

Chronic pancreatitis
Postoperative (traumatic)
Sclerosing cholangitis

Carcinoma head of pancreas
Cholangiocarcinoma
Metastases in porta hepatis (no palpable gall bladder unless cystic LN of Lund is involved)

Surgery

Surgery

less than 100 i.u./l). Alkaline phosphatase has four sources—liver, bone, intestine and placenta. It is therefore high in liver diseases (including jaundice), bone diseases (and growing children), intestinal lymphoma and pregnancy.

(c) Prothrombin time—prolonged but correctable (with vitamin K) in obstructive jaundice; prolonged uncorrectable in hepatocellular jaundice; and normal in haemolytic anaemia.

(d) Australian antigen (HB_s Ag) indicates viral hepatitis. Spherocytosis (full blood count), red cell fragility, reticulocytosis, positive Coomb's test and absent haptoglobins indicate haemolysis. Reversed albumin/globulin ratio (normally 2:1) in chronic hepatocellular jaundice.

Auto-antibodies (especially antimitochondrial) indicate primary biliary cirrhosis.

A provisional diagnosis should be made now. If the above clinical and laboratory assessment points to a hepatocellular jaundice then radioactive (e.g. gallium) liver scan and liver biopsy are indicated. If the provisional diagnosis is obstructive jaundice (surgical jaundice) then proceed as follows:

4. Ultrasound scan to illustrate intrahepatic bile ducts, biliary stones and the state of the liver and pancreas. If there is any suspicion of pancreatic disease or if the ultrasound scan is inconclusive, as in obese patients or because of excess overlapping bowel gas, then CT scan is used as its resolution is better.

5. The next step is percutaneous transhepatic chol-

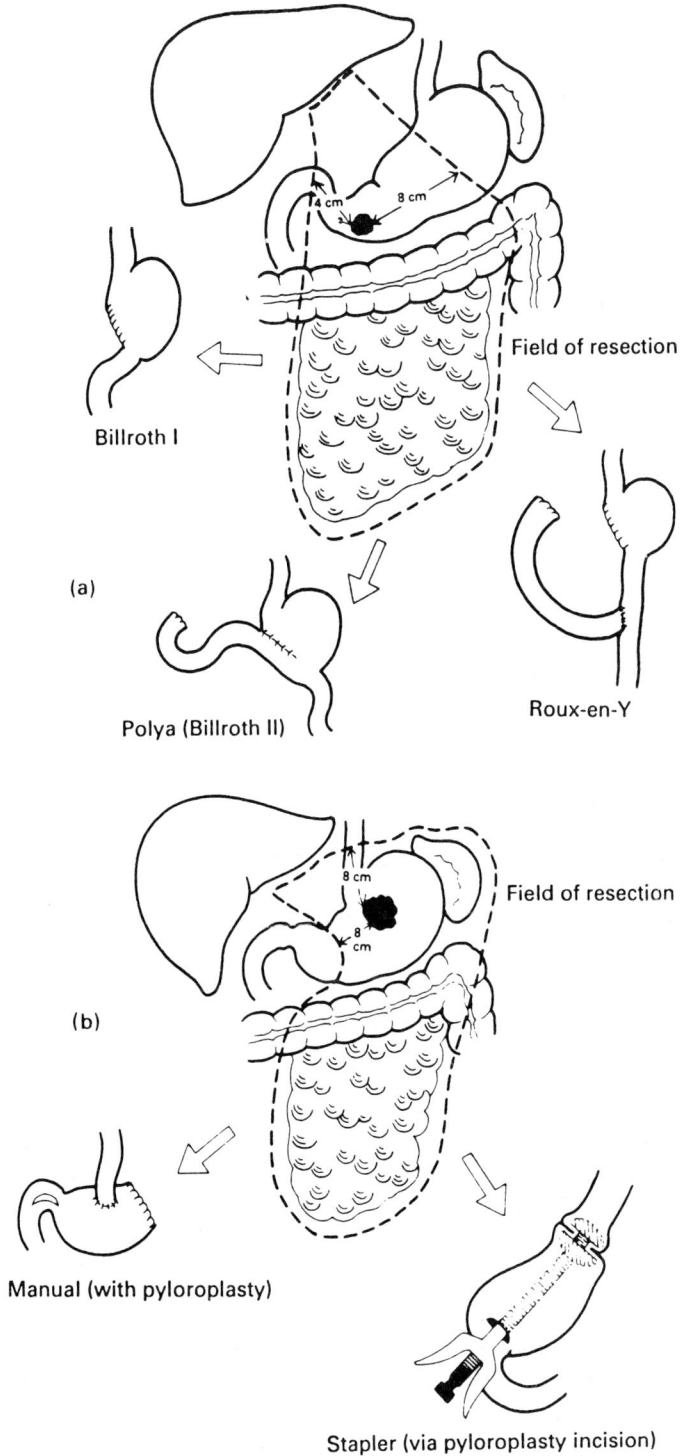

4 cm   8 cm

Field of resection

Billroth I

(a)

Polya (Billroth II)

Roux-en-Y

(b)

8 cm

8 cm

Field of resection

Manual (with pyloroplasty)

Stapler (via pyloroplasty incision)

Fig. 6 (a) Distal gastrectomy (antral tumour) and (b) proximal gastrectomy (fundus tumour), showing alternative methods of repair

emptying and resuscitation of the patient. Up to 48 h, OGD gives a satisfactory diagnostic rate and after 72 h the diagnostic yield falls. The commonest lesion in the UK is duodenal ulcer (up to 35 %), followed by gastric ulcer (up to 20 %), erosions (up to 15 %), and Mallory–Weiss tears (up to 13 %). Bleeding varices (3–5 %) are uncommon in the UK but carry 50 % mortality.

Therapeutic

- Eder–Puestow dilatation of oesophageal strictures (e.g. peptic and corrosive strictures, achalasia).
- Insertion of oesophageal tubes for inoperable carcinoma, injection of sclerosants for varices, removal of ingested foreign bodies, polypectomy, guided small bowel biopsy and laser photocoagulation or electrocoagulation of bleeding or potentially bleeding lesions.
- Local application of drugs (by spraying clotting factors or tissue adhesive; or intralesional injection, e.g. noradrenaline).
- Application of arterial clips.
- Placement of Teflon feeding tubes for enteral nutrition under vision if the pylorus cannot be passed by the usual methods.
- Sphincterotomy for gall stone removal and papillary stenosis as well as palliative intubation.
- Biliary drainage of the bile duct after sphincterotomy and dilatation of the stricture.

Lasers

LASER (light amplification by stimulated emission of radiation) is basically a high-power source of light energy leading to coagulation or destruction of tissue protein on striking human tissues.

Endoscopic electrocoagulation requires direct contact between the coagulating probe and the bleeding vessel in the ulcer base; furthermore the depth of thermal injury is difficult to control and coagulum is easily dislodged when the probe is removed. By contrast, endoscopic laser photocoagulation performs its function without touching the lesion. However fresh blood and clot should be cleared from the lesion by using sucking and a high-power water jet so that the bleeding vessel in the ulcer base can be identified and to enable the beam to penetrate to the bleeding vessel. Firing the laser through clots destroys the fibre tip and prevents effective photocoagulation. Coaxial inert gas keeps the tip free from blood and the vessel relatively clean. Photocoagulation should be aimed around

the base of the bleeding vessel to produce thrombosis and shrinkage, thus achieving permanent haemostasis. A dual-channel endoscope is especially valuable to allow for continuous lavage during photocoagulation.

There is no irradiation hazard from laser beams but they may cause skin burns if directed at close range. As viewing the laser beams during coagulation is potentially dangerous to the viewer's retina, all laser systems incorporate a fail-safe shutter filter attached to the endoscope eyepiece. Observers should wear protective goggles. A fully installed laser system of any type costs around £30 000.

Laser photocoagulation can be used therapeutically for active peptic ulcer and oesophageal bleeding and prophylactically for those with endoscopic evidence of visible vessels in the ulcer base or stigmata of recent haemorrhage (the two indicators of the risk of recurrent bleeding). Haemostasis is achieved in over 90 % of cases and is usually permanent. The risk of perforation is rare.

Laser photocoagulation is also used in the treatment of gastrointestinal vascular malformations, e.g. haemangiomas, colonic angiodysplasia and gastroduodenal telangiectasia as in hereditary haemorrhagic telangiectasia.

Many tumours take up haematoporphyrins preferentially and porphyrins are powerful photosensitising agents which sensitise cells so that exposure to light induces damage. Therefore i.v. injection of tumour sensitiser, e.g. haematoporphyrins, followed by endoscopic photocoagulation can lead to destructive treatment of early tumours in the upper gastrointestinal, bronchial and urinary bladder regions.

There are three types of laser system used currently in medical practice:
1. Neodymium Yttrium Aluminium Garnet (Nd-YAG) is the most versatile and the one currently used for gastroenterology and experimental surgery.
2. Argon for gastroenterology and ophthalmology.
3. Carbon dioxide for surgery.

Research

No clinical trial of a drug claimed to have ulcer-healing properties would be complete without serial endoscopic control.

Screening

Japanese and, recently, European experience has shown that superficial 'early' gastric carcinomas may be diagnosed by endoscopy and that the prognosis of patients who have such lesions operated on is excellent.

Hazards of OGD

Include erroneous diagnosis, complications of medication (e.g. dysrhythmias, apnoea and sudden death), perforation (incidence 0.01–0.1%), pulmonary aspiration, cardiovascular complications induced by medication and instrumentation (e.g. ECG abnormalities during endoscopy), bleeding due to clot dislodgement or biopsying a lesion likely to bleed and rarely the introduction of hepatitis. The overall morbidity is 0.05–0.35% and mortality is 0.01–0.025%. Special risk factors include old age, degree of illness, emergency endoscopy.

ENDOSCOPIC RETROGRADE CHOLANGIOPANCREATOGRAPHY

Endoscopic retrograde cholangiopancreatography (ERCP) is a combined endoscopic (side-viewing duodenoscope) and radiographic technique which can demonstrate the anatomy of the pancreatic and biliary duct systems, obtain pure pancreatic juice for biochemical and cytological examination and permit non-operative removal of gall stones from the common bile duct. It is a difficult and costly procedure which should not be undertaken when simpler methods can provide the same information.

Indications

Diagnostic

- Investigation of pancreatic disease either neoplastic or inflammatory. Grey scale ultrasonography or computerised tomography are complementary and provide information about pancreatic size.
- Investigation of jaundice, especially when the biliary system is thought to be normal. Percutaneous transhepatic cholangiography (PTC) is simpler when there is dilatation of the biliary system. Preliminary ultrasonography is helpful in deciding which is the more suitable technique. ERCP is safer when percutaneous cholangiography is prevented by a coagulation disorder.
- Suspected biliary disease when cholecystography or i.v. cholangiography is unsatisfactory.

- Postcholecystectomy problems when intravenous cholangiography is unhelpful or when there is an allergy to i.v. contrast materials.
- Preliminary to endoscopic papillotomy for retained common bile duct stones.

Therapeutic

Includes sphincterotomy for papillary stenosis, stone extraction, dilatation of biliary strictures, transnasal biliary drainage and endoprosthesis insertion.

Complications—specific to ERCP

Occur in approximately 2% of examinations; much more common with inexperienced endoscopist or when contraindications are ignored.
- Acute pancreatitis—very rare unless previous acute pancreatitis existed. More likely after overfilling of pancreatic duct or extravasation. Simple hyperamylasaemia is common but of no consequence.
- Infection of pancreatic pseudocyst—a dreaded complication. Avoid if possible by detecting cysts by ultrasonography. If pseudocyst is opacified urgent surgical drainage should be considered.
- Cholangitis—associated with anatomical abnormalities of biliary system, especially stones. Prevented by giving appropriate antibiotic before or immediately after ERCP.
- Bacteraemia and septicaemia as a consequence of cholangitis—prevented by antibiotics.
- Perforation of passages with cannula or by overdistension with contrast.
- Wrong diagnosis due to inadequate filling of ducts or poor radiology.
- Mucosal dissection of duodenal wall—a nuisance as it may produce swelling and prevent adequate cannulation.

The current place of ERCP in jaundice

First establish:
- Whether the bile ducts are dilated.
- The anatomy of the lesion.

Current methods

Non-invasive
- Grey scale ultrasonography.
- Computerised axial tomography.

- Recurrent ulcer rate is less (7% versus 11%).
- Less bile reflux, thus possibly lessens the chance of cancer of the stomach.
- There may be problems with afferent loop and dumping.
- Diarrhoea may follow.

PERFORATED DUODENAL ULCER

Conservative treatment

This consists of continuous suction, i.v. fluids and antibiotics. It is indicated in old patients unfit for operation, in cases of cardiovascular insufficiency or shock and is also used on board a ship or in remote parts of the world. It is not recommended because:

- The underlying cause of the perforation is left undiagnosed and could be gastric ulcer, carcinoma of the stomach or colonic carcinoma.
- No peritoneal toilet means a high risk of abscesses.
- It makes great demands on the time of the nursing and medical staff.

Operative treatment

After preoperative preparation of analgesia, nasogastric suction, i.v. fluids, CVP line and urinary catheter. This is the main method of management and there are two alternatives.

Simple closure and peritoneal toilet

Operative mortality is 7%. Recovered patients require postoperative cimetidine and careful follow-up.

Advantages
- Quick simple procedure.
- Can be done by Senior House Officers and Registrars.
- Healed ulcer already (in minority of patients).

Disadvantages
- Leaves an untreated vicious and dangerous ulcer.
- An overlooked kissing ulcer posteriorly caused by the stress of peritonitis and operation may bleed and lead to death in 2% of cases.
- Reperforation due to friable oedematous tissue.
- Gastric outlet obstruction.
- Long-term complications (30% develop further complications, 40% continue to have sympto-

matic peptic ulcer and in 30% the peptic ulcer remains silent). Follow-up required.

Definitive treatment at the time of perforation

TV + P converts the actual perforation into a Finney or Mickulicz repair. If perforation is large, PG may be necessary. HSV is hardly ever used as an emergency. Cimetidine 400 mg nightly should be given for 12 months postoperatively.

Disadvantages
- Difficult.
- Higher operative mortality.
- Mobilisation of distal oesophagus in the presence of peritonitis may lead to mediastinitis (theoretical).

PERFORATED GASTRIC ULCER

This is more dangerous than duodenal ulcer because of the advanced age and poor health of the patients, the large perforation, gross peritoneal contamination, haemorrhage from ulcer and ulcer-cancer in 10% of cases. It is treated by:

- Partial gastrectomy (Billroth I) in chronic cases and suspected carcinoma.
- Simple closure with multiple biopsies (if acute).
- Biopsy and closure with TV + D in selected cases.
- Wide ulcer-bearing segment resection, which is both diagnostic and therapeutic.

BLEEDING PEPTIC ULCER

Chronic peptic ulcer represents 60% of bleeding cases, acute gastric erosions represent 10–20%, while varices and the Mallory-Weiss syndrome account for the remainder. Unlike perforated ulcer, bleeding ulcer must *always* be treated by a definitive ulcer-curing procedure, however ill the patient may be. Generally the operative mortality is 10% and the surgeon must be an expert. After first aid treatment, a full history is taken, and the patient is managed as follows.

1. Resuscitation by blood transfusion until skin is warm and pink, blood pressure is stable and urinary output is good. Four units of blood are reserved.
2. Cimetidine is given intravenously.
3. The source of bleeding is identified using:

- Emergency oesophagogastroduodenoscopy. This is diagnostic and can be therapeutic (electrocautery, laser photocoagulation, variceal sclerotherapy or polypectomy according to the nature of the bleeding lesion).
- Radiography (double contrast).
- Angiography. This is sometimes done and is diagnostic of the site and therapeutic (selective injection of vasopressin and therapeutic embolisation).

4. Central venous pressure (CVP) line, two i.v. cannulae, nasogastric suction, urinary catheter, ampicillin or cephalosporin with good anaesthesia are required (since hypotension and arrhythmias during induction are common).

5. The operation is via a midline incision (palpate the stomach and duodenum). Adhesions indicate the ulcer site and duodenotomy is performed and the bleeding ulcer is underrun by X-stitches of 00 Dexon or vicryl absorbable suture. TV + P is carried out by suturing the gastroduodenotomy transversely, producing a Mickulicz repair. The recurrent ulcer rate is 13% and mortality is 8% (about half that of the alternative Polya PG, which is 15%). In the absence of adhesions, separate duodenotomy and/or gastrostomy (without damaging the pyloric sphincter) and underrunning of the bleeding points with HSV are performed.

In bleeding gastric ulcer, a PG (Billroth I) is done with operative mortality of 20%; however, if the patient is unfit, the ulcer should be underrun, biopsied or excised with vagotomy. The ulcer base could be excluded by leaving it attached to the pancreas. Acute gastric erosions are better treated conservatively. However, if bleeding continues, then operation can be done—either TV + P or HSV. Subtotal Billroth I is another option.

In stress ulcer, operation should be avoided in often septic, seriously ill patients. However, if required, TV + P with underrunning of bleeding points can be performed, but this carries high mortality in a sick patient.

Mallory-Weiss syndrome rarely requires a relatively simple underrunning of the tear via gastrostomy.

PYLORIC STENOSIS

This may be due to fibrosis and/or oedema and/or spasm. Clinically there is copious vomiting, succussion splash and stomach compensation by hyperperistalsis.

Gastric outlet obstruction secondary to peptic ulcer is differentiated from carcinoma by barium meal, gastroscopy and biopsy, BAO and MAO (the latter is normal or high in peptic ulcer and low in carcinoma). Treatment is by repeated gastric lavage, correction of anaemia, dehydration and electrolyte imbalance, with chest physiotherapy, vitamin C supplement and treatment of dental caries; followed by total vagotomy + Finney's pyloroplasty or highly selective vagotomy + digital or Hegar (size 16) dilatation via a gastrostomy or highly selective vagotomy + duodenoplasty.

RECURRENT PEPTIC ULCER

Peptic ulcer is a disease with recurring symptomatic periods. Postoperative symptomatic recurrence can take one of three forms.
- Ulcer dyspepsia with endoscopically proven ulcer.
- Ulcer dyspepsia without endoscopic evidence of peptic ulcer.
- Endoscopic silent recurrence.

There is no relationship between preoperative gastric acid output and subsequent recurrence.

Causes of recurrence (in order of frequency)

1. Technical errors: incomplete vagotomy; insufficient gastric resection; poor antral drainage.
2. Failure in the choice of operation.
3. Ulcerogenic drugs, e.g. aspirin, steroids, phenylbutazone (Butazolidin) NSAIDs and others.
4. Others: Zollinger–Ellison syndrome (ZES), G-cell hyperplasia, parathyroid adenoma, multiple adenoma syndrome, rarely polycythaemia and liver cirrhosis.

Diagnosis (history of symptoms after operation)

- Endoscopy (to confirm peptic ulcer and to see whether gastric or duodenal).
- Barium meal to evaluate gastric emptying rate only; it cannot confirm peptic ulcer in an operated case because of deformity and scarring.
- Insulin test.
- If the ratio of basic acid output (BAO) to maximal acid output (MAO) is more than 1:3 then ZES is not present.
- If BAO/MAO is 1:1 then do: basal and food-stimulated gastrin level (possibility of ZES), serum calcium and phosphate (parathyroid adenoma) and blood glucose (hypoglycaemia) with

ation or poor technique, or because of one of the contraindications mentioned above. There may be blind spots at the splenic or hepatic flexure, in the caecum and sigmoid colon, or behind prominent haustral folds. It may not be possible to intubate all strictures or to obtain adequate biopsies at these sites.

Complications

The procedure is an invasive technique. Complications are those associated with medication and those directly due to the procedure.
- Perforation may be due to direct instrumentation, air pressure, biopsy or diathermy.
- Vagal reflex may be caused by traction on the mesentery and result in hypotension which may be associated with myocardial infarction.
- Bacteraemia and retroperitoneal emphysema have also been recorded.
- Polypectomy may be complicated by perforation, haemorrhage or a transmural burn which may lead to the postpolypectomy coagulation syndrome.

Colonoscopy is an accurate diagnostic tool but has not replaced the barium enema. It has, however, replaced diagnostic laparotomy and surgical polypectomy.

1.17. Bleeding in Surgery

Bleeding during or after an operation is due either to local causes or to a haemostatic failure.

Local causes (and their brief treatment)

- Slipped ligature: controlled with artery forceps and religation (or diathermy coagulation applied to small bleeding vessels).
- Profuse bleeding of scalp: direct forcipressure (applying and everting a series of forceps to the epicranial aponeurosis).
- Cerebral or lumbar vessels: silver Cushing clips.
- Uncontrollable bleeding: may be underrun or transfixed and sutured in a figure-of-8 knot; if the continuity of a main vessel is to be restored then 4/0 silk or Prolene mounted on an atraumatic needle is used.

- Bleeding after embolectomy or vascular grafting: pack pressure using rolls of gauze or peanut gauze held by forceps for a few minutes. Sometimes a piece of muscle is cut, hammered (to release thromboplastin) and used to seal bleeding from arteriotomy.
- For continuous oozing: Oxycel or Surgicel (gelatin absorbable sponge providing a mesh upon which fibrin and platelets can be deposited) or gauze soaked in adrenaline 1:1000 solution.
- Oozing bone: dealt with by bone wax.
- Bleeding spleen (ruptured) is controlled by splenectomy while bleeding liver or kidney is treated conservatively.

General causes of bleeding

Purpura due to vascular defects

- Henoch–Schönlein (anaphylactoid purpura).
- Scurvy.
- Severe infections (e.g. Waterhouse–Friderichsen syndrome) complicating meningococcal and rarely staphylococcal, *Eschirichia coli* and *Haemophilus influenzae* septicaemia.
- Abdominal rose spots in typhoid fever.
- Splinter haemorrhages of the nail beds in subacute bacterial endocarditis.
- Purpura in many viral diseases such as smallpox, measles, and chicken pox.
- Drug side-effects (e.g. aspirin, belladonna and snake venom).
- Macroglobulinaemia and hereditary haemorrhagic telangiectasia (generalised hemartomatous dysplasia, pulmonary arteriovenous fistulae and splenic artery aneurysms).

Purpura due to platelet abnormalities

- Primary idiopathic thrombocytopenia.
- Secondary thrombocytopenia—seen in blood dyscrasias (leukaemia and aplastic anaemia), as a side-effect of drugs (sedormid, sulphonamide, quinidine), in thrombotic thrombocytopenic purpura (triad of thrombocytopenia, purpura and acute haemolytic anaemia along with transient neurological signs), in systemic lupus erythematosus in acute infections (infectious mononucleosis and rubella), in extensive haemangiomas in infants and following massive blood transfusions.
- Thrombocytopathic purpura due to defective platelet function (normal count) as seen in renal and hepatic failures and in macroglobulinaemia.

- Thrombocythaemic purpura due to excessive platelet count with some dysfunction causing severe gastrointestinal tract and postoperative bleeding. The condition occurs in a rare disease—haemorrhagic thrombocythaemia.

Defects in the clotting mechanisms

- Haemophilia (VIII deficiency), Christmas disease (IX deficiency), Von Willebrand's disease (VIII and platelet abnormalities).
- Hypoprothrombinaemia (V, VII and X deficiencies) occurs either as an inherited autosomal recessive disease or as an acquired disease, with the primary problem of vitamin K deficiency; seen in liver failure, malabsorption syndrome, obstructive jaundice, haemorrhagic disease of the newborn and anticoagulant therapy.
- Hypofibrinogenaemia—congenital or acquired. The acquired cases are seen in the defibrination syndrome, which is encountered in the fibrinolytic syndrome and in disseminated intravascular coagulation.

Fibrinolytic syndrome Activation of the plasmin system when large amounts of tissue activator are released into the blood, e.g. in cardiopulmonary operations, abruptio placentae, prostatic carcinoma, acute leukaemia, liver disease and congenital heart disease. In these conditions, the plasmin digests fibrinogen, making the blood unable to coagulate, resulting in bleeding from an operation site. Fibrin degradation products can be detected in blood. The platelet count is normal. Treatment consists of eliminating the cause, replacing clotting factors and giving a fibrinolytic inhibitor, e.g. epsilon aminocaproic acid (EACA).

Disseminated intravascular coagulation (consumptive coagulopathy) Occurs as a result of the release of clotting factors into the bloodstream and/or extensive endothelial damage leading to fibrin formation which produces vascular obstruction and microinfarction and activates the fibrinolytic system. The extensive intravascular coagulation consumes the clotting factors, leading to afibrinoginaemia, thrombocytopenia and microangiopathic haemolytic anaemia seen in the blood film. The final two paradoxical effects are infarction and bleeding respectively.

Disseminated intravascular coagulation is seen in abruptio placentae, intrauterine retention of a dead fetus, incompatible blood transfusion, after severe trauma, fat embolism, open-heart surgery with extracorporeal circulation and extensive lung operations, in the newborn (after abruptio placentae, birth asphyxia, hypothermia and rhesus immunisation), in severe infections (as in Waterhouse–Friderichsen syndrome and generalised Shwartzman reaction after endotoxin blockage of reticuloendothelial cells), in purpura fulminans, metastatic cancer (especially prostate), thrombotic thrombocytopenia purpura, malignant hypertension.

Clinically there is postoperative bleeding, ecchymosis and bleeding from the orifices. Treatment is with platelet and fresh blood and/or fibrinogen. Heparin should be given as a continuous infusion of 10 unit/kg. EACA is contraindicated since clots are unlysable and bilateral renal necrosis can occur in disseminated intravascular coagulation treated with EACA.

- Circulating anticoagulants (antithromboplastins): encountered in patients with haemophilia and Christmas disease who have developed antibodies after repeated transfusions of Factors VIII and IX respectively. Also found in pregnancy, systemic lupus erythematosus and with ionising radiation.

Practical points

Clinical assessment

Is important. Past history of bleeding from the umbilicus after childbirth or after circumcision, tooth extraction or tonsillectomy for 48 h postoperatively suggests a bleeding disorder. Other factors are family history (of clotting defects and hereditary haemorrhagic telangiectasia) and drug history. Examination can reveal petechial haemorrhages or purpura (suggests platelet/generalised vascular disorder) or ecchymoses and/or haemarthrosis (suggests VIII or IX clotting defects).

Laboratory investigations

Include platelet count, prothrombin time (which tests extrinsic system, i.e. factor VII and common pathway, i.e. factors X, V and prothrombin) and partial thromboplastin time (which tests intrinsic system, i.e. factors XII, XI, IX, VIII and common pathway). If prothrombin time and partial thromboplastin time are normal, the defect is probably in

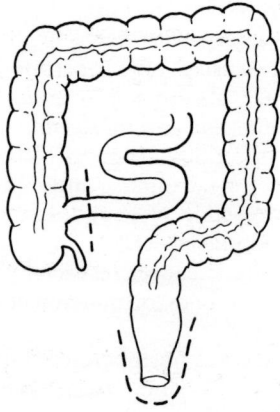

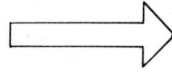

Proctocolectomy and ileostomy

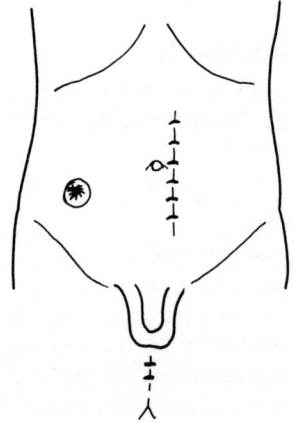

With ileorectal anastomosis (elective)

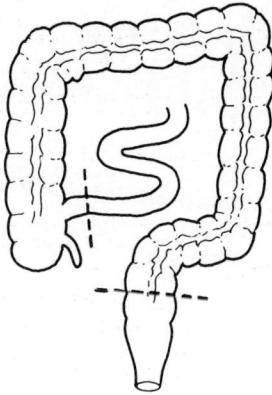

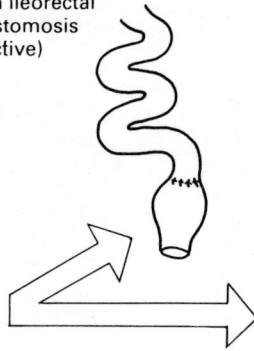

With ileostomy and rectal mucous fistula (emergency)

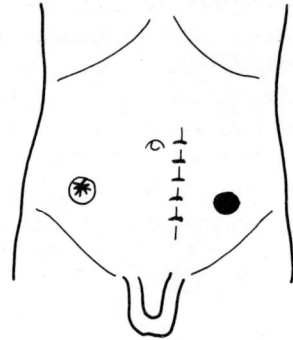

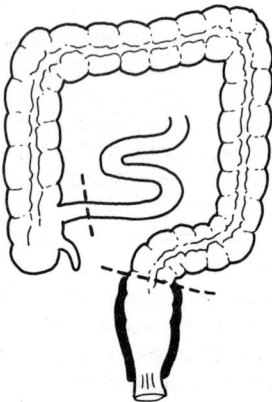

Subtotal colectomy

Colectomy, rectal mucosectomy, ileoanal anastomosis and pelvic ileal pouch (with temporary proximal loop ileostomy)

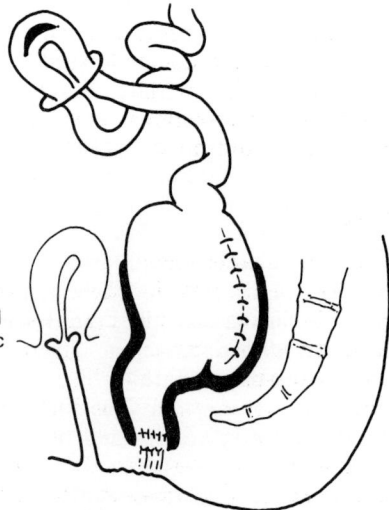

Fig. 9   Surgical options in ulcerative colitis

Surgical options

Gastroduodenal disease

Gastroenterostomy or duodenoenterostomy with vagotomy are indicated only in severe stenosis (never resect).

Small bowel disease

Crohn's disease is precancerous and has a tendency to recur. Therefore, resection is generally better than exclusion surgery. Resection also avoids the risk of the blind loop syndrome. However, resection should be restricted to the diseased segment in order to leave the small bowel for normal absorption and secretion:

- Resection (including lymph nodes) is performed in complicated Crohn's disease, i.e. obstruction, abscess, fistula, perforation, bleeding and carcinoma.
- Resection should always be avoided in diffuse small bowel disease and in acute florid non-obstructive ileal disease. Acute ileitis may be due to *Yersinia enterocolitis* and even if not recurrence is rare if acute ileitis is treated medically.
- Emergency appendicectomy can be performed if the caecum is intact, since postoperative fistulae are rare.
- If both the terminal ileum and caecum ± appendix are involved by the chronic process then ileocaecal resection (limited right hemicolectomy) is done.
- In multiple skip lesions if intervening segments of macroscopically healthy bowel are less than 10 cm apart they can be sacrificed and if the segment is less than 20 cm from the ileocaecal valve then resection should include the caecum.
- If longer segments of intervening bowel are present, multiple small resections or frequent stricturoplasty may be indicated.

Large bowel disease

The indications are less precise here:

- Defunctioning loop ileostomy: in the hope that colonic disease will be improved by faecal diversion in acute active colonic disease not responding to medical treatment.
- Defunctioning split ileostomy: Faecal diversion is better than the above.
- Colectomy and ileorectal anastomosis: there is a risk of recurrence in rectal mucosa and life-long sigmoidoscopic and barium follow-up is required.

- Proctocolectomy.
- Abdominoperineal excision of rectum.

Perineal disease

- Drainage of abscesses.
- Strictures dilated.
- Fistulae are left alone (spontaneous healing occurs in 50% of cases).
- However, low fistulae could be laid open safely.

1.14. Critical Review of Abdominal Stoma

Abdominal stoma include:

- Surgically designed gastrointestinal stoma constructed percutaneously, i.e. gastrostomy, jejunostomy (for feeding in e.g. proximal advanced malignancies), ileostomy and colostomy (intestinal content diversion) whether temporary or permanent, terminal end or looped fashion.
- External stoma. Include fistulae due to a variety of causes (diseased bowel such as Crohn's or diverticular disease, following penetrating abdominal trauma, postoperatively after resection and primary intestinal anastomoses, following radiotherapy and rarely congenital umbilical fistula).
- Urostomy in urinary diversion, i.e. ileal conduit. We will deal here only with ileostomy and colostomy problems, abdominal fistulae and urostomy.

ILEOSTOMY AND COLOSTOMY

Stoma site

Preoperatively the intended site of the stoma should be marked on the skin of the abdominal wall while the patient is standing. The selected site should be visible to the patient and should take account of the proposed site of the laparotomy incision. To ensure that the appliance sits squarely on the skin the opening should be sited away from the umbilicus and bony points, and as far as practically possible should avoid previous abdominal incisions. The patient should try out an appliance before the operation and should meet the stoma therapist who will help with after-care.

outflow from the liver and pressure in the inferior vena cava. In portal hypertension it reaches 400 mmH$_2$O or more. Bleeding from oesophageal varices starts when portal pressure exceeds 250–300 mmH$_2$O. The portal vein is formed of two main vessels—the superior mesenteric and splenic veins. It has no valves. As a result of portal hypertension, extrahepatic portasystemic anastomotic channels become engorged and dilated (i.e. oesophageal varices with profuse painless haematemesis, caput medusae around umbilicus and haemorrhoids). Hypersplenism with pancytopaenia, stasis in the portal circulation with portal vein thrombosis and infarction of the intestine, as well as ascites, also result.

Causes of portal hypertension

- Prehepatic presinusoidal (liver is normal) include umbilical sepsis (neonatal), clotting diathesis (polycythaemia), malignant portal vein obstruction and idiopathic causes.
- Intrahepatic presinusoidal (liver is diseased) include schistosomiasis, congenital hepatic fibrosis, sarcoidosis and liver intoxication.
- Intrahepatic postsinusoidal group includes cirrhosis and veno-occlusive disease (Jamaican bush tea).
- Posthepatic postsinusoidal include hepatic vein obstruction (Budd-Chiari syndrome) and constrictive pericarditis.

Schistosomiasis and cirrhosis are the commonest causes of portal hypertension world-wide.

Indications for elective surgery in portal hypertension

Bleeding oesophageal varices (once they have bled they will bleed again) is an absolute indication. Hypersplenism and ascites are relative indications.

Diagnosis and assessment of portal hypertension

Liver function tests; chest X-ray; barium swallow (soap-bubble appearance of varices); barium meal; i.v. urography to evaluate left renal function (for lienorenal shunt); splenoportography and ultrasound (may show patent or obstructed portal vein); transhepatic venography and endoscopy especially in emergency bleeding to confirm the site of bleeding from chronic peptic ulcer or erosive gastritis which may account for 40% of misdiagnosed bleeding varices. Peptic ulcer is more common in cirrhotics and the presence of varices does not necessarily mean that they are the source of upper gastrointestinal tract bleeding. The severity of liver disease is graded according to Child's classification into A, B and C and modified into a flexible system using points.

Serum bilirubin	
(mg/100 ml)	< 2 (1), 2–3 (2), > 3 (3)
(μmol/l)	< 34 (1), 34–51 (2), > 51 (3)
Serum albumin	
(g/100 ml)	> 3.5 (1), 3–3.5 (2), < 3 (3)
Prothrombin time	
(seconds prolonged)	< 2 (1), 3–5 (2), > 5 (3)
Ascites	None (1), Mild/moderate (2) Gross (3)
Encephalopathy	None (1), Minimal (2), Moderate/severe (3)

The added points are classified as follows:

A = 5–7 points
B = 8–9 points
C = 10–15 points

A liver biopsy is essential and liver scan may be required to exclude hepatomas. The ideal patient for a shunt operation should be under 45 years of age, category A or B, with inactive liver disease and should look and feel well.

Elective treatment of portal hypertension

Surgical (shunts) (Fig. 10)

The most effective method of permanent control. Includes portacaval, lienorenal, mesocaval (jump graft or graft interposition) shunts and selective decompression (Warren's operation—distal lienorenal shunt and gastrosplenic isolation with spleen left *in situ*).

Non-surgical approach

- Injection sclerotherapy of oesophageal varices, via rigid and flexible endoscope.
- Percutaneous transhepatic embolisation of varices.
- Propranolol for prevention of recurrent haemorrhage (not fully established).

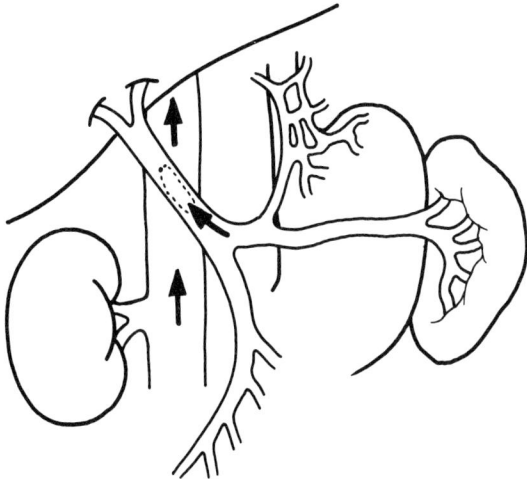

Side-to-side portacaval

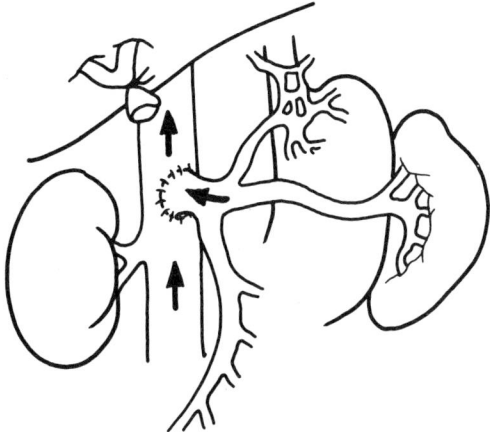

End-to-side portacaval

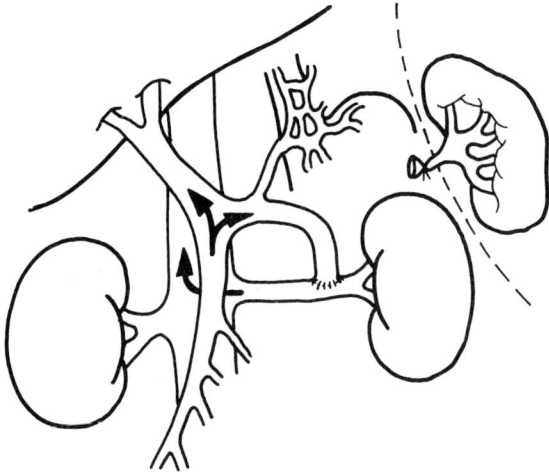

Lienorenal with splenectomy

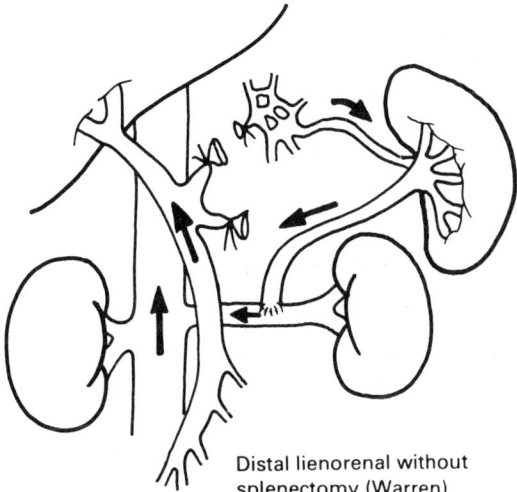

Distal lienorenal without
splenectomy (Warren)

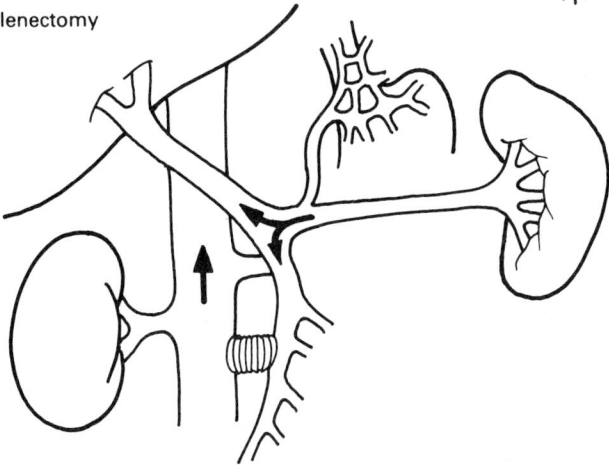

Mesocaval graft interposition

Fig. 10 Shunting procedures in portal hypertension

Prolapse

Colostomy

Prolapse is a much commoner complication of loop colostomies than of end colostomies. Once a colostomy prolapses it becomes oedematous and the mucosa splits. It may also become abraded by the stoma appliance and bleed. Most prolapses cause little discomfort but may make changing the bag difficult or cause the bag to be pushed off the abdominal wall. The bulk of a prolapsed colostomy may be a social embarrassment.

With a right transverse loop colostomy prolapse of the distal loop is usually more troublesome than prolapse of the the proximal loop. Prolapse of the proximal loop can be avoided by making the colostomy as far to the right of the middle colic vessels and as near to the hepatic flexure as possible. For the same reasons, when fashioning a defunctioning loop left iliac colostomy, the stoma should be placed as near to the descending colon as possible.

An oedematous prolapsed colostomy can be left alone if it is small and not troublesome. A large problematical prolapse can usually be reduced on the ward by patient gentle digital manipulation. Closure of a loop colostomy is the best method of cure but if restoration of the continuity of the bowel is not contemplated, it may be necessary to convert the loop into a single barrel provided there is no distal obstruction. If there is distal obstruction a divided colostomy or double-barrelled colostomy can be fashioned. If it is not possible to close a right transverse loop colostomy on its own, it can be closed if a defunctioning loop ileostomy is constructed proximally at the same time. The prolapsed problematical end colostomy may need to be revised. This is usually a simple matter of amputating the redundant bowel.

Ileostomy prolapse and recession

When the ileostomy is being fashioned, approximately 8 cm of terminal ileum is brought through the abdominal wall uneverted at the site of election. The inner tube of bowel is fixed either by suturing the mesentery of the bowel to the abdominal wall from within the abdominal cavity or by suturing it to the anterior rectus sheath from without. Alternatively, very superficial sutures are passed directly between the ileal serosa and the rectus sheath. The ileum is then everted and the distal mucosa sutured directly to skin. The final ileostomy bud should project between 2.5 and 4 cm.

A fixed excessive projection of the bud may force the appliance off the abdominal wall, while fixed inadequate projection predisposes to seepage of efflux onto the skin, leakage and skin problems.

Failure to secure the inner tube of ileum to the abdominal wall or subsequent collapse of the fixation may result in a sliding prolapse of the ileostomy or a sliding recession. Leakage of the appliance becomes a problem.

Fixed excessive projection can be treated by straightforward amputation of the stoma bud to the desired length. Alternatively, all of these stoma problems can be dealt with by revising the stoma completely. The mucocutaneous junction is circumcised and adhesions between the two limbs of the bud broken down. The outer tube is uneverted, the bowel is amputated to the desired level, the inner tube of ileum is fixed to the rectus sheath, the spout is everted and the mucosa sutured to skin. The presence of a large defect at the level of the posterior rectus sheath which predisposes to prolapse may have to be closed at laparotomy and the ileostomy resited—possibly even in the left iliac fossa.

Parastomal hernia

Para-ileostomy and paracolostomy hernia result from making too large a hole in the abdominal wall. The extent of the hernial bulge is variable but large bulges result in problems with the appliance. In a large number of instances the herniation can be controlled by the fitting of a surgical corset with an aperture for the stoma. Should this be insufficient, then a repair of the hernia may have to be carried out. This may be difficult. The operation may entail merely the tightening of the abdominal wall around the stoma or it may necessitate a major repair using non-absorbable mesh and the resiting of the opening.

Recurrent Crohn's disease

The recurrence of Crohn's disease in the spout of an ileostomy may be associated with the formation of fistulae. The extent of the diseased segment will have to be gauged and the offending segment resected with the fashioning of a new stoma.

Stone formation

Ileostomy diarrhoea (due to resection of halting ileocaecal valve, or to diseased or resected terminal ileum with consequent cathartic action of unabsorbed bile salts) and loss of bile salts interfere with enterohepatic circulation of bile salts. This disturbs the cholesterol/bile salts ratio, ultimately leading to gall stone formation. Dehydration and selective uric acid and oxalate absorption are also claimed to cause renal stones.

The quest for continence

The search for reliable methods to establish continent stomas has had more success in relation to the small bowel than the large. A number of mechanical devices have been invented to achieve a continent colostomy but they are not particularly successful. These include the implantable Erlangen magnetic closing device, hinged clips and the implanted Silastic cuff. A method of constructing a new sphincter for the emergent colostomy limb from transplanted colonic muscle has also been described.

Some patients prefer the method of colostomy irrigation to control the efflux from the bowel. Each morning the patient irrigates the colostomy with 1.5 litres of warm water, and the colostomy is drained into a collecting bag. For the rest of the day the patient wears a vented cap over the stoma and can dispense with the use of a cumbersome appliance. The problem with this method is that it is time-consuming.

Reservoir ileostomy

A reservoir is constructed within the abdomen from loops of terminal ileum. A small bowel loop from the reservoir to the abdominal skin is intussuscepted to produce a nipple. This projects into the reservoir and acts as a valve. The emergent limb from the valve is fashioned flush with the abdominal wall. The initial reservoir is constructed with a capacity of approximately 200 ml but with the passage of time its capacity increases to 1 litre. The reservoir can be emptied via a catheter introduced through the valve and into the liquid stool. The construction of such a device is not without its problems: extrusion of the valve results in incontinence; necrosis of the reservoir can result in the loss of a large absorptive surface area of small bowel; and perforation of the reservoir is possible by the passage of the catheter.

INTESTINAL FISTULAE

We deal here briefly with the principles of management of intestinal fistulae. Broadly speaking fistulae can be divided into two large groups. In those that arise due to an *underlying intestinal disease* with the diseased segment of bowel remaining *in situ*, treatment should be aimed at the underlying pathological lesion—the bowel needs to be removed before the fistula will heal. Fistulae that arise as a result of the *dehiscence of an intestinal anastomosis* following the removal of a diseased segment of bowel can be expected to close spontaneously provided there is no distal obstruction and the fistula has not become epithelialised.

Small bowel fistulae

Small bowel fistulae present a greater challenge in management than do those arising from the large bowel. The efflux of a small bowel fistula contains proteolytic enzymes which can cause severe skin problems, and the daily losses from the fistula cause metabolic and nutritional disturbances. The higher the fistula the greater are the associated metabolic problems. Fluid and electrolyte and acid-base disturbances rapidly follow gastric, duodenal and jejunal fistulae. Ileal fistulae do not as a rule cause marked metabolic upset.

Initially, the daily losses from the fistula need to be calculated accurately. The volume of the efflux and its electrolyte content are estimated and the acid-base status and nitrogen balance of the patient monitored. Appropriate replacement of the losses is required with maintenance of the nutritional status of the patient being of paramount importance. A regimen of total parenteral nutrition is instituted with the patient kept in positive nitrogen balance. Provided there is no distal obstruction, spontaneous closure of the fistula is expected.

Operative intervention to close a persistent fistula is done when the patient is fit.

Small bowel fistulae discharge their liquid efflux containing proteolytic enzymes directly onto the skin. In the problem patient there may be multiple openings onto the abdominal wall at points where it is difficult to fit collecting appliances. Stomahesive is now available in large sheets and its use in such a form has considerably aided in the management of these stomas. Irregularities in the abdominal skin can be filled with Stomahesive or karaya gum before placement of the Stomahesive square into which apertures have been cut to conform exactly to the site and shape of the fistulous openings. Collecting bags can be attached to the square and changed without disturbing the skin. Transparent tubed covers can allow irrigation of large defects without disturbance.

Retrospectively, acute pancreatitis can be regarded as severe if it necessitates more than 14 days' hospitalisation and/or results in severe complications (renal or respiratory failure, pancreatic abscesses and pseudocysts) and/or death (Michael *et al.*, 1980).

N.B. Investigations should include blood (as above), urine (for amylase and to monitor volume), X-rays (chest to see any evidence of respiratory failure, abdominal erect and supine to elucidate gall stone aetiology), abdominal ultrasound (to reveal gall stones or pancreatic oedema, and pseudocysts or abscess 2 weeks later especially in the presence of low-grade fever), HIDA biliary scan (non-functioning gall bladder strongly suggests biliary disease; a normal scan does *not* exclude gall stones). CT scan may localise pancreatic slough and necrotic tissues accurately.

III Elucidation of aetiology and treatment according to severity

Mild cases

All mild cases irrespective of aetiology need peripheral i.v. infusion, nasogastric suction (to prevent the release of pancreozymine and cholecystokinin which stimulate the diseased pancreas), nil by mouth, urinary catheter and subclavian catheter *if necessary* (i.e. in the presence of myocardial insufficiency), regular analgesia (if narcotic drug is used it should be administered with an anticholinergic drug, e.g. atropine or hyoscine butylbromide (Buscopan) to counteract the spasm of sphincter of Oddi). Once the patient has recovered, operation for gall stones should be carried out within 1 week.

Severe cases

Should be admitted to the intensive therapy unit and given peripheral i.v. infusion, with nasogastric suction, urinary catheter, ECG monitoring, subclavian CVP line and peritoneal dialysis (claimed to be of therapeutic value). Good analgesia (pethidine and Buscopan) and total parenteral nutrition are required. The current trend is to investigate such cases extensively and if they are proved to be acute pancreatitis with gall stones endoscopic papillotomy is recommended within the first 48 h for

stone retrieval (Carter, 1984). Surgery in severe alcoholic pancreatitis is highly debatable.

Indications for laparotomy

- Diagnostic uncertainty: if the pancreas is normal treat other causes as appropriate. Where acute pancreatitis is diagnosed feel for gall stones and if found proceed to cholecystectomy and exploration of the common bile duct. If acute pancreatitis is not due to gall stones close the abdomen, leaving a catheter inserted through the foramen of Winslow into the lesser sac for peritoneal lavage.
- Patients with acute pancreatitis and multisystem failure who do not respond to intensive treatment within 48 h (especially alcoholic patients), or those with extensive retroperitoneal slough who decline over a period of 5–7 days despite intensive treatment.
- Increasing jaundice and biliary sepsis.
- Late complications of pseudocysts or abscesses.

IV Follow-up

Since the operative treatment of severe alcoholic acute pancreatitis is debatable, follow-up should be regular and might include social and psychiatric follow-up. All patients with acute pancreatitis should be followed for life.

Questionable therapeutic manoeuvres

- Do not routinely give aprotinin or glucagon (they are expensive and of no proven value). Aprotinin is *only* indicated in patients undergoing surgery following which there is a risk of pancreatitis, i.e. sphincteroplasty or common bile duct exploration. Give 500 000 units i.v. in theatre and continue with 200 000 units 6-hourly. Review after 24 h and stop if the amylase is normal.
- Antibiotics are of no proven value in routine management. They are indicated in:
  —Patients with suspected cholangitis.
  —Patients undergoing surgery—give routine prophylactic preoperative cover.
- Nasogastric aspiration is under review and may be unnecessary in mild cases with normal bowel sounds on admission.

1.20. Clinical Aspects of Obstructive Jaundice

Jaundice is clinically detected when serum bilirubin is greater than 40 mmol/l with yellowish discoloration evident mainly in the skin and the sclera. Normal serum bilirubin is 3–17 mmol/l. Extrahepatic jaundice is due to mechanical obstruction of the common bile duct (CBD) which can be corrected surgically. Obstructive or surgical jaundice, as it is termed, may be a life-threatening condition because of the interplay of various factors, e.g. ascending cholangitis, acute renal failure, hampered defence mechanisms with poor antibiotic penetration, high serum fibrinogen/fibrin degradation products, peripheral and portal endotoxaemia. Biliary operative decompression is, therefore, important and also relieves the attendant unpleasant symptoms. Recently, non-operative decompression has been performed with prostheses via percutaneous transhepatic or endoscopic retrograde routes.

Common causes

The pathological distribution of obstructive jaundice in a district general hospital represents a more natural cross-section (among the population) than that seen in specialised centres in which the pathological distribution is skewed as a result of selective referral patterns. Thus in a district general hospital the common causes are:

Benign	CBD Stone	(38%)
	Chronic pancreatitis	(8%)
Malignant		
Primary	Carcinoma of head of pancreas	(30%)
	Extrahepatic CBD carcinoma	(8%)
	Carcinoma ampulla of Vater	(6%)
	Primary duodenal carcinoma	(2%)
Secondary	Portahepatis obstruction	(8%)

Other miscellaneous causes such as traumatic CBD stricture, hydatid disease, chronic duodenal ulcer and sclerosing cholangitis are rarely seen in UK surgical practice.

Diagnosis

Clinical assessment

1. *History*. Age, occupation (hydatid disease in farmers), surgery (stricture), alcohol intake (cirrhosis), drugs and contraceptive pill, biliary colic with fever and jaundice (Charcot triad), injections or transfusions (hepatitis B). Family history of anaemia, splenectomy and gall stones (hereditary spherocytosis). History of present illness, e.g. fluctuating obstructive jaundice (CBD stone and ampullary carcinoma) or progressive obstructive jaundice (other malignant causes), the sudden onset (gall stones) or gradual onset (cirrhosis or malignancy), painful (CBD stone) or painless obstructive jaundice (malignancy or viral hepatitis), fever and rigor (cholangitis in CBD stone and rarely in ampullary carcinoma), dark-coloured urine and clay-coloured stool, pruritus due to irritation of cutaneous nerves by raised bile salts, weight loss (suggests malignancy) or weight gain (suggests gall stones).

2. *Physical examination*. The depth of jaundice, signs of liver failure (spider naevi, ascites, fetor hepaticus, gynaecomastia, testicular atrophy, flapping tremor, clubbing, ankle oedema, palmar erythema and ecchymoses), scratches (due to pruritus), xanthomas (primary biliary cirrhosis), supraclavicular lymph nodes (metastatic carcinoma) and fever (due to cholangitis or viral hepatitis). Notice also abdominal scars from previous operations, palpable gall bladder (carcinoma pancreas), hepatomegaly (slight in obstructive jaundice, hard nodular in secondaries and fine nodular in cirrhosis), splenomegaly (in portal hypertension or haemolytic anaemia), caput medusa (portal hypertension), abdominal mass (malignancy), ascites and rectal examination (remember LUMPS; *see* Section 2, A1.).

Investigations (Table 4)

Start with the cheapest, simplest relevant non-invasive tests:

1. Urine. Absent urobilinogen in obstructive jaundice and absent bilirubin in haemolytic jaundice.

2. Stool. Colour, absent bile pigment in obstructive jaundice, occult blood in ampullary carcinoma.

3. Blood.

(a) High serum bilirubin confirms jaundice and its level gives an idea of severity.

(b) Alkaline phosphatase can differentiate obstructive jaundice (greater than 100 i.u./l) from hepatocellular and haemolytic jaundice (raised but

Drugs Contraceptive pill has been reported to cause liver cell adenomas, hepatoblastomas and hepatocellular carcinoma. This depends on the duration and the dose of both oestrogen and progesterone. However, there is no statistical back-up and it is currently agreed that the contraceptive pill may cause benign hepatic tumours only. Androgen/anabolic steroids can cause benign hepatomas and hyperplasia.

Mycotoxins Are toxic metabolites of fungi and include sterigmatocystin, luteoskyrin and the best known aflatoxins, a group of compounds produced by *Aspergillus flavus*.

Hepatitis B There is a significant association between HB_sAg with both cirrhosis and hepatocellular carcinoma and with α-fetoprotein production.

Pancreas

Diet While fruits and vegetables have a protective value, a high fat diet stimulates bile and increases the availability of bile acids, cholesterol and their metabolites, thus increasing the pancreatic cell multiplication (via cholecystokinin) and causing hyperplasia and possibly carcinoma. While tea consumption was found to be associated with a reduced risk of pancreatic carcinoma, coffee consumption, in contrast, was found to correlate with pancreatic, prostatic carcinomas and leukaemia in males only. Even decaffeinated coffee was found to be associated with pancreatic carcinoma. Later studies were equivocal and the relationship remains to be confirmed (coffee drinkers are usually smokers and the blame probably lies with smoking rather than coffee consumption).

Smoking Increases the risk of pancreatic carcinoma as documented by the high incidence of pancreatic hyperplasia and atypia in autopsies of smokers. The risk is directly proportional to the amount smoked.

Alcoholism Predisposes to oral, pharyngeal, oesophageal, laryngeal, hepatic and possibly pancreatic malignancies (weak relationship).

Familial predisposition Is very rare but definite. It is associated with Gardner's syndrome and hereditary pancreatitis (both autosomal dominant). In multiple endocrine neoplasm (MEN-I), which is also autosomal dominant, the pancreatic neoplasm is usually islet cell functional insulinoma, glucagonoma or gastrinoma and is associated with adenocarcinoma of the pituitary, parathyroid and adrenal cortex. Pancreatic carcinoma is 15 times more common in ataxia telangiectasia than in control relatives. Occult pancreatic adenocarcinoma is also associated with Lindau's disease and with neurofibromatosis.

Diabetes There is a statistically significant excess of deaths in diabetics due to pancreatic carcinoma in both sexes.

Chronic pancreatitis Pancreatic carcinoma develops in 30 % of families with chronic pancreatitis, but it is probably related to the associated alcoholism or the biliary tract disease (or both).

Small bowel

Coeliac disease Significantly associated with intestinal lymphoma and lymphosarcoma.

Peutz–Jeghers syndrome Usually benign but very rarely the polyps undergo malignant changes.

Crohn's disease Rarely may be complicated by malignancy.

Neural crest remnants (Apudoma or carcinoid tumours or argentaffinoma.)

Large bowel

Multiple primary cancers occur in 5–20 % of cases.

Diet There is sufficient evidence to indicate that patients with large bowel cancer have a greater consumption of fat or meat than controls. Beer consumption was also associated markedly with colorectal cancer. Vegetables have a protective value.

Burkitt (1971) stressed that the low-fibre content of Western diets may be responsible for the higher incidence of colon cancer and other diseases in the West than in Africa. He rightly suggested that the longer intestinal transit time and the lower stool weight associated with a low residue would tend to increase both the concentration of any faecal carcinogens and their period of contact with colonic mucosa.

Fibre is a group of structural substances present in the plant cells. Crude fibre signifies the heterogeneous residue remaining after plant foods have been treated successively with dilute acid and dilute alkali. Dietary fibre includes all structures of plant foods that are not digested by human digestive enzymes, e.g. cellulose, hemicellulose, lignins and all indigestible plant polysaccharides. There is sufficient epidemiological evidence to indicate that

angiography (PTC) if the intrahepatic ducts were dilated, or endoscopic retrograde cholangiopancreatography (ERCP) if the intrahepatic ducts were not dilated. Both PTC and ERCP are invasive techniques and need expertise. PTC necessitates a normal clotting screen, prophylactic antibiotics and a Cheeba fine pliable needle inserted under local anaesthesia with injection of contrast medium for diagnosis. Therapeutically PTC external biliary drainage is used in the elderly or as preoperative biliary decompression.

Surgical treatment of obstructive jaundice

Preoperative preparations are essential and include vitamin K injection, correction of prolonged prothrombin time (subsequent bleeding is rare), and infusion of 500 ml of 10% mannitol pre- and peroperatively (with urinary catheterisation). Perioperatively the fluid balance is controlled to maintain a high urine flow (and prevent hepatorenal shut down), and external intermittent pneumatic calf compression (rather than Minihep injection) is used to prevent deep venous thrombosis. Prophylactic antibiotics are also required, and a blood sample is grouped, crossmatched and saved.

The treatment protocol depends on the cause of the obstructive jaundice and is summarised as follows.

CBD stone Cholecystectomy and stone extraction via exploration of the CBD supraduodenally, transduodenally or both. In cases with multiple stones packed in the CBD and in primary biliary stone (i.e. CBD stone developing after 2 symptom-free years following cholecystectomy with no evidence of cystic duct stump or distal CBD stenosis and the stone morphologically is soft, crushable and brown), a choledochoduodenostomy is the prophylactic permanent drainage procedure of choice. CBD stones with carcinoma of head of pancreas may be treated by cholecystectomy and choledochoduodenostomy or choledochojejunostomy (if the CBD is dilated) or extraction of the stone with cholecystojejunostomy without gall bladder removal (if the CBD is not dilated).

Chronic pancreatitis Supraduodenal exploration and dilatation or preferably transduodenal sphincterotomy to treat CBD stenosis. Cholecystectomy is performed routinely.

Early traumatic CBD damage End-to-end reconstruction over a T-tube is recommended. Late strictures are managed with reconstruction and Roux-en-Y hepaticojejunostomy, splinting the anastomosis with a latex tube brought out via the anterior abdominal wall through jejunum or liver.

Pancreatic carcinoma Whipple's operation (radical pancreatoduodenectomy) is performed in early cases (with operative mortality approaching 34% in good centres) although palliation by bypass is preferable, i.e. cholecystojejunostomy + gastrojejunostomy + jejunojejunostomy (triple, double or single bypass does not make much difference and the rationale for constructing an enteroenterostomy to prevent food entry via the cholecystojejunostomy with subsequent ascending cholangitis is theoretical).

Carcinoma of ampulla of Vater and primary duodenal carcinoma Whipple's operation.

Extrahepatic CBD carcinoma and porta hepatis obstruction Hepaticodochojejunostomy (± prosthetic tube insertion). In advanced cases, laparotomy and biopsy are the only practical procedures.

Advanced cases or in ill patients Non-operative biliary decompression via endoprosthesis insertion or external biliary drainage are now used more frequently.

Comments

The overall postoperative mortality (16%) of operated obstructive jaundice cases is directly related to preoperative serum bilirubin (especially greater than 250 μmol/l). Age, coexistent cardiac or respiratory disease and the magnitude of operation performed are important contributory factors. However, most if not all operative deaths usually occur in the malignant group.

The bile culture state (e.g. infection) is intimately related to the morbidity, i.e. postoperative complications, rather than to the operative mortality.

Recently eight useful parameters were viewed collectively in the prediction of risk in biliary surgery and correlate well with mortality, i.e. serum creatinine (more than 130 μmol/l), serum albumin (less than 30 g/l), serum bilirubin (more than 100 μmol/l), WBC (more than 10 000 cells/mm^3), haematocrit (less than 30%), malignancy, serum alkaline phosphatase (more than 600 units/l), and age (more than 60 years).

1.21. Restorative Resection of Carcinoma of the Rectum

PERSPECTIVES IN COLORECTAL ANASTOMOTIC LEAK

Anastomotic leak or dehiscence remains the most challenging mortality and morbidity problem in restorative rectal resection. Although minimal leaks, especially after high anterior resection, often pursue an innocuous, subclinical course, major leaks are life-threatening and prolong convalescence. Anastomoses between the colon and extraperitoneal rectum, classified as 'low', leak more readily than intraperitoneal 'high' ones when the rectum has a serous peritoneal coat. The lower the anastomosis, therefore, the greater the likelihood of leakage. The mortality is 20–22% in leaking cases compared with 7% when the anastomosis is intact. The anastomotic leak is a spectrum and diagnosed clinically (postoperative faecal fistula, local or general peritonism), radiologically (suture line barium enema—diluted barium under low pressure performed towards the end of the second postoperative week can diagnose silent subclinical leaks), rectally (the examining finger reveals pus or feels the anastomotic gap) or sigmoidoscopically. Radiological evidence varies from 6 to 35% and is higher than the clinical evidence (2–18%).

Anastomotic healing

Intestinal anastomotic healing passes through the same phases of wound healing as occur elsewhere in the body. In general, first-intention wound healing consists of three distinct phases:
1. The lag or substrate phase (occurs within the first 4–6 postoperative days), when fluid containing plasma, blood cells and fibrin exudes from tissue into the wound.
2. The healing or proliferation phase (6th–14th postoperative day), when fibroblasts multiply rapidly, bridging wound edges and restoring continuity. Collagen is secreted from cells and formed into fibres. Healing begins rapidly and terminates about the 14th day.
3. The maturation phase (14th–21st postoperative day), when there is sound scar formation.

The collagen concentration in the large bowel is low in the immediate postoperative period and does not increase subsequently (in contrast to that of the small bowel). Mucosal collagenase activity increases after surgery and in the colon there is a predominance of collagen breakdown during the first 4 postoperative days, whereas synthesis predominates in the second week. Factors influencing collagenase activity are: infection, a collagenase inhibitor in plasma and intestinal obstruction.

Decisive factors in anastomotic leak

These can be divided into general and local factors.

General factors

Age (over 60 years), malnutrition and vitamin C deficiency, severe protein malnutrition, zinc depletion, jaundice, uraemia, diabetes, immunosuppression and large doses of steroids all have adverse effects, enhancing anastomotic dehiscence. These factors are patient-related and of no great interest surgically.

Local factors

Colonic contents and infection

About 40% of the dry weight of faeces consists of bacteria and 97% of this is obligatory anaerobes. Without antimicrobial prophylaxis a 50% abdominal wound infection rate can be expected. Combined metronidazole-cefuroxime prophylaxis (i.v. 500 mg and 750 mg respectively three times a day starting with premedication and continued for 24–48 h postoperatively) is effective enough to abolish abdominal wound sepsis. It can improve anastomotic healing although not eliminate complications completely. Attempts to sterilise the faeces are impossible and dangerous. However, mechanical colonic emptying before surgery is essential. Whole gut irrigation was found popular neither with patients nor nurses but 500 ml of 20% mannitol given orally as an osmotic laxative may be used (can lead to explosion if diathermy is used). However, Picolax (two sachets) given orally 1 day before surgery was found to be very successful. (Laxatives are principally of four types: stimulant, e.g. Picolax, cascara, senna; osmotic, e.g. oral mannitol, lactulose, magnesium sulphate; faecal softners, e.g. liquid paraffin, acting by lubrication; and finally bulk-forming drugs, e.g. bran, spaghula husk, methylcellulose.) Rectal enema (phosphate retention or soap water), suppository (Dulcolax) or washout (using a lavage tube with syphon principle) should be done routinely. In the event of occasional failure, peroperative on-table irrigation is done.

Shape of the pelvis

The low anastomosis lies in the presacral space which is deep (especially in males) and has a rigid curved posterior wall. Blood and exudate accumulate here easily and become infected resulting in an abscess bursting through the suture line. Drainage of the presacral space is therefore important (for 5 days using a sump drain or Redivac). In high anastomoses the dead space should be filled with living tissues, e.g. small intestine or omental wrap, to seal any possible leak.

Suturing techniques

Staplers undoubtedly make the operation quicker and easier and are very practical in low anastomoses. However, the overall results are only slightly better than those of hand suturing and the radiological leak rate is not altered.

There was no difference clinically between single- and two-layer hand suturing in high intraperitoneal anastomoses.

Single-layer anastomoses, however, were superior when constructed below the peritoneal reflection. The inverted interrupted serosubmucosal (partial-thickness) single-layer hand technique was found to be simple and effective for difficult anastomoses low in the pelvis (circular staplers can give a comparable result in such cases and may be even simpler in difficult access). Experimentally, the single-layer technique provides a larger lumen (no stenosis), minimal tissue strangulation (mucosal sloughing occurs with two-layer technique) and better anastomotic strength. The inverted technique was superior to everted techniques when performed expertly in a clinical situation.

Whichever technique is used, the anastomosis should be gas-tight, not strangulating and there should be no mesocolic vascular tension.

Suture materials

The ideal suture does not exist; however in colonic anastomoses a suture should not potentiate infection, it should be non-braided, dissolve slowly, exhibit low irritancy, and should knot easily and securely. Monofilaments, either absorbable (PDS) or nonabsorbable (polypropylene or nylon) are possibly the sutures of choice and should be incorporated into one layer of any sutured colonic anastomoses. However it is the handling properties rather than any other factor that determines the surgeon's choice of a particular material.

Blood supply

There should be pulsatile extramural blood flow. The documented avascular critical points of Sudeck (1907), Toupet (1951) and Griffiths (1956) at the rectosigmoid junction (between the last sigmoidal and superior rectal arteries), the sigmoid colon (between the sigmoidal arteries) and the splenic flexure respectively are merely extramural macroscopic points with no intramural microscopic counterparts. The terminal colorectal vessels constitute minicollateral vessels easily compromised by intramural haematoma or complete transmural suturing. Therefore intramural haematoma necessitates re-resection and re-anastomosis. There are two primary transmural plexuses—at the subserosal and submucosal (the most important and extensive) sites—with two subsidiary plexuses at the intermuscular (fed by subserosal) and mucosal (fed by submucosal) sites. Single-layer (hand) suturing, therefore, should be partial (seromuscular) and from the outside-in, using submucosal grooves as landmarks for entry or exit bites. The mucosal layer is optional; although it reinforces the gas-tight barrier, careless deep strangulating suturing predisposes to leakage and also leads to late stenosis. As the cut ends of the intramural transverse vascular circles have variable shapes, there is an unavoidable percentage of leakage, theoretically caused by microvascular mismatch between the uncompensated vascular circles in the free cut ends of the anastomosed segments.

The physiological properties of the colonic microcirculation are important—shock, haemorrhage and hypotension during anaesthetic induction may predispose to leakage. Lowering of the systolic blood pressure by more than 50 mmHg below the base line for 15 min or longer during the operation results in a 150% increase in the rate of leakage. Homeostatic visceral vasoconstriction usually occurs to preserve cerebral and coronary blood flow at the expense of intestinal blood flow. A loss in blood volume of 10%, while producing only small changes in blood pressure and cardiac output, can reduce colonic blood flow and oxygen availability by 28%, as shown in dogs. The worst possible clinical combination is inadequate volume replacement using only blood (dextran or Hartmann's solution should be used instead—*see below*). Measured haemodilution, done by withdrawing blood and replacing with Hartmann's solution until haemoglobin is around 11 g/100 ml, was found to decrease viscosity and improve oxygen transport at the microcirculation level. Anastomotic leak was found to be associated with a mean haemoglobin level of 14.6 g/100 ml as compared to 12.5 g/100 ml when leak was not present. Furthermore, perioperative blood transfusion is associated with significant colorectal recurrences and bad long-term prognosis.

Intra-abdominal sepsis

In the absence of infection leak occurred in about 7.9% of cases while it occurred in 20.5% when infection was encountered during the operation. This represents a 150% increase in the incidence of postoperative leak. Primary colostomy, therefore, is required in the presence of local, general or spreading peritonitis.

Emergency operation

Increases the leak rate by 150% as compared to elective operation (due to poor bowel preparation).

Anastomotic rest

Intracolonic pressure is generated by colonic segmentation and peristalsis. The latter are activated by neostigmine (used to reverse the effects of relaxants in the recovery from anaesthesia—some advocate the use of pyridostigmine instead), morphine (as a postoperative analgesia), metoclopramide (Maxolon; as a postoperative antiemetic), food ingestion and emotion and these should be avoided. However colonic segmentation is paralysed by propantheline bromide and reduced by pethidine (safe postoperative analgesic). Immediate postoperative anal digital stretch may be practised or a rectal tube may be used to overcome any anal sphincteric spasm that might strain the anastomosis by high colonic pressure (not proven).

Other factors

● Colostomy does not influence the incidence of leak but it is supposed to be life-saving if leakage occurs. The current trend is to carry out primary anastomosis with no primary colostomy, reserving colostomy as a secondary procedure should a

leak occur (usually 1 out of 10 postoperative patients will leak clinically).
● Preoperative radiotherapy mitigates against primary healing. Radiation causes intestinal microcirculatory changes which are dose-dependent.
● Drains in general potentiate infection (demonstrated experimentally and clinically). Closed suction drains after low anastomoses have some complications and probably do not serve the drainage function as was expected.

SPHINCTER-SAVING RESECTION

The majority of large bowel growths are found in the lower sigmoid colon and upper rectum. Sphincter-saving resection has stood the test of time and is comparable in results to abdominoperineal excision of the rectum with permanent colostomy. For Duke's B and C tumours of average malignancy, there was no difference between sphincter-saving resection and abdominoperineal excision of the rectum in terms of 5 year survival. If the rectal stump was well irrigated at operation (sphincter-saving resection), malignant implantation in the suture line was very rare. It was thought that the possibility of recurrence was higher in sphincter-saving resection because it is less extensive than abdominoperineal excision of the rectum.

While both operations deal with upward spread it was the distal and lateral spread of tumour cells which led to the debatable 5 cm distal clearance rule in sphincter-saving resection. However, distal intramural spread is rare and usually extends for less than 1 cm. Spread greater than this indicates advanced C or D with poor prognosis and patients usually die of distant metastases before they develop local recurrence. Distal extramural lymphatic spread was found less than 2 cm from the distal margin of the tumour. The amount of tissue that can be removed laterally is just as extensive in radical sphincter-saving resection as in abdominoperineal excision of the rectum. The minimal 2 cm distal clearance from the tumour is therefore adequate.

For anorectal function 6–8 cm anorectal preservation was thought necessary but studies showed that very low colorectal or even coloanal anastomoses will achieve continence and sensation after a period of 18 months' adaptation. The quality of life is certainly better in sphincter-saving resection because the social and/or psychological trauma of permanent colostomy is avoided.

In terms of operative mortality and morbidity sphincter-saving resection is probably safer. The morbidity of permanent colostomy in abdominoperineal excision of the rectum is comparable to that of anastomotic leak in sphincter-saving resection.

SOME PRINCIPLES IN COLONIC SURGERY

- Sigmoidoscopy and biopsy are the keystone investigations in both emergency and elective cases. Emergency barium enema is indicated in acute cases (to identify the level of colonic obstruction) when emergency operation is contemplated on the day of admission.
- Bowel preparation should be perfect in the partially obstructed bowel: use laxatives (Picolax), enema, suppositories or rectal washout preoperatively; and if the bowel is still not clean, use operative on-table antegrade colonic irrigation.
- Do not operate without antibiotic cover or prophylaxis (start i.v. or i.m. with premedication and continue for 24 h, e.g. metronidazole, cefuroxime).
- Full mobilisation is essential, especially of the splenic flexure, to cut the congenital bands so that anastomosed segments are floppy and tension-free; otherwise ischaemia and/or leak may occur.
- Early vascular interruption to prevent intravascular dislodgement of tumour cells.
- Always identify the ureter in left colonic surgery (no need for preoperative IVU). In right colonic surgery identify the ureter operatively as well as preoperatively (IVU).
- Recurrence in anterior restorative rectal resection or sphincter-saving resection is higher than in abdominoperineal excision of the rectum owing to intraluminal exfoliation of malignant cells; therefore, always irrigate the rectal stump operatively (prior to anastomosis) with 1% noxythiolin (Noxyflex) solution. This minimises suture line recurrence.
- The anastomosis should be made gas-tight, not strangulating and with no tension using a single- or double-layer (hand) technique in high anastomosis and a single-layer (hand) or stapler technique in low anastomosis. It should be covered by living tissue such as the small intestine or omentum.
- In low colorectal anastomosis drainage of the presacral space is important to prevent haematoma bursting through the suture line (drain is removed on the fifth day). Mobilised splenic flexure area may necessitate another drain because of excessive exudation (such a drain does not influence the anastomotic integrity).
- Colostomy does not influence the anastomotic leak but is certainly a life-saving procedure when the leak occurs. Therefore a primary anastomosis can be constructed without protective primary colostomy, but in this case the surgeon should be prepared to perform secondary colostomy when the leak occurs (roughly in 1 out of 10 cases postoperatively). A primary colostomy is indicated, however, in the presence of intraperitoneal sepsis or when a low anastomosis is insecure because of difficult suturing or unavoidable tension.
- Postoperative anal digital dilatation is recommended (though not proven) to decompress the intracolonic pressure. Similarly drugs increasing intracolonic pressure or enhancing peristalsis should be avoided, e.g. neostigmine, narcotic analgesia (morphine) and Maxolon.

1.22. Surgery for Incontinence

FAECAL INCONTINENCE

The involuntary loss of faeces is a distressing social disability. Normally the anorectal mechanism is made up of two tubular-shaped parts, one ensheathing the other. The innermost structure is the termination of the gut (*visceral* part); this is surrounded by pelvic floor *skeletal* muscles, the lower part of which form the *external anal sphincters*. The lower rectum and anal canal are innervated by the autonomic nerves and are therefore not subject to voluntary control. It is the surrounding skeletal muscle sphincter that is essential for establishing normal continence. The upper part of the visceral component is lined by unstratified, mucus-secreting columnar epithelium which is almost devoid of sensory receptors. Fortunately, the terminal 2 cm is atypical in that the visceral mucosa has been replaced by squamous epithelium which does not secrete mucus; the perineum is therefore not continuously soiled by mucous discharge.

This lower 2 cm is supplied with somatic sensory nerves which supply information to the spinal centres and is a valuable part of the mechanism of continence. The terminal part of the circular muscle is greatly enlarged to form the *internal sphincter muscle*. Its visceral tone is the most important factor in maintaining a closed anal canal, but it is autonomically supplied and there is no control over it. Outside this there is a relatively thin layer of longitudinal muscle that has no significant function in this area.

The external sphincter muscles maintain control over the outlet. In addition they have an antigravity function in maintaining a closed pelvic outlet against the forces of abdominal pressure. However, surgical division of the internal sphincter rarely results in any serious disability. Similarly extensive division of the external sphincter (in anal fistulae) leads to only a slight disability. The forward pull of the fibres of the puborectalis muscle creates an *anorectal angle* (normally 60–105°) which is maintained involuntarily by a spinal reflex; once this angle is exceeded, faecal incontinence occurs. *Faecal continence therefore appears to be related principally to the preservation of a normal anorectal angle which in turn is dependent on a normally functioning puborectalis muscle with a flap-valve mechanism accentuated by the intra-abdominal pressure.*

The sensation of continence is conducted through receptors lying within the rectum and the nearby pelvic floor muscles which cradle it (and therefore coloanal anastomosis does not interfere with this sensation).

Diagnosis

A careful history (current complaint and duration, gastrointestinal symptoms, neurological symptoms, past history of congenital defect, operative trauma or neurological disease), rectal examination (to exclude rectal neoplasm, assess sphincteric function and test anal skin sensation) and sigmoidoscopy. Intra-anal pressure recording and preoperative electromyographic exploration of the perineum may be helpful in mapping out the deficient skeletal muscles.

Classification of causes with treatment

True incontinence

Partial incontinence

This occurs in the presence of partial or complete rectal prolapse or commonly as a complication of minor surgery, e.g. sphincterotomy, fistula surgery, haemorrhoidectomy or manual dilatation of the anus. There is normal function within the pelvic floor muscles and external anal sphincter.

This group may need no treatment or simple conservative treatment (constipating agents). Complete rectal prolapse, however, may need a purse-string procedure or even rectopexy.

Complete incontinence

Usually there is a normally functioning internal anal sphincter and a markedly deficient or dysfunctioned skeletal muscle component.

Idiopathic No apparent underlying neurological or anatomical causes. However denervation of pelvic floor muscles and the external sphincter with anal reflex delay is thought to be the cause as proved by microscopic and special histochemical examination of muscle biopsies (*localised neuronal damage*). Spontaneous occurrence of incontinence in women is due to a prolonged second stage of labour with possible perineal tears. Prolonged straining at defaecation may lead to the *descending perineum syndrome* due to pudendal nerve stretch injury. There may be pudendal nerve entrapment within Alcock's canal (comparable to carpal tunnel syndrome).

Postanal repair (muscle-tightening procedure) may be indicated in which the levator ani, puborectalis and external sphincter muscles arc apposed behind the anorectal ring. The gracilis sling procedure or free autotransplantation of the palmaris longus or sartorius muscle placed as a U-shaped sling around the rectum may also be used.

Traumatic Due to anal injury, fistula surgery damaging the integrity of the puborectalis sling and abolishing the anorectal angle; treatment is by sphincteroplasty (*see* comment below) which necessitates a temporary defunctioning colostomy.

Neurological As in tabes dorsalis or multiple sclerosis, paraplegia and cauda equina. Conservative measures may be used (not very effective) and include pelvic floor faradism, external sphincter stimulation by direct electrode implantation and external anal plug stimulation.

Congenital As in anorectal agenesis and anal ectopia. This needs accurate siting of the *neoanus* and rectum in relation to the pelvic floor and necessitates preoperative electromyography.

False incontinence

Incontinence may be secondary to organic colo-rectoanal disease or occur in severe diarrhoea. The commonest cause in the elderly is dyschesia; this is a spurious diarrhoea due to liquefaction of impacted faeces. Treatment is that of the primary cause.

Comment on sphincteroplasty

Surgical repair of the injured sphincter basically includes apposition, overlapping and reefing. In principle the surgeon usually attempts to repair the external sphincter muscle or puborectalis sling or both. Gracilis muscle transposition or a Dacron-impregnated Silastic sheet sling can be used to supplement the sphincter mechanism.

URINARY INCONTINENCE

The involuntary loss of urine is the most distressing disability in urological practice. Successful storage of urine demands that the bladder does not contract inappropriately (remains stable) and that the sphincter mechanism be competent. These two criteria differentiate non-surgical from surgical urinary incontinence. In the former, which affects up to 10% of the population, there is *idiopathic instability* or *urgency incontinence* (though uninhibited detrusor hyperreflexia also occurs in neurological bladder). The latter is genuine *stress incontinence*—the involuntary loss of urine due to a sudden rise in intra-abdominal pressure. It is an exceedingly common condition affecting up to 50% of young healthy nulliparous women. However 80% of incontinence cases are in the perimenopausal age group, especially multiparous women.

Under normal conditions urine is retained in the bladder because the intravesical pressure is very much less than the intraurethral pressure. This is achieved by suppression of the sacral reflex arc by the higher centres which prevents detrusor contractions occurring during filling of the bladder.

The urethral lumen is kept occluded at a higher pressure than the bladder by a combination of the actions of the smooth- and striated-muscle components and the engorgement of the venous plexuses and elastic tissue around the bladder neck. The urethra is also held forwards and upwards by the pubourethral ligaments so that rises in intra-abdominal pressure are equally transmitted to the bladder and upper third of the urethra, which lie above the pelvic floor, thus maintaining the pressure gradient between the two. In addition a reflex contraction of the levator ani compresses the mid-urethra.

Diagnosis

A careful history (current complaint with urological symptoms, duration and severity, neurological symptoms, gynaecological symptoms integrated with urological complaint, medical disorders, psychiatric disorders and drug therapy; also past history of urinary operations, drugs, obstetric history (in females), enuresis, retention and urinary tract infections), examination (general, neurological, vaginal examination in females and rectal examination in males) and investigations (intravenous urography, voiding cystourethrogram, rarely ascending urethrogram which may demonstrate urethral stricture, cystourethroscopy and particularly urodynamic studies in the form of cystometry, voiding cystometrogram or urethrocystometry) are important.

Male urinary incontinence

Causes and treatment

Congenital

- Ectopia vesicae: treated by re-forming the bladder and the abdominal wall and constructing a *neourethra*; however urinary diversion may be required.
- Ectopic ureter: inserted into the urethra below the sphincter. Can be divided and reimplanted into the bladder; in the presence of ascending kidney infection a nephroureterectomy is preferable.

Postprostatectomy urinary incontinence

This occurs in up to 1% in prostatectomy and 20% in radical prostatectomy. The risk is minimised by removal of adenomatous tissue leaving no residual tags behind. In open prostatectomy the urethral mucosa at the apex should be severed sharply and well above the urogenital diaphragm.

During transurethral resection (TUR) it is important to avoid resecting or coagulating extensively at or below the verumontanum. With established mild postprostatectomy urinary incontinence, expectant therapy (time will cure or ameliorate a percentage of all types of urinary incontinence) and possibly pharmacological manipulation (Table 5) are of value.

Table 5. Pharmacological manipulation of postprostatectomy urinary incontinence

Action	Drug
Acting on the bladder	
Stimulation (used in retention)	Bethanechol (Myotonine Chloride)
	Distigmine (Ubretid)
	Phenoxybenzamine (Dibenyline)
Inhibition (used in frequency, enuresis and incontinence)	Atropine
	Propantheline (Pro-Banthine)
	Methantheline (Banthine)
	Oxybutynine (Ditropan)
	Dicyclomine (Bentylol)
	Flavoxate (Urispas)
	Imipramine (Tofranil)
	Emepronium (Cetiprin)
Acting on the bladder and proximal urethra	
Stimulation	Ephedrine
	Pseudoephedrine (Sudafed)
	Imipramine (Tofranil)
	Phenylpropanolamine (Eskornade)
Inhibition	Phenoxybenzamine (Dibenzyline)
	Guanethidine (Ismelin)
	Methyldopa (Aldomet)

In severe cases, urodynamic studies are needed to ascertain whether the patient has an unstable detrusor. A stable detrusor can be treated by passive urethral compression (detachment and crossing of penis crura to compress bulbous urethra—*Kaufman I*; approximation of crura together in the midline with the aid of Teflon mesh tape placed around them to compress bulbous urethra—*Kaufman II*; or placement of silicone-gel prosthesis to compress bulbous urethra with the aid of Dacron straps passed around crura—*Kaufman III*). An unstable detrusor can be managed by use of an implantable inflatable *Rosen compression prosthesis* or an implantable inflatable *Brantley–Scott hydraulic cuff prosthesis*. Electric and electronic stimulation of the pelvic floor (similar to that used for faecal incontinence) may also be used. Other surgical methods include urethral reconstruction, urethral angulation, suspension and sling procedure (not as successful as in females).

The prostheses and devices generally give a success rate of at least 60%, although morbidity may occur in the form of infection, fistula or device failure, and reoperation may be required. Nevertheless they have superseded urethral reconstruction operations.

Neuropathic bladder (*with urge or overflow urinary incontinence*)

● Spina bifida, myelomeningocoele.
● Spinal trauma causing paraplegia or tetraplegia. The bladder is either spastic (upper motor neuron lesion with involuntary detrusor contractions, high pressure and hypertrophy, and reduced capacity) or flaccid (lower motor neuron lesion with infrequent detrusor contraction, low pressure and large capacity). Spastic bladder is managed satisfactorily by regular manual squeezing of the abdomen, genitalia or thighs. A large capacity bladder (whether flaccid or spastic) requires intermittent self-catheterisation (with Texas condom catheter) or regular intermittent catheterisation (with silicone Foley catheter). Pharmacological manipulation can be tried. TUR sphincterotomy (of bladder neck, or internal or external sphincter) is used to overcome the spastic obstructing outlet. Ileal conduit diversion is the final answer.

Established urinary incontinence

Can be treated by:

● Texas condom catheter with collecting bag tied to the thigh or calf.
● Drainage with indwelling Foley catheter with small balloon or fine 8 Fr Gibbon catheter.
● Cunningham or Baumrucker penile clamps.
● Absorbent pads.

Remember that overflow urinary incontinence is a false incontinence since it is due to urinary retention, the underlying causes of which should be treated on their merit.

Female urinary incontinence

Causes

Urethral

● *Stress urinary incontinence* (surgical) due to urethral sphincter incompetence following childbirth trauma, cystocoele, TUR of bladder neck, denervation in hysterectomy or sphincter atrophy.
● *Overflow urinary incontinence* due to outflow obstruction (surgical fibrosis or elevation of

bladder neck and urethral stricture) or neurological lesions (spinal shock, cauda equina, tabes dorsalis, poliomyelitis and diabetes).

- *Urge urinary incontinence* (non-surgical) due to detrusor instability because of impaired corticospinal inhibition of the sacral reflex (normally a result of stress, but can also result from psychosis, nocturnal enuresis, congenital defects such as spina bifida, trauma, multiple sclerosis, stroke, or intracranial or spinal malignancy).
- *Reflex urinary incontinence* occurs in spinal cord lesions and trauma and prevents sensation of the bladder filling and involuntary control of micturition.

Extraurethral urinary incontinence (surgical)

- *Ureterovaginal fistula* due either to congenital ectopic ureter (draining upper kidney moiety and inserted into vaginal vault or close to external urethral meatus) or traumatic pelvic surgery, e.g. hysterectomy in which case the ureter is injured by direct trauma and/or pressure necrosis from a ligature and/or avascular necrosis particularly after pelvic irradiation.
- *Vesicovaginal fistula* due to obstetric cause in developing countries (obstructed labour, associated with infection and pressure necrosis of bladder base) or to gynaecological surgery in developed countries (during abdominal or vaginal procedures especially where there has been distortion of the anatomy by either infection or irradiation).

Treatment

Stress urinary incontinence

- *Pelvic floor strengthening* Physiotherapy and electrical stimulation can be tried first.
- *Urethral suspension*
  —Fascial sling using pyramidalis, rectus muscle, Mersilene mesh, Teflon strips.
  —Marshall–Marchetti–Krantz cystourethropexy.
  —Burch retropubic bilateral colposuspension.
  —Anterior colporrhaphy.
  —Modified Peyrera needle suspension procedure with cystoscopic Stamey modification.
- *Urethral lengthening* Urethroplasty, urethral narrowing and plication of bladder neck have all been tried.
- *Periurethral Teflon paste injection*

- *Prosthesis surgery* The Brantley–Scott sphincter hydraulic inflatable cuff, with many modifications, has been used for female urinary incontinence.

Overflow urinary incontinence

The aim is to reduce the urethral obstruction and enhance detrusor activity. Urethral dilatation or Otis urethrotomy to a depth of 2 mm at 3 and 9 o'clock is recommended. To promote bladder-emptying, detrusor activity can be stimulated electrically or by a parasympathomimetic drug such as Ubretid. Intermittent self-catheterisation is also recommended.

Urge urinary incontinence

With unstable bladder is treated by one of the following:
- Drugs, e.g. anticholinergic or sympathomimetics (orciprenaline and propantheline) or prostaglandin inhibitors (indomethacin, aspirin and flurbiprofen) are used to subdue detrusor instability with symptomatic amelioration in 50% of cases.
- Cystodistension under epidural anaesthesia.
- Bladder training—intensive bladder drill.
- Bladder denervation.

Ureterovaginal fistula

May close spontaneously; however treatment should be monitored by IVU. Surgical treatment should aim at reimplantation of the ureter with possible Boari flap or psoas hitch or even by an intervening ileal conduit between the ureter and the bladder.

Vesicovaginal fistula

Preoperatively, urinary infection treatment with antibiotics, indwelling urethral catheterisation and treatment of vaginal mucosal ulceration with stilboestrol are recommended. The aim of surgery is to excise the fistula tract completely and to close the bladder and the vaginal defect in layers without tension preferably with an intervening mobilised omentum pedicle graft (or labium majus mobilised subcutaneous fat or mobilised gracilis muscle) to promote healing in such extensive tissue devitalisation. Gynaecologists use the vaginal approach while urologists prefer the retropubic extraperitoneal intravesical approach.

Comment on vesicointestinal fistulae

These are due to diverticulitis, colorectal carcinoma, bladder carcinoma, Crohn's disease and trauma in this order of frequency. Common findings are faecaluria, recurrent urinary tract infections and pneumaturia. Cystography or barium enema and cystoscopy may reveal the fistula. In other cases the diagnosis is very difficult to prove. The fistulae rarely close spontaneously, though they may be symptom-free. Preoperative sterilization of urine and bowel contents with antibiotic and bowel preparation are needed.

The decision whether to perform a single-stage or a multistage operation can only be made during operation. If there is a walled-off abscess associated with the fistula or a very large inflammatory mass, then preliminary faecal diversion by transverse colostomy may be wise (with excision of the fistula-bearing segment of the bowel and bladder, intestinal anastomosis and closure of the bladder). This can be followed later by colostomy closure and restoration of bowel continuity (two-stage procedure, used especially in colonic malignancy which is treated occasionally by faecal diversion alone if inoperable). If the surgical situation looks relatively simple, bowel excision, intestinal anastomosis, closure of fistula, closure of the bladder and diversion of the urine by suprapubic cystostomy and urethral catheterisation may be performed (one-stage). Use of pedicled omental flap is often desirable. The decision whether to perform a protecting colostomy after bowel excision and fistula closure should be made by the surgeon in the course of the operation.

1.23. Surgical Treatment of Obesity

Severe obesity is a life-threatening condition and is associated with:
- Increased mortality due to cardiovascular, respiratory, hepatobiliary complications and suicide; a 20% weight excess raises the mortality rate by 15%.
- Obesity-related diseases, e.g. gall stones, hiatus hernias, osteoarthritis, varicose veins, thrombophlebitis and gravitational oedema, fractures and severe limb injuries, prolapse and cystocele, maturity-onset diabetes, arterial diseases and renal calculi (surgically treated diseases) as well as chronic obstructive airway diseases, dermatological problems and infertility.

Overeating is often compulsive and addictive and is commonly associated with little or no physical activity. Dietary energy restriction with increased physical activity should be tried first but diet, drugs, in-patient starvation, hypnotism and psychiatric therapy have only a short-term effect and are usually unsatisfactory since the weight lost is rapidly regained after termination of the programme.

The rationale for surgery is based on two facts:
1. Severe obesity is associated with high mortality and morbidity.
2. Long-term medical treatment often fails.

On the other hand, obesity influences surgery in two ways:
1. Obesity-associated diseases (treated surgically, *see above*).
2. Adverse effects on surgical management preoperatively causing late diagnosis, e.g. hidden carcinoma in a fatty breast and difficult diagnosis of intra-abdominal masses. Postoperatively wound sepsis, haematoma, burst abdomen, respiratory insufficiency and atelactasis, deep venous thrombosis and pulmonary embolism occur more frequently and the results of varicose vein or hiatus hernia surgery are poorer in obese patients.

Indications for surgery

- Morbid or massive obesity defined as at least twice or 45 kg over the ideal weight (matched for age, sex and height) of at least 5 years' duration.
- Failure of standard medical dietary treatment and/or patient failure to adhere to prescribed dietary regimen.

Criteria of suitability for surgery

- Absence of correctable endocrine abnormality which might be a cause of the obesity (e.g. Cushing's syndrome, myxoedema).
- Absence of unrelated diseases which might increase the operative risk.
- Absence of excessive alcohol intake.
- Presence of certain obesity-related complications which might be improved by a significant weight loss, e.g. hyperlipidaemia, maturity-onset diabetes, hypertension or Pickwickian syndrome (cardiorespiratory embarrassment due to excessive obesity).

- Assurance of patient cooperation both in preoperative assessment and in prolonged postoperative management.

Preoperative measures (especially in intestinal shunts)

1. High-protein diet for 3 weeks.
2. Bowel preparation (e.g. oral neomycin and metronidazole), elemental diet, mechanical cleansing and washout.
3. Low-dose heparin subcutaneously started with premedication until the patient is mobile postoperatively (to prevent thromboembolism).
4. Prophylactic antibiotics to prevent wound infection.

Surgical procedures

Historical (not recommended)

Truncal vagotomy without drainage To decrease gastric emptying (pylorospasm) and therefore limit the transit time of food, reducing the intestinal absorption accordingly.

Lipectomy (apronectomy or panniculectomy) Surgical elliptical excision of the large apron of fat that forms the anterior abdominal wall as it interferes with ventilation and causes intertrigo and mechanical impairment with walking. It was widely practised and removal of up to 26 kg was reported. It does not contribute significantly to obesity control. Furthermore, repair of coexisting umbilical hernia is frequently followed by bleeding, haematoma and wound sepsis.

Dental splintage Cap splints or interdental wiring are used to restrict the patient to a fluid diet (e.g. milk or soup with iron and vitamin supplements). The wiring is released monthly for 2–3 days at a time to prevent trismus and to facilitate adequate dental hygiene. Fifty per cent of patients could not tolerate the procedure and only 10% allowed the procedure to continue long enough for satisfactory weight loss in spite of short-term good results. The long-term results are no better than those of conservative medical means.

Current (recommended)

Gastric operations (Fig. 11)

(a) Subtotal gastrectomy (small gastric fundic pouch and large stoma): causes dumping syndrome with decreased food intake and weight loss (unsatisfactory, with high mortality).
(b) Gastroplasty: by incision partially traverses the stomach from the lesser curve, leaving a small channel intact along the greater curvature. Weight loss occurs only during the first 6 postoperative months.
(c) Gastric bypass (large gastric pouch and small stoma).
(d) Gastric bypass (small gastric pouch and small stoma): bypasses 90% of stomach, leaving a 12 mm gastroenterostomy stoma.
(e) Gastroplasty: a stapler is used, without division of the stomach, to create a 10% fundic pouch and 1 cm stoma on the greater curve (easy, safe and reversible).

Results: Operative mortality is 2.8% and total mortality is 5.1%. Although the immediate weight loss is rapid, the majority of patients will not reach their ideal weight. Fistulation and gastroenterostomy anastomotic disruption is the most important complication (reduced by careful technique and prolonged postoperative nasogastric decompression). Other non-specific complications, e.g. thromboembolism, respiratory failure and wound infection, are common.

Dumping syndrome is severe in 20% of patients. Oedema, diarrhoea and syncope are other side-effects. Stomal ulceration is low in the gastric exclusion operation but significant in gastroenterostomies. Such gastric operations are probably not the operation of choice in morbidly obese patients wishing to return to their ideal weight and therefore should be reserved for moderately obese patients (after failure of conservative means) who will be content to lose 36 kg.

Intestinal bypass or shunt

The operation of choice. The idea was conceived after the survival of a patient following massive small intestinal resection for volvulus and mesenteric thrombosis. The length of the anastomosing parts of the bowel is the most decisive factor in the success of the operation. Types of operation include (Fig. 12):

(a) Jejunocolic bypass: anastomosis of proximal 38 cm of jejunum with transverse colon (end-to-side). Dramatic weight loss occurred but due to the prohibitive morbidity of severe diarrhoea, electrolyte disturbance and hepatic failure, the operation was condemned and abandoned in favour of jejunoileal shunts.

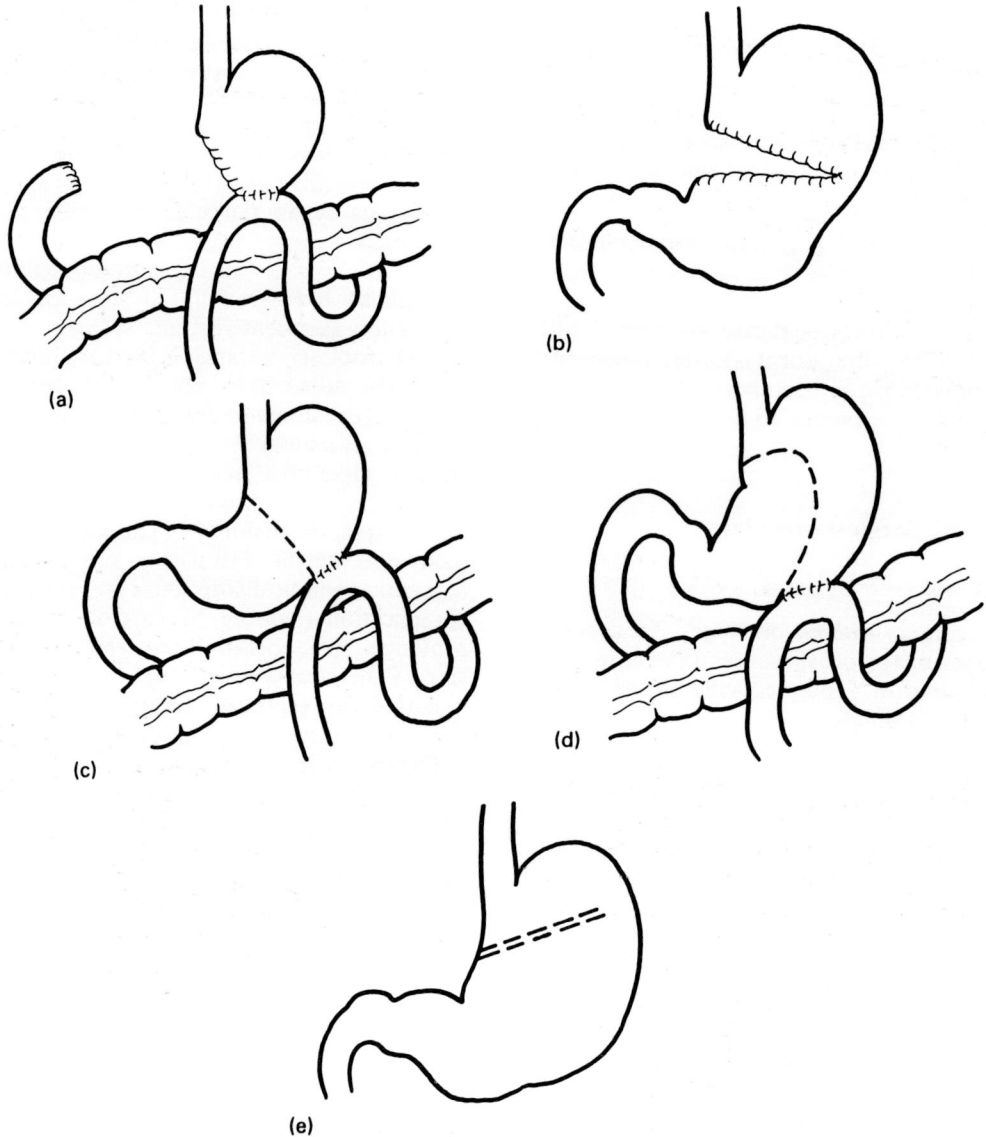

Fig. 11 Gastric operations

(b) Jejunoileal shunt (Payne, 1969): anastomosis of 35 cm of proximal jejunum end-to-side with the terminal 6.5 cm of ileum. Weight loss was inadequate owing to extensive reflux of food into the bypassed blind loop which was still able to absorb the food.

(c) Jejunoileal shunt (Scott, 1971): anastomosis of the proximal 30 cm of jejunum end-to-end to the terminal 15–30 cm of ileum. The bypassed small intestine is vented into either the transverse or sigmoid colon.

The *results* are classified into:

Good: satisfactory weight loss, no diarrhoea and no metabolic deficits.

Fair: weight loss not ideal, mild diarrhoea and minimal metabolic deficits.

Poor: unsatisfactory weight loss and/or persistent diarrhoea and/or severe metabolic deficits.

The majority of Payne end-to-side shunts were poor while the majority of Scott end-to-end shunts were good.

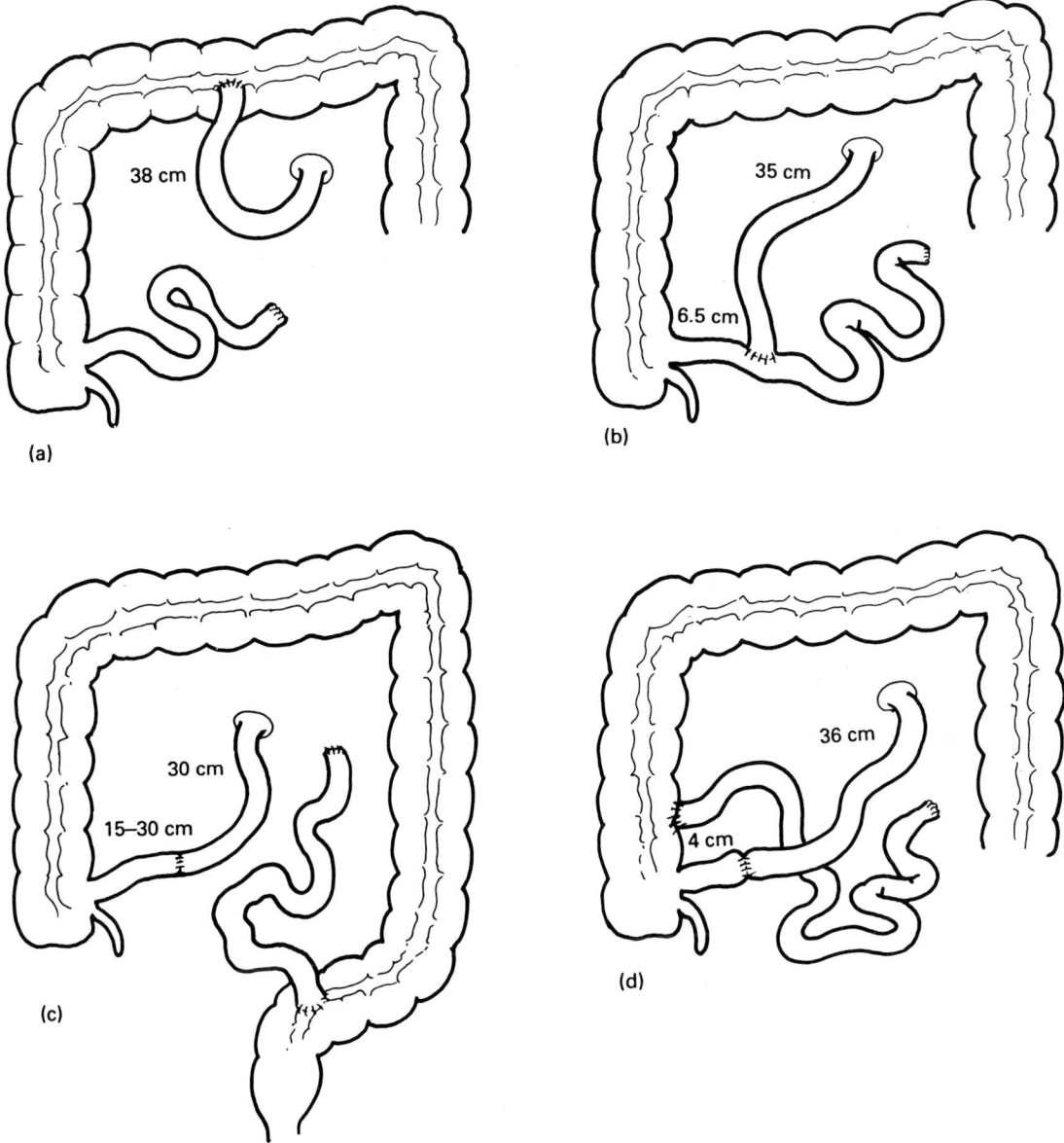

Fig. 12 Intestinal shunts

(d) Jejunoileal shunt (Joffe, 1979): anastomosis of the proximal 36 cm of jejunum to the last 4 cm of ileum, end-to-end (two layers). The bypassed small intestine is drained end-to-side to the ascending colon. Liver biopsy is performed routinely (the operation is conducted via a transverse supraumbilical incision).

Postoperative complications

- Diarrhoea for a few weeks.
- Fatty liver: a serious complication as it may eventually lead to hepatic coma and death. Preoperative baseline liver biopsy and liver function tests follow-up are essential to detect this problem (confirmed by needle liver biopsy).

- Malabsorption, metabolic and electrolyte deficits.
- Anastomotic blockage, bleeding and leakage.
- Wound dehiscence and incisional hernia.
- Operative mortality due to burst abdomen, myocardial infarction, pulmonary embolism and acute fatty liver.

Postoperative care and follow-up

1. Respiratory intensive care unit with ventilation for 48 h.
2. Nasogastric suction for 5 days followed by Gastrografin follow-through before oral feeding is commenced.
3. Diarrhoea control with Lomotil and codeine phosphate.
4. Regular follow-up, monitoring the body weight, liver function and recurrence of diarrhoea, is essential.

1.24. Multiple Injuries

GENERAL PRINCIPLES

Trauma ranks behind cardiovascular disease and cancer as a cause of death. It is the number one killer under the age of 40. The management in the first few minutes is crucial for the final outcome. The luxury of obtaining a clinical history may not be possible because of clinical urgency or the absence of witnesses at the time of the accident. The surgeon, therefore, should assume the worst and proceed as if the airway is compromised, the neck fractured, the intravascular space contracted and the stomach full. The 3 R general management plan is useful: resuscitate, review, then repair.

Management plan

Resuscitation

First aid measures on the spot or on arrival in the Accident and Emergency Department done within the first minute.
- Ensure patent airway (intubation or tracheostomy may be needed).
- Breathing (occlude sucking chest wounds quickly or assisted ventilation may be required).

- Circulation (check blood pressure and pulse and establish an i.v. life-line for fluid replacement, crossmatch blood and save).
- Stop severe external bleeding.

Review

Includes assessment and monitoring, history, physical examination, special tests.

A detailed relevant history is essential paying special attention to the exact time and mechanism of accident and the presence of concomitant diseases for which the patient may be receiving treatment. Physical examination (include vital signs, general and special examinations) should be quick, thorough and methodical, e.g. in systems or anatomical order (no orifice should be left unchecked). Special tests include:
- Full blood count grouping and crossmatch, urea and electrolytes.
- X-ray of suspected fractures, chest and deep lacerations with foreign bodies.
- Specific tests according to injury.

Tests must not interfere with life-saving treatment. The aim of such assessment is to identify the injuries as precisely as possible and to determine which systems need to be monitored later on. Arrangement of injuries in order of priority in management is essential.

Highest Priority

- Cervical spine injuries (immobilisation).
- Respiratory impairment (thoracic injuries).
- Cardiovascular insufficiency.
- Severe external bleeding.

High Priority
- Intraperitoneal and retroperitoneal (abdominal) injuries.
- Brain and spinal cord injuries.
- Severe burns or extensive soft tissue injuries.

Low Priority
- Lower genitourinary tract injuries.
- Peripheral vascular, nerve and tendon injuries.
- Fractures, dislocations.
- Facial and soft tissue injuries.
- Tetanus prophylaxis.

Shocked patient
The following procedures are required for differential diagnosis of shock and monitoring:
- Wide-bore i.v. cannulae.
- CVP line.
- ECG monitoring.

- Bladder catheterisation.
- Core/peripheral temperature.

Further monitoring in an intensive therapy unit (ITU) should continue when necessary.

Repair (definitive treatment)

The aims are to:
- Restore intravascular volume.
- Restore cardiac output and ensure its distribution.
- Ensure adequate gas exchange and protect lungs from excessive fluid loading, aspiration and infection.
- Ensure renal perfusion and output.

General measures

- Fluid replacement and blood transfusion.
- Immobilise fractures with splints until specific treatment is performed by orthopaedic team.
- Analgesia should not be withheld from injured patients. In the absence of head injury, judiciously administered narcotic analgesics do not mask the signs or symptoms of skeletal or visceral trauma and where pain is the limiting factor pulmonary ventilation may be improved. Pethidine, buprenorphine and morphine could be given i.v. to provide a steady level. Nerve or plexus block is recommended in rib fractures, and upper and lower limb injuries.
- Assisted ventilation is required when there is excessive respiratory work or ventilatory inadequacy with hypercapnoea. Hypoxia (Pao_2 less than 65 mmHg) demands positive end-expiratory pressure (PEEP) ventilation. In coincidental head injury, ventilation should be considered in certain situations.
- Continuous monitoring recording in ITU:
  —Conscious level.
  —Heart rate and rhythm and blood pressure.
  —Respiratory rate and rhythm and blood gas analysis.
  —Core/peripheral temperature difference (non-invasive indication of peripheral perfusion adequacy and reflects changes in cardiac output).
  —Urine output through urinary catheter (indicative of total renal blood flow).
  —Abdominal girth.
  —Haemoglobin/haematocrit (PCV).
  —Electrolytes/acid-base balance.
  —Chest X-ray.
- Antitetanous prophylaxis.

- Antibiotics (prophylactically).
- Care of comatose patient (patent airway, position, feeding, bed sores, urination, defaecation and temperature control).

Special measures

The specific injuries—head, cervical, thoracic, abdominal and hand injuries—should be treated on their merits.

PULMONARY CONSIDERATIONS IN TRAUMA

All severely injured patients suffer from hypoxia to varying degrees and immediate oxygen administration is indicated. Hypoxia may be central (in head injury and injudicious morphine overdose) or peripheral (airway obstruction, pneumo- or haemothorax), anaemic (from blood loss) or stagnant (due to associated shock). The precise causes of hypoxia in multiple trauma are:

Respiratory system:
- Head injury (central respiratory depression).
- Maxillofacial trauma (asphyxia, aspiration of blood, teeth, bone, debris and vomitus).
- Rib cage trauma (pneumothorax, haemothorax, subcutaneous/mediastinal emphysema).
- Ruptured diaphragm (abdominal contents herniation and compression collapse of lung).
- Ruptured oesophagus (mediastinitis, pleural effusion and sepsis).
- Tracheobronchial trauma (ruptured bronchus, trachea with massive air leak—subcutaneous/mediastinal emphysema, pneumothorax).
- Pulmonary trauma (contusion, haematoma, laceration).
- Increased capillary permeability (non-cardiogenic pulmonary oedema, injury oedema, chemical pneumonitis, acid aspiration, smoke injury, disseminated intravascular coagulation, fat embolism).
- Left ventricular failure (cardiogenic pulmonary oedema).
- Adult respiratory distress syndrome.

Cardiovascular system
- Hypovolaemic hypotension, e.g. bleeding, burns (decreased preload, increased afterload, decreased cardiac output).
- Tension pneumothorax, mediastinal emphysema, pericardial bleeding (cardiac tamponade).

- Myocardial injury, contusion ischaemia, acidosis, valve injury (pump failure, conduction defects).

Respiratory management

The first priority is to ensure that the patient's airway is free and his or her ventilation is unimpaired.

1. Obstructing elements should be removed under direct vision using a laryngoscope and low-vacuum sucker, e.g. dentures, broken teeth, debris, foreign bodies, blood or vomitus.

2. If laryngeal and pharyngeal reflexes are present, forward tongue retraction by insertion of an oral mouthpiece or nasopharyngeal tube may suffice.

3. If reflexes are absent then low-pressure cuffed endotracheal intubation is needed.

4. Tracheostomy is rarely needed as an emergency procedure unless intubation is impossible because of pharyngolaryngeal obstructing injury.

5. Laryngotomy is an alternative to tracheostomy.

6. Thorough tracheal and bronchial toilet should be performed. An asphyxiating plug may require emergency bronchoscopy.

7. Large-bore nasogastric tube aspiration of gastric contents may be needed but should be performed cautiously (or even abandoned) in CSF rhinorrhoea to avoid infection. Extreme care must be taken in intubation of patients with unstable cervical fractures.

8. In pneumothorax, an apical chest drain should be inserted through the second anterior intercostal space (*above* the third rib border to avoid injury of subcostal neurovascular structures) in the midclavicular line. An additional large drain is inserted through the fifth, sixth or seventh intercostal space (depending on the position of the spleen) in the midaxillary line in haemothorax.

9. In rib fractures with or without pneumothoraces, chest drainage on the fracture side is mandatory prior to artificial ventilation and advisable prior to general anaesthesia. In bilateral fractures with haemothoraces, bilateral apical and basal drains must be inserted.

10. In tension pneumothorax the use of intermittent positive pressure ventilation can kill a patient in seconds. This should be relieved temporarily by a wide-bore i.v. cannula (inserted through the second anterior intercostal space in the midclavicular line) until a chest drain is available. Respiratory distress and cyanosis should always raise suspicion and on examination shifted positions of trachea and apex beat are confirmatory.

The choice between crystalloids (water and electrolyte solutions) and colloids (plasma, albumin, gelatins, dextrans) and their effect on pulmonary gas exchange is controversial. Those who favour colloids claim that colloid osmotic pressure (COP) is maintained and any extravasated albumin is cleared quickly by pulmonary lymphatics while crystalloids reduce COP and increase pulmonary extravascular water and pulmonary oedema. Those favouring crystalloids maintain that with colloids pulmonary lymphatic drainage is rapidly overwhelmed and extravasated albumin increases extravascular COP and oedema (wet lungs are infected lungs since macrophages lose their antibacterial effect).

1.25. Abdominal Trauma

GENERAL CONSIDERATIONS

Often combined with multiple injuries which tend to be more obvious than abdominal ones. They are either penetrating (open—after gunshot or knife stabbing) or blunt (closed—usually after road traffic accidents). The management starts with first aid resuscitation (for shock or associated injuries— *see* Section 1.24), followed by clinical assessment, then definitive treatment (whether conservative or operative intervention).

Clinical assessment

History

In penetrating injuries ascertain the nature and direction of penetration (e.g. knife or bullet) as well as patient position at the time of injury. Pathological visceromegaly should be asked about (e.g. in tropical areas—malaria, hepatitis or Kala Azar) as well as drug treatment (e.g. steroids). Shoulder pain is deliberately asked about in splenic injuries.

Examination

For vital signs of revealed or concealed haemorrhage and shock (hypotension, tachycardia and decreased CVP). Obvious cutaneous bruising from a seat belt or underwear may indicate deep injury. Other signs are abdominal distension, tenderness guarding, rigidity, flank fullness and dullness on percussion, hyperaesthesia over the shoulder (referred pain due to subdiaphragmatic irritation by blood—Kehr's sign). The abdominal girth is measured and the abdomen marked with indelible pen for repeated measurements. The pelvis is sprung to detect fracture. Rectal examination to detect the prostate position (normal or floating) and abnormal swellings; note whether there is any blood on the finger. Failure to pass urine may indicate urethral injury. Physical examination may be difficult in comatose patients.

Ancillary procedures and investigations

- Erect chest X-ray to show:
  - —Diaphragmatic injury.
  - —Rib fractures close to liver or spleen.
  - —Subphrenic gas due to ruptured abdominal viscus.
- Supine abdominal X-ray to show:
  - —Splenic, hepatic, renal shadows.
  - —Outline of psoas muscle (masked in retroperitoneal haematoma and splenic injury).
  - —Gastric bubble shape and situation (deviated medially in splenic injury).
  - —Ground-glass appearance of intra-abdominal bleeding.
  - —Pelvic fractures.
- Four-quadrant tap (needle paracentesis) is a quick test for intra-abdominal bleeding and is done with a wide-bore needle and syringe.
- Peritoneal lavage: more sensitive but time-consuming; carried out if the tap is negative in suspected intra-abdominal bleeding. The bladder should be empty (e.g. via a catheter), then a peritoneal dialysis catheter is inserted subumbilically via a trocar stab or a small incision under direct vision with local anaesthesia. One litre of normal saline is passed intraperitoneally and siphoned out into a plastic bag (with gentle abdominal palpation). A false positive may be due to traumatic instrumentation.
- Urgent intravenous urography (IVU) may show:
  - —Presence or absence of functioning kidney on each side.
  - —Hitherto unexpected pathology, e.g. horseshoe kidney or tumour.

When IVU reveals a non-functioning kidney, renal arteriography should be carried out immediately to detect the remediable damage to the renal vascula-

ture in time to save the kidney; otherwise renal transplantation should be considered.

Continuous monitoring

Two days of continuous monitoring in hospital followed by re-examination at intervals is an absolute necessity in abdominal trauma. Nasogastric aspiration is done to prevent acute gastric dilatation (may occur in trauma even without viscus rupture). Blood pressure, pulse rate, abdominal girth, CVP, and i.v. fluid balance are monitored. A decision on whether to pass a urinary catheter is made carefully, in the presence of urethral injury; however, a urethral catheter is needed in all cases of severe urethral injuries and shock to monitor urinary output.

Definitive treatment

Conservative treatment

This is all that is required for the majority of cases after careful monitoring.

Laparotomy

Indicated in:
- All eviscerations (even with a small tag of protruding omentum). The wound itself should be enlarged via laparotomy and protruding viscus (covered with sterile wet dressing preoperatively) replaced, followed by methodical exploration for visceral injuries.
- All gunshot wounds.
- Some stab wounds selectively. A separate laparotomy incision is indicated when there is significant blood loss and peritonitis (otherwise treatment is conservative).
- Some closed abdominal injuries when:
  - —Frank blood detected by four-quadrant tap and/or peritoneal lavage.
  - —Persistent signs of peritonitis, e.g. tenderness, guarding and loss of bowel sounds or signs of spreading peritonitis.
  - —Signs of internal bleeding.
  - —Urinary damage as revealed on urgent IVU.
  - —Blood in stomach, bladder or rectum.

Operative intervention should only be considered after adequate haemodynamic resuscitation and stabilisation except in:
- Horrendous bleeding outstripping all attempts at fluid and blood replacement.

- Evisceration with obvious strangulation of the protruding viscus.

The abdominal incision may be a quick midline or paramedian. Can be extended into a thoracoabdominal or into the flank by a T-shaped lateral extension. Generous access with good exposure is essential. A transverse supraumbilical incision is useful only in children under the age of 5 years. Exploration should proceed methodically with examination of spleen, liver, diaphragm (in that order) then stomach (anterior and posterior wall through a window in the lesser omentum or gastrocolic ligament), duodenum, pancreas, small and large bowel, rectum and bladder (and uterine tubes and ovaries in female) and kidneys, recording the findings of each organ. Quick mass closure, leaving a drain behind, is best.

SPECIAL CONSIDERATIONS

Liver

The largest organ in the abdomen (1.5 kg). The liver and the spleen are the most frequently injured abdominal organs. Many studies point out that the incidence of liver injuries is almost the same as that of splenic injuries. The overall mortality rate for hepatic trauma is 15 % (20 % from blunt trauma and 2 % from penetrating injuries). A combination of injuries involving the gut often results in death from sepsis and/or multiple organ failure. Conservative management is the rule.

- Liver injuries that are not bleeding at the time of laparotomy are best left alone, clots should be evacuated and the perihepatic area drained.
- Large bleeding lacerations: suturing of bleeding points and/or ligation of isolated bleeding points. Deep sutures should not be tried first since they cause local ischaemia, necrosis and infection. For temporary haemostasis Pringle's manoeuvre (compressing the lesser omental free edge between finger and thumb) should be maintained for 15 min only. For longer periods gauze packing may be required for 48 h with generous drainage. Ligation of the main hepatic artery (healthy liver can survive on portal blood alone) or one of its branches is the last resort in controlling active bleeding.
- Debridement of devitalised liver is necessary in 10 % of cases.
- Lobar or sublobar hepatic resection may be required in 5 % of cases and reserved for bursting injuries and those with hepatic venous and intrahepatic vena caval injuries. Hepatic lobectomy has a 50 % mortality rate. Adequate blood and platelet transfusion, monitoring of coagulation parameter, parenteral nutrition and prophylactic antibiotics are needed. Hepatic lobectomy is a formidable operation and is not advised for hepatic injury unless there is no alternative. The bile duct should not be drained unless it is injured (T-tubes cause stenosis in normal-calibre common bile duct).

Spleen

Injuries are dealt with routinely by splenectomy. Lethal postsplenectomy sepsis and pneumococcal infection in children have lead to more conservative approaches in such injuries of children and adults below 40 years of age. Blunt abdominal trauma often results in a subcapsular haematoma, cracks in the parenchyma and fragmentation of the pulp.

- Attempts should be made to preserve the splenic tissue by suturing lacerations with mattress sutures supported by pledgets of Teflon felt or omental tissue (splenorrhaphy).
- In fragmentation, partial splenectomy is carried out by ligating the artery that supplies the damaged sector and removing the part of the spleen that subsequently becomes devascularised.
- If splenectomy must be done, spleniculi should be sought and carefully preserved because they may undergo hyperplasia with eventual preservation of splenic function. Pneumococcal vaccine and long-term oral prophylactic penicillin may be administered postoperatively.
- Autotransplantation of splenic tissue into muscle, omentum or retroperitoneal tissues is technically feasible (but still experimental).

Colon

Mortality is high and is related to associated organ injuries, to faecal peritonitis, and postoperative incisional and intra-abdominal complications due to faecal contamination. Preoperative preparation consists of i.v. fluid, nasogastric suction and various monitoring procedures with prophylactic metronidazol and cephuroxime antibiotics. Treatment is as follows.

- Caecal injuries: caecostomy.
- Right colon injuries: right hemicolectomy with primary ileocolic anastomosis.

- Perforated transverse, splenic flexure and descending colon: primary closure with proximal protective colostomy, which is later closed.
- Large sigmoid lacerations: Hartmann's operation, bringing up the damaged colon as a terminal left iliac end-colostomy and closing the rectal end. They are reanastomosed together later as a cold operation.
- Rectal wounds: proximal colostomy, perirectal drainage and irrigation of faeces from rectum. The rectal perforation should be closed if accessible.

No wound of the colon should ever be closed if there is:

- Profound hypovolaemic shock (blood pressure of less than 60/40 mmHg).
- Blood loss of more than 25% of anticipated blood volume.
- Massive faecal contamination.
- Eight hour delay after injury.
- Destructive bowel wound demanding bowel resection.

Instead, the primarily repaired colon is temporarily exteriorised as a potential colostomy. It should be kept moist with frequent dressing changes. The exteriorised segment is resected after 48 h and closed after 6 weeks.

Small bowel

Double-layer inverting sutures are used.

- Perforation: closed transversely to avoid stricture.
- Mesentery damage: bowel resected with end-to-end anastomosis.
- Difficult duodenal injuries: Kocherisation and closure of small rent transversely.
- Larger duodenal tears: a Roux loop is brought up to anastomose the defect, and feeding jejunostomy or even gastrojejunostomy bypass of the pancreatic duct is performed.
- Pancreatoduodenectomy: rarely used as it carries a high mortality.

Kidneys

Exploration is indicated in bleeding open wounds involving the kidney, expanding perirenal extravasation (with progressive swelling) or massive haematuria. Treatment is according to the urgent IVU results and operative wound findings. Polar or partial nephrectomy is always preferred. A tense retroperitoneal haematoma may be ignored lest the incision and drainage lead to uncontrollable bleeding. Such a conservative approach produces good results with further follow-up.

Bladder

Injury is diagnosed later but fortunately mortality is low. Urethral catheterisation with closure of the vent via laparotomy is indicated.

Urethra

Treatment is debatable (see Section 1.24).

Diaphragm

Injury occurs in 4–5% of patients with blunt or penetrating trauma and mainly on the left side as the liver protects the right hemidiaphragm. The mechanism in blunt injury is sudden intrathoracic or intra-abdominal force applied against the fixed diaphragm. The injury is often masked by associated injury of the stomach, spleen and/or splenic flexure and sometimes overlooked during exploration. Blunt chest injuries with an elevated or obscured hemidiaphragm or penetrating wounds below the nipple should raise suspicion. The patient may experience shortness of breath and chest pain, or there may be no signs or symptoms at all. As the injury may be difficult to repair from the abdomen the abdominal incision is converted into a thoraco-abdominal one. It is not advisable to repair purely through the chest unless the surgeon is experienced because of the possibility of contaminant intra-abdominal injury. Once the abdominal exploration is finished interrupted figure-of-8 non-absorbable sutures are applied through the chest followed by chest tube drainage with underwater seal. Chronic diaphragmatic injury with diaphragmatic herniation is approached through the chest because the herniated viscera are adherent to the lung in most cases.

Pancreas

The main operative principles are:

- Complete haemostasis.
- Removal of devitalised tissue.
- Drainage of pancreatic juice.
  Pancreatic trauma is classified into four types:
1. Superficial non-ductal.
2. Deep lacerations (involving duct).
3. Severe transection of the head.
4. Combined pancreaticoduodenal injury.

If the tail is injured simple closure or resection is done. A Roux loop of jejunum may be used to anastomose the cut end. Partial pancreatectomy and very rarely total pancreatectomy are required.

1.26. Thoracic Trauma

GENERAL PRINCIPLES

Approximately 25% of trauma deaths are due solely to thoracic injuries and 50% of patients who die from multiple injuries have significant thoracic injury. They are either penetrating (open—by gunshot, knives or other weapons) or blunt (closed) injuries. The mortality rate from penetrating chest wounds was 56% in World War I, decreasing to 8% during World War II and to 3% in the Vietnam War as a result of improved transport systems which enabled critically injured patients to reach medical care alive. Generally, mortality ranges between 4% and 12% and increases to 12–15% if extrathoracic regions are involved.

Initial steps in the treatment of penetrating chest injury are:
- Securing an airway and ventilation (occlude sucking chest wound and establish artificial endotracheal ventilation if necessary).
- Restoring circulation and stopping obvious bleeding.
- Tube thoracostomy (chest tube) if necessary— *see below*.

The above measures are all that are required in 70–85% of patients with open chest trauma.

A brief history is taken from the patient or witnesses about time of injury, weapon type and its direction, the patient's position at the time of injury and the patient's progress during transport. On examination the medicolegal aspects of trauma should be considered. All physical evidence of the weapon should be preserved and neither fingerprints nor adherent tissue, hair or clothing should be removed from the weapon. A quick thorough examination of the anterior and posterior aspects of the chest for associated injuries is carried out, and vital signs and breathing sounds on the side of injury are looked for.

The amount of initial chest tube drainage is recorded and the decision for thoracotomy is based on subsequent drainage rather than the initial amount. *Thoracotomy* is indicated in:
- Persistent bleeding (more than 100 ml/h).
- Exsanguinating bleeding.

If the patient is *haemodynamically unstable* (tachycardia, hypotension and there are no breathing sounds on side of injury) then:
- Insert large-bore chest tube (underwater drainage) immediately on the side of injury without prior chest X-ray (under local anaesthesia in the seventh intercostal space immediately above the eighth rib—to avoid injury of the seventh subcostal neurovascular structures) at the midclavicular line and push the tube upward (apical—in pneumothorax), or keep it low (basal—in haemothorax), or both (in pneumohaemothorax).
- Insert at least two large-calibre i.v. cannulae for rapid fluid replacement. Simultaneously blood is aspirated for a baseline PCV, grouping and crossmatching.
- Arterial blood gases if ventilation is compromised.
- Obtain upright posteroanterior chest X-ray during inspiration (only when the patient is haemodynamically stable).
- In addition to chest X-ray, an aortogram should be obtained if:
  —The missile traversed or passed close to the mediastinum.
  —Absent or decreased pulse or bruit.
  —Wide mediastinum on chest X-ray.
- Thin barium swallow should be obtained if:
  —Missile traversed mediastinum.
  —Mediastinal emphysema.

Abdominal injuries are investigated on their merit (*see* p. 82).

SPECIAL CONSIDERATIONS

Penetrating heart wounds

Only 20% of such patients reach hospital alive and gunshot wounds are responsible for 80% of deaths due to intracardiac injuries, e.g. valve disruption, septal defects and major coronary transections. Patients present with either haemorrhagic shock (hypotension, tachycardia, low CVP and brisk bleeding through the wound or via tube thoracostomy, which demand immediate thoracotomy on the wound side) and/or cardiac tamponade (triad of paradoxical pulse, high CVP and muffled heart sounds).

CVP is the most reliable test for determining

whether the shock is due to blood loss, cardiac tamponade or both. It is essential that the zero level of the manometer be at the midaxillary line in the fourth intercostal space: the saline column in a manometer fluctuates freely during respiration and blood flows back if the bottle is positioned below the heart level. Measurement is obtained while the patient is quiet and if the pressure is above 12 cm of saline a diagnosis of tamponade is fairly certain. However false high CVP is frequently present as a result of:

- Shivering.
- Straining from pleural or peritoneal irritation.
- Malpositioning of CVP catheter.

On balance, patients with any mediastinal wound, high CVP and hypotension should be assumed to have cardiac tamponade until proven otherwise.

Pericardiocentesis with a large-gauge needle may be used diagnostically and therapeutically initially. However, as clotted blood often leads to a false negative result the best way of accomplishing decompression is subxiphoid pericardial exploration (diagnostic and therapeutic) under local anaesthesia—while the patient is breathing spontaneously to avoid profound hypotension and a drop in cardiac output which accompany general anaesthesia and endotracheal intubation. If blood is found in the pericardium the tamponade is relieved, the patient is given a general anaesthetic and intubated with controlled ventilation. The incision is extended into a standard median sternotomy and the heart wound is repaired with simple techniques (ventricular wounds are controlled with large mattress sutures reinforced with Teflon felt atrial or great vessel wounds can be controlled with a partially occluding clamp and then sutured at leisure with a running vascular suture). The venae cavae may need to be compressed digitally to decompress the heart and control bleeding. Cardiopulmonary bypass may be used selectively but is never necessary routinely as it necessitates prolonged hospital stay and undesirable heparinisation.

Blunt cardiac injury occurs in 20 % of cases and produces either cardiac rupture and tamponade or myocardial contusion (ECG reveals ST elevation and sometimes Q wave with arrythmia and the patient has chest pain). They are rarely fatal and treated like myocardial infarction.

Penetrating transmediastinal injuries

A rapid systemic approach is adopted to detect structural damage by:

- Bilateral tube thoracostomy.
- Oesophagoscopy or contrast study of oesophagus.
- Bronchoscopy.
- Aortography.

Intrathoracic aorta injury (in penetrating or blunt chest injuries)

Occurs mainly in high-speed road traffic accidents and usually results in immediate death. In 50 % of cases there is no external sign of injury and therefore traumatic aortic rupture should be highly suspected when any of the following is present:

- Pulse amplitude difference between the upper and lower extremities (as in coarctation of aorta).
- Upper hypertension.
- Widening of superior mediastinal shadow seen in chest X-ray. Other radiological signs are obstructed aortic knob, deviation of oesophagus or trachea to the right, downward displacement of left main stem bronchus, hemithorax and fractured ribs.

Rupture at the isthmus (ligamentum arteriosum) is responsible for 90 % of aortic injuries and is possibly caused by horizontal deceleration of the aorta with its fixation at the ligamentum arteriosum. Vertical deceleration (e.g. falls) cause rupture of the ascending aorta as a result of aortic lengthening. Thoracic aortography by the femoral or brachial route is essential. In the treatment, associated abdominal injury may take precedence because of continuous bleeding from visceral tears. Aortic rupture is treated by direct repair or restoration of continuity by a tube graft without or with (rarely) cardiopulmonary bypass (or femoral artery-to-vein cardiopulmonary bypass).

Subclavian and innominate artery injuries

Injuries can be penetrating or blunt (blunt rupture with dissecting haematoma or false aneurysm is rare). In penetrating injuries, audible bruit, absent pulse, widening of the superior mediastinum, expanding haematoma, brachial plexus injury or haemodynamic instability are confirmatory signs. Aortography is essential in the presence of these signs.

Proximal vascular control (via median sternotomy for subclavian, innominate and left common carotid injuries) and distal control (incision in the deltopectoral groove for subclavian vessels and extension of the sternotomy incision in a 'hockey stick' fashion along the anterior border of the sternomastoid muscle for innominate arterial branches) are essential. Excision of part of the clavicle may be required for repair of the subclavians. Direct repair or use of a tube graft is recommended.

Oesophageal injury

Although rare, this is a rapidly progressive and fatal injury because of mediastinal contamination by saliva and gastrointestinal contents. There is a high incidence of associated injuries, e.g. trachea and vessels. The *causes* generally are:
- Iatrogenic perforation during endoscopy or dilatation.
- Spontaneous rupture during emesis (called Boorhavee's syndrome—a longitudinal mucosal tear of the gastro-oesophageal junction during emesis is called the Mallory-Weiss syndrome).
- Ingestion of a foreign body with immediate perforation or erosion.
- Blunt or penetrating external trauma (discussed here).
Oesophageal injury results in either:
- Fulminating mediastinitis (if mediastinal pleura is intact); or
- Fulminant pleuritis with massive pleural effusion and hypovolaemia (if mediastinal pleura has ruptured). The effusion results in hypovolaemia, sepsis and cardiorespiratory embarassment due to mediastinal shift.

Cervical oesophageal perforation is confined by the deep cervical fascia. The upper two-thirds of the intrathoracic oesophagus perforates and drains into the right pleural space. The distal one-third perforates and drains into the left pleural space only if the mediastinal pleura is not intact. Rarely the last 4 cm of the intra-abdominal oesophagus perforates and drains into the peritoneal cavity. The most common site of injury is at the tracheal bifurcation—rarely traumatic tracheoesophageal fistula results. Clinical features are fever, tachycardia, hypotension, leucocytosis and pain, deep subcutaneous emphysema confined to deep cervical fascia from the mandible to the clavicle. Mediastinal emphysema on chest X-ray is highly suggestive. Diagnosis is confirmed with a thin barium swallow with immediate and delayed films in the posteroanterior and lateral views. Early recognition with urgent operative intervention is mandatory. Secured two-layer closure (continuous non-absorbable mucosal suture followed by continuous non-absorbable muscular suture) with

drainage is essential. Late perforations of the intrathoracic oesophagus may best be treated by oesophageal exclusion rather than by primary intrathoracic repair.

Tracheobronchial injuries

Classified into three groups:
- 'Straddle' injury in which the main-stem bronchus (usually the right) is avulsed at the carina, caused by anteroposterior compression of the chest.
- Tracheal blow-out fractures, caused by a sudden increase in endotracheal pressure against the closed glottis.
- Transverse lacerations, caused by rapid deceleration.

These are rapidly fatal and only a few patients reach hospital alive. Mainly caused by road traffic accidents. Signs and symptoms of tracheobronchial injuries are similar to those of oesophageal perforation depending on the site and nature of the injury and the degree of obstruction of the airways. However, dysphagia and hoarseness as well as cervical emphysema from the mandible to the clavicle (confined to the distribution of the deep cervical fascia) also occur in tracheal injury. Distal blow-out fractures cause massive mediastinal emphysema (if the mediastinal pleura is intact) or right pneumothorax (if the mediastinal pleura is ruptured). In straddle injury of the main-stem bronchus at the carina there is minor haemoptysis, but massive air leak through the chest tube drain with lobar atelectasis is common. Bronchoscopy is both diagnostic and therapeutic to retain control of the airway. Primary repair is achieved with interrupted non-absorbable sutures (e.g. 3/0 Prolene). It is important to debride all fractured tracheal cartilages and suture the intact cartilaginous ring. Pneumonectomy may be required for straddle injury of the main bronchus. Minor lacerations may require only a tracheostomy (through the penetration itself or distal to it) for decompression of the tracheobronchial tree.

Chest wall trauma

Either crushed (closed) or penetrating (open). In both cases the outcome depends on the severity and extent of the underlying structural damage.

Respiratory insufficiency

Caused by:
- Pain interfering with coughing.

- Instability or chest wall deformity.
- Presence of blood or secretions in the bronchial tree.
- Underlying pulmonary contusion.
- Associated haemo- or pneumothorax.
- Associated head injury and depressed respiration. Chest X-ray in two views is essential in all cases and blood gas analysis (and sometimes bronchoscopy) is required in complicated cases.

Rib fractures

Simple isolated

Commonly affect the fourth to the ninth and more often occur on the left than on the right side. Usually result from road traffic accidents, falls or beatings.
- First rib fracture is a hallmark of severe thoracic trauma and multiple system injuries in road traffic accidents. Locally it can produce injury to the brachial plexus or subclavian artery, Horner's syndrome, or thoracic outlet syndrome. The aorta is injured in 7.8 % of first rib fractures and arteriography is indicated.
- Sternum fracture, usually caused by steering wheel trauma. Cardiac contusion or rupture is the most life-threatening associated injury. A displaced sternum should be stabilised by suturing. Careful observation, chest X-ray (especially lateral view) and ECG are important.
- Scapula fracture: indicates severe thoracic trauma (like first rib) with significant associated injuries (e.g. rib, clavicular, pulmonary, brachial plexus, vertebral), and even abdominal injuries. Local pain and tenderness and chest X-ray confirm the diagnosis. Immobilisation of the arm in a sling is important for a few weeks until the fracture is stable and the pain resolves. Treatment of associated injuries may take priority.

Complicated fractures
- Multiple fractured ribs in a row on one hemithorax.
- Stove-in-chest multiple rib fractures with permanent indentation and depression of the chest wall.
- Flail chest with a flaccid unstable anterior chest wall (sternum) caused by bilateral multiple fractures or two rows of fractured ribs on one hemithorax with unstable segment, accompanied by paradoxical breathing.

- Traumatic pneumothorax with a sucking chest wound and late tension pneumothorax (total lung collapse and mediastinal shift towards the opposite side detected by tracheal and apex beat shift and manifested by acute cardiorespiratory failure. It is fatal if not relieved by immediate occlusion of the sucking wound and urgently by chest tube underwater drainage.)
- Traumatic haemothorax or haemopneumothorax.
- Pulmonary contusion and laceration.

Complicated fracture is managed in the following way.
1. Stabilisation of chest wall (strapping or internal fixation with wires or better still tracheostomy).
2. Artificial ventilation via tracheostomy or endotracheal tube.
3. Pain relief, using injectable analgesics (e.g. small doses of morphine) or intercostal nerve block.
4. Pleural decompression of blood and air via chest tube underwater drainage.
5. Tracheobronchial secretions are aspirated bronchoscopically or via tracheostomy.
6. Exploratory thoracotomy following primary chest drainage is indicated in:
- Blood loss sufficient to cause shock (more than 200 ml/h over 4 consecutive hours) or if haemothorax is clotted.
- Massive air leak (tracheobronchial injury).
- Tamponade in most cardiac wounds.
- Oesophageal injury indicated by surgical emphysema or thin barium swallow.
- Open sucking wounds, if skin loss has occurred, as they lead to tension pneumothorax.
7. Treatment of shock lung by colloid replacement for blood, restricting crystalloid solutions, and giving i.v. diuretic (e.g. frusemide 20 mg twice daily for 3 days, and methylprednisolone 30 mg/kg).

1.27. Craniospinal Trauma

HEAD INJURY

Head injury is the cause of 9 deaths/100 000 of the population each year in the UK and 22 deaths/100 000 in the USA. About half the deaths occur before arrival at hospital. Most of these have overwhelming multiple injuries or irreparable brain damage. Over half the head injuries are in those less than 30 years of age (head injury is the commonest cause of death in the 15–24-year-old population). Much of the mortality and morbidity (potentially preventable) is attributable to secondary brain damage after the patient reaches hospital.

Causes

The major ones are:
1. Road traffic accidents—the commonest.
2. Assaults—in Scottish men aged 15–25 years assault is as common as road traffic accidents as a cause of head injury.
3. Falls.
The minor ones are:
4. Sporting injuries.
5. Birth trauma.
6. Industrial accidents.

Compulsory use of seat belts in Australia has resulted in 50% less brain damage and 40% fewer fatalities in car occupants involved in road traffic accidents. Very occasionally a disease may precipitate head injury, e.g. myocardial infarction, collapse or epileptic fit. Ingestion of alcohol is a common associated factor and 50% of head injuries were found (in some studies) in drunk pedestrians and those involved in assault.

Pattern of injury

1. Adult pedestrians tend to suffer from more limb, pelvic and femoral injuries, while small children are more likely to be run over and suffer injury to the trunk.
2. The highest incidence of head injury, whiplash neck injury and chest trauma occurs in car drivers and front seat passengers. Twenty per cent of in-car deaths include fatal cervical spine injuries.
3. Domestic trauma (falls in the home): high incidence of limb fractures with 40% sustaining head injuries.
4. Industrial trauma: the head is involved in less than 2% of cases.

Classification

Minor

No or a very brief loss of consciousness and no fracture (clinically or radiologically).

Severe

Prolonged or profound loss of consciousness or post-traumatic amnesia or lucid period of consciousness (as in intracranial haematoma). Fracture may or may not be present.

Closed   Intact scalp with no communication between intracranial contents and the exterior but often associated with fairly diffuse brain damage. Fracture may or may not be present.

Open   Communication between intracranial contents and the exterior and often associated with focal brain damage. It is caused by a small sharp object, e.g. a stone, bottle or missile. Fracture is always present and is usually of the depressed compound type.

The Glasgow Coma Scale is the proper charting for quantifying the severity of injury (*see* p. 92). A patient who is alert and fully orientated as regards place, person and time scores 15 while one with severe head injury scores 7 or less.

Pathology

A combined pathology is commonest (e.g. contusion and laceration or contusion and intracranial haemorrhage or subdural haematoma and contusion with laceration).

Immediate impact injury (at the moment of injury)

Scalp   Bruises and laceration.

Skull   Fractures in vault or base, fissure or depressed, closed or open (compound). The fracture itself is of no consequence unless it is compound.

Brain
- Concussion (transient loss of consciousness with diffuse neuronal damage with quick recovery—this is a clinical rather than a pathological term).
- Contusion (bruised brain with oedema later on).
- Lacerations (cerebral tear).
- Diffuse white matter damage.

Cranial nerves   Any may be involved but I olfactory is the commonest and XII hypoglossal is the rarest. Paralysis is due to laceration by fractured ends (immediate and permanent) to blood clot compression (after a few days with recovery), or to scar or callus (after weeks and permanent).

Blood vessels   Vessels torn at the time of injury give rise to bleeding with later formation of pressing expanding haematoma.

Extracranial injuries
- Very common (neck, chest, abdomen and limb fractures).
- Metabolic (fat embolism).

Primary complications

Although initiated by head injury they develop some time after the injury and are distinguished by their amenability to treatment.
- Intracranial haemorrhage (intracerebral, subdural and extradural haematoma) with brain shift and herniation due to a space-occupying lesion.
- Brain swelling (brain swells first because of increased blood volume due to cerebral autoregulation in traumatic shock and second because of cerebral waterlogging with oedema fluid due to contusion).
- *Cushing* stress peptic ulcer (extracranial).

Intracranial haematoma accounts for one-third of the deaths of patients who have talked at some stage after head injury. These deaths are due to delayed evacuation of an intracranial haematoma as a result of late diagnosis. Haematoma is also a common source of disability in survivors. Occurrence of intracranial infection after head injury (*see below*) is also often a consequence of delayed or inadequate initial care. Such mortality and morbidity are preventable with better management.

Secondary complications

- Brain damage secondary to raised intracranial pressure.
- Hypoxic brain damage (less obvious but disastrous—it is found in 90 % of patients who die in hospital after head injury. It is due to inadequate cerebral perfusion secondary to systemic hypotension and/or raised intracranial pressure).
- Infection (meningitis and cerebral abscesses).

Other complications

- Late bleeding (chronic subdural haematoma due to osmotic expansion of a trivial surface clot).
- Permanent cerebral damage (local signs of hemiparesis, hemiplegia, dysphasia, and blindness). In mid-brain (signs of ataxia, tremor, rigidity, dysarthria). Measured sometimes by post-traumatic amnesia:

0–1 h (slight)
1–24 h (moderate)
1–7 days (severe)
over 7 days (very severe).

About 70 % of patients with less than 24 h post-traumatic amnesia return to work in 8 weeks.
- Retrograde traumatic amnesia.
- Epilepsy (early 5 % and late 5 %). Presents as a fit within the first 24 h (due to brain oedema), as true post-traumatic epilepsy occurring between 6 months and 21 years after injury (due to contracted scar) or idiopathic epilepsy which becomes evident within days or weeks of head injury. Diagnosed clinically and by EEG and encephalography. If the scar is focal it should be excised, and the dura grafted with fascia or sutured with nylon membrane to prevent more fibrosis. Anti-epileptic drugs are needed.
- Coma causes many problems but the Mendelson (1946) syndrome is fatal. This is fulminating aspiration pneumonia caused by inhalation of irritant vomit (containing hydrochloric acid) during coma or induction of anaesthetic. Dyspnoea, cyanosis and tachycardia with adventitious lung sounds and bronchospasm are followed by gross pulmonary oedema and death. X-ray shows irregular mottling scattered through lung fields but no lung collapse. Small quantities of free hydrochloric acid may be responsible for death.
- Psychiatric disturbance (postconcussional syndrome—lack of concentration, and defective memory and emotional control).
- Post-traumatic hydrocephalus.
- Diabetes insipidus.
- Inappropriate ADH secretion.
- Pneumatocele, meningocele, CSF leaks and carotid–cavernous fistula.

MANAGEMENT

First aid measures

Airway, breathing, circulation and stoppage of external bleeding.

Assessment and monitoring

A. History

Precise mechanism of injury, patient status after injury, duration and presence of any previous diseases, and whether patient is an alcoholic.

B. Examination

General examination

For lacerations, CSF or blood leak from the nose or ear—periorbital haematoma, retromastoid bruising. Associated injuries should be looked for, particularly of the cervical spine. Neck stiffness (meningism) indicates subarachnoid bleeding caused by trauma, ruptured Berry's aneurysm or spontaneous intracerebral haematoma. Signs of malignancy may indicate intracranial metastases.

Neurological examination

Consciousness Degree and duration is the best index of the amount of diffuse damage caused by acceleration–deceleration forces. Changes in consciousness level in the first few hours provide the most reliable guide to whether recovery will occur or whether intracranial complications will develop.

The Glasgow Coma Scale (GCS) is the best means of assessing, recording and displaying the level of consciousness. The score ranges between 3 and 15 when the full scale is used. A score of 7 or less indicates severe head injury, while a score of 15 indicates minor head injury. The parameters with response and score are as follows:

Eye opening

Spontaneous	(4)
To speech	(3)
To pain	(2)
None	(1)

Best verbal response

Orientated	(5)
Confused conversation	(4)
Inappropriate words	(3)
Incomprehensible sounds	(2)
None	(1)

Best motor response

Obeys commands	(6)
Localises	(5)
Flexes: Normal	(4)
Abnormal	(3)
Extends	(2)
None	(1)

The scale is charted so that medical and nursing staff can readily see the changes (this is particularly important since personnel change many times a day).

Pupil size and reaction Light reflex tests optic (II) and oculomotor (III) nerves. Failure of pupil to react to both direct and consensual light implies a III lesion. Reaction to consensual light only implies II or retinal lesion. III lesion is the most useful indicator of an expanding intracranial lesion. Increased intracranial pressure leads to bilateral fixed dilated pupils. An ipsilateral dilating pupil is a sign of extradural haemorrhage. However, a fixed dilated pupil in coma is not pathognomonic of an intracranial lesion (and mid-brain compression due to uncal herniation from a tentorial hiatus). Since direct eye injury leads to traumatic mydriasis, associated hyphaemia (blood effusion in the anterior eye chamber) should be looked for. An epileptic fit can also produce transient fixed dilated pupils. Bilateral pinpoint pupils are due either to drug overdose or pontine haemorrhage.

Eye movements Abnormal eye movements indicate structural damage.

- Conjugate deviation to the right indicates damage to the right frontal visual field (Brodmann's area 8) or left pontine gaze centre and vice versa.
- Oculocephalic (doll's eye) reflex: head movement in a comatose patient produces transient reflex eye movements in the opposite direction. Normally visual fixation prevents this reflex. Failure to elicit this reflex in coma carries a grave prognosis and implies severe brain-stem damage.
- Oculovestibular reflex (caloric test): in coma with intact brain-stem the eyes drift slowly towards the side of injection of ice water in the external auditory meatus when the head is elevated 30°. Persistent absence of this reflex in coma implies brain-stem damage with poor prognosis. The normal response is nystagmus with fast eye movement away from the injected area.
- Dysconjugate eye movement (eyes do not move in parallel): especially in upward gaze may indicate compressing intracranial lesion.

Limb deficit (assessed as part of GCS). Asymmetrical weakness, hemiparesis or hemiplegia occurs in limbs contralateral to lesion side. However, ipsilateral weakness may be due to uncal herniation pushing contralateral cerebral peduncle onto opposite edge of tentorium cerebelli (termed a false localising sign).

More neurological signs
- Systemic hypertension, reflex bradycardia (dissociated signs), papilloedema are indicative of raised intracranial pressure.
- Localising signs apart from pupil and fracture/bruise site include:
  — Jacksonian epilepsy.
  — Hemiparesis/hemiplegia.
  — Dysphasia or aphasia (clot pressing over left dominant hemisphere in right-handed patient).
  — Homonymous hemianopia of half visual field opposite to the visual cortex or optic radiation compressed by expanding haematoma.
- Low temperature may be due to shock (rarely due to intracranial bleeding but usually due to associated injuries, e.g. thoraco-abdominal or fractures) but a high or progressively rising temperature (in the absence of infection) indicates damage to the thermostatic centre of the hypothalamus and should be kept below 38.5°C (by fan, ice bag and chlorpromazine).
- Impaired facial movements on one side in response to a bilateral supraorbital pain stimulus indicates VII facial nerve weakness.
- Corneal reflex (tests V and VII nerves): loss of blink response in both eyes indicates V lesion on the stimulated side, while loss of blink in one eye irrespective of the side stimulated indicates VII lesion.
- Cerebral lesion may produce slow respiration or Cheyne–Stokes periodic respiration. Drug overdose, respiratory failure and CO_2 narcosis may also be responsible and blood gas analysis is indicated.

Investigations

Skull X-ray A well penetrated AP skull, true lateral skull and cervical spine and AP chest X-rays are essential in all coma cases. The presence of one or more of the following clinical criteria indicates a need for skull X-ray in patients with a history of recent head injury.
- Loss of consciousness or amnesia at any time.
- Neurological symptoms or signs.
- Cerebrospinal fluid or blood from the nose or ear.
- Suspected penetrating injury or scalp bruising or swelling. Simple scalp laceration is not a criterion for skull X-ray.
- Alcohol intoxication.
- Difficulty in assessing the patient (e.g. the young, epilepsy).

However, many advocate routine skull X-ray in all cases of head injury for medicolegal reasons.

CT scanning A non-invasive facility which should not be used as a substitute for clinical assessment. It is done after resuscitation is complete, in selected cases:
- Deteriorating, fluctuating or prolonged unconsciousness.
- Localising signs (including focal epilepsy).
- Severe head injury (GCS 7 or less) in the absence of localising signs.
- Penetrating head injury.
- Differential diagnosis of coma.
- Head injury with known intracranial pathology.
- Late indications (CSF fistula, infection, hydrocephalus, chronic subdural haematoma).

Intracranial pressure (ICP) monitoring Used by some neurosurgeons (*see* Section 3.7). The difference between ICP and systemic arterial pressure (the cerebral perfusion pressure) has an important influence upon the maintenance of cerebral blood flow. An extremely high ICP can shut off cerebral blood flow. ICP is a good indicator of a space-occupying lesion, e.g. intracranial haematoma.

Echo encephalography Simple, non-invasive method of detecting a shift in the cerebral midline.

Multimodality evoked electrical potential (by computer) To record visual, somatosensory and auditory near-field and brain-stem reflexes. It provides a prognostic index (limited use).

The last three investigations have practical limitations and are used only when clinical assessment is impossible as in comatose patients under controlled ventilation.

Continuous monitoring of the clinical state

- GCS.
- Pupil size and reaction.
- Limb movements.
- Vital signs (blood pressure, pulse rate, temperature, respiratory rate).

Definitive treatment

Minor head injury

Patients with no fracture, who are walking and talking (orientated) can be allowed home provided the relatives are warned to return the patient to hospital if headache, vomiting, drowsiness, visual disturbance or coma occurs.

Hospital admission after recent head injury is indicated in the presence of one or more of the following:

- Confusion or any other depression of the level of consciousness at the time of examination.
- Skull fracture.
- Neurological signs or headache or vomiting.
- Difficulty in assessing the patient, e.g. alcoholics and epileptics.
- Other medical conditions, e.g. haemophilia.
- Unsuitability of the patient's social conditions or lack of responsible adult/relative.

Note
- Post-traumatic amnesia with full recovery is not an indication for admission.
- Patients sent home should be given written instructions about possible complications and appropriate action.

Head injury with expected risk of complications

Patient should be hospitalised for observation as described (admission is indicated for all vault and basal fractures, all closed head injuries with altered consciousness or localising signs, multiple injuries with coexisting medical diseases (e.g. diabetes), known intracranial pathology (e.g. tumour, alcohol or drug ingestion), absence of responsible adult relatives or friends and if clinician is in doubt). If a patient deteriorates and an obvious extracranial cause such as hypoxia, hypotension or dehydration cannot be found, intracranial bleeding should be suspected and transfer arranged to a neurosurgical unit.

Consultation with and referral to a neurosurgical unit is indicated in the presence of one or more of the following:

- Skull fracture in combination with:
  — Confusion or other depression of the level of consciousness;
  — Focal neurological signs; or
  — Fits (including epilepsy).
- Confusion or other neurological disturbance persisting for more than 12 h even if there is no skull fracture.
- Coma continuing after resuscitation.
- Suspected open injury of the vault or the base of the skull (risk of CSF leak, meningitis).
- Depressed fracture of the skull.
- Deterioration.

In these cases decompression is required in the form of burr hole(s) or craniotomy (osteoplastic flap is preferred since it provides wider exposure and better decompression).

Head injury with coma
(but without intracranial haematoma)

- Patient needs special care (to keep airway open with tracheostomy care if applicable, positioning, nutrition, urination and defaecation). Medical management of severe head injury is the only treatment for those in whom there is no intracranial lesion.
- Respiratory function is of the utmost importance. Controlled ventilation is indicated in the following groups:
  —Missile head injury.
  —Head injury associated with severe respiratory trauma.
  —Head injury with pulmonary pathology, e.g. pneumonitis.
  —Head injury with severe generalised brain swelling especially in children.
  —Status epilepticus.
  —Acute reduction of intracranial pressure during coning or brain shift.
  —As part of anaesthesia for all urgent surgery in injured patients.
  —For all investigations requiring immobilisation, e.g. CT scanning.
- Steroids (dexamethasone) have been used in closed head injury but there is no substantial clinical or experimental evidence as to their efficacy.
- Mannitol and other osmotic diuretics could be given as a bolus 1.5–2 g/kg body weight in the early post-injury period. *N.B.* Many centres prohibit the use of steroids and mannitol for reduction of cerebral oedema since possible associated subclinical intracranial haemorrhage may expand when the brain shrinks (they also lead to false interpretation of CT scans by masking the magnitude of brain swelling). They should therefore be used only after strong confirmation of absence of intracranial bleeding and when there is no indication for CT scanning.
- Cimetidine 200 mg three times a day with 400 mg at night is effective in controlling gastric acid output and possibly preventing stress ulcer.
- Broad-spectrum antibiotics are given only in pulmonary complications, compound fracture or CSF leak.
- Anticonvulsants are given for fits and prophylactically for extensive open head injury (risk of future epilepsy is more than 50 %): phenytoin 300 mg or phenobarbitone 60 mg three times a day orally or i.v. is recommended. Acute epilepsy requires i.v. diazepam. Status epilepticus needs controlled ventilation.

Prognosis

The majority of head injuries are trivial. Of patients with severe head injuries 50% die, 10–12% are severely disabled or vegetative and 40% make a good recovery or have only a moderate disability.

The Glasgow Outcome Scale provides a practical means of classifying the outcome in terms of overall social disability:
- *Death*.
- *Vegetative*: sleep/wake cycles with eyes open but no sentient activity.
- *Severely disabled*: dependent, physically or intellectually, on another person at some point in every day.
- *Moderate disability*: independent but unable to resume fully their previous activities.
- *Good recovery*: may have residual neurological signs.

There is correlation between such outcome with the initial scoring of head injury by the GCS: a score of more than 11 is associated with 87% moderate disability or good recovery and 12% dead or vegetative while a score of 3–4 is associated with 87% dead or vegetative and 7% moderate disability or good recovery.

CERVICAL SPINE INJURY

The commonest vertebral column injury and the most dangerous when associated with spinal cord damage. Such injury is often missed or misdiagnosed because of:
- Pre-existing medical problem, e.g. rheumatoid arthritis.
- Multiple injuries (diverting attention from the neck).
- Head injury with unconsciousness making the clinical assessment difficult (in which case cervical X-ray is the only means of assessment and should be done routinely).
- Alcohol/drug abuse.
- Mild weakness and lack of physical signs (painful movement limitation, tenderness, retropharyngeal haematoma seen through the open mouth in Cl or C2 injuries and head rotation to one side in unilateral dislocation, all rarely present).
- Lateral cervical X-ray visualisation is often incomplete in the upper or lower parts of neck.

Therefore a *lateral complete cervical X-ray* (while the arms or shoulders are pulled down and the head is steadied with a halter) is the keystone of diagnosis and should be practised routinely (in addition to X-ray of the odontoid process taken through the open mouth). Myelogram is indicated in neurological deterioration and in stable but incomplete deficit due to cord compression.

Classification

Either dislocation or fracture (complete or incomplete with or without interruption to cord continuity respectively and stable or unstable).

Stable injuries

When bones will not displace further in the course of ordinary nursing care. They require neither reduction nor immobilisation (for bone healing) but may require a collar or skull traction to control pain.
- Whiplash injury in acceleration–deceleration head injury (extensor–flexor strain) leading to soft tissue injury, rarely with fracture or dislocation manifested by severe pain and stiffness. Treatment is by collar and gentle massage.
- Central cord syndrome due to forward fall with extension strain in elderly patients leading to paralysis of all four limbs (tetraplegia). Paralysis is greatest in the arms and least in the legs with flaccid hand paralysis and spastic leg paralysis. The bladder is paralysed. The syndrome is due to haemorrhage and oedema in the central area of the cervical spine over several segments (involving the anterior horn cells). Treatment is the same as for body paralysis. The neck requires no treatment. The condition is not painful.
- Simple extension lesion with a flake fracture of the inferior edge of the body.
- Fractures of atlas (spinal cord injury uncommon).

Unstable injuries

Require reduction of any displacement, and immobilisation which should continue until spontaneous healing of fractures and torn ligaments occurs.
- *Dislocation* following hanging: occurs between the atlas and axis with forward displacement of the atlas after transverse ligament rupture.
- *Hangman's fracture* at C2–C3 by direct extension: caused by hanging or lifting the head with the hands encircling the neck from behind.

In both the above cases death is immediate as a result of brain-stem injury and paralysis of the respiratory muscles.

- Axis fractures (X-ray through open mouth) with the odontoid process displaced forward or backward. Forward displacement of the odontoid may press on the brain stem and kill the patient immediately. Endotracheal intubation (for respiratory paralysis) may accentuate the cord compression and should be done with great care by an expert anaesthetist.
- Burst fractures (C3–C7): caused by vertical compression (due to diving into shallow water and striking the head on the bottom).
- Fracture–dislocations.

Cord injury

Produced by three factors:
- Long axis stretch causing concussion or rupture of nerve fibres and vessels within the cord.
- Nipping of the cord between the fractured bony edge and vertebral lamina.
- Disc protrusion leading to compression.

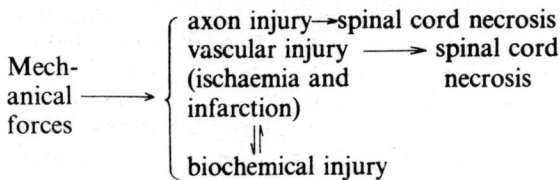

Mechanical forces →
{
axon injury→spinal cord necrosis
vascular injury ——→ spinal cord necrosis (ischaemia and infarction)
⇅
biochemical injury
}

The cord traumatic haemorrhage may be:
- Intramedullary (haematomyelia).
- Extramedullary into CSF (haematorrachis), either:
  —Extradural: with progressive cord compression and paraplegia (Thorburn's gravitation paraplegia); or
  —Intradural: with root irritation (blood detected in lumbar puncture).

Segmental injury

Upper cervical injury Cl–C4 →	Respiratory paralysis (since phrenic nerve is derived mainly from C4) with tetraplegia.
C5 ———→	Tetraplegia only (breathing OK).
C6 ———→	Tetraplegia but patient can abduct shoulder by deltoid muscles.
C7 ———→	Paraplegia with triceps paralysis in upper limbs.
T1 ———→	Paralysis of small hand muscles and Horner's syndrome.

All cord injuries result in spinal shock (complete flaccid paralysis below the level of the lesion with urinary retention). In cord contusion this lasts for 48 h followed by return of reflexes (recovery), followed by a third stage of septic complication. If no recovery is seen after 48 h, the injury may be either partial cord lesion (spastic paralysis in extension appears and urinary retention continues) or complete cord lesion (spastic paralysis in flexion appears with mass reflex).

Treatment

Management includes four phases:
1. Injury—first aid means.
2. Transport—immobilisation of neck.
3. Diagnosis (usually radiological though suspected clinically).
4. Treatment. The treatment aims are:
- To avoid incidents that could cause fresh damage to the spinal cord.
- To promote recovery from the damage already sustained.

Accurate clinical assessment of the severity of the damage may be impossible in the first few hours because of spinal shock. Radiological assessment (lateral and transoral X-ray and sometimes myelogram) is therefore essential. Reduction of unstable fractures is done by simple traction with skull calipers and graded increments in weight (also constitutes immobilisation if maintained until bony union occurs). The patient should be confined to bed. A minerva jacket (or halo vest) may be required for ambulant immobilisation. Reduction may be done quickly by closed manipulation under anaesthesia. Once reduction has been achieved spontaneous stabilisation by bony fusion is anticipated in 90 % of cases over 9–10 weeks. If by that time X-rays do not show stability on flexion or extension, the patient should undergo an internal fixation with bone grafting. Laminectomy or decompression is not beneficial as cord compression occurs at the time of injury.

Early management of paraplegia and rehabilitation

- High-protein diet (to compensate serum exudation from bed-sores).
- Positioning to prevent bed-sores.
- Intermittent urinary catheterisation—to prevent urinary infection (retention is present only initially).
- Active and passive movements and splints (quadriplegia).
- Treatment of respiratory failure.

1.28. Hand Injury and Infections

HAND INJURY

Main causes are:
- Industrial accidents (machinery in 40% of cases).
- Home accidents.
- Transport accidents.

Contributory factors include age (usually young in work-related accidents) and experience. The effects of severe hand injury are:
- Economical.
- Personal.
- Psychological.

Types of hand injury

- Incised wound (treated with primary suture).
- Crush injury with oedema, either open (treated with secondary suture) or closed (necessitates decompression incision).

The aim of treatment is to achieve the best possible result in the shortest possible time.

Assessment

1. The injury sustained (*see below*).
2. The functional loss.
3. The functional requirement of the patient.

Assessment of the injury sustained

- Is there any tissue loss? (e.g. bone, tendon, muscle).
- What structures are exposed?
- Viability of the skin.
- What structures are damaged?
  - Tendon injury is assessed by finger movements.
  - Nerve injury is assessed by sensation (not the motor power which is impaired already).
  - Bone injury by X-ray.
  - Joint stability only under general anaesthesia.

Treatment priorities

1. Skin cover.
2. Tendon repair.
3. Nerve repair.
4. Bone and joint injury treatment.

Principles of skin loss repair

1. Free partial thickness skin graft.
2. Free full thickness skin graft.
3. Local skin flaps
   - Rotation flap
   - Cross finger flap
   - Advancement flap
   - Neurovascular island flap.
4. Pedicle grafts.
5. Vascularised free grafts.

Principles of tendon repair

Tendons heal rapidly when held in apposition and strong union occurs at 4 weeks. Tendons easily become adherent to surrounding tissues, limiting their gliding movement. Such adhesions can be reduced by using *Klinert's traction*. The fingertip, e.g. nail, is attached by a rubber band to the plaster splint of the forearm. Because of rubber band recoil, the patient can actively extend his finger with a passive flexion. A reflex antagonistic relaxation of the flexor hand muscles prevents any mounting tension on the repaired tendon.

The results of immediate repair of extensor tendons are better than those of flexor tendons (due to flexor sheath in the latter).

Flexor tendons are sutured with primary repair or secondary late repair using tendon graft from palmaris longus or plantaris.

Extensor tendons are sutured with primary repair (in open wounds) or treated conservatively by immobilisation (in closed wounds).

Nerve injury

Should be treated by primary immediate repair and tested by nerve conduction study.

Hand bones fractures

K-wire internal fixation is indicated in:
- Fractures involving a joint surface.
- Metacarpal and proximal phalangeal fractures causing shortening, rotation or malalignment.
- Multiple fractures.

Principles of hand surgical technique

1. Tourniquet is essential to provide an adequate bloodless field; good light is important.

2. Anaesthesia—general is better than regional and local. If the latter is used, adrenaline is contra-indicated.

3. Careful wound toilet and cleansing.

4. Excision of devitalised tissue and haemostasis of bleeding vessels after release of the tourniquet.

5. Antibiotic and antitetanus toxoid should be administered routinely.

6. After treatment:
- Position of function (not ease) (i.e. flexion of metacarpophalangeal joints, extension of inter-phalangeal joints, abduction of thumb and dor-siflexion of wrist).
- Elevation of the hand.
- Proper Cramer wire splintage.
- Early physiotherapy.

Cut flexor aspect of the wrist

- Quick assessment with fluid replacement if still bleeding from cut arteries.
- Immediate repair of at least one artery (radial and/or ulnar artery) with 7/0 Prolene.
- Venous injury, however, can be ignored and the vein ligated.
- Immediate primary nerve repair (nearly always median nerve) should always be attempted (*see* 'Nerve injury'). Secondary nerve repair is rarely done (because of poor results).
- Immediate primary tendon repair should always be performed as there is abundant areolar tissue which prevents adhesions (providing the conditions permit). End-to-end repair should be carried out using Bunnell (criss-cross) stitch or Kessler (grasping) stitch (Fig. 13). All tendons should be sutured with the exception of palmaris longus which can be resected to reduce bulky scarring and prevent gross adhesions.
- Skin closure is essential as raw areas (uncovered by skin) predispose to infection and fibrosis.
- Antibiotics and antitetanus toxoid should be administered routinely.

Tendon injuries on the hand palmar aspect

Zone 1 (from the wrist to the distal palmar crease). Both flexor digitorum profundus and superficialis are repaired primarily (if conditions permit).

Zone 2 (from the distal palmar crease to the proximal interphalangeal joint) is called '*no man's land*' or '*the danger area*'. Traditionally if both flexor tendons are divided, close the skin alone. At the second operation resect flexor digitorum superficialis and repair flexor digitorum profundus by tendon graft. If only flexor digitorum profundus is divided, disregard lest repair endanger flexor digitorum superficialis. However, in expert hands, good results have been achieved after primary repair of both flexor tendons when combined with Klinert's postoperative rubber band traction.

Zone 3 (distal to proximal interphalangeal joint). Divided flexor digitorum profundus is repaired primarily (if conditions permit); otherwise flexor tendon graft via terminal phalanx with a pull-out wire is performed.

If flexor tendon injuries in the wrist and palm, Zones 1 and 3, cannot be repaired primarily, then secondary repair, tendon grafting or arthrodesis of the distal interphalangeal joint is performed later.

HAND INFECTIONS AND TREATMENT

Hand infections are either superficial, deep or unclassified.

Superficial (Fig. 14)

Nail fold infection (paronychia)

Can be complicated by chronic paronychia or pulp space infection.

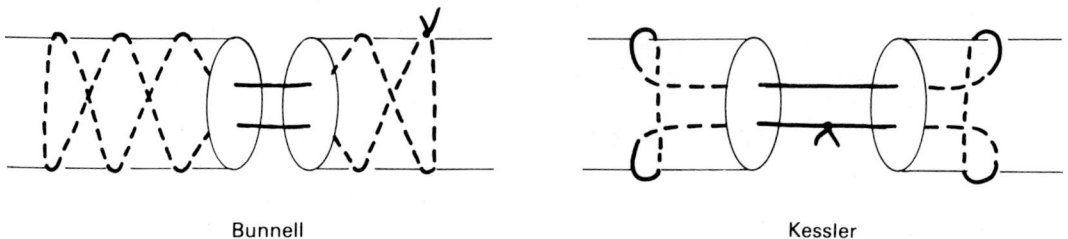

Bunnell   Kessler

Fig. 13 Tendon repair

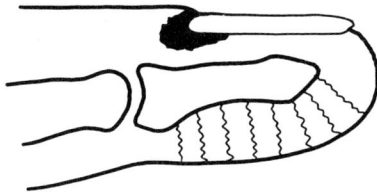

Paronychia

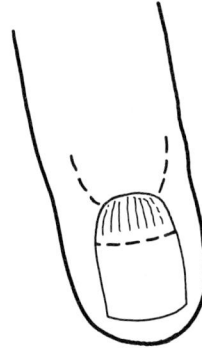

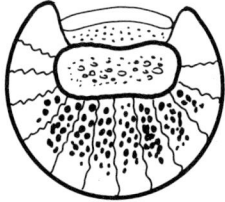

Pulp space infection

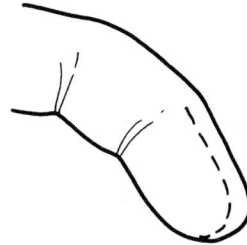

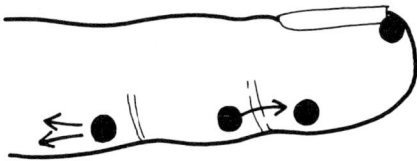

Subcutaneous infections

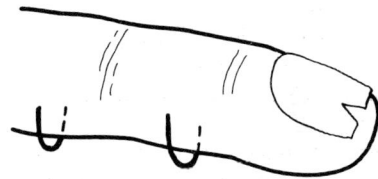

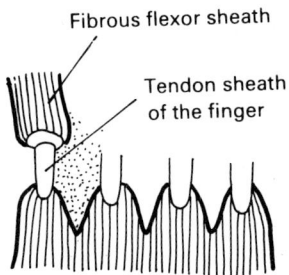

Fibrous flexor sheath

Tendon sheath
of the finger

Web space infections

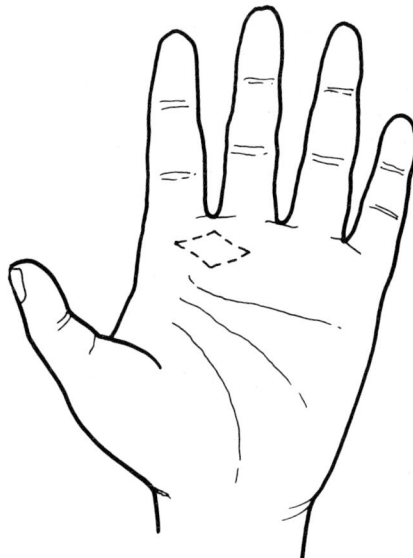

Fig. 14 Superficial hand infections: incisions and drainage

Pulp space infection (whitlow, felon)

Due to fibrous bands intersecting the space between the phalanx, tendon sheath and the skin; pus collection is rapid and painful leading to necrosis of the pulp tissue and the skin. Untreated it leads to osteomyelitis, pyogenic arthritis and even flexor tenosynovitis.

Subcutaneous infections

Apical subungual abscess and volar space infections.

Web space infections

Occur between the dorsal and volar skin. Spaces are filled with loose fat bulging between divisions of palmar fascia and straddling the deep transverse ligament. Treated by a diamond-shaped incision over the affected web space.

Deep (Figs 15–17)

Thenar space infection

The thenar space lies deep between adductor pollicis behind and flexor tendon of the index finger in front. It is separated from the mid-palmar space medially by the intermediate palmar septum (extending from palmar fascia) and laterally by the thenar eminence muscles. True infection of this space is rare and is usually an extension of a web space infection.

Mid-palmar space infection

The mid-palmar space lies between the interossei and metacarpal bones behind and the flexor tendons of the middle, ring and little fingers in front. This infection is usually an extension of subcutaneous palm abscesses. In deep palmar spaces lymphangitis occurs.

Tendon sheath infections (tenosynovitis) (Fig. 17)

There are three classical signs:
- Symmetrical swelling of the entire finger.
- Flexion of the finger (Hook sign) with exquisite pain on extension.
- Tenderness over the infected sheath.

Each tendon infection is treated with two incisions. It is a very serious condition and is complicated by:
- Forearm infection after ulnar or radial bursa rupture into the space of Parona between pronator quadratus and interosseous membrane dorsally and flexor digitorum profundus ventrally.
- Chronic tenosynovitis.
- Pyogenic arthritis.

A stiff digit is treated by amputation. Paralysis of

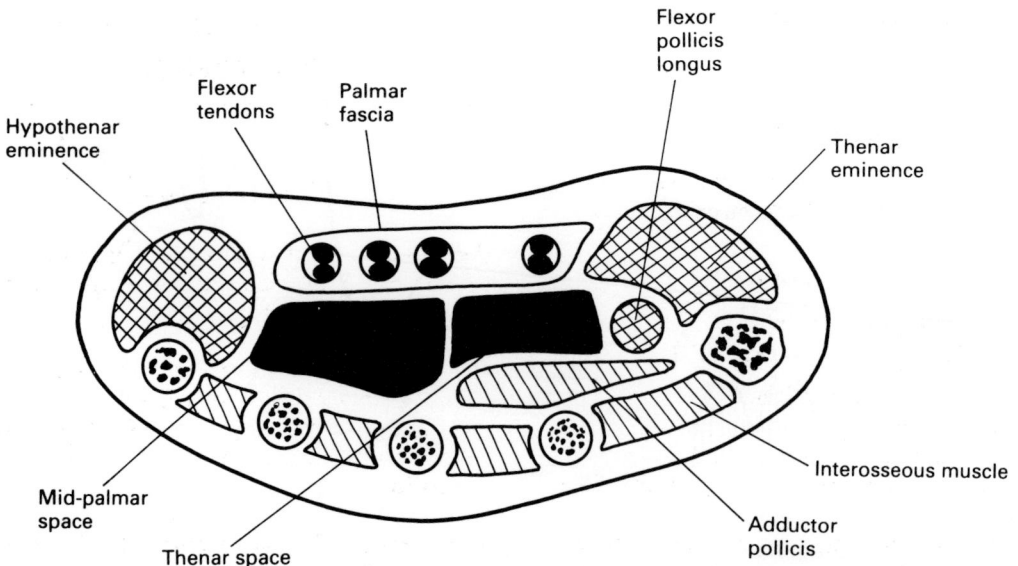

Fig. 15 Deep hand infections: anatomy (transverse section of hand)

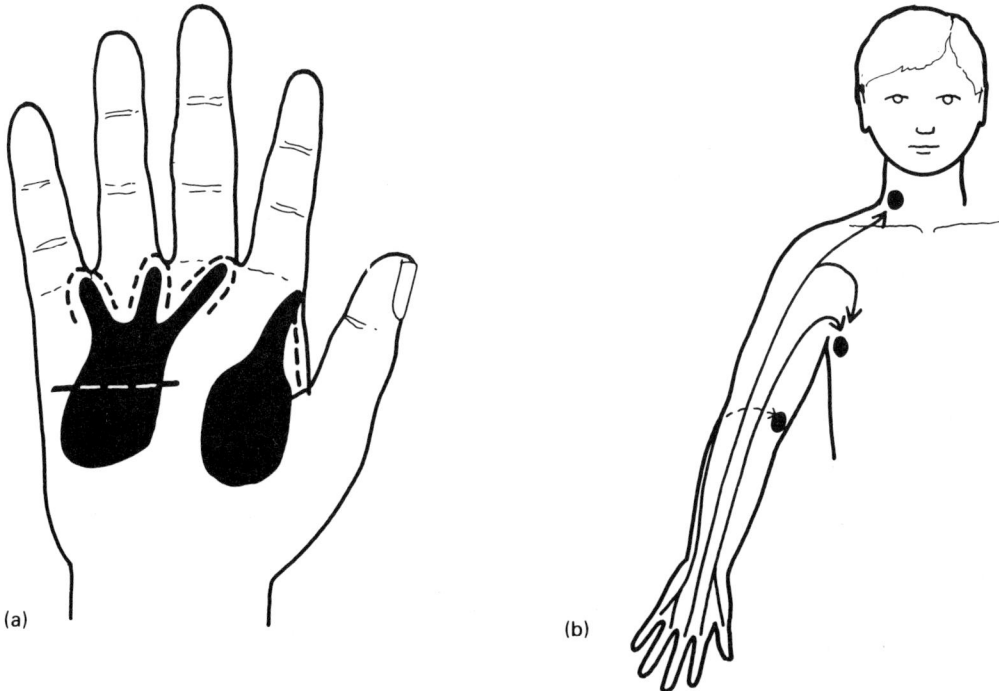

Fig. 16   Deep hand infections: (a) drainage sites; (b) lymphangitis

the median nerve requires urgent decompression (similar to carpal tunnel syndrome).

Unclassified infections

Include human bite, orf (contagious pustular dermatitis of sheep) and Barber's pilonidal sinus.

General principles of hand infection treatment

1. Antibiotics e.g. flucloxacillin.
2. Rest and elevation.
3. Diagnosis and localisation of pus.
4. Evacuation of pus and/or debridement of abscess cavity wall.
5. Adequate after-treatment (position of function, dry dressing and change of wet dressings, physiotherapy and rehabilitation).

1.29. Nerve Injury and Entrapment

Types of injury

Neurapraxia   Physical paralysis of conduction due to stretching or distortion without any organic rupture. Recovery is complete.

Axonotmesis   Intrathecal rupture of nerve fibres within an intact sheath. Wallerian degeneration and slow but good recovery by proliferating axons and intraneural fibrosis with fusiform neuroma formation.

Neurotmesis   Partial or complete division of the nerve sheath and fibres due to penetrating wounds; central and/or lateral neuroma with retrograde

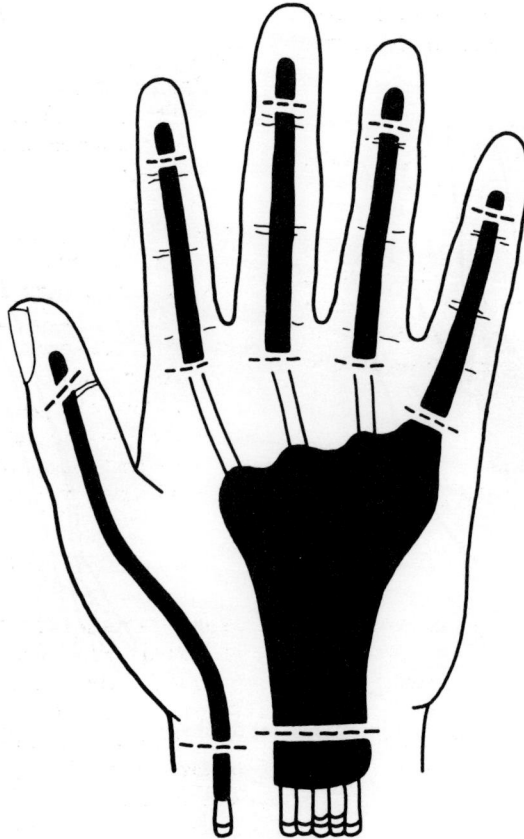

Fig. 17 Sites of tendon sheath infections

Wallerian degeneration and Schwann cell proliferation. Recovery is poor without nerve repair. Even accurate nerve suture may lead to an imperfect result owing to wastage of axons in scar tissue at the suture line and maldistribution of those fibres reaching the distal segment (maldistribution is greatest in mixed nerves and motor nerves supplying a large number of small muscles). The density of scar tissue at the suture line is increased by local sepsis and inflammation and by tension at the suture line.

NERVE REPAIR

Immediate primary suture is the ideal treatment for a divided nerve in tidy clean incised wounds (no sepsis and no tension). In untidy contaminated wounds, early secondary suture 3–4 weeks after injury is recommended for the following reasons.

● Primary suture requires enlargement of the wound to mobilise the nerve ends without tension. Since the wound is potentially infected, exposure of previously uncontaminated tissues should be avoided.

● Normally the nerve sheath is a delicate structure which is easily torn by the slightest tension. The sheath is also weakened by longitudinal tears but 3 weeks after the injury, epineural fibrosis occurs resulting in a thicker and tougher sheath and accurate coaptation of nerve ends by that time is greatly facilitated.

If a divided nerve is encountered accidentally in an open untidy wound it should be marked with fine silk for future identification but on no account should an attempt be made to identify or scrutinise a nerve.

Technique

After adequate exposure, the two ends of the nerve are identified, freed and freshened with a scalpel until projecting fibres are seen and blood oozes freely from the cut surface. Apposition of the two ends is accomplished by:

- Mobilisation.
- Relaxed position of the limb.
- Transposition, e.g. of ulnar nerve in front of the medial epicondyle and the radial nerve in front of the humerus.
- Nerve anchoring with tension stitches.

(Resection of bone is rarely required.) The sheath is sutured with non-irritant material, e.g. 7/0 Prolene mounted on an atraumatic needle or tantalum wire. Catgut should never be used. Tension or torsion should be avoided.

Principles of neurorrhaphy

- Elimination of tension.
- Use of atraumatic technique.
- No tourniquet.
- Proper mapping and aligning of fascicles.
- Prevention of fascicular gaps.
- Avoidance of lengthy mobilisation which has a devascularising effect.
- Use of meticulous intraneural haemostasis.
- Minimisation of foreign body reactions.

Aids in the repair

- Microsurgery of at least × 4 magnification with straight microsurgical forceps held in the left hand and curved microsurgical forceps (also acting as a needle-holder) or microscissors in the right hand. Interfascicular nerve repair is now the treatment of choice in cleanly incised fresh nerve injuries in which correct fascicular matching is feasible (90% of cases); by checking the rotational orientation of the alignment of the longitudinally running blood vessels in the epineurium, the corresponding fascicular groups can be readily identified.
- Nerve electrostimulation.
- Nerve glues (thromboplastin).
- Nerve wrapping, e.g. tantalum foil, Silastic or Millipore to prevent epineural fibrosis and the spurting of axons from the suture line which may produce a painful local lesion.
- Embedding—sutured nerve may be embedded among muscle fibres through an opening in the muscle sheath.
- Plaster cast—advisable after placing the limb in a suitable position to prevent any nerve strain.

Results

Depend on:
- Preoperative factors
  —The nerve affected: maldistribution is great in mixed nerve repair.
  —Infection.
  —Time.
  —Preoperative management of injured muscles and tendons.
- Operative technique
- Postoperative factors
  —Absence of infection.
  —After treatment, maintenance of relaxation of paralysed muscles, massage, electrical treatment and muscular effort.
  —Patient cooperation.
  —Vicarious movements of other muscle groups.

IRREMEDIABLE INJURY

When primary neurorrhaphy is impossible, owing to actual loss of the nerve substance, one of the following procedures is advisable.

- Nerve grafting from autogenous sural or lateral cutaneous nerve of the thigh to bridge the gap created by the injured nerve.
- Nerve anastomosis, e.g. part of the hypoglossal nerve to the distal end of the facial nerve.
- Tendon transplantation, e.g. in radial paralysis.
- Arthrodesis.
- Amputation.

Compression–entrapment nerve injury

May include:
- Root lesion, e.g. cervical spondylosis and intervertebral disc protrusion.
- Plexus lesion, e.g. thoracic outlet syndrome.
- Cranial nerves (rarely), e.g. conductive deafness in Paget's disease due to bony entrapment of facial nerve.
- Peripheral nerves (commonly).

The compression is either external (e.g. cast, plaster and bandage) or internal (e.g. haematoma due to anticoagulant therapy). The entrapment is the compression in the natural pathways in fascial planes or fibro-osseous tunnels especially during movement. Examples of nerve entrapment are:

Median nerve

- Pronator syndrome (between pronator teres heads): causes signs of median nerve palsy confined to the hand.

- Anterior interosseous syndrome (via interosseous membrane): affects pinch grip with severe pain.
- Carpal tunnel syndrome: acroparaesthesia, tingling and burning pain worse at night and wasting of thenar muscles. The pain is relieved by hanging the hand from the bed. Commonly affects females, usually in the dominant hand. Predisposing factors act either via carpal tunnel narrowing (e.g. rheumatoid arthritis, wrist fracture, tenosynovitis, gout and ganglion rarely) or via enlargement of tunnel contents (e.g. venous engorgement due to dialysis and shunt, contraceptive pill, pregnancy, myxoedema, acromegaly). However, commonly carpal tunnel syndrome is idiopathic. Treatment is by deroofing of the median nerve (decompression via longitudinal incision of flexure retinaculum).

Ulnar nerve

- Old supracondylar fracture of humerus with cubitus valgus leads to tardy ulnar nerve palsy. Fixation of the nerve (due to adhesions following osteoarthritis) or injury can occur in the cubital tunnel (i.e. elbow tunnel syndrome) after it passes behind the medial humeral epicondyle under the arcuate ligament into the forearm between flexor carpi ulnaris and flexor digitorum profundus. There is sensory loss of the medial one and a half fingers and wasting of the hypothenar, interossei and medial two lumbrical muscles (claw hand). Treatment is by anterior transposition of the nerve to the front of the medial epicondyle.
- Entrapment at wrist, palm or in Guyton's canal towards the little finger (no sensory loss). The small intrinsic muscles of the medial aspect of the hand are affected.

Radial nerve

- In the spiral groove of the humerus due to heavy sleep with the arm over the sharp back of a kitchen chair (Saturday night paralysis).
- Posterior interosseous nerve (entrapped between two heads of the supinator muscle). The extensors of the wrist and fingers are affected.

Thoracic outlet syndrome

Due to cervical rib in 0.5–1 % of the population. Fibromuscular band may cause the same syndrome. C8/T1 (lower trunk of brachial plexus) is affected with selective wasting of hand muscles (neurological). The vascular component is due to thromboembolism of the poststenotic dilated segment. The pain does not wake the patient at night. Electromyography (EMG) can determine whether the pain is due to cervical rib or to carpal tunnel syndrome.

Meralgia paraesthetica

Entrapment of lateral cutaneous nerve of the thigh as it passes through the inguinal ligament leading to hyperaesthesia and tingling in the lateral aspect of the thigh.

Anterior tibial compartment syndrome

Due to common or lateral peroneal nerve entrapment as the nerve winds around the fibular neck deep to the tendinous arch of the origin of peroneus longus. The condition occurs after unusual exercise, trauma (fracture, soft tissue injury or bandage) and arterial thromboembolism of the iliac, femoral or anterior tibial artery. Treatment is by fasciotomy through a 5 cm longitudinal incision of the lateral aspect of the leg.

Tarsal tunnel syndrome

The tibial nerve is entrapped in a fibro-osseous tunnel deep to flexor retinaculum behind and below the medial malleolus. Clinically, the condition is equivalent to carpal tunnel syndrome. A sphygmomanometer cuff inflated up to systolic blood pressure, applied around the calf for 1 min may reproduce the symptoms. Treatment is by decompression.

Morton's metatarsalgia

Due to neuroma (intermetatarsal bursitis) on the interdigital nerve between the metatarsal heads. Treatment is by excision of bursa.

1.30. Surgery in Ischaemic Heart Disease

Ischaemic heart disease is responsible for 150 000 deaths each year in the UK and is the commonest cause of death in the world. (By the age of 65 years, 45% of all men will have some form of ischaemic heart disease.)

Patients with stable or unstable angina are clinically assessed followed by exercise testing to identify those with serious coronary disease. Coronary arteriography is an essential part of cardiac catheterisation which, together with echocardiography and radionuclide scan, can assess the cardiac function preoperatively.

Coronary transluminal angioplasty

Indications

- Clinical, i.e. short history of angina resistant to medical management with objective evidence of myocardial ischaemia and relatively normal ventricular function.
- Anatomical, i.e. *severe proximal* single-vessel coronary artery disease. *Proximal* two- and even three-vessel disease can now also be treated.

Contraindications

- Diffuse or calcified stenoses.
- Left main coronary disease.
- Previous coronary spasm and occluded coronary arteries.

Procedure

Is done with a guide catheter and steerable wire introduced intra-arterially percutaneously via the femoral route by the Seldinger technique. Contrast injections are used to reveal the anatomy under fluoroscopic control after local anaesthesia and premedication.

Complications

Include local trauma, coronary dissection, occlusion, rupture of the coronary arteries, myocardial infarction and delayed restricture. Emergency surgery may be required in 5–7% of patients undergoing angioplasty. The hospital mortality is around 1%.

Coronary artery bypass grafting

Indications

- Angina unmanageable by medical treatment.
- The quality of life is adversely affected by long-term administration of drugs.

- Significant stenosis of the left main coronary artery (50% stenosis) regardless of left ventricular function or the degree of angina.
- Three-vessel disease.
- Unstable angina but without evolving infarction.

Procedure

Generally coronary artery bypass grafting is done within 6 months of coronary arteriography. Prior to surgery, smoking should be stopped, obesity should be reduced, and diabetes and hypertension controlled. The long saphenous vein must be carefully examined. In the presence of varicose veins and/or bilateral stripping, the cephalic vein or the internal mammary artery should be used instead. Coronary artery bypass grafting is done under general anaesthesia, using a median sternotomy approach. The long saphenous vein (from the leg) is excised and reversed before grafting. The bypass is controlled with an infusion of nitroprusside or nitroglycerine.

Complications

Include perioperative infarction and operative mortality in the region of 1%. Immediate and complete relief from angina occurs in 80% of patients. Graft patency after 12 months is 70–90%. Graft occlusion due to thrombosis or fibrosis may occur. A late closure rate of 2–3% per year is generally reported. Up to 30% of patients develop recurrent angina over a 5 year period. Good quality of life postoperatively is the rule in terms of less medication, improved exercise, symptomatic relief and return to work.

Other surgical procedures for ischaemic heart disease

- Left ventricular aneurysm (postinfarction) may be symptomatic (left ventricular failure) and may or may not have associated angina. In symptomatic patients, aneurysmal resection can improve left ventricular function. However the long-term results depend on the quality of the residual contracting myocardium and the extent of coronary disease progress.
- Postinfarction ventricular septal defect with subsequent rupture occurs in 1% of myocardial infarctions and carries a grave prognosis. The development of a pansystolic murmur (of ventricular septal defect) after myocardial infarction is an indication for urgent cardiological assess-

ment with a view to emergency surgery (if treated conservatively, 85% of patients die within 2 months).
- Mitral regurgitation following myocardial infarction is due to papillary muscle rupture or dysfunction. Acute rupture is usually fatal within 24–48 h if not corrected. The chronic form is due to dysfunction or partial rupture and needs mitral valve replacement.
- Inferior myocardial infarction may be complicated by heart block necessitating a permanent epicardial or intravenous endocardial pacemaker implantation.
- Ischaemic heart disease with advanced heart failure in suitably selected patients may be treated with heart transplantation.

1.31. Burns Management and Principles of Skin Grafting

BURNS MANAGEMENT

Burns present clinically in four stages:
1. Shock.
2. Infection.
3. Healing.
4. Contracture and scarring.

Generally burns are classified according to their depth into partial thickness (pin-prick pain sensation is present) or full thickness (pain sensation is lost) irrespective of the cause (whether thermal, electrical, chemical or radiation burns). Mortality depends on the percentage of burned surface area (Rule of Nine), patient age and the efficiency of the treatment. Generally, if the age + the percentage area affected is over 100, the chances of survival are very poor.

Treatment

General

- Ensure non-obstructed airways and remove clothes.
- Estimate the percentage of surface burns (Rule of Nine) and the body weight (in kg).

- Via an i.v. or venous cut-down a transfusion of Dextran 110 or plasma solution is given to all adults with 15% burn and all children with 10% or more burn. Deep burns require blood transfusion in addition. In 10–25% burn, the second ration is replaced by blood transfusion, while in 25–50% burn the second and sixth rations are replaced by blood transfusions (*see below*).
- The volume to be transfused is six equal rations over six consecutive periods of 4, 4, 4, 6, 6 and 12 h.

$$1 \text{ ration (ml)} = \frac{\% \text{ surface burn} \times \text{weight (kg)}}{2}$$

- The need and rate of infusion subsequently depend on clinical and laboratory observations, e.g. blood pressure, pulse rate, CVP (should be 10–15 cmH$_2$O), urine output (via a catheter), vomiting and packed cell volume (PCV).
- Analgesic morphine 10–20 mg i.v. (as required).
- Oral fluids are given as 60 ml/h increased to 100 ml/h (if there is no nausea). Burn of 35% or over needs nasogastric suction hourly.
- Curling peptic ulcer and the possible need for cimetidine therapy should be remembered.
- Antibiotics are required, particularly against Pseudomonas, the main intensive therapy unit microorganism (e.g. gentamicin and carbenicillin).

Local

The aims are to achieve skin cover and prevent infection and further skin loss.
- Exposure treatment (after skin cleansing with cetrimide–chlorhexidine solution) is practised in head and neck burns and those on a single surface of the trunk or limbs.
- Antiseptic dressing (after skin cleansing) is used in other burn sites. It is done in three layers, i.e. silver sulphadiazine (Flamazine) ointment with Soframycin is placed immediately next to the skin, followed by cotton gauze then absorbent wool held in place with crêpe.
- In full thickness burns the black slough is separated in 3 weeks through frequent baths and hypochlorite solution (EUSol). Recently there is a tendency to use early excision and skin grafting to speed up the healing and to reduce the risk of infection. Then a split skin graft (autograft) is used for cover; alternatively lyophilised skin (xenograft) or amnion dressing is used.
- Deep localised burns, e.g. electrical, need early local excision and grafting.

Complications

1. Respiratory damage due to smoke inhalation (requires oxygen therapy and/or tracheostomy).
2. Infection, especially Pseudomonas.
3. Anaemia due to deep burns (destroying red cells) and/or gastrointestinal tract bleeding due to curling ulcer.
4. Acute renal failure due to hypovolaemic shock.
5. Metabolic complications, e.g. hypokalaemia, hyponatraemia (sick cell syndrome)—treated with dextrose solution, insulin and potassium chloride. Also hypoxia and acidosis (due to tissue underperfusion, lung atelectasis—smoke inhalation and immobility—and increased oxygen needs). Glycosuria and hyperglycaemia can also occur.
6. Burn encephalopathy due to water intoxication, hypertension (caused by stress) and pyrexia.
7. Late burn contractures and deformities.

PRINCIPLES OF SKIN GRAFTING

Indicated in:
- Trauma (fingers and skin).
- Burns.
- Certain diseases (e.g. varicose ulcer).
- Surgical excision of a neoplasm (e.g. malignant melanoma).

The aim is to cover the raw area and obtain healing in order to limit deformity and/or disability.

Free skin grafts

Are used when the raw surface is healthy vascularised tissue (e.g. subcutaneous tissue, deep fascia, paratenon) or clean granulations.

Split thickness graft (Thiersch) Consists of one-third to two-thirds of skin thickness. The skin is usually taken from the thigh by a Humby's knife or dermatome. The graft is taken easily and can be fixed by sutures, but it has a tendency to shrink. After being taken, the graft is placed on a wood board and covered with tulle gras. It is then applied to the area with a pressure dressing to secure cohesion between the two surfaces and prevent oedema, haematoma or seroma formation. A split graft can be punctured to spread it over a wide area (*Mesh graft*), e.g. in extensive burns. When cut into postage stamp size pieces it is called a 'patch graft' and this is done to ensure escape of exudate without hindrance and facilitate the take.

Full thickness graft (Wolfe) Consists of full skin thickness, which is defatted (no subcutaneous fat). It is not easy to take but has no tendency to shrink and is of a better colour and texture than a split skin graft. May be taken from the postauricular area to cover excised rodent ulcer of the face; from the supraclavicular area again for use on the face; or from the groin to use on the hand. Cone-shaped pieces (*pinch grafts*) can be taken, providing a hardy graft with better survival in sepsis but with slow healing, scarring and poor cosmetic results.

Pedicle flaps (Fig. 18)

Indicated to cover areas with exposed cartilage, open joints, bare cortical bone or bare tendon, and if the vitality of the recipient area has been depressed by scarring or radiotherapy. Also in defects involving a cavity, e.g. full thickness excision of the lip or cheek. The flap is skin with subcutaneous tissue which remains attached to the body by one end to maintain its blood supply.
Types include:
- *Local flaps* to repair skin defects by *local V-Y* or *Z-plasty adjustment*, by *skin transposition* or by *rotational flaps*.
- *Direct flaps*, e.g. *cross-finger flap*, *cross-leg flap* and *abdomen-to-hand flap*.
- *Indirect flap via an intermediate carrier site*, e.g. from the abdomen to the face or to the lower limb using the wrist as a carrier.
- *Pedicle vascular flap* (retaining its vascular or neurovascular axial pedicle) e.g. *island flaps* of amputated finger tip.
- *Myocutaneous flap* is another modification, e.g. *latissimus dorsi flap* for postmastectomy reconstruction, *tensor fasciae latae flap* used for closure of defects overlying the greater trochanter.

Free vascular transplant

Necessitates microvascular reanastomosis of the skin flap artery to the recipient artery.

Tissue expanders

Recently developed tissue expanders are being increasingly used to repair local defects. These are prostheses implanted adjacent to the defect and inflated gradually over a 2–3 week period to expand the overlying tissue which can subsequently be used to close the defect.

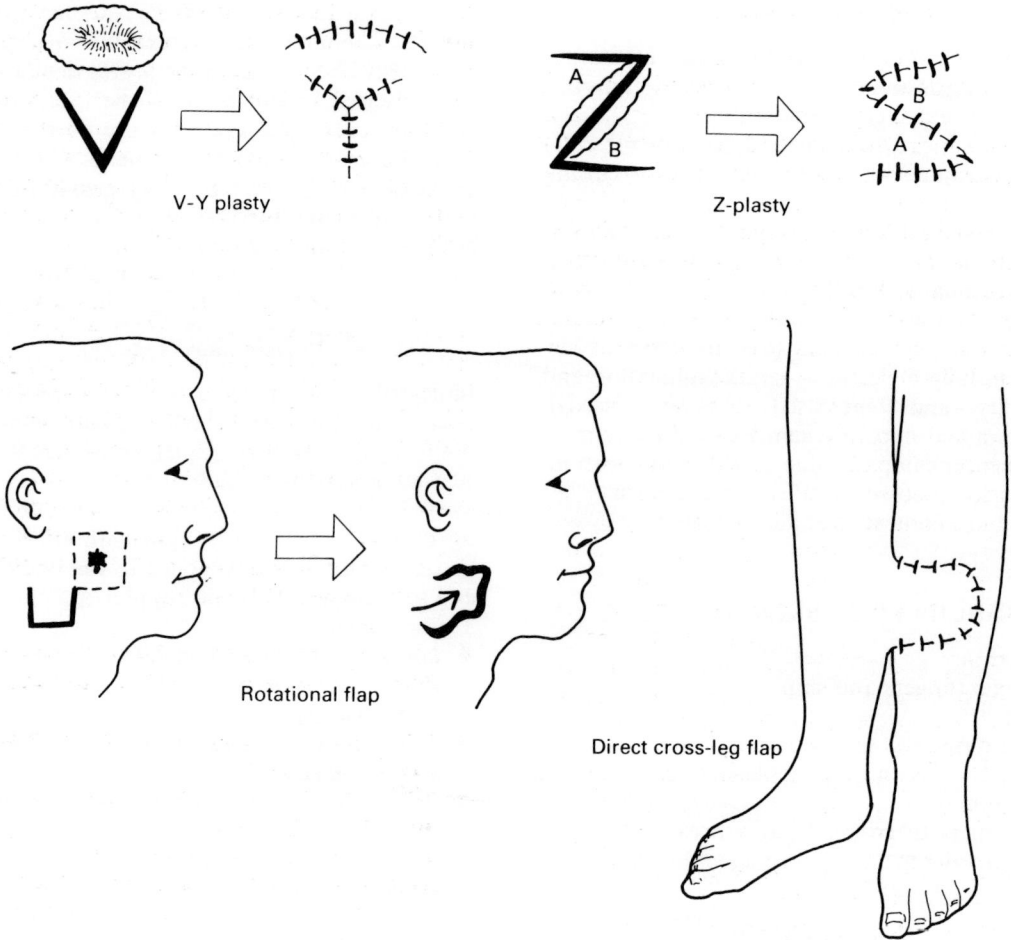

Fig. 18   Some pedicle flaps

Factors affecting take

- Recipient site nature (e.g. cartilage, bone or bare tendon), vitality (e.g. depressed by radiotherapy) and type of defect (e.g. involving a cavity).
- Technique (proper graft for proper area).
- Ischaemia.
- Infection.
- Haematoma or seroma formation.
- Mobility damages graft take.

1.32. Diabetes and Surgery

Surgical procedures are more common in diabetics than non-diabetics because:

- Eighty per cent of diabetics are over 40 years of age and surgical procedures are more common in this age group.
- Diabetes and its complications predispose to a variety of surgical disorders:
  —Large blood vessel diseases (macroangiopathy) including peripheral vascular insufficiency and gangrene.
  —Cardiac (ischaemic and hypertensive) disorders.
  —Eye (proliferative and non-proliferative retinopathies and cataracts).
  —Renal (uraemia and hypertension).
  —Infections: skin boils and abscesses, moniliasis (vulvitis and balanitis) and tuberculosis, as well as urinary tract infections.

The current high standard of surgical and anaesthetic technology make the surgical outcome in diabetics comparable to that in non-diabetics.

Preoperative assessment

The aims are to prevent ketosis and avoid hypoglycaemia. Medical evaluation of diabetic control is carried out and the presence of any complication noted, e.g. neuropathy, retinopathy and hidden infections as well as autonomic neuropathy (postural hypotension, gastroparesis and, in men, erectile impotence). Renal complications and electrolyte disturbances must be recognised, with serum creatinine and potassium respectively. Hypokalaemia is not uncommon in those receiving diuretics for essential hypertension or congestive heart failure and, if it occurs during anaesthesia, induction, may be dangerous (arrhythmias). Furthermore, hypokalaemia may worsen hyperglycaemia, and therefore it must be corrected preoperatively. The elective cases should be admitted 2 days prior to surgery; blood sugar should always be measured serially; oral hypoglycaemic agents, e.g. chlorpropamide, should be stopped 36 h before surgery (because of its long half-life) and replaced with insulin during the intra- and postoperative period. However, in hospitalisation for urgent surgery, regular insulin should be administered immediately until hyperglycaemia is reduced and the required surgery then undertaken (*see below*).

Preoperative medications are the same as for non-diabetics. The patient should never fast for prolonged periods before surgery. Scheduling of the operation for the morning hours is recommended, so that the first glucose infusion replaces breakfast energy. Intravenous feeding (rather than oral liquid breakfast) is advisable even for those scheduled for the afternoon, since surgery may be moved up if an earlier operation is cancelled.

Intraoperative management

Anaesthesia combined with surgical stress has a definite hyperglycaemic effect. Local, field block, spinal or epidural anaesthesia produces little metabolic disturbance; therefore the spinal approach is recommended whenever feasible. General anaesthesia, however, is well tolerated by most diabetics.

Hypotension (postural) and hypoglycaemia should be monitored throughout anaesthesia.

A. Elective surgery in insulin-dependent diabetics

The complications of hypoglycaemia and hypokalaemia are less likely to occur following infusion of low physiological doses of insulin than following therapy for diabetic ketoacidosis or hyperosmolar non-ketotic coma with the traditional higher (pharmacological) doses of insulin. Continuous intravenous infusion of insulin coupled with a separate infusion or piggybacked into the same vein as dextrose/water is recommended for ketosis-free patients. The infusions can be initiated preoperatively or intraoperatively and continued postoperatively. The recommended infusion is 50 units of insulin in 500 ml of normal saline, giving an insulin concentration of 1 unit per 10 ml/h, via an accurate infusion pump such as IVAC, coupled with 5% dextrose infusion at a rate of 100 ml (5 g glucose)/h to maintain the blood glucose in the desired range of 8.5–14 mmol/l. This regimen is very safe even if it is started on the evening before surgery. Blood glucose levels should be determined in the operating room and measured at 2 h intervals postoperatively. Adjustment in the rate of insulin and/or glucose infusion should be made according to the blood glucose results.

Note that:

- The postoperative fluid replacements should be dealt with separately from glucose and insulin infusions.
- Urine glucose estimation (even via a catheter) should be avoided.
- This method should continue until the patient is able to take fluids orally.
- This method can lead to insulin-induced hypoglycaemia (more dangerous than hyperglycaemia) if the i.v. glucose infusion line is kinked or extravasated (tissuing).

B. Emergency surgery in insulin-dependent diabetics

Acute surgical emergencies are likely to cause rapid diabetic ketoacidosis and dehydration, and ultimately death. Insulin-dependent (Type 1) diabetes is not uncommonly first manifested at the time of acute illness, e.g. perforated peptic ulcer, abscesses or acute cholecystitis, and delay in its recognition is fatal. Examination of blood and urine specimens will reveal diabetes which should be treated immediately. An i.v. normal saline infusion should be administered rapidly over a 4 h period. A 10 unit bolus of insulin is given i.v. followed by continuous infusion of 10 units insulin for 1 h from an independent reservoir (50 units insulin in 500 ml saline). Potassium chloride should be added if the initial serum K^+ is subnormal. This should be measured periodically since insulin (even in low doses) can cause hypokalaemia. Frequent monitoring of serum electrolytes and acetone is necessary. Blood glucose should be determined at the bedside at 2 h intervals using Dextrostix with a glucometer. The basic saline infusion should be changed to Dextrose/saline (5 % glucose + 0.45 % saline) once the blood glucose level has fallen to 14 mmol/l. Nasogastric suction is used if there is vomiting or gastroparesis, and antibiotics should be given when appropriate. A period of 4–8 h of rapid fluid and insulin infusion should be sufficient to improve the metabolic situation so that the patient can safely undergo emergency surgery. It is futile to delay such surgery further while attempting to eliminate ketosis completely, since the underlying acute progressive surgical condition, if uncorrected, will lead to rapid deterioration. (Thereafter careful monitoring of the patient during and after surgery is as for elective surgery.)

Note that:

- The sliding scale of insulin based on the colour of urine treated with Clinitest reagent tablets (rainbow method) should be abandoned.
- The Biostator (Miles Laboratory) is a recently developed automatically computerised instrument which continuously displays the blood glucose concentration. It is programmed to maintain normal blood glucose levels by infusing either 5 % glucose or insulin, according to the desired glucose level selected by the doctor.

C. Surgery in non-insulin-dependent diabetics

This type of diabetes (Type 2) is the most common form of the disease. Most patients are over 40 years of age. Diabetic ketoacidosis is rare because of limited reserves of endogenous insulin, but the stress of major surgery may sometimes push patients into ketoacidosis.

1. For minor operations: Whether patients are controlled with diet only, oral hypoglycaemic or insulin, they should be observed and these agents withheld until after the procedure.
2. For major operations: Patients controlled with diet only should be observed. Oral hypoglycaemic agent should be discontinued from those previously controlled with it and replaced with 10 units insulin in 1 litre of 5 % dextrose. Those previously controlled with insulin should be treated like insulin-dependent diabetics. If the postoperative blood glucose is above 14 mmol/l, 10 units of subcutaneous insulin + 20 units of insulin increment in subsequent infusion (in persistent hyperglycaemia) should be administered.

Postoperative management

In (A) as before but each litre of postoperative i.v. infusion should contain 5 % glucose, 0.45 % saline and 44 mEq of potassium chloride. Extrarenal fluid losses from drainage and suction should be replaced independently (with potassium chloride). The postoperative goal for the blood glucose level is between 8.5 and 14 mmol/l. Oral fluids, once started, should be followed by a soft diet then a diabetic diet. The usual daily insulin dose can be resumed according to 3-hourly blood glucose estimation.

In (B) as before. Once blood glucose falls below 14 mmol/l, insulin is administered i.m. or subcutaneously adjusted according to serial blood glucose estimations. Thereafter the patient is stabilised by changing to an intermediate acting insulin, e.g. Lente with a soluble insulin.

In (C) preoperative therapy should be resumed.

Hyperosmolar non-ketotic coma

This syndrome is increasingly recognised in surgical patients (iatrogenic). Delay in diagnosis and therapy is fatal. Preoperative dehydration and surgical stress with postoperative hyperglycaemic drugs predispose to hyperosmolar non-ketotic coma. It has also been observed in burns, following hyperalimentation, following i.v. dextrose infusions (exogenous glucose loads), and complicating cardiopulmonary bypass as well as haemodialysis and peritoneal dialysis. Vascular thromboses (e.g. mesenteric thrombosis) are a major complication of hyperosmolar non-ketotic coma. Surgical intervention may be needed when such patients develop signs of acute abdomen—more frequent than in those with diabetic ketoacidosis. Thromboses may also block lower limb vessels, necessitating amputation.

Diabetes management during open heart surgery

These patients need a glucose/insulin/potassium infusion with much greater amounts of insulin (1 unit/g of glucose) than non-cardiac diabetics (0.3 unit/g or 3 units with 10 g glucose) to cope with extra trauma, hypothermia and glucose loading when cardiopulmonary bypass begins.

1.33. Common Surgical Conditions Affecting the Hip Joint

CONGENITAL DISLOCATION OF THE HIP

True dislocation of the hip at birth is rare. The condition referred to as congenital dislocation of the hip (CDH) is a dysplastic condition of the joint which predisposes to dislocation.

Incidence

Examination of the newborn in the UK reveals unstable or subluxating hips in 1.7%. However, 68% of these will stabilise within a week and 88% by the end of 2 months. After this time 1.5 per 1000 will have a true dislocation.

The incidence is affected by a number of factors.

Sex Higher incidence in girls (7:1).

Epidemiology The variable incidence in different population groups may have a genetic basis:

UK	1.5/1000
Sweden	1/100
Lapps/North American Indians	5/100
Chinese	Very low incidence

This may be explained by nurture. The higher incidence groups tend to swaddle babies with their hips extended and adducted, while the Chinese carry their children with hips spreadeagled in flexion-abduction.

Familial Ten times higher incidence than general population in siblings of affected children. Incidence of 40% in second monozygous twin if first affected. There may be familial joint laxity.

Joint laxity In boys there may be a genetic basis. In girls there may be a hormonal basis. Circulating maternal relaxins may be responsible.

Fetal position In one series 16% of CDH were breech born. In another study 50% of breeches had CDH. Extended breech births have a still higher incidence.

Aetiology and pathogenesis

The two constant features of CDH are acetabular dysplasia and ligamentous laxity, but the relationship between the two in the initiation of the process which leads to dislocation and how much instability itself contributes remain unknown.

Anteversion of the femoral head accompanies dysplasia of the acetabulum and the two worsen the longer the joint is unstable or dislocated. It is thought that anteversion and acetabular dysplasia contribute in a complementary fashion to the pathogenesis of the condition.

Primary acetabular dysplasia in a typical case may be evidenced at birth. There is osseous hypoplasia of the roof of the acetabulum but the cartilagenous contribution is intact. Provided concentric pressure from the femoral head can be applied to the cartilage, it responds by ossification and spontaneous correction. In the majority this does not occur and the acetabulum remains hypoplastic. The femoral head migrates upwards and outwards and the femoral neck becomes anteverted. An anteverted head applies pressure to the anterior part of the acetabulum and flattens and everts the fibrocartilagenous limbus. The acetabular cartilage deforms. As the socket flattens its ossification becomes delayed. Actual dislocation of the hip occurs when the femoral head passes over the fibrocartilagenous rim and the head loses contact with the acetabular floor. The limbus inverts as a result of its inherent elastic recoil. Reduction of the femoral head is prevented by the secondary soft tissue changes which occur.

Pathology

The head of the femur is in a 'false acetabulum' on the outer surface of the ilium with capsule interposed between it and periosteum. The cartilagenous head is large in comparison with the empty acetabulum, and flattened medially and posteriorly. Its ossification is delayed. The femoral neck may be anteverted up to 90°.

The acetabular floor and outer surface of the ilium lie in a straight line. The floor of the acetabulum becomes overgrown with fibrocartilage to which capsule often adheres. The ligamentum teres is either attenuated or hypertrophied. At the point where the psoas tendon crosses the capsule, it becomes constricted and resembles an hour glass;

the head of the femur is in the upper chamber and the lower one contains the acetabular contents. The muscles attached to the femur either lengthen, resulting in their mechanical disadvantage, or shorten, so that they act as blocks to reduction of the head.

Clinical presentation and radiological features

Neonatal period

All neonates should be examined for abnormalities of the hip joint. The examiner should note assymetry of the skin folds of the thigh, eccentricity of the labia and widening of the perineum (bilateral CDH). An adduction contracture may or may not be present. Shortening of the femur may be apparent (Galeazzi's sign) and the trochanter of the affected side will be above Nélaton's line. On testing movements abduction is limited while internal rotation is often increased. Ortolani's manoeuvre may reveal subluxation of the hip as a 'click' or jerk as the femoral head rides over the acetabular margin and goes back into the socket. On the basis of Barlow's test the severity of the instability of an abnormal hip can be graded (Fig. 19). Hips will generally be normal, minimally unstable, severely unstable or truly discolated.

In the neonatal period radiological screening for CDH is generally of no value. However, signs that may be of value include increase in the acetabular

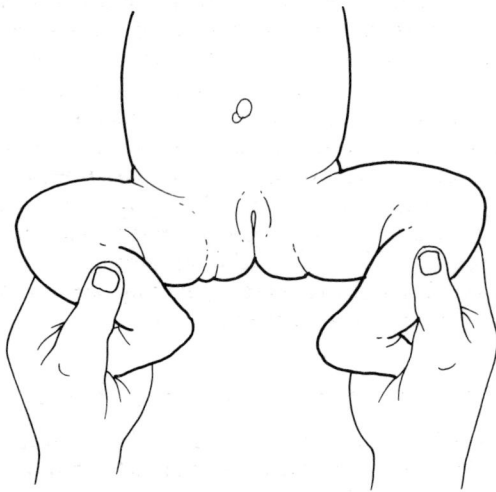

Fig. 19 Ortolani–Barlow test (abduction of flexed hip and knee joints)

angle and lack of definition of the lateral lip of the acetabulum. A line drawn along the shaft of the femur should pass through the triradiate cartilage (Von Rosen's line) but in CDH it does not. X-rays of the femur in different positions should show the depth from the ossified femur to the acetabular floor to be the same; if not, subluxation can be inferred.

Infants

A dislocated hip may be suspected in the presence of assymetry, clicking of the hip or difficulty in putting the child in nappies because of limitation of abduction on the affected side. When the child starts to walk, assymetry may become more obvious and the child may limp (Trendelenburg gait). In bilateral CDH a 'rolling sailor's gait' is observed and lumbar lordosis is exaggerated. Normally, the secondary ossification centre for the femoral head appears between age 4 and 6 months, but in CDH its appearance is delayed, sometimes up to the age of 12 months. Drawing vertical lines from the lateral edge of the acetabulum and horizontal lines through the triradiate cartilages (Perkin's lines), the secondary ossification centre of the femoral head should be located inferomedially. In CDH the ossification centre lies superolaterally. The acetabulum is obviously shallow and anteversion of the femoral neck may be obvious. A false acetabulum, seen as a shallow depression in the ilium, is sometimes visible. The labrum is folded in the acetabular shallow cavity, the ligaments are lax, muscles are shortened and the capsule is elongated.

Management

The majority (90%) of clicking hips at birth stabilise within 2 months. For minor instability double nappies worn for 2 weeks will normally suffice. More severe instability at birth or persistent minor instability beyond 2 weeks warrants application of an abduction splint. If at the end of a 3 month period the hip is stable and developing normally, as judged by X-rays, the splint can be restricted to use at night only. Follow-up is for 18 months and frequent out-patient checks are made in this period.

Residual instability at 3 months or the discovery of an unstable hip beyond the neonatal period requires concentric reduction of the femoral head. This can usually be achieved by gentle traction and closed reduction. The child's hip is held in a 'frog plaster' in abduction until stability is achieved.

Secondary changes in the soft tissues as described above may prevent concentric reduction, in which case operative treatment is indicated. Soft tissue release and derotation osteotomy will usually suffice in children up to the age of 3 years, but beyond this age an additional innominate osteotomy is usually required.

Operative treatment

Soft tissue procedures

Release of the psoas tendon may be sufficient to allow concentric reduction of the femoral head. However, excision of the joint capsule, removal of the acetabular contents, including the ligamentum teres, or an inverted limbus may be required.

Derotation osteotomy

Approximately 80% of cases of CDH diagnosed late have significant anteversion of the femoral neck. Concentric reduction of the femoral head and abduction in a frog plaster will result in spontaneous correction of anteversion in some cases. Persistent anteversion exceeding 60% requires subtrochanteric derotation osteotomy. This may also be required if the femoral head displaces after closed reduction.

Innominate osteotomy

CDH presenting between the ages of 18 months and 6 years is associated with the complete gamut of soft tissue and bony problems and requires operative intervention. In addition to soft tissue release and removal of interposed soft tissues plus derotation osteotomy, innominate osteotomy is required to ensure concentric reduction of the femoral head. The Salter osteotomy swivels the acetabulum to cover the anterolateral defect. The Pemberton osteotomy or acetabuloplasty rotates the anterosuperior acetabulum laterally and downwards and has the advantage over the Salter osteotomy of not creating a defect posteriorly. The Chiari osteotomy displaces the acetabulum medially and creates an extension to its root laterally.

PERTHES' DISEASE

Aetiology

This condition of the hip joint affecting children between the ages of 3 and 10 years is not an inflammatory condition but is considered to have an ischaemic aetiology resulting in the upper capital epiphysis becoming wholly or partially avascular. Depending upon the extent of the avascular necrosis the capital epiphysis becomes deformed and the hip dysplastic. The average duration of the disease is between $2\frac{1}{2}$ and 4 years.

The aetiology of the condition is unknown but genetic, anatomical and environmental factors have been implicated; 80% of those affected are boys. The sharply defined age range correlates well with a period when the capital epiphysis is nourished principally by a precarious blood supply from vessels crossing the lateral epiphyseal line. Four per cent have associated major genitourinary abnormalities (the hip and genitourinary system are derived embryologically from the mesonephric ridge). The skeletal maturity of children with Perthes' disease is delayed.

Clinical presentation and radiological features

Clinically the child presents with pain in the hip and a limp. There may be limitations of hip movements, muscular wasting of the buttock and thigh, and shortening of the limb if the femoral head collapses.

Radiological studies indicate that changes occur in the femoral epiphysis and metaphysis, the acetabulum and joint cavity. The earliest feature is flattening and sclerosis of the lateral anterosuperior quadrant of the epiphysis associated with translucency of the adjoining metaphysis. As the head undergoes avascular necrosis it becomes dense, flattened and broader, and a linear translucency can be seen within it. As revascularisation takes place the epiphysis assumes a fragmented appearance with translucent areas. The metaphyseal area of the femur is also affected: it becomes broader and rounded off and the neck of the femur shortens relatively. Cysts often appear on the metaphysis. Within the acetabular cavity the distance between the medial side of the capital epiphysis and the acetabulum appears increased, owing to an increase in thickness of the articular cartilage. The acetabulum becomes dysplastic, adapting itself to the changes in the head of the femur.

Radiological classification and prognosis

Perthes' disease is a self-limiting condition with an overall fair prognosis which is better in boys and the younger child. The problem has been to identify those children with the disease likely to have a poor outcome if untreated.

A radiological classification based upon the extent of involvement of the femoral head and identifying the 'head at risk' has been made by Catterall. Using this classification treatment is reserved for those children with 'head at risk'.

Group I	Only anterior epiphysis involved. No collapse of the femoral head occurs.
Group II	More of anterior epiphysis involved with appearance of a dense oval collapsed sequestrum. As this sequestrum is absorbed collapse of the head occurs. Metaphyseal cysts may be seen.
Group III	Only a small part of epiphysis not sequestrated. As collapse occurs lateral segment displaces and metaphysis broadens.
Group IV	Whole epiphysis sequestrated. Mushrooming of femoral head. Extensive metaphyseal changes.
'Head at risk'	Small V-shaped osteoporotic defect of lateral epiphysis accompanied by similar defect in metaphysis—Gage's sign. Lateral calcification. Lateral displacement of the femoral head. Diffuse or extensive metaphyseal changes. Horizontally disposed growth plate.

Management

- Rest for the irritable hip.
- Careful supervision and radiological follow-up until revascularisation complete.
- Treatment for 'head at risk' aimed at containment of the femoral head concentrically within the acetabulum.

OSTEOARTHROSIS OF THE HIP

The nomenclature of this condition is disputed. It is primarily a degenerative disease of the joint and therefore some clinicians use only the term osteoarthrosis. Others prefer the term osteoarthritis since they argue that it only becomes symptomatic when secondary inflammatory changes take place in the soft tissues.

Secondary osteoarthrosis can follow trauma, inflammatory and pyogenic arthritis, haemophilia, gout and avascular necrosis.

Primary osteoarthrosis is used to describe the degenerative joint disease where none of the above factors apply. In this condition, a myriad of clinical syndromes have been described but its aetiology is ill-understood. Occupation and obesity are implicated and there are poorly defined genetic factors. There is a rising non-linear relationship with age. Fifty per cent of all adults have at least one joint affected and 7% are disabled by osteoarthrosis. Between the ages of 55 and 65, 80% have radiological evidence of the condition and this rises to 98% between the ages of 65 and 74 years.

Pathology

Osteoarthrosis is not primarily an inflammatory condition but a degenerative one. The primary lesion is in the articular cartilage with secondary inflammation in the soft tissues.

In the hip joint it has been demonstrated that in 71% of joints the primary degeneration of the articular cartilage occurs in the non-weight-bearing areas, in 3% it starts in the pressure areas and in 26% in a combination of both. The cartilage receives its nourishment by intermittent compression causing imbibition of synovial fluid. The absence of this pumping mechanism in the non-weight-bearing areas would support the theory that the lack of nutrition begins the degenerative process.

The non-weight-bearing cartilage becomes soft, heaps up and undergoes fibrillation. In response the subchondral blood vessels hypertrophy and invade the cartilage which then undergoes calcification with osteophyte formation. The loss of cartilage results in fissuring and cleft formation, and also exposes the underlying bone which becomes dense and eburnated. Cysts form beneath the pressure areas; their enlargement is probably caused by synovial fluid being forced into them through cracks in the cartilage as a result of pressure from joint movement. Trabecular fatigue fractures result in decrease in bone height and irregularities of the articular surface. Areas of hyperaemia with venous stasis develop in the bone ends and venous engorgement is said to contribute to night pain which is a feature of the disease.

Biochemical changes in the cartilage precede the visible changes. There is a loss of matrix proteoglycans and collagen. Death of chondrocytes occurs in the degenerating areas. Increased cell division in the cartilage that is left and increased glycoaminoglycan synthesis cannot maintain cartilage repair. Release of enzymes from the chondrocytes into the synovial fluid aggravates the process and, together with the detritus of cartilage flakes, causes synovitis. The synovium undergoes hyperplasia with villous formation. The cartilage flakes and small pieces of bone enter the synovium and the underlying joint capsule becomes involved in the inflammatory process. The capsule and synovium thicken and become fibrosed with consequent shortening and reduction in the range of movement of the joint.

Loose body formation occurs as a result of detachment of osteophytes and pieces of bone and cartilage from the joint surface and shedding of cartilagenous synovial polyps into the joint space. These further damage the joint and give rise to locking.

Clinical features

Aching is usually the first sign of the disease and is probably due to synovitis. It gradually becomes severe and constant. Night pain prevents the patient from sleeping. Pain may be referred to the knee.

Stiffness is a prominent symptom and is worse after resting. It is due to fibrosis and oedema in the capsule. Deformity arises from muscular spasm and capsular fibrosis. The patient limps as a result of a fixed flexion deformity associated with adduction and external rotation of the femur.

The patient walks with an antalgic or a Trendelenburg gait and the affected limb may be obviously adducted and externally rotated with a fixed flexion deformity. Quadriceps wasting may be noted.

The examiner should note old scars and sinuses around the hip joint. Apparent shortening of the limb is greater than true shortening. Thomas' test may uncover a fixed flexion deformity.

The classic X-ray features of osteoarthrosis are joint space narrowing, osteophyte formation, subchondral sclerosis and subchondral cyst formation.

Management

Conservative measures result in improvement in approximately one-third of sufferers. Weight loss is to be encouraged. A walking stick held in the opposite hand should be used. A heel raise may prevent pain and limping. Short-wave diathermy is often helpful and non-steroidal anti-inflammatory drugs are indicated.

Surgery is principally reserved for pain relief but other indications include stiffness and deformity. Age is an important consideration in patient selection. The older patient with a more sedate life-style will do well. However, total hip replacements are carried out in younger age groups.

Total hip replacement

Total hip replacement (THR) has revolutionised the treatment of arthritis of the hip, superceding arthrodesis, femoral osteotomy and excision arthroplasty. THRs have given some patients 15 years of service and those being inserted now are expected to last over 20 years.

The THR prosthesis consists of:
- A femoral component—made of stainless steel, titanium or cobalt-chrome. The head size varies between 22 mm and the natural size. The smaller the head the lower the friction, but the larger ones have a greater range of movement.
- An acetabular cup—utilises high-density polyethylene or ultra-high molecular weight polypropylene which minimises friction at the joint surface.
- The components are fixed into place using methylmethacrylate. This is prepared just before insertion as a putty which hardens into a cement by an exothermic reaction once inside the body. Certain cements are antibiotic-loaded.

Operative technique

To minimise complications of THR—infection, dislocation, loosening of the components and fracture of the stem of the femoral component or fracture of the shaft of the femur—scrupulous attention to insertion technique is mandatory.

The patient should have no focus of infection. Preoperatively a prophylactic antibiotic is administered. The operation should be conducted in an ultra-clean laminar flow enclosure. The surgeon and all assistants wear Ventile gowns with an exhaust system.

In the preparation of the bone surfaces, the acetabulum is reamed so that it will accommodate the largest available cup and it is cleared entirely of all soft tissue, cartilage, fibrocartilage and osteophytes. Keying holes for the cement are drilled into the ilium, pubis and ischium. The acetabular component is cemented into position 40° to the horizontal and in a neutral position.

The femoral head is removed with a Gigli saw. If an oscillating power saw is used the blade should be cooled with saline to prevent heating with consequent thermal destruction of osteocytes. The femoral shaft is reamed and cleared of all cancellous bone. A trial femoral component is inserted and reduction attempted. The prosthesis must not sit in a varus position. The trial prosthesis is removed, a cement restrictor placed in the femoral shaft and cement introduced into the reamed femur. The definitive prosthesis is inserted and held until the cement has cured, after which reduction is effected.

Revision arthroplasty

Revision of hip prostheses with complications are being carried out in increasing numbers. Loosening of the prosthesis and infection are the two major indications for revision surgery.

Revision arthroplasty should be regarded as a salvage operation.

TRAUMATIC DISLOCATION OF THE HIP

Posterior dislocation of the hip

The majority of posterior dislocations of the hip result from the 'dashboard' injury—force along the long axis of the femur while the thigh is adducted and flexed. Some arise as a result of blows to the back with the person stooping or kneeling, e.g. mining accidents.

Clinically the limb is adducted, medially rotated and shortened. It is important to exclude an injury to the sciatic nerve.

Radiographs may show a concomitant fracture of the posterior lip of the acetabulum.

The majority of these dislocations can be managed by closed reduction. Under a general anaesthetic using muscle relaxants, one of two manoeuvres can be used to reduce the dislocation:
- The hip is flexed, abducted, laterally rotated and then brought into extension in a neutral position (Bigelow's manoeuvre); or
- The hip is flexed, brought into a neutral position and the head of the femur lifted gently into the acetabulum.

Then, Hamilton–Russell traction is applied for 3 weeks, after which the patient is allowed up on crutches. Full weight-bearing is allowed at 6 weeks.

Anterior dislocation of the hip

Posterior dislocation of the hip is 20 times more common than anterior dislocation.

High type

As a result of forced external rotation and abduction of the extended hip, the head of the femur comes to lie on the pubic ramus opposite the iliopectineal eminence.

Clinically the hip is held in full extension, slightly flexed with up to 60° of abduction.

Low type

An external rotation and abduction force on the flexed hip results in the head of the femur coming to lie near the obturator foramen. Clinically, the limb is externally rotated in extension with some abduction. Reduction is effected by adducting the femur and medially rotating it. The head of the femur can be gently lifted into the acetabulum.

Dislocation of the hip associated with fractures of the acetabular rim

Posterior dislocation of the hip may be associated with a marginal fracture of the posterior lip of the acetabulum. The fragment is usually held closely to the head of the femur and reduction of the dislocation usually results in accurate replacement of the fragment. Occasionally if a large fragment is not reduced and the hip remains unstable in flexion, adduction and internal rotation, then operative reduction and fixation of the fragment with a single screw is indicated. Stable hips are treated as ordinary dislocations.

Complications of dislocation of the hip

Sciatic nerve palsy

Ten per cent of dislocations of the hip are associated with sciatic nerve palsy and in 80% of these the lesion is incomplete, affecting only the peroneal division. A nerve injury is much more common if there is an associated marginal fracture of the acetabulum. Operative intervention to decompress an injured sciatic nerve is reserved for those cases with an associated fracture. Straightforward dislocations with sciatic nerve injury are managed conservatively with expectation of recovery of function.

Irreducible dislocations

It is rare not to be able to reduce a hip. Inability to reduce the dislocation with a satisfying clunk or a non-concentric reduction on the 'post-reduction' film means that there must be soft tissue or interposed bony fragments. In these cases the hip must be explored and the offending impediments to reduction dealt with appropriately.

Avascular necrosis of the head of the femur

This is a late complication of dislocation of the hip affecting 10 % of uncomplicated dislocations, 25 % of cases with an associated fracture of the acetabulum and 50 % of cases where there is also a fracture of the femoral neck.

Indications for operation

- Failure of reduction or non-concentric reduction of the hip because of soft tissue or bony interposition.
- Sciatic nerve injury in dislocations associated with a marginal fracture of the acetabulum.
- The unstable hip with a posterior acetabular fracture. The fragment of the acetabulum needs to be fixed with a screw.

Central fracture-dislocation of the hip

These are often part of a multiple injury and can easily be missed.

Group 1   This is a result of a 'dashboard and sideswipe' injury—pressure along the axis of the femur plus a blow to the greater trochanter. The weight-bearing portion of the acetabulum remains intact. Most commonly the head of the femur is medially displaced or posteriorly dislocated. Less often it is dislocated anteriorly.

Group 2   Direct injury to the greater trochanter and the pelvis results in a true central dislocation of the hip with comminution of the acetabulum including the weight-bearing area and the head of the femur pushed centrally through into the pelvis. A genitourinary injury is often associated with this fracture.

Management

Initially the patient is resuscitated and the affected limb placed in Hamilton–Russell traction. Associated injuries that have priority are treated.

Group 1 fracture-dislocations   Open reduction and fixation is required:
- When the head of the femur is completely displaced from under the weight-bearing area and there is only one large bony fragment.
- When the head of the femur is partially displaced, lying partly in contact with the weight-bearing area and partly in contact with the displaced fragment.

Group 2 fracture-dislocations   Treated conservatively with Hamilton–Russell traction for 6 weeks. Full weight-bearing is achieved by 3 months.

FRACTURES OF THE NECK OF THE FEMUR
(intracapsular and extracapsular fractures)

Most patients who sustain this injury are elderly females. However, no age or sex is exempt. In children and young adults the treatment of choice is internal fixation.

Treatment of fractures of the neck of the femur in the elderly is surgical if cardiac and pulmonary problems related to prolonged recumbency are to be avoided.

Intracapsular fractures

A lateral rotation strain to the lower limb transmitted to the femoral neck fractures it at or near the subcapital level. The problems of non-union and late avascular necrosis associated with this fracture are due to disruption of the retinacular blood vessels which cross the fracture. This may result in ischaemia to the femoral head.

Garden's classification (Fig. 20)

Grade I   Incomplete fracture of the femoral neck. The inferior cortex is not breached.
Grade II   Complete fracture of the femoral neck including the inferior cortex. No displacement has occurred.
Grade III   Complete fracture in which partial displacement has occurred. The distal fragment rotates laterally while the proximal fragment rotates medially and is

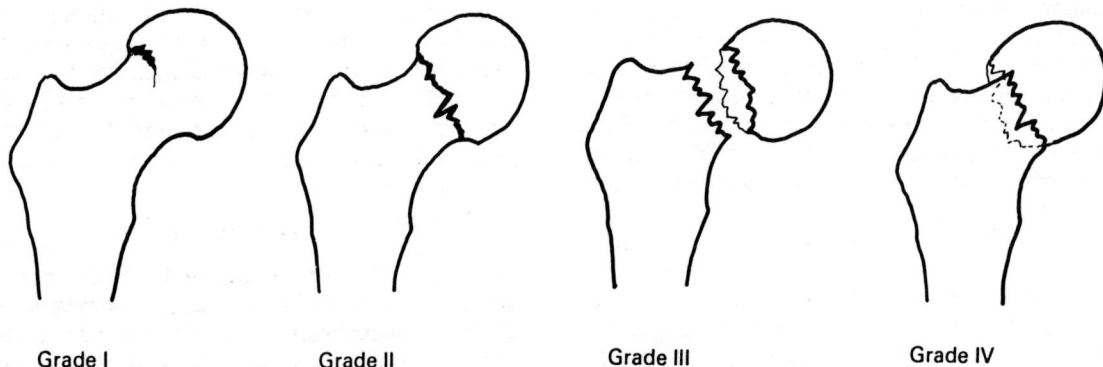

Grade I   Grade II   Grade III   Grade IV

Fig. 20 Garden's classification of intracapsular fractures

abducted. In clean breaks the posterior retinacular attachment remains intact.

Grade IV   Complete fracture with full displacement. Contact between the fragments is lost. The distal fragment is laterally rotated. The proximal fragment resumes its normal position within the acetabulum.

Treatment

Grades I and II

Internal fixation is the treatment of choice either by crossed screws or by closed nailing under image-intensified X-ray control. A sliding nail plate is preferable to a single pin. The incidence of avascular necrosis in these groups is low since the blood supply to the head of the femur is only minimally disturbed.

Grades III and IV

In these groups the incidence of avascular necrosis is high. This is thought to be due to a severe valgus deformity of the head of the femur.

Some surgeons maintain that the fractures in these groups should be perfectly reduced and internal fixation achieved with a sliding nail plate. Others advocate prosthetic replacement of the head of the femur (e.g. with a cemented Thompson prosthesis) in order to avoid the complication of avascular necrosis and the subsequent necessity for a second operation.

Extracapsular (or trochanteric) fractures

In this type of fracture, union can usually be relied upon. To enable the early mobilisation of the patient and to avoid union with a coxa vara deformity, some form of internal fixation is necessary.

Classification and treatment

Stable fractures

Type I   The proximal fragment consists of the head and neck of the femur alone. Having no muscular attachments, the proximal fragment lies in the neutral position except in the slightly displaced fracture when it rotates laterally with the distal fragment. The fracture can be anatomically reduced by internally rotating the leg.

Type II   The proximal fragment consists of the head, neck and major part of the greater trochanter. The proximal fragment is laterally rotated and the fracture can only be reduced by external rotation of the leg.

Treatment is accurate anatomical reduction followed by internal fixation with a nail plate.

Unstable fractures

These are fractures with loss of continuity of bone cortex between the opposing surfaces of the proximal and distal fragments, either as a result of complete separation of the posterior trochanteric fragment or comminution of the calcar femorale medially.

Classically four fragments are seen: the head and neck of the femur, the greater trochanter, the lesser trochanter and the shaft of the femur. The problem with this fracture is that, despite anatomical reduction and internal fixation, a high percentage of the internal fixation devices fracture or migrate, resulting in union with a varus deformity of the neck of the femur.

The high failure rate has led to modifications of the traditional pin and plate fixation since it does not restore stability to the fracture. One modification is fixation of the fracture with medial displacement of the distal fragment followed by the insertion of a nail plate. Another method is to use curved intramedullary nails. These are introduced through the medial condyle of the femur and guided across the fracture into the femoral neck under image-intensified X-ray control.

1.34. Peripheral Vascular Disease

Acute or chronic limb ischaemia is the usual mode of presentation of peripheral vascular disease. However, it must be stressed that peripheral perfusion is related not only to the patency of the arterial tree, but also to the efficiency of the cardiac and venous pumping mechanisms, and to the quality and viscosity of the blood.

ACUTE ISCHAEMIA

Sudden main artery blockage leads to immediate pallor, loss of distal pulses, progressive cooling, sensory loss commencing distally, rest pain, and muscle weakness and tenderness. Progression to limb death may occur within 6 h, but this period may be much longer, depending on collateral flow; spontaneous recovery occurs in some cases.

Causes

Arterial trauma, embolism, thrombosis and dissection. Rarer causes are severe vasospastic disease, frostbite and ergot. The usual problem is to distinguish between embolism and thrombosis. Thrombosis may be precipitated by a hypotensive episode or heart failure and is suggested by a history of claudication and evidence of atherosclerosis elsewhere; the clinical picture is less dramatic than that of embolism. Embolism is suggested by dramatic onset, atrial fibrillation, mitral stenosis, recent myocardial infarct, subacute bacterial endocarditis or proximal aneurysm.

Management

Intravenous heparin immediately on diagnosis of acute occlusion. Full cardiovasular assessment and ECG. If thrombosis is the likely cause, a short period of observation with the bed head elevated and use of plasma expander, e.g. Dextran 40, may be justified. Persisting peripheral sensory loss indicates the need for intervention. Major embolism must be treated with an emergency embolectomy as soon as possible provided the limb is still judged to be viable. Cardiac output should be improved first if possible. Most lower limb emboli can be removed through one or both common femoral arteries under local anaesthesia, using Fogarty catheters. Wide below-knee fasciotomies may be advisable after restoration of flow. If the major vessels cannot be cleared with Fogarty catheters, arteriography should be performed immediately in order to assess the feasibility of arterial reconstruction.

CHRONIC ISCHAEMIA

Causes

Arteriosclerosis obliterans is by far the commonest cause. Others include Buerger's disease, popliteal entrapment, cervical rib, arteritis and vasospastic conditions. Diabetes is an important contributory factor.

Arteriosclerosis obliterans

Affects mainly males and older females. Intimal deposits become widespread in large and medium-sized arteries, leading to progressive narrowing. Final occlusion is followed by secondary thrombosis proximally and distally to the next sizable branch. Aetiological factors include smoking, hypertension, hyperlipidaemia, diabetes and heredity.

Distribution of atheroma is widespread but patchy with predilection for certain sites (related to haemodynamic factors). Peripherally it affects particularly the femoropopliteal segment, distal aorta and iliac arteries and the lower leg arteries, with a tendency to spare the profunda beyond its origin and the distal popliteal artery. Arteriosclerosis may weaken the media and lead to aneurysm, particularly in the infrarenal aorta and the popliteal arteries. Diabetes leads to premature onset of arteriosclerosis and a tendency to small vessel involvement, as well as to neuropathy and liability to spreading infection in the feet.

Clinical picture of peripheral ischaemia

Intermittent claudication

Femoropopliteal disease leads to calf claudication; aortoiliac occlusion causes claudication pain in buttock, hip, thigh or calf and is often associated with impotence (Leriche syndrome).

Severe ischaemia (rest pain and gangrene)

May be caused by repeated minor embolism by thrombotic material from more proximal ulcerated plaques or stenoses, or more often by multiple levels of occlusion usually including at least two of the three main below-knee arteries. It is particularly common in diabetics, although gangrene in diabetes is often precipitated by infection in a neuropathic foot rather than main vessel ischaemia. Drugs such as β-blockers may precipitate ischaemia by reducing the heart rate so that it is unable to cope with exercise (relative ischaemia). The intake of these drugs should therefore be terminated.

Examination

Assess patient's 'biological' age. Look at cardiovascular system as a whole, including blood pressure, search for carotid bruit, upper limb pulses, abdominal aorta for aneurysm. In affected limb(s) look for colour changes, wasting, loss of hair, trophic lesions, venous guttering on elevation, and dependency rubor. Feel for temperature changes; assess and record all pulses. Listen for bruits and measure ankle/brachial systolic pressure index. In claudicants measure walking distance and re-examine the limb at the onset of claudication; this will help distinguish ischaemic from neurogenic claudication due to spinal stenosis.

Investigations

Should include full blood count, erythrocyte sedimentation rate (ESR), serum lipids, fasting blood glucose, ECG and ultrasound. The Doppler ultra-

sonic probe is placed over the posterior tibial or dorsalis pedis and pneumatic cuffs are placed around the thigh, calf and ankle. The cuffs are inflated one at a time to record the lower limb cuff occlusion pressure, which is compared with the brachial artery upper limb pressure and expressed as a ratio (pressure index). Normally the ratio is more than 1 but in ischaemia it is less than 1 and can give a numerical assessment of the impedance to flow at different levels down the limb as well as indicating the level at which the pressure gradient is steepest.

Aortography is only considered when surgery is contemplated. Surgical intervention is indicated in:
- Disabling intermittent claudication
- Rest pain
- Distal gangrene (due to distal embolisation from a proximal disease)

Management

For claudication immediate management should be conservative with advice to stop smoking, modify diet, if necessary, and to exercise to encourage collateral development. Reassurance that only some 10% eventually come to amputation should be given. Progress should be observed over several months, after which those whose enjoyment of life or ability to work is seriously impaired may be considered for reconstructive surgery, provided they have stopped smoking. Aortography then becomes essential, and this must be done without delay in those presenting with limb-threatening ischaemia, so that a limb-saving procedure can be undertaken if feasible. In patients with multiple levels of occlusion it is essential to deal with the proximal lesion first. For example, in aortoiliac cases restoration of good pulsatile flow to the profunda is usually effective in the presence of a femoropopliteal block.

BUERGER'S DISEASE (THROMBOANGIITIS OBLITERANS)

This affects younger, mostly male, patients who smoke, often with a history of thrombophlebitis migrans. Thrombosis and inflammation commence in the smaller arteries of the hands or feet and spread proximally. Foot claudication, rest pain and gangrene may develop. Distal pulses are lost first. Cessation of smoking is vital and will stop progression of the disease. Lumbar sympathectomy may help and conservative amputation may be successful for gangrene. Prostaglandin E_2 infusion may help the patient during an exacerbation.

RAYNAUD'S PHENOMENON

Attacks of digital ischaemia are provoked by exposure to cold or emotion.

Primary (Raynaud's disease)

Occurs mostly in young women, is bilateral and unassociated with other disease. Tissue loss rarely occurs. Treatment is by reassurance and advice on avoidance of exposure to cold. Sympathectomy is rarely of more than temporary benefit.

Secondary

Usually starts later in life and sooner or later an underlying disease becomes manifest particularly scleroderma or CREST syndrome (calcinosis, Raynaud's phenomenon, oesophageal involvement, sclerodactyly and telangiectasis). It also occurs in other collagen diseases, with long use of vibrating tools, as a complication of certain drugs, in polycythaemia and dysproteinaemias and as a manifestation of proximal arterial lesions such as those caused by cervical rib. In severe cases plasma exchange often produces great improvement for a few months, perhaps by lowering blood viscosity.

SURGICAL METHODS IN PERIPHERAL VASCULAR DISEASE

Transluminal angioplasty

Forcible balloon dilatation via the common femoral artery appears to be a useful method, best suited for stenoses and short occlusions in the iliac artery. Long-term results are uncertain but the procedure is simple for the patient and does not prejudice later open reconstruction.

Thromboendarterectomy

Mainly used for short blocks in large arteries.

Bypass graft

The method of choice for long occlusions. A preclotted knitted Dacron graft is best for aortoiliac or aortofemoral bypass, the latter often combined with profundoplasty. Autogenous reversed saphenous vein is best for femoropopliteal bypass with umbilical vein homograft or PTFE as an alternative when the patient's saphenous vein is absent or less than 4 mm in diameter. Profundoplasty can be done if femoropopliteal bypass is impossible. An alternative is femorodistal bypass, using *in situ* saphenous vein after destroying the valves. Grafting should never be undertaken in the presence of more proximal obstruction, and in claudicants only if the run-off is good. In limb salvage procedures a poor run-off may be acceptable.

Extra-anatomical grafts

Femorofemoral cross-over graft is useful in poor-risk subjects with unilateral iliac block. Axillobifemoral grafting can be used in similar subjects for aortic or bilateral iliac occlusions, or for replacement of an infected aortic graft.

Lumbar sympathectomy

Unlikely to benefit claudication but useful for mild ischaemic rest pain and small areas of skin necrosis. Chemical destruction of the chain by phenol injection under X-ray control is a useful alternative to surgical sympathectomy, particularly in the elderly.

Amputation

Required for intractable rest pain and gangrene when reconstruction is not feasible or has failed. Below-knee amputation using a long posterior flap should always be preferred when the blood supply permits, i.e. in many patients with obstructions below the common femoral.

For patients unsuitable for below-knee amputation, knee disarticulation or Gritti-Stokes amputation is preferred in elderly patients because of the longer lever provided. Standard above-knee amputation permits better fitting of a knee joint mechanism and is used in younger patients. Prophylactic penicillin should be used for all amputations for ischaemia.

1.35. Stroke and Surgery

Stroke is a disturbance of cerebral function which occurs in vascular disease. It results from inadequate blood flow or microembolism caused by atheroma which has become detached from the carotid bifurcation. When the focal neurological defect lasts only a few minutes and does not persist for more than 24 h it is called a *transient ischaemic attack*; when the attack lasts more than 24 h but is reversible it is called *reversible ischaemic neurological defect*. *Stroke in evolution* denotes the step-like development of a focal neurological defect occurring over a few hours or for up to several weeks. *Completed stroke* is the stable end stage. Stroke is the third largest killer (after heart disease and cancer) in those over 50 years of age and is the most crippling of disabilities. Patients with carotid disease and transient ischaemic attack, who are treated medically with aspirin and dipyridamole (Persantin) have a stroke risk of 15–20 %, but when treated surgically (e.g. endarterectomy) the stroke risk becomes 4 %, indicating the significance of surgical treatment in stroke.

Aetiology

- Atherosclerosis mainly affects the carotid bifurcation in more than 50 % of cases. Other sites in decreasing order of frequency are the vertebral, left subclavian, external carotid, innominate, right subclavian and left common carotid arteries.
- Aneurysms of the brachiocephalic system may be post-traumatic, mycotic, syphilitic, post-radiotherapeutic or dissecting as well as atherosclerotic.
- Arteriovenous fistulae (congenital or acquired).
- Congenital malformations, kinks, coils and bands occur in the carotid region.
- Rare arterial conditions, i.e. fibromuscular hyperplasia, medial wall necrosis, diffuse arteritis, giant cell arteritis, scleroderma, drug-induced stenoses and adjacent inflammatory cervical nodes.
- Carotid body tumours.
- Extracranial factors, e.g. hypercoagulability, severe hypertension, thrombosis due to, e.g. pregnancy, contraceptive pill, polycythaemia.

Indications for investigations

- Transient motor or sensory disturbance
- Transient speech impairment
- Visual disturbance and amaurosis fugax
- Stroke
- *Hollenhorst* plaques in retina
- Asymptomatic bruit

Investigations

- Oculoplethysmography and Doppler ophthalmic test
- Non-invasive Doppler scanner
- Digital subtraction venous angiography
- Direct selective arch arteriogram

Surgical treatment

General anaesthesia with induced *hypo*carbia. This protects damaged cerebral tissue by the so-called Robin Hood effect since *hyper*carbia increases the cerebral blood flow to normal tissue at the expense of any damaged areas (intracerebral steal). Regional or local anaesthesia may also be used.

There are three operative choices, selected according to the level of the disease.

Disease of aortic arch and its branches

Dealt with by bypass procedures using a graft with or without endarterectomy, e.g. aortic bifurcation graft, corticosubclavian, axilloaxillary, subclavian-subclavian, corticoaxillary, axillofemoral bypass. The vertebral artery needs endarterectomy via a longitudinal arteriotomy in the subclavian artery.

Carotid artery disease

1. Endarterectomy is the commonest procedure. The patient is placed in the supine position with the head rotated and flexed towards the opposite side; a sand-bag is placed under the shoulders.
2. Incision along the anterior border of the sternomastoid muscle. Dissection, exposure and mobilisation of the external and internal carotid arteries away from the common carotid bifurcation, using sharp dissection, in a plane close to the vessel wall (in this way the carotid chemo- and baroreceptor regions and the carotid sinus nerve are not damaged). Do not manipulate or compress the junction to avoid dislodgement of atheroma into the internal artery; this will cause embolism and stroke in the same way that trash foot is caused in abdominal aortic manipulation. Proximal and distal control using slings then follows.
3. Heparin 7000 units i.v. is given before the three carotid vessels are clamped; then the longitudinal arteriotomy across the bifurcation is extended into the internal carotid artery.
4. The use of shunt is controversial. Some argue that one should *never use shunt* (due to air embolism); others that you should *always use shunt*; and a

third group maintains that shunting should be *selective*.

5. Endarterectomy is performed followed by closure of arteriotomy.

6. Suction drain and closure.

Other operative choices for carotid disease include caroticocarotid saphenous vein bypass with bilateral endarterectomy of carotid bifurcation. For kinks, loops and coils of the internal carotid artery various angioplastic techniques are available.

Intracranial disease

Cerebral revascularisation is needed for persistent neurological damage. Extracranial intracranial anastomosis is used. The superficial temporal artery is anastomosed to a branch of the middle cerebral artery via a single burr hole or craniotomy using a microsurgical technique.

1.36. Critical Review of Early Breast Carcinoma Management

At presentation, 20% of breast cancer cases represent advanced disease (M_1) and 80% are potentially curable (by surgery) = early breast carcinoma (Stage I and II or T_1, T_2, N_0, N_1, M_0). At least 40% of the latter become advanced after 10 years. Thus, about 60% end finally with an advanced disease.

Early breast carcinoma (T_1, T_2)	Advanced breast carcinoma (M_1)	
80% at presentation	20% at presentation	
40% (N_0)→20% =	8% after 10 years	60%
40% (N_1)→80% =	32% after 10 years	total

Thus early diagnosis and treatment are essential. Breast cancer is the commonest cause of death in females between 35 and 55 years of age, and over 10 000 females per year die from breast carcinoma in the UK.

Diagnosis

The usual work-up includes:
- Clinical examination and staging.

- Good mammography (for patients over 35 years of age, should include two views oblique and craniocaudal showing all the beast tissue). Signs of malignancy include microcalcification, increased density and architectural disturbance.
- Aspiration to differentiate between solid or cystic lesions (outpatient).
- Fine needle aspiration biopsy-cytology (FNABC), or Tru-cut needle biopsy under local anaesthesia (if FNABC not available), is a desirable outpatient procedure for preoperative diagnosis of solid tumours. This approach is much better than the policy of 'excisional biopsy—frozen-section—? proceed with mastectomy' because one can tell the patient in advance whether she is going to have a mastectomy or not.

The above four methods are done routinely. However, one can also search for distant metastases: up to 25% of early breast carcinomas diagnosed clinically show skeletal metastases on bone isotope scanning, leading to the belief that the breast cancer is a systemic disease from the start. The search includes:

Physical means
- Conventional chest X-ray.
- Skeletal survey.
- Skeletal isotope scan. Metastases show as 'hot spots' and so does a healed fracture, Paget's disease of bone and degenerative osteoarthritis; X-ray of doubtful areas may resolve this ambiguity.
- Isotope-labelled colloid scanning for liver secondaries—if hepatomegaly present.
- Grey scale ultrasonography.
- CT scan for mediastinal and retroperitoneal masses, if suspected.

Biochemical markers
- Alkaline phosphatase and glutamyl transaminase—raised in liver metastases.
- Urinary calcium and hydroxyproline—raised in bone metastases.
- Calcitonin, carcinoembryonic antigen (CEA), specific milk protein—may indicate residual tumour after mastectomy.

Comment

- FNABC is becoming a very popular means of diagnosis of almost all solid tumours (e.g. thyroid, breast, lymphadenopathy, salivary tumours, prostate, testis) with no documented risk of tumour spread into blood vessels. The procedure is very simple. A 20 ml plastic disposable syringe with a No. 1 or 21 gauge needle is inserted into the tumour after skin cleansing with an injection swab. Then suction is applied while the syringe is passed into the mass of the tumour in three or four directions to disturb and dislodge tumour cells. The syringe is withdrawn and the contents are blown onto a clean slide which is dried in air, labelled and fixed in ethanol and stained by Papanicolaou or haematoxylin and eosin for direct microscopic examination. The remaining tumour fragments and tissue juice in the syringe can be mixed with saline and injected into a test tube for cytological examination of the floating cells. Remember that in splenic, hepatic and abdominal puncture, clotting factors should be normal and local anaesthesia is required. There is no need for prophylactic antibiotics.

- Any discrete breast mass or mammographic abnormality is best removed so that the surgeon is certain that it has been removed and it can be examined histologically. Also psychologically, the patient is happier without it.
- Breast lipoma should not be trusted—perform mammography since it may be a pseudolipoma with underlying breast carcinoma (producing a fibrofatty mass due to infiltration along Cooper's ligaments).

Current concepts of surgical treatment

- Breast carcinoma gains direct access to blood and to vital organs early in the course of its development (systemic disease).
- Tumour cells reaching a lymph node (LN) are not necessarily trapped there but can either traverse the LN intact or bypass the LN via lymphovenous communications.
- Internal mammary LNs are involved in 28 % of all breast cancers, 25 % of laterally placed cancers and 50 % of medially placed cancers; in 5–10 % of cases they are involved before axillary LNs.
- If axillary LNs are involved, 40 % of internal mammary glands are involved already.
- Lymph nodes themselves are regarded as actively hostile to the proliferation of tumour cells owing to the inherent tumoricidal capacity of immunologically competent host cells in these lymph nodes. Therefore if lymph nodes are not involved, this represents a favourable tumour-host relation which may be unbalanced by

removal or radiation of such immunologically competent lymph nodes. If lymph nodes are involved, this indicates that the disease is already widely disseminated owing to exhaustion of host-restraining factors and in this case the treatment of lymph nodes is important for symptomatic relief, but it does not increase the cure rate. Lymph nodes are not a nidus for secondary spread and their involvement is merely a sign of poor prognosis. The outcome of treatment is predetermined by the extent of micrometastasis at the time of diagnosis and not influenced by the extent of local therapy.

- The breast should be removed for the following reasons:
  - To prevent local recurrence.
  - To control the disease locally so that at the very least if the patient dies of her metastases, she is not also troubled by an ulcerating, painful, offensive lesion on her chest which may be further complicated by lymphoedema of the arm due to malignant infiltration of axilla.
  - In order not to leave the patient in doubt.
  - Removing the bulk of the tumour and involved regional lymph nodes leaves a sufficiently small tumour burden for which host defence factors may be adequate, and gives radiotherapy a better chance of achieving palliation. Recently wide excision of a tumour followed by radiation of the breast and draining lymph node areas has given promising results with minimal disfiguration (see Table 6).

Current concepts of radiotherapy

- Normal tissues should never be irradiated prophylactically because of X-ray complications:
  - Skin reaction.
  - Lung fibrosis.
  - Painful bone atrophy, joint destruction and stiffness.
  - Lymphoedema.
  - Decreased immunity, which may accelerate the appearance of metastasis and reduce survival.

As a primary modality in early breast cancer, radiotherapy alone has been used with cure in some cases but the uncertainty about the long-term outcome compared with surgery (no controlled trials) and the danger of radiation-induced neoplasia make such an approach unwise.

- Aims of radiotherapy are:
  - To control possible residual disease at the margins of a surgical resection.
  - To destroy cells implanted or seeded in the operative field.
  - To sterilise lymph nodes not removed at operation.
- Postoperative radiotherapy does protect against local and skin recurrence but treatment of recurrence by radiotherapy when it appears is equally effective. The number of patients with local recurrence persisting until death is the same in the two groups.
- Ten-year survival is identical in extended radical mastectomy and simple mastectomy; thus the extension of treatment by surgery or radiotherapy beyond the breast and axillary lymph nodes does not improve survival.
- Recurrence-free survival rate is identical in simple mastectomy and radical mastectomy when both are followed by radiotherapy, indicating that surgery and radiotherapy are equally effective in treating axillary lymph nodes when these are involved by metastatic disease.
- It is important not to irradiate the axilla after radical or modified radical mastectomy because the combined treatment is a major cause of clinically significant arm lymphoedema.

Table 6. Treatment policies for early breast carcinoma (modified from Forrest, 1969)

Surgery	Radiotherapy	Reference and remark
Supraradical mastectomy (clavicle and supraclavicular LN removal + as below)	— —	Wangensteen, 1950 Andreassin and Dahl-Iversen, 1949 (abandoned)
Extended radical mastectomy (internal mammary LN removal + as below)	—	Urban and Baker, 1952 (abandoned)
Radical mastectomy (breast + axillary LNs + pectoral muscles)	Variable	Halsted, 1894 (uncommon)
Extended simple mastectomy = modified radical mastectomy (as above leaving pectoralis major)	Variable	Patey and Dyson, 1948 (common)
Simple mastectomy (breast only)	— Postop. X-ray	Crile, 1961 McWhirter, 1955
Subcutaneous mastectomy + breast reconstruction	—	Watts, 1976 (limited use)
Simple mastectomy with pectoral or lower axillary LN sampling	Variable, depending on LN involvement	Forrest and Kunkler, 1968 (very common)
QUART = QUadrantectomy + Axillary dissection and Radio Therapy	Postop. X-ray	
Extended tylectomy	Postop. X-ray	Atkins, 1972 (common)
Lumpectomy or tumorectomy	Radium implant Postop. X-ray	Keynes, 1930 Porritt, 1964 (common)
—	Radiotherapy alone	(uncommon)
Surgery + adjuvant chemotherapy CMF (cyclophosphamide, methotrexate and 5-fluorouracil) or tamoxifen	—	Milan Study, 1981 (Rossi *et al.*, 1981)
—	Tamoxifen alone	Preece *et al.*, 1982 (common in women over 70 years of age)

Treatment rationale (Table 6)

The aim is to achieve local control of the disease with minimal morbidity. The principles are:

- Surgery or radiotherapy should be given only to sites of proven involvement.
- Excessive removal or radiotherapy of normal tissues which are not involved by tumour increases morbidity but not cure.
- The presence of substantial axillary lymph node involvement indicates that the disease is incurable.
- Involved lymph nodes are equally well treated by radiotherapy as by surgical clearance of axilla.

The most commonly used policy is simple (total) mastectomy with axillary sampling (followed by radiotherapy if nodes are involved). This prevents intraclavicular hollowing and lymphoedema. The disadvantages are false negative axillary sampling (inadequate staging) and a high local recurrence rate; postoperative radiotherapy may therefore be required.

Patey's modified radical mastectomy is also employed and has the advantage of no infraclavicular hollowing. Intramuscular recurrence is rare, and leaving the pectoralis major gives a better cosmetic result with no bridle-like tight scar. With an axillary clearance as good as in radical mastectomy this procedure represents a good compromise and avoids the need for postoperative radiotherapy. Local excisions of macroscopic tumour (lumpectomy, tylectomy), formal quadrantectomy, or partial mastectomy with or without axillary sampling can all have a beneficial cosmetic and psychological result. Since breast cancer is multifocal in 30% of cases the recurrence rate is high and unacceptable without routine postoperative radiotherapy in local approaches. Adjuvant early radiotherapy or chemotherapy (CMF or perioperative cyclophosphamide) or hormonal therapy (Tamoxifen) could be used in addition to the surgical treatment—trials are awaited.

1.37. Urinary Stone

Stones are formed as Carr concretions or Randall's plaques. They are either primary (metabolic in origin in a normal urinary system and normal acidic urine pH) or secondary (non-metabolic in origin; due to infection, dehydration and alkaline urine pH).

There are four types of urinary (or renal) stones according to composition:

- Calcium oxalate—mulberry calculi (80–85%).
- Triple phosphate, i.e. calcium, magnesium and ammonium phosphate—staghorn calculi (10%).
- Uric acid stones (10%).
- Cystine calculi and xanthine stones (1%).

Urinary stones are classically radiopaque in 90% of cases. Uric acid and xanthine stones are radiolucent (10%).

Aetiology

Metabolic causes

- Hypercalcaemia in primary hyperparathyroidism, sarcoidosis, vitamin D intoxication, milk-alkali syndrome and ectopic parathormone secretion, e.g. hypernephroma and bronchogenic carcinoma.
- Primary hyperoxaluria.
- Hyperuricaemia in gout, protein catabolism, e.g. leukaemia, and in cytotoxic drug therapy.

Non-metabolic causes

- Dehydration in tropical areas (e.g. Burma) and chronic diarrhoea cases (e.g. Crohn's disease and ileostomy).
- Infection with urea-splitting organisms, e.g. *Eschirichia coli*, *Bacillus proteus*, streptococcus and staphylococcus, leads to alkaline urine and stone formation which leads to obstruction, stasis and perpetuation of infection (vicious circle).
- Residual stagnant urine (stasis) due to immobilisation or distal obstruction leads to infection and stone formation, e.g. a stone-causing pelviureteric junction obstruction and hydronephrosis can lead to a secondary stone in the proximal urine (different in composition from the primay one).
- Congenital, e.g. medullary sponge kidney with congenital calyceal cystic calcification (a similar condition is papillary necrosis which occurs in drug abuse and other, rare, conditions).
- Diet (e.g. excess milk or oxalate-containing food) or deficiency of urinary inhibitors of crystallisation (decreased acid mucopolysaccharides or increased uric acid) together with less fluid intake may lead to supersaturation of urine with crystalloids (increased calcium, oxalate, pH or decreased volume).

Clinicoradiological grading (Fig. 21)

Grade 1 A small stone usually metabolic (Mulberry spiky stones) subdivided into: (A) immobile, e.g. asymptomatic stone in lower calyx (no need for surgery); or (B) mobile (surgery indicated if over 0.5 cm in diameter or symptomatic, i.e. causes haematuria or is intrapelvic with ball-valve obstruction).

Grade 2 Usually metabolic in origin causing pelviureteric junction obstruction possibly with haematuria, backache and urinary tract infection (minimal symptoms). Pyelolithotomy is required.

Grade 3 Usually infective in origin; occasionally metabolic with multiple calculi in pelvicalyceal system of the kidney (soon forms staghorn calculus). Nephrolithotomy is required.

Grade 4 Infective in origin. The staghorn calculus moulded to the shape of the pelvicalyceal system with kidney calcification as an end-result of Grade 3. Nephrectomy is required.

Investigations

● Abdominal plain X-ray, intravenous urethrography to see function and whether one or two

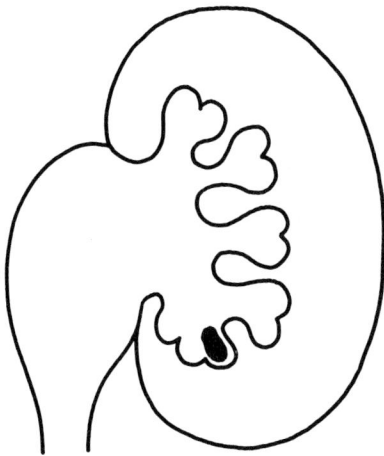

Grade 1

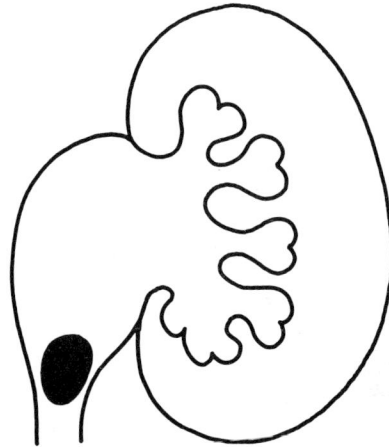

Grade 2

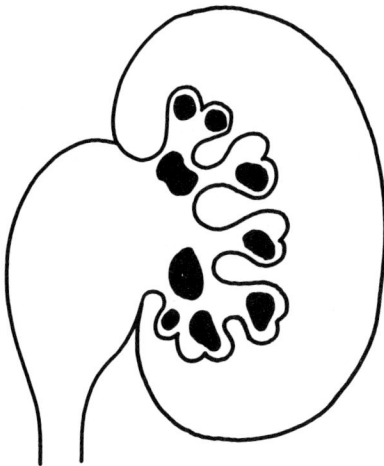

Grade 3

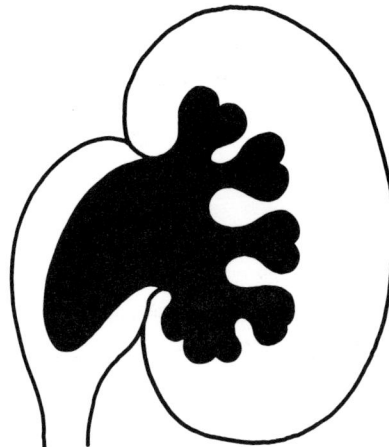

Grade 4

Fig. 21 Clinicoradiological grading of renal stones

kidneys are present (urgent IVU in renal colic), MSU (look for red blood cells—microscopic haematuria) with culture and sensitivity.

- Blood urea, creatinine and serum electrolytes, calcium and phosphorus with blood protein (low proteins lead to false low calcium level).
- Alkaline phosphatase and acid phosphatase (in case of skeletal metastases from prostatic carcinoma with hypercalcaemia), uric acid and 24 h urinary calcium (normally 2.5–7.5 mmol/24 h urine collection) phosphate, urate and oxalate.
- Parathormone (PH) assay is required in suspected primary hyperparathyroidism (increased PH and increased Ca^{2+}).
- Radioactive isotope scan (renogram) to assess bilateral renal function is important.

Types of treatment

Prophylactic conservative

Used in small (less than 0.5 cm in diameter) asymptomatic stones. Includes:
- High fluid intake achieving high daily urine output.
- Dietary advice (avoid excess milk and oxalate-containing food). In areas with hard water supplies, ask patients to use water softener before drinking. (Hard water is bad for the kidneys but claimed to be good for the heart and cancer, i.e. the incidence of coronary heart disease and cancers is low in hard water areas.)
- Treatment of urinary tract infection (combined high fluid intake, urinary antiseptic and urinary alkalinisation).
- Thiazide diuretics—useful hypocalcaemic agents in recurrent calcium-containing stones. Allopurinol is used in hyperuricaemia and uric acid stone prophylaxis.

Surgical treatment

Prophylactic

- Correction of hyperparathyroidism by removal of parathyroid adenoma because in these cases the nephrocalcinosis is irreversible. The patient feels better and further stones are prevented (hyperparathyroidism is a disease of stones, bones, abdominal groans—peptic ulcer and pancreatitis and psychic moans).
- Correction of any distal urinary obstruction responsible for proximal stone formation.

Similarly, prostatic obstructive uropathy should receive treatment priority over associated renal stones.

Therapeutic

Surgery is indicated:
- For obstruction. Manifested clinically by pain, chemically by high urea and creatinine, and radiologically by impaired renal function both on IVU and renogram.
- For infection. Especially in obstructed cases since the change of hydronephrosis into pyonephrosis has a grave outcome.
- For stones over 0.5–1 cm in diameter, whether symptomatic or not, and below that if symptomatic, causing severe pain and/or haematuria. All staghorn calculi should be operated on once diagnosed.

Principles of surgery

To preserve as much as possible of the functioning renal tissue and to prevent complications (e.g. obstruction, infection and severe pain, malignancy and rarely stricture formation).

Anaesthesia (by induction, halothane) may lead to decreased urine output after renal surgery in an already dehydrated patient. Thus, there is no place for hypotensive anaesthesia in renal surgery.

Special considerations

- In bilateral kidney stones, operate on the most painful side first then on the other side.
- In bilateral kidney stones with one non-functioning (bad) kidney, operate on the healthy side first then perform nephrectomy on the bad kidney.

Available approaches (Fig. 22)

A lateral approach through a subperiosteal 12th rib excision or lumbotomy (lumbar sympathectomy-like incision) provides direct posterior intrarenal access for stone removal (impossible anteriorly owing to the renal vessel). One of three methods can be used (the functional renal reduction is expressed in percentage terms).
- Simple or extended sinus pyelolithotomy of Gil-Vernet, 1965 (0%). Extended pyelolithotomy is done by dissecting through the renal sinus and lifting the kidney substance from the renal pelvis.

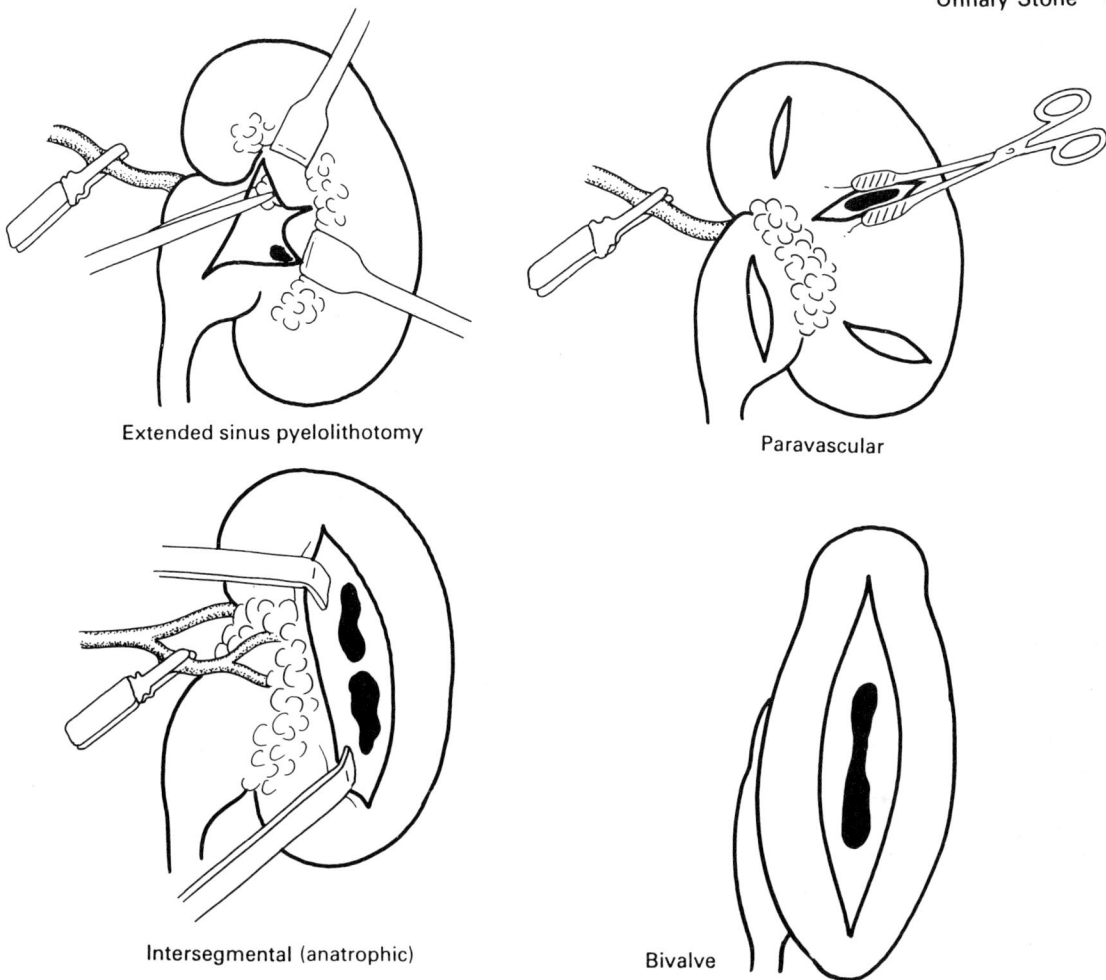

Fig. 22 Approaches for nephrolithotomy

- Paravascular radial approach of Wickham *et al.*, 1974 (20%).
- Intersegmental anatrophic approach of Boyce and Elkins, 1974 (30%).

The bivalve approach (50%) is very traumatic and should not be used. While the operation is in progress, vascular arrest may be necessary and hypothermic preservation is achieved with slush ice, external coils or by the intra-arterial method. Sometimes systemic i.v. inosine is used. Arterial clamping is used frequently while cooling the kidney and the clamp should be released every 10 min (a 1 h operation therefore requires six clamping releases and applications). An ischaemic time of 60 min leads to 70% intrarenal depression which will return to normal in 14 days; 120 min ischaemia leads to 100% depression with only partial re-

covery; 180 min ischaemia leads to 100% depression and no recovery.

After stone extraction (in order that all residual stone fragments are discovered and extracted):

- Carry out a contact nephrogram on the table checking the preoperative IVU on the viewing box from time to time.
- Use syringe and good irrigation with saline.
- Use finger manipulation.
- Carry out pyeloscopy on table (like choledochoscopy).
- Rarely coagulum pyelolithotomy is used. A material is injected that sets and moulds with the stone pieces and can then be extracted in one large piece (the pelviureteric junction should be secured beforehand).

Percutaneous nephroscopy

Used in intrapelvic primary renal stones or residual recurrent ones. A good interventional radiologist is needed to create the track into the renal pelvis using IVU and ultrasound guidance. A fascial dilator is used followed by an angioplasty balloon catheter and then rigid concentric rods to prepare for the nephroscopic stone retrieval. Direct stone extraction is done by:

- Ultrasonic disintegration 27 000/s (lithotripsy denotes crushing stone *in situ* while litholapaxy denotes crushing the stone, and washing it out)
- Extracorporeal electrohydraulic spark shock wave destruction with the patient lying in a water bath under general anaesthetic.

A Malecot catheter is left *in situ* (like a T-tube left after biliary stone extraction) and a nephrostogram is done 24 h later so that any remaining fragments can be seen and removed. The procedure may lead to residual renal stones, retroperitoneal extravasation and bleeding from the renal artery (requires renal arterial embolisation or even nephrectomy if bleeding is uncontrollable) and ureteric obstruction by fragmented stone. Contraindicated in:

- Staghorn calculus.
- Higher stones under 12th rib.
- Embedded peripheral calyceal stones.
- Impacted pelviureteric or high ureteric stone.
- Stones in solitary or horseshoe kidney.

Recurrent renal stone

Usually due to a missed metabolic cause (hyperparathyroidism) or persistent urinary tract obstruction or infection. The patient should be investigated thoroughly, e.g. stone screen including serum, calcium, phosphorus urate, oxalate and alkaline phosphatase as well as 24-h urine collection for calcium, phosphate and urate. Prophylactic conservative and surgical treatment should be stressed. Percutaneous nephroscopy has a place in the treatment.

Ureteric stones

Upper ureteric and pelviureteric junction: approached like kidney stones.

Mid-ureter: iliac lumbotomy (like lumbar sympathectomy).

Lower ureter: approached either cystoscopically (using Collin's knife meatotomy and manipulation with ureteric catheter or Dormia basket extraction) or through a suprapubic open approach.

Recently, flexible fibreoptic ureteroscopy has been introduced for intraureteral litholapaxy, biopsy and fulguration of ureteric transitional cell carcinomas.

1.38. Urinary Diversion

Indications

- To maintain renal function by relieving the obstructive uropathy and clearing the infection.
- To improve urinary continence, e.g. in cystectomy, ectopia vesicae, neurological bladder and an incurable vesicovaginal fistula.
- When sphincteric mechanism is diseased or removed.

Types

Temporary diversion

Nephrostomy Indicated in:
- Uraemia or acute obstruction in a solitary kidney.
- Pelvic or gynaecological operation with ureteric damage—percutaneous nephrostomy.
- Congenital urethral valves in male children (Foley's or Malecot's catheter could be inserted through the thin cortex of the kidney).

Percutaneous nephrostomy can: serve as a temporary or permanent urinary diversion; provide diversion to allow distal fistula to heal; provide a route for splinting the ureter as well as extracting renal stones.

In adults, kidney mobilisation and opening through the kidney pelvis (not cortex) are important. There are two types of nephrostomy in adults—percutaneous and ring nephrostomy. The catheter in the latter can be changed and irrigated easily and works very well.

Pyelostomy

Ureterostomy (not very satisfactory) Constructed as loop or Y-shaped in children. In adults a ureterostomy *in situ* is used (via an appendicectomy-like muscle-cutting incision and ureteric catheterisation).

Suprapubic bladder drainage

Urethral drainage

Permanent diversion

Reservoir Includes ureterosigmoidostomy with various modifications, trigonosigmoidostomy and rectal bladder. Ureterosigmoidostomy could be done with a colonic conduit or rectal bladder (and permanent colostomy). It is contraindicated in the presence of:
- Upper urinary tract dilatation.
- Urinary incontinence (neurological problem) since this leads to faecal incontinence.

Complications include:
- Infection. If there is increased pelvic colonic pressure, longitudinal colonic myotomy is indicated together with the treatment of infection with antibiotics.
- Ureteric obstruction with recurrent pyelonephritis.
- Troublesome diarrhoea with hyperchloraemic hypokalaemic metabolic acidosis (with vomiting, thirst, acidotic breathing and coma). Hypokalaemia damages the kidney further.
- Development of malignant disease is not uncommon in diversion. In rectal bleeding therefore one should not do a barium enema (causes ascending infection) but colonoscopy to see and biopsy the possible bleeding rectal polyp.

External stoma Includes cutaneous ureterostomy in children, vesicostomy (difficult to attach bag to) and anterior transposition of urethra in females (rarely done).

Intestinal conduit Using ileal, colonic or ileocaecal segment. Most common is the ileal conduit formed by anastomosing the two ureters to one end of the segment and bringing the other end to the surface as a spouting ileostomy (or urostomy).

Complications are:
- Stomal stenosis, needing revision (since increased intraureteric pressure eventually leads to kidney infection).
- Pyelonephritis (in 18% of cases).
- Renal stone formation (in 10% of cases), due to urine stagnation and kidney infection.
- Intestinal obstruction—early postoperative complication in up to 15% of cases.
- Pyocystis is a problem in neurological bladder cases, if the bladder is not removed.
- Hyperchloraemic acidosis in ileal conduit—may occur but rarely.

Criteria for successful ideal diversion

- Continence with voluntary control of urine and faeces.
- Complete separation of urinary and faecal streams.
- Functioning urinary reservoir without absorptive problems.
- Absence of unnatural or artificial orifices.
- Accessible to endoscopic assessment.

1.39. Urothelial Tumours, Kidney Tumours, Testicular Tumours

UROTHELIAL TUMOURS

Include tumours arising from the transitional cell epithelium of the urinary tract, i.e. transitional cell carcinoma of the urinary bladder, renal pelvis and ureter. Rarely urothelial metaplasia with subsequent squamous cell carcinoma occurs in the urinary bladder (due to bilharziasis) and in the renal pelvis (due to chronic irritation of a renal stone). They generally present with haematuria and are diagnosed by midstream urine examination (MSU), urine cytology, intravenous urography (IVU) and cystourethroscopy.

Aetiology

Occupational, e.g. aniline dye workers exposed to α- or β-naphthylamine, benzidine, auramine or magenta dyes (carcinogenic).

Inflammatory, e.g. bilharziasis (*Schistosoma haematobium* infestation) or chronic inflammation due to bladder stone.

Congenital, e.g. urinary diverticulum or adenocarcinoma developing in the urachus (remnant attaching bladder fundus to umbilicus).

Miscellaneous, e.g. smoking and abnormal tryptophane metabolism (leading to a carcinogenic metabolite). Benign bladder papillomas are rare and may transform into the usual malignant tumours by the time of presentation.

Histological grading

G1   Well differentiated.
G2   Moderately undifferentiated.
G3   Highly undifferentiated (or dedifferentiated or anaplastic).

Staging

Determined by a combined clinical (bimanual examination under anaesthesia), cystoscopic evaluation and histology (Fig. 23).

T_{IS} Flat carcinoma *in situ* confined to the epithelium.

T_a Papillary carcinoma confined to the epithelium.

T_1 Papillary carcinoma involving the epithelium and invading lamina propria.

T_2 Tumour has invaded detrusor muscle layer.

T_3 Tumour has extended into the perivesical fat but is still mobile.

T_4 Tumour has infiltrated into the contiguous structures and is fixed.

Lymph node spread is only assessed during operations on bladder tumours (N_1: regional lymph nodes involved; N_2: juxtaregional or bilateral lymph nodes involved; N_3: fixed). Metastasis in bladder tumours is uncommon. The prognosis depends on *staging* and *histological grading*.

Salient features of bladder tumours and management

T_{IS}

There is no exophytic tumour, but abnormal mucosa with positive cytology. Occurs mostly in males and presents mainly with unusual symptoms (e.g. frequency, dysuria, urethral and/or perineal pain). Haematuria is not a predominant presentation. If T_{IS} is localised diathermy is required but if

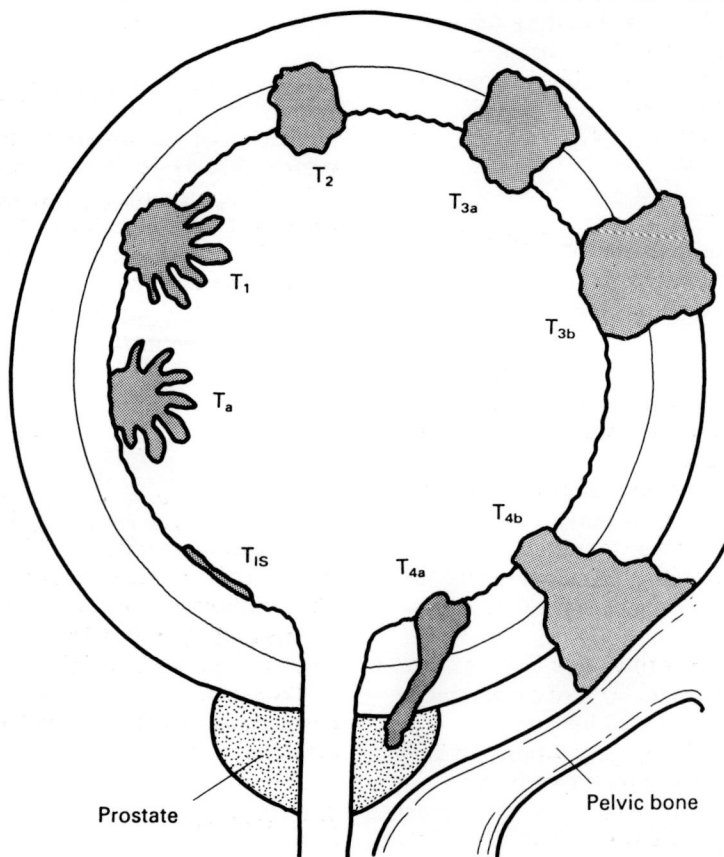

Fig. 23   Bladder cancer—staging

widespread then cystourethrectomy is necessary. There is a role for intravesical adriamycin or i.v. cyclophosphamide (but not for radiotherapy).

Superficial tumours (T_a, T_1)

- Are the commonest and respond best to treatment.
- Usually well differentiated and do not invade beyond the lamina propria.
- Sometimes invasion is limited to the core of the papilla but may be deeper.
- Have tendency to recur rather than to invade.
- Overall 5 year survival is 80%.
- Treatment is by any of the following approaches:
  - Endoscopic diathermy (destruction) or resection (TUR) are the commonest treatments.
  - Open excision.
  - Partial cystectomy.
  - Cystourethrectomy.
  - External radiotherapy.
  - Intracavitary radiotherapy.
  - Intracavitary chemotherapy, e.g. thiotepa, ethoglucid (Epodyl), can give 60% of patients a disease-free period of 1 year.
  - Helmstein balloon therapy (cystodistension under epidural anaesthesia for half an hour) is rarely successful.
  - Hyperthermia.
  - Mucosal stripping.

Invasive tumours T_2, T_3, and T_4

T_2

- Difficult to diagnose (since the invasion may be superficial and just beyond lamina propria).
- Tumour less than 2 cm and G1 or G2 is treated endoscopically (TUR).
- Tumour greater than 2 cm or G3 is treated with radiotherapy.
- There is a role for partial cystectomy.
- 5 year survival is 50%.

T_3

- Incidence of positive lymph node at operation.
- Cystourethrectomy alone (5 year survival is 25%).
- Radical deep X-ray therapy (6000 rad) + salvage cystourethrectomy (5 year survival is 40%).
- Preoperative deep X-ray therapy (4000 rad) + radical cystourethrectomy (5 year survival is 38%).

- Flash deep X-ray therapy (2000 rad) + radical cystourethrectomy (5 year survival is 40%).
- Urethra must be removed because:
  - It is involved in 18% of bladder tumours (urothelial tumour is multiple).
  - Carcinoma *in situ* risk.
  - Poor prognosis in urethral recurrence.

T_4

Inoperable, poor prognosis. Treated with:
- Palliative radiotherapy or
- Chemotherapy (methotrexate or cis-platinum).

Renal pelvis tumour

When the *pelvicalyceal system* is involved the tumour tends to be more invasive and highly malignant. Treatment is by partial nephrectomy or even more radical excision, i.e. nephroureterectomy with sleeve resection of the bladder.

When the *pelviureteric junction* is involved, treatment is by radical excision, i.e. nephroureterectomy with partial cystectomy.

Ureteric tumours

Midureter: treatment is local resection with end-to-end anastomosis or cross-ureteroureterostomy.

Lower end of ureter: the treatment is by local excision, opening the bladder and making a Boari flap or transureteroureterostomy especially if a long segment is involved.

Upper end of ureter: nephroureterectomy and partial cystectomy.

KIDNEY TUMOURS

Wilms' tumour of children
(10% of renal tumours)

A connective tissue tumour accounting for 20% of all malignancies in children, usually within the first 7 years of life (adult Wilms' tumours are very rarely reported); presents mainly as a loin mass and less frequently as haematuria. Should be differentiated from hydronephrosis, multicystic kidney and neuroblastoma.

Investigations

- IVU shows grossly distorted kidney. Bilateral kidney involvement occurs in 10% of cases.

- Abdominal ultrasound is helpful in children.
- Chest X-ray (and no further investigation).

Management (depends on age of child)

Below 2 years of age Adjuvant chemotherapy within 24 h before surgery. The tumour should be removed via the anterior abdominal approach to allow for extension (into a long subcostal or thoracoabdominal incision in case the intestine is stuck to the tumour when performing nephrectomy) and also for examination of the other kidney which if involved requires partial nephrectomy. Postoperative adjuvant radiotherapy is also used.

Over 2 years of age Combined chemotherapy using two agents, actinomycin D and vincristin, is curative in 80% of cases.

Clear cell carcinoma or adenocarcinoma (75% of renal tumours)

A common tumour that originates from cortical proximal tubular cells (adenocarcinoma) and affects males over 40 years of age. Usually mixed and its presentation is disguised in a number of ways.

Loin pain, lump and haematuria Occur in a third of cases and should be differentiated from splenomegaly or hepatomegaly and, if the pain is diffused, from renal stones.

Systemic manifestations Due to immunological reaction provoked by kidney tumour, e.g. profound anaemia (6–9 g/dl), increased ESR (greater than 100), pyrexia of unknown origin, abnormalities in liver function tests such as high alkaline phosphatase or high calcium. The patient may be intolerably ill and miserable (carry out IVU to reveal renal cancer).

Endocrinal manifestations Due to hormonal secretion (normal or ectopic), i.e. renin (secreted by ischaemic part of the kidney distal to the tumour) leads to hypertension, abnormal ectopic parathormone secretion leads to hypercalcaemia and erythropoetin secretion leads to polycythaemia (though generally anaemia is commoner).

Metastatic manifestations for the first time e.g. backache, collapsed vertebra, fractures (skeletal); or lung (solitary usually) or brain deposits.

Rare presentations e.g. Budd-Chiari syndrome and left testicular varicocele.

Investigations

- IVU especially its nephrogram phase in 1 min film. If inconclusive then 1–2 ml/kg contrast medium is needed with tomography to see the outline of the kidney showing a lump at one pole.
- Abdominal ultrasound can confirm whether the lump is solid or cystic with 95% accuracy; if cystic can be aspirated for cytology followed by injection for cystogram to see its outline (ultrasonic guided aspiration leads to 99.9% cure of simple benign cysts).
- If the lump is solid, or the cystic aspirate is bloody, the surgeon can proceed with operation without the need for arteriography (and its complications). However CT scan is now regarded as the third step to produce the final diagnosis (CT scan has replaced arteriography).
- Venogram (rather than arteriography) is sometimes needed to see if the vena cava is involved, especially in right renal tumours.
- Chest X-ray to discover any solitary metastasis (relevant to the management since lobectomy could be performed).

Treatment

Mainly surgical. Nephrectomy via the anterior abdominal approach is preferred. However, subperiosteal lateral extraperitoneal approach is recommended if it is certain that the inferior vena cava is clear of tumour lumps. Pulmonary lobectomy is practised in solitary metastasis.

Radiotherapy and chemotherapy are useless but hormonal therapy is worth trying by giving Provera 100 mg three times daily—response is good in 30% of males and 5% of females. If there is no response testosterone 100 mg three times weekly can be given.

The prognosis is directly related to the stage of spread (Stage 1: kidney; Stage 2: perinephric fat; Stage 3: vascular/lymphatic involvement; Stage 4: distant spread). In Stage 1, 5 year survival is 65%.

Renal pelvis tumours (10% of renal tumours)

See Urothelial tumours.

TESTICULAR TUMOURS

Usually occur in men under the age of 40 years. They are fortunately rare as there are no benign testicular tumours (all are malignant). The types are closely related to age: in babies—orcheoblastoma; in young men (20–30 years)—teratoma; in middle-aged men (30–40 years)—seminoma; and in the elderly—lymphoma. The germinal group represents 96% of all testicular tumours (seminoma and teratoma) while the non-germinal group (Sertoli cell, Leydig cell tumours) and paratesticular tumours (lipo-, lienomyo-, fibro-, neuro- and rhabdomyo- sarcomas) together constitute less than 4%.

There are various types of teratoma, named differently according to the British and American classification:

Teratomas (British)	Non-seminomas (American)
Malignant teratoma differentiated (MTD)	Teratoma
Malignant teratoma undifferentiated (MTU)	Embryonal carcinoma
Malignant teratoma intermedia (MTI)	Teratocarcinoma
Malignant teratoma trophoblastica (MTT)	Choriocarcinoma

Chemotherapy is effective and can change MTT into MTI and MTI into MTU.

Local spread of testicular tumour is exceptionally rare because of encapsulation within tunica albuginea. However, it spreads to iliac, para-aortic, mediastinal and supraclavicular lymph nodes and sometimes to lung (extralymphatic).

Testicular tumours are staged accordingly into:

Stage I   Tumour is confined to testis.
Stage II Para-aortic abdominal lymph node involvement.
Stage III Supraclavicular (thoracic supradiaphragmatic) lymph node involvement.
Stage IV Lung involvement (extralymphatic).

Carcinoma in situ has recently been recognised in infertile males (found in testicular biopsy), in males with undescended testicles, in contralateral testis of patients with testicular tumours and in intersex patients.

Diagnosis

- Painless rapid testicular enlargement (heavy with increased size and same shape).
- Painful testis in 15% of cases after minor trauma.
- Secondary hydrocele in 5% of cases.
- Advanced spread, e.g. para-aortic abdominal masses, supraclavicular lymph nodes, haemoptysis (lung metastasis).
- Gynaecomastia.

Clinical examination with fingers is the most reliable method of detection.

Investigations

- Blood for β-human chorionic gonadotrophin and α-fetoprotein (tumour markers).
- Chest X-ray.
- IVU to exclude ureteric displacement by para-aortic lymph node enlargement.
- Urine examination and full blood count are sent routinely to differentiate testicular tumour from epididymo-orchitis. Post-traumatic haematocele is difficult to differentiate since testicular tumour may also start after trauma; exploration will therefore be the final answer.
- Early exploration via inguinal incision (never scrotal since this leads to local spread). A soft clamp is applied to the cord at the internal inguinal ring, the testis delivered and examined (any procedure can be freely carried out after clamping with no risk of blood-borne metastases). If it is obviously cancer then carry out orchidectomy; if in doubt, slice open and send for a frozen section taken from the cut surface (if proved to be cancer carry out orchidectomy but if a benign lesion is discovered then tunica albuginea incision can be sutured with no risk of atrophy). The scrotum remains untouched.
- Once the histological confirmation is obtained, a meticulous search for metastases is to be followed by lymphangiography and CT scanning of retroperitoneal tissues and mediastinum as well as whole lung tomography (staging for proper treatment).

Treatment

In seminomas (always treat one stage ahead, i.e., therapeutic treatment of the clinical stage plus prophylactic treatment for possible subclinical microscopic spread):

Stage I   Orchidectomy and prophylactic retroperitoneal radiotherapy.

Stage II   Orchidectomy and prophylactic retroperitoneal and mediastinal radiotherapy.

Stage III   Orchidectomy with combined (retroperitoneal and mediastinal) radiotherapy and chemotherapy.

Stage IV   Orchidectomy and chemotherapy.

The common agents are cis-platinum, vinblastine and bleomycin. The 5 year survival in Stage I is 90%.

In teratomas the treatment is similar but prophylactic chemotherapy is given first and if it fails then radiotherapy. (If radiotherapy is given first, it may damage the bone marrow and restrict the dosage of chemotherapy that can be given subsequently.) Surgery (thoracotomy or laparotomy) is needed for removal of bulky masses and for radical retroperitoneal lymph node dissection (marginally better than retroperitoneal radiotherapy). It is acceptable now that the cure rate is 90% in stage I and 80% in the presence of metastases.

1.40. Prostatic Carcinoma

Includes three main groups:

Clinical carcinoma: diagnosed clinically on the basis of combined obstructive uropathy and findings (on rectal examination) of hard, irregular prostate with obliteration of sulcus or with a nodule. The clinical diagnosis is confirmed histologically.

Latent carcinoma: found incidentally with no clinical evidence of the disease.

Occult carcinoma: the primary tumour manifests itself by secondaries in its first presentation.

The incidence of prostatic carcinoma is low in populations with short life expectancy (it is rare before the age of 40 years). It is claimed to be greater in married men and urban people, less in Jews. There is evidence for a hormonal association, based on:

- Regression following castration or oestrogen therapy.
- Multiple endocrine changes in postmortem specimens.
- Correlation with male breast carcinoma.
- Biochemical studies.
- Incidence of prostatic carcinoma in cirrhotics.

The carcinoma usually arises from the peripheral prostatic zone; thus, open prostatectomy (for benign glandulocystic fibromuscular prostatic hyperplasia which arises from the central zone) does not guarantee against future development of carcinoma.

Staging is based on T (primary tumour) progress:

T_0 No palpable tumour. Includes cases with incidental finding of carcinoma in an operative or biopsy specimen (also called Stage A).

T_1 Intracapsular tumour nodule surrounded by palpably normal tissue.

T_2 Tumour is still confined to prostate with smooth nodule deforming the contour of prostatic lobe or lobes but lateral sulci and seminal vesicles are not involved.

T_1 and T_2 are termed Stage B. Early cancer includes Stages A and B only.

T_3 Extraprostatic spread ± involvement of lateral sulci ± involvement of seminal vesicles.

T_4 Tumour is fixed and invading nearby tissues.

T_3 and T_4 are Stage C in the absence of metastasis and Stage D in the presence of distant metastasis. C and D are advanced cancer stages.

Such minimum requirements for assessment expressed by T_x cannot always be met and further investigations are required:

- Rectal ultrasound probe can assess the size, site and nature of the tumour. Ultrasound scanning can be done per urethram or transabdominally.
- Plasma biochemistry, i.e. urea, electrolytes, creatinine, acid and alkaline phosphatases.
- Radiology, i.e. chest X-ray, intravenous urogram, and skeletal survey.
- $^{99}Tc^m$ – polyphosphate bone scan.
- Cystourethroscopy and examination under anaesthesia.
- Biopsy (fine needle or Tru-cut punch needle via perineal (better) or transrectal routes) or transuretheral resection (TUR) biopsy (of prostatic chippings). Needle biopsy may lead to infection, bleeding, bacteraemma and septic shock. A prophylactic antibiotic is therefore recommended especially for the transrectal route.

Treatment options

Radical prostatectomy + radical inguinal lymphadenectomy   Popular in USA (not UK); used for

Stages A and B and claimed to have very good long-term results but with permanent impotence and urinary incontinence.

Radiotherapy Popular in UK and used alternatively for Stages A, B and C. The current trend is to use interstitial radioactive isotope therapy via needles inserted under ultrasound guide into the tumour area (after first being diagnosed with rectal ultrasound and then confirmed by biopsy). The prostatic carcinoma is a slow radiosensitive tumour, necessitating prolonged local radiotherapy applied to the disease area.

Hormonal therapy For advanced Stage D. This is the treatment of choice since skeletal metastases melt away and prostatic obstructive uropathy improves. Anti-androgen therapy is either medical or surgical. Medically, stilboestrol is commonly used initially in a low dose (e.g. 2–3 mg daily for 1 week) followed by a maintenance dose of 1 mg/24 h indefinitely. Alternatively, TACE (Tripara-Alnisil-ChlorEthylene) fosfestrol sodium (Honvan), or cyproterone acetate (testosterone antagonist) could be used in the presence of some stilboestrol side-effects (*see* Section 1.47). However, in patients with thromboembolic complications of stilboestrol or with a history of myocardial infarction, stroke or deep venous thrombosis (due to lymphatic or venous obstruction of the lower limbs or as a thrombotic complication of prostatic cancer *per se*) a surgical approach is preferred in the form of bilateral subcapsular orchidectomy.

Others TUR may be diagnostic, therapeutic (if 25% of the resected prostatic chippings prove to be cancer) or palliative in prostatic obstructive uropathy. On occasions no treatment is required apart from indefinite indwelling urinary catheterisation.

Currently there is emphasis on early diagnosis using ultrasound rectal probe and prostatic biopsy followed by curative treatment with radiotherapy or radical prostatectomy. Hormonal therapy is used less frequently.

Prostatic TUR versus open prostatectomy

TUR is indicated commonly in benign prostatic hyperplasia and in carcinoma when there is:
- Acute urinary retention. ⎫ Obstructive
- Chronic retention with ⎬ indications
  overflow. ⎭
- Prostatic bleeding.

Poor selections for TUR:
- Recent cardiovascular accident, Parkinsonism and neurological deficiency.
- Abdominoperineal resection of rectum (rectal examination is impossible for assessment of size or lifting the prostate during TUR).
- History of urinary frequency (nocturia, urgency and enuresis) due to detrusor instability which may become worse after TUR.
- Patients under age 55.

Open prostatectomy is indicated in:
- Very large prostate. May be best treated by an open operation, although an experienced surgeon (who can resect more than 1 g/min) can treat almost any size by TUR.
- Bilateral hip osteoarthritis or arthroplasty making lithotomy position of the patient impossible.
- Large bladder stones, which are impossible to crush and wash out endoscopically (litholapaxy).
- History of urethral stricture (relative).
- Bladder diverticula which require excision during operation (relative).
- Very long penile urethra (relative).

Complications of TUR

Bleeding May be primary (due to large gland or bleeding disorder). This should be treated by:
- Gauze tamponade on catheter pulled snugly on bladder neck.
- Local hypothermia.
- EACA (aminocaproic acid) intravesically to prevent further bleeding or intravenously.
- Hydrostatic pressure using continuous irrigation to wash out bladder clots (which encourage further bleeding).
- Evacuation of clots and blood transfusion.
- Bimanual pressure, e.g. one hand suprapubically and another rectally pressing against each other.
- Traction on the catheter to pull the balloon against resected prostatic bed (pressure haemostatic effect).
- Occasionally exploration ± direct intravesical pressure packing (removed after 48 h). Antibiotic prophylaxis is required.

Bleeding may be secondary due to: increased venous pressure on the 10th to 21st day postoperatively; bleeding prostatic bed granulations; or infection. This requires catheterisation with irrigation (*see above*) and antibiotics. Sometimes, endoscopy may be needed to diathermise the bleeding vessels.

Infection ($\pm$ septicaemia)   Originates from either the surgeon or the patient himself (either from pre-existing intravesical bacteria, bladder tumour or stone).

Epididymitis   May occur. Prophylactic vasectomy is recommended for repeated TURs.

Incontinence   Caused by sphincteric damage. Rare when special attention is given to the verumontanum. More common after open prostatectomy than TUR.

TUR syndrome   Dilutional hyponatraemia due to water intoxication secondary to excessive fluid absorption leading to decreased level of consciousness, fits and cardiac arrhythmias. Treated by decreasing the irrigation rate (with limited resection time and positioning the irrigating reservoir from less than 60 cm above the symphysis pubis), thiazide diuretic and Digoxin. TUR syndrome occurs even though the irrigating fluid is 1.5% glycine solution—a natural isotonic amino acid which does not conduct electrical current and does not affect the patient when absorbed (NaCl conducts and dissipates the electrical current, making electrical resection impossible).

Bladder wall perforation with extravasation of urine   Requires urethral catheterisation for at least 7 days, decrease or stoppage of continuous irrigation and prophylactic antibiotics. Also nasogastric suction and i.v. fluids in intraperitoneal bladder perforation (with signs of peritonism).

Urethral stricture and bladder neck stenosis (rare)

Prophylactic antibiotics in urology are indicated in:
- Urological conditions, i.e. bladder stone, large bladder tumour and preoperative urinary tract infection.
- Non-urological conditions, i.e. heart valve diseases, prostheses (including pacemakers) and immune suppression cases.

1.41. Introduction to Clinical Oncology

Neoplasia (or tumour) is defined as 'an abnormal mass of tissue, the growth of which exceeds and is uncoordinated with that of the normal tissues and persists in the same excessive manner after cessation of the stimuli which evoke the change'. It can be benign (localised, encapsulated, slowly growing by expansion and not fatal unless it causes mechanical obstruction or hormonal imbalance) or malignant (rapidly proliferating and locally invasive with systemic metastatic potential and fatal if not treated early). Histologically a benign tumour is similar to normal tissue while cancer is not. Neoplasia has to be differentiated from:

Hypertrophy—increased organ growth due to an increase in the size of its constituent cells (e.g. prostate).

Hyperplasia—increased organ growth due to an increase in cell number (e.g. thyroid).

Metaplasia—replacement by a cell type not normally present in an organ (e.g. inflammation and squamous cell metaplasia in urinary transitional epithelium).

Wound healing—although the actual mechanism is unknown, the rate of cell and tissue production exceeds that seen in most cancers; however, the presence of chalones, the local inhibitory factors, will prevent further cell division once the wound is healed. Absence of chalones could be a factor in neoplasia.

Development of cancer

Cancer passes through a four-phase evolution (chronic process).
1. Induction phase (15–30 years) with exception of radiation-induced leukaemia (2 years) and genetically determined cancers of infancy (shortly after birth).
2. *In situ* phase (5–10 years).
3. Phase of invasion—aided by cell multiplication, increased amoeboid cell motility, decreased cell cohesiveness, elaboration of lytic substances and lack of intercellular bridges found in all normal cells (e.g. hyaluronidase).
4. Phase of dissemination—by regional invasion (treated surgically and/or by X-ray therapy) and metastases which initially are micrometastases (treated by chemotherapy).

Types of cancer

The commonest cancers in the UK are, in order of frequency:
Solid tumours (over 90% of all cancers)
　　Lung
　　Colon and rectum

Breast
Stomach
Bladder
Prostate
Pancreas
Cervix
Non-solid tumours (haematogenous)
Hodgkin's lymphoma
Non-Hodgkin's lymphoma
Leukaemias
In females, breast and cervix uteri cancers are the leading malignancies.

Incidence

Varies according to the following factors.

Age

Cancers develops at any age but the risk increases with age, with the exception of early childhood cancers (leukaemia and central nervous system tumours) which carry a higher risk in the first 5 years of life than in the following 10 year period.

Sex

Average incidence is similar in both sexes, although the mortality in men is higher. However, under 10 years of age it is higher in males, between 20 and 60 years of age it is higher in females (due to breast and cervix uteri cancers), and over 60 years of age, the incidence tends to be higher in men.

Site of origin

- The rates for cancers of the upper gastrointestinal and of the respiratory tract are strikingly higher in men.
- The rates for gastric, reticuloendothelial and hematopoietic cancers are higher in men but not as markedly so as in the previous group.
- Cancers of the breast, reproductive organs and thyroid are more common in women.
- For all other sites the rates between sexes are similar.

Environmental factors

- Life habits, e.g.
  —Age at marriage, number of pregnancies, breast feeding—breast cancer
- Dietary and smoking habits, e.g.
  — Alcohol consumption—gastric cancer
  — Smoking—lung cancer
  — Reverse smoking (ignited end in mouth)— oesophageal cancer in South America
  — Bush tea drinking—hepatic carcinoma in Africa
- Socioeconomic status

Race

Cancers occur more frequently in non-Caucasian than in Caucasian people. Coloured males have more oesophageal, gastric, pancreatic, lung and prostate cancers and myelomas, while white males have more colonic and bladder cancers, melanomas, lymphomas and leukaemias. Coloured females have more oesophageal, gastric and pancreatic cancers and markedly increased rates of cervical cancer while white females have more breast, endometrium and ovary cancers.

Geographical distribution

May be specific to certain cancers although some have world-wide distribution. The following areas of predilection represent the highest incidences:
- Oesophagus (Central Asia)
- Stomach (Eastern Europe, USSR, Japan and Latin America)
- Large bowel (industrialised societies and Hawaiian Chinese)
- Liver (Africa and South East Asia; ? Europe)
- Pancreas (as large bowel)
- Larynx and hypopharynx (Western Europe, Assam, Burma, North Thailand and Egypt)
- Breast (developed communities and Hawaiian whites)
- Cervix uteri (Asia, Latin America and Africa)
- Prostate (Sweden)
- Urinary bladder (Egypt, South Iraq and Sudan)
- Melanoma (Australia)

Prognosis

Not only the length of survival but the quality of life after treatment must be considered. The average cancer mortality rates in developed countries are higher in men than in women. This is due to anatomical differences—in men there is a higher incidence of cancer of low curability (e.g. lung and gastric cancer) whereas in women the most common cancers are reasonably curable (breast and cervix cancers).

The arbitrary '5 year survival rate' is reasonably satisfactory. It includes patients both with and without residual or recurrent cancer; '5 year cure', however, includes only those patients apparently free of disease at the 5 year mark. The 5 year cancer-survival rates (in their localised stage and with regional involvement) are as follows. (These figures should be remembered at least approximately for the final FRCS examination):

Gastric	Early 63 %; advanced 10 %
Bladder	Early 72 %; advanced 21 %
Breast	Early 85 %; advanced 56 %
Colon and	
rectum	Early 71 %; advanced 44 %
Larynx	Early 79 %; advanced 37 %
Lung	Early 33 %; advanced 11 %
Oral	Early 67 %; advanced 30 %
Prostate	Early 70 %; advanced 61 %
Uterus	Early 83 %; advanced 46 %
Thyroid	Early 90 %; advanced ?

In fact, only 5 % or less of people with cancer of the lung, stomach, oesophagus or pancreas will be alive after 5 years. Factors bearing on prognosis include sex, age, pregnancy, hormone-dependence, histological grade, lymph node metastases, distant metastases and the interval between treatment and local recurrence or metastases.

The nature of the tumour is another factor (spontaneous regression and cure as well as multiple primary cancers). Spontaneous cure is an extremely rare phenomenon seen in neuroblastoma (children), bladder and renal cell carcinoma and malignant melanoma.

Multiple primary cancers may occur at the same time (synchronous) or at different times (meta-chronous). These are due to pre-existing multiple foci. This phenomenon is extremely common in skin colon and breast cancers, the incidence possibly rising to 20 % in patients cured 20 years earlier. In smokers, cancers of the mouth, larynx and lung are frequently multiple and development of cancer at one of these sites indicates an increased risk of cancer at the other site. Papillary thyroid carcinoma is also multifocal. Treatment itself (especially multi-modal) may result in a second primary cancer (both radiation and cytotoxic therapy are carcinogenic). However, certain genetic and immune deficiency states are the predisposing factors.

Tumour spread

Tumour is spread by direct invasion along lines of least resistance in surrounding normal tissues or by infiltration into epithelial structures, e.g. ductal carcinoma infiltrates the overlying epidermis leading to Paget's disease of the nipple. Local invasion without distant metastases occurs in basal cell carcinoma, craniopharyngioma, glioma and well-differentiated fibrosarcoma. Tumour spread occurs via:

- Lymph nodes by embolism or permeation; when lymph nodes are infiltrated and obstructed a retrograde spread occurs. Lymphatic spread becomes haematogenous when cancer cells enter the blood stream through the thoracic duct. Malignant melanoma and tongue cancer invade the lymphatics very early. Squamous cell carcinoma of the skin or lips spreads rather late. Basal cell carcinoma of the skin does not spread to lymph nodes.
- Blood by infiltration through small veins or vascular spaces of the tumour itself or following lymphatic spread. It is the common route in sarcomas. Lung, breast, kidney, prostate and thyroid cancers spread via blood early and lymphatically later. Body tissues have different affinities to metastasis. Liver, lungs, bone, brain and adrenal glands are common sites in that order. By contrast spleen, skeletal muscle and skin are very rarely involved. This selective affinity may be specific, e.g. metastases to spine and pelvis in prostatic carcinoma whilst a solitary lung metastasis would point to a renal carcinoma.
- Implantation, as in serous cavities when cancer cells gravitate to and land in the rectovaginal or rectovesical pouch. Cerebrospinal fluid (CSF) may act as a carrier in brain tumours. Urine may do the same in the spread of renal pelvis carcinoma to the bladder (although the theory of multicentric origin refutes this). Even the surgeon's knife may implant the cells in the operative wound causing recurrence later on.

Tumour structure

Macroscopic (gross) features

Benign tumours may be deep (solid or cystic) or epithelial. The projectile epithelial nodule is morphologically a polyp (pedunculated or sessile); if the epithelium is secretory it is called an adenoma. Cancers may be intraluminal, extraluminal or transmural (according to the direction of growth) and may be fungating (cauliflower), ulcerative (excavating) or annular (stricture) in hollow viscera, e.g. the gastrointestinal tract. In compact organs cancers may be solid (scirrhous) or cystic.

Microscopic (histopathological) features

According to the Broder classification, cancer can be well-differentiated (Grade I), moderately differentiated (Grade II) or undifferentiated (dedifferentiated, anaplastic; Grade III).

Tumour-host relationship

Benign tumours can cause serious mechanical obstruction of natural passages, e.g. trachea, ureter, intestine, intracranial and intraspinal sites. Endocrine tumours (phaeochromocytoma, Zollinger–Ellison syndrome) may also affect the host. Cancers can cause local destruction as well as haemorrhage, ulceration and secondary infection.

Systemically, cancers can cause: anaemia as in gastrointestinal tract cancer (e.g. gastric and caecal) as a result of chronic blood loss, malabsorption and bone marrow replacement; thrombophlebitis migrans in pancreatic cancer; afibrinogenaemia in prostatic cancer (haematological); central nervous system; demyelination, peripheral neuritis, myopathic weakness and dermatomyositis (neuropathic). Non-endocrine cancers, e.g. lung, may produce Cushing's syndrome, hypoglycaemia, hypercalcaemia and hyponatraemia (hormonal). Pulmonary osteoarthropathy could be produced by lung cancer. Immunologically, Hodgkin's lymphoma produces delayed cell-mediated hypersensitivity while lymphosarcoma induces a humoral immunoglobulin-induced hypersensitivity.

Cancer causes death in 50% of patients by virtue of its complications (e.g. ureteric obstruction and anuria in 50% of pelvic cancers, fulminating haemorrhage in cancers of the upper airways and upper gastrointestinal tract, intercurrent infection in cancers of airways, gastrointestinal tract and haematopoietic system). Few patients die from the consequences of the treatment (operative mortality is 25% in oesophageal cancers; operative or radiotherapy mortality is 3–4% in pelvic cancers due to late urinary complications or prolonged radiation of the lumboabdominal region with renal and digestive complications).

Cancer cachexia is the classic cause of death; it is a vague term covering a complex biological course (cancer cells concentrate alanine, methionine, histidine and isoleucine and thus compete with intestinal and hepatic cells leading ultimately to negative N_2 balance ending in death). Other causes of death are cardiac metastases due to direct invasion from primary lung and oesophageal cancers or to secondaries from lymphoma and melanoma. Major endocrine infiltration (e.g. adrenal and hypophyseal) is found in 30–35% of autopsies. Cerebral metastases inducing coma can cause sudden or rapid death.

Diagnosis

Early diagnosis of a cancer is directly related to the educational level of the public. Whether it is done on an individual basis (by history, physical examination and selected investigations, depending on the particular cancer) or on a population basis (mass screening), the aim is to detect early cases for successful treatment. The extent of the disease is evaluated by clinical staging, using either the TNM system or the traditional system (early—Stage 0 *in situ*; Stages I and II; and advanced—Stages III and IV). A treatment strategy is then planned.

Treatment

The therapeutic armamentarium includes single or multimodal treatment of surgery, radiotherapy and chemotherapy.

Surgical treatment

The major treatment (for most solid tumours). Its main limitation is that it is a localised treatment for a disease which may be systemic at the time of presentation, e.g. carcinoma of bronchus and breast. In early cancer, adequate radical surgery which eradicates the tumour with margins of normal tissue and regional draining lymph nodes is curative (while inadequate initial surgery leads to local recurrences). Surgery may be palliative (prolonging comfortable life), e.g. removal of gastrointestinal tract cancers causing bleeding and obstruction, amputation of limbs with painful bleeding sarcomas, mastectomy of ulcerating bleeding fungating breast, endocrine ablation, arterial infusion of cytotoxics (hepatic and carotid artery), urgent decompression of spinal cord tumours.

Surgery, however, has three other therapeutic aspects:

Preventive: by removal of premalignant and *in situ* lesions, e.g. familial polyposis coli and *in situ* carcinoma of cervix uteri.

Reductive or debulking: in the hope that chemotherapy and/or deep X-ray therapy may be able to contain or cure the micrometastases, e.g. childhood tumours.

Reconstructive: for those parts destroyed by initial therapeutic procedures (e.g. plastic procedures to restore the results of aggressive ENT surgery and prosthetic bone replacement for bone tumours).

Diagnostic: (e.g. staging laparotomy in Hodgkin's disease, mini laparotomy, exploratory laparotomy and various types of biopsies) should be distinguished from therapeutic surgery.

1.42. Radiotherapy

Ionised radiations damage both normal and neoplastic tissues (DNA strand breaks). However, normal tissues recover while neoplastic tissues do not, resulting in therapeutic benefit. A radiation dose is defined as the energy absorbed per unit of mass and is expressed in rads or in Grays (1 Gray = 1 joule/kg = 100 rad). Radiotherapy is used mainly for malignant tumours and rarely in benign tumours (e.g. thyrotoxicosis and some skin conditions). It may be palliative or radical.

Cancer response

Varies according to the following.

Type of cell May be very radiosensitive (e.g. reticulosis group, Wilms' tumour and seminoma), moderately sensitive (e.g. rodent ulcer, squamous epithelioma and transitional cell carcinoma) or variable (e.g. melanoma, thyroid carcinoma and osteogenic sarcoma). Sarcomas and recurrent tumours following previous irradiation are generally radioresistant. Note that while seminoma needs 2000 rad, Hodgkin's disease requires 4000 rad and squamous cell carcinoma of the larynx needs 6000 rad.

Differentiation of cells Radiosensitivity is directly proportional to reproductive activity and inversely proportional to the degree of cell differentiation; thus, germinal cells and spermatogonia are very sensitive while neurones are resistant (except medulloblastoma). Anaplastic cancers are generally radiosensitive.

Blood supply Anoxic cells are radioresistant, e.g. in large rapidly growing cancers or in association with syphilis or post-inflammatory scarring.

Hyperbaric O_2 increases the radiosensitivity of cancer.

Localisation The more localised the cancers the easier they are to control (e.g. basal cell carcinoma, carcinoma of the cervix) and the better the results (provided they are radiosensitive).

Assessment of tumour

Radiation is administered after the extent of the cancer has been accurately assessed by diagnostic radiography, surface anatomy, examination under anaesthesia and preoperative insertion of radiopaque markers around the target. Radiation dose depends on age, condition of patient, type of cancer and the target volume (the larger the cancer, the greater the number of radiation fractions). Deep-seated cancers are most often treated by multiple convergent beams or by rotational therapy.

Irradiation effects (total body)

Immediate
- Very high dosage (over 5000 rad single exposure) produces cerebral syndrome (nausea, vomiting, tremor, convulsions and death).
- Moderate dosage (800–5000 rad single exposure) produces gastrointestinal syndrome (nausea, vomiting, diarrhoea, dehydration and death).
- Low dosage (under 800 rad single exposure) produces haematological syndrome (mild initial nausea and vomiting but mainly bone marrow aplasia with panocytopenia manifested by infection and bleeding).

Late
- Premature ageing
- Cataract
- Sterility
- Fetal abnormalities
- Malignant disease
- Genetic effect

Local irradiation effect on skin (in chronological order)

1. Erythema followed by pigmentation.
2. Fibrinoid necrosis with vessel thrombosis leading to radionecrotic ulcer (painful, indolent, sloughing base, clean-cut edge).

3. Fibrosis with absent hair follicles and accessory glands (delayed healing in injury). Skin becomes atrophic with telangectasia.

Types of radiotherapy and administration

External beam irradiation

- Conventional X-ray therapy (orthovoltage 10–500 kV)—either superficial or deep.
- Megavoltage (1.2–40 MV) from:
  (a) γ sources ^{60}CO, ^{137}CS teletherapy.
  (b) X-ray sources from linear accelerator giving sharper, deeper but more expensive radiation.
  (c) Particle beam (electrons) from linear accelerator.
  (d) Betatrons (circular electron accelerators).
  (e) Cyclotrons and synchrotrons producing heavy particles, e.g. neutrons.
  (a) and (b) are electromagnetic radiations while (c), (d) and (e) are particle radiations.

Brachytherapy

Radioactive sources are inserted within or close to the cancer.

Intracavitory

Used mainly in gynaecology for treatment of carcinoma of cervix and corpus uteri. Radium, ^{137}Cs, ^{90}Y (bladder carcinoma) and ^{198}Au colloid (in malignant effusion—ascites or pleural) are used. One method involves insertion of a special applicator (under anaesthesia) which is left in for 24 h; this procedure should be repeated many times. The cathetron technique involves inserting a shielded ^{60}Co source holder under general anaesthesia after loading it mechanically from another room.

Interstitial

Involves application of moulds under general anaesthesia (e.g. radium and ^{137}Cs needles, ^{192}Ir, ^{192}Ta and ^{90}Y wires; ^{198}Au grains; and radon seeds). Used in tongue and bladder carcinoma. Can be used with surgery (unresectable tumour) in parotid and apical lung cancers.

Systemic radiotherapy

Uses ^{131}I (for thyrotoxicosis and thyroid carcinoma) and ^{32}P (for polycythemia rubra vera). It is given i.v. The materials are taken up preferentially by malignant cells in much higher concentrations than by normal cells.

Clinical uses

Radical radiotherapy (alone), with the aim of cure, e.g. squamous cell carcinoma of skin and oral cavity, vocal cord and laryngeal carcinoma and carcinoma of cervix uteri.

Planned combination of *surgery with radiotherapy*, e.g. seminoma (with improved 5 year survival of from 50% to 80%) and carcinoma of pharynx. Radiotherapy can be preoperative (as in hypernephroma) but is more commonly postoperative (as in breast carcinoma).

Planned combination of *cytotoxic therapy with radiotherapy*, e.g. late stage malignant lymphoma and head and neck tumours.

Palliative radiotherapy, e.g. in bronchogenic carcinoma to control profuse haemoptysis, bone pain, dysphagia, and obstruction of bronchus (dyspnoea) and superior vena cava; in breast carcinoma to control bone pain (due to metastases) and retrobulbar deposits causing proptosis.

Future advances in radiotherapy

Include administration of chemical and physical radiosensitising procedures such as:
- Hyperbaric oxygen.
- Hyperthermia (lethal to malignant cells).
- Misonidazol (with conventional X-ray).
- Use of particle radiation, e.g. fast neutrons, protons and negative pimesons (O_2 independent).

Special indications for surgery

When complete excision is possible, surgery is preferred to radiotherapy under the following conditions:
- Site is vulnerable to friction (sole of foot), moisture and infection (axillae), which favour radionecrosis.
- Underlying tissue is cartilage or bone, e.g. dorsum of hand, shin and pinna.
- Peritumour area is prone to malignant change so wide excision is indicated, e.g. vulva.
- Peritumour area is already damaged (e.g. by burns, scars, syphilis or previous irradiation) with anoxia prevailing, and radionecrosis of normal tissues is likely.

1.43. Chemotherapy

Drug treatment of cancer is varied. It includes:
- Cytotoxic, antineoplastic, or anticancer drugs.
- Endocrine therapy.
- Immunotherapy.
- Retinoid.
- Interferon.
- Systemic (metabolic) radiotherapy (i.v. radioisotopes).
- Supportive therapy (e.g. nutrition, antibiotics, analgesics).

CYTOTOXIC THERAPY

Cancer can be completely excised *en masse* (surgery) or it can be covered by a field of radiation (both means are localised and have limited value when the disease has disseminated). Cytotoxics may be used for both local and metastatic cancer. These agents affect both cancer and normal cells and are always cidal drugs unlike antimicrobial agents (affect bacteria only and are either bacteriostatic or bactericidal).

Cytotoxic therapy aims to bring about cure or prolong survival. These aims have been partially achieved in haematological and childhood cancers. Cure by cytotoxics alone has been reported in acute lymphatic leukaemia (children), Hodgkin's disease, Burkitt's lymphoma, Wilms' tumour, Ewing sarcoma and rhabdomyosarcoma. Prolonged survival has been demonstrated in acute leukaemia (adults), lymphocytic lymphomas, multiple myeloma and neuroblastoma. Among adult solid tumours the picture is far less encouraging. Cure has only been seen in relatively uncommon cancer, e.g. chorion carcinoma and seminoma. Prolonged survival has been claimed in ovarian and breast cancers.

Cytotoxics are given either as adjuvant 'prophylactic' chemotherapy over a prolonged period of time for patients presumably cured (by surgery and/or radiotherapy) to counteract subclinical microscopic micrometastases, e.g. early breast carcinoma, or as an aggressive multimodal therapy for certain disseminated cancers (e.g. childhood cancers which are relatively anaplastic and rapidly growing with high growth fraction); hence, a combination of radical chemotherapy, surgery and radiotherapy is used. Such carefully designed multimodal protocols (to treat other solid cancers in adults) are becoming more popular throughout the world.

Tumour growth (Fig. 24)

Synthesis of DNA occurs in a relatively short interval in the 'cell cycle', the pattern of which was revealed by radioactive labelled thymidine. Tumour growth in relation to DNA synthesis in the cell cycle is called tumour kinetics. The cycle passes through the following phases:

G_0	Some cells have division capacity but are temporarily removed from the cycle; suitably stimulated they move to G_1
G_1	Apparent metabolic rest
S	Synthetic period (of DNA)
G_2	Premitotic period
M	Mitosis (cell division)

A normal cell divides only to replace a lost cell (total cell number is constant). A cancer cell divides and adds to existing cells (total cell number is continually increasing). Tumour growth is the outcome of three combined parameters and is expressed as tumour doubling time (T_D) (the time it takes a given amount of tumour tissue to double its own volume). $T_D = 4-500$ days. Leukaemia and lymphoma have the shortest T_D followed by sarcoma with carcinoma having the longest T_D.
- Growth fraction (G_f) = the ratio of actively dividing cells to resting cells.
- Cell cycle time (T_c) = (for human cells) 40–80 h.
- Cell loss coefficient = the ratio of cells lost to cells produced. It is 100% for normal tissues (zero growth) and 95–99% in cancer. Reduced cell population is due to tumour cell loss caused by exfoliation by friction (skin and gastrointestinal tract), central necrosis, biologically inadequate cells, metastases (washed away) and destruction by host defences, or to the presence of resting cells (Table 7).

A cancer may therefore be viewed not as a mass of very rapidly dividing cells but as a tissue dividing at an approximately normal rate but failing to lose cells in the normal fashion and therefore gradually increasing in size. T_D is constant for any tumour, i.e. a cancer that can double its size in 2 days will have quadrupled its size in 4 days and be eight times its original volume in 6 days (such proportional increase in size with unit time is termed 'exponential growth'). The human body contains 5×10^{13} cells; a tumour is clinically detectable when it reaches 10^9

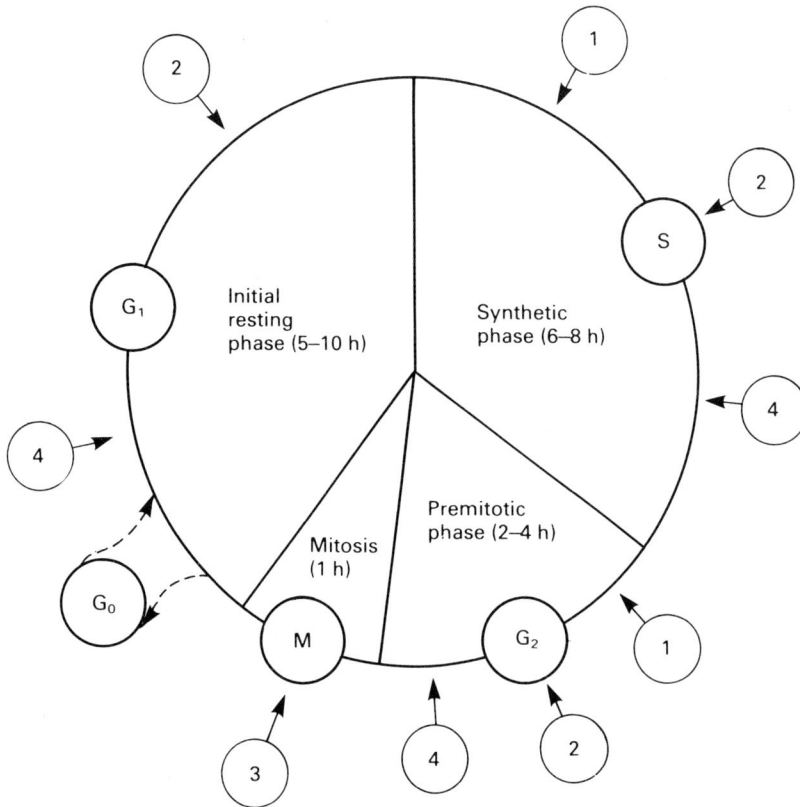

Fig. 24 Tumour cell growth cycle and sites of action of cytotoxics. 1—polyfunctional alkylating agents; 2—antimetabolites; 3—mitotic spindle inhibitors; 4—antitumour antibiotics

Table 7. Tumour cells

Dividing	Non-dividing
Tumour stem cells ⇄ Resting tumour cells	
Doomed cells (divide 4–5 times and then stop for biological reason)	End cells (though alive never divide)

cells $= 1$ g $= 1$ cm in size and when it reaches 10^{12} $= 1$ kg the patient is near death. A tumour is therefore clinically detectable and treatable during the last 10–14 of its 35–40 doubling times.

Classification of cytotoxic drugs

This is according to their chemical structure and mechanism of action (Fig. 24).

1. *Polyfunctional alkylating agents* Interfere with cross-linkage of DNA, e.g. nitrogen mustards (mustine, cyclophosphamide, chlorambucil, melphalan), thiotepa, busulphan and piposulfan.

2. *Antimetabolites* Interfere with nucleic acid synthesis because they are analogues of normal metabolites and act by competition, e.g. folic acid antagonist (methotrexate), purine antagonist (6-mercaptopurine), pyrimidine antagonist (cytosine arabinoside), halogenated pyrimidine (5-fluorouracil) and glutamine antagonist (Azaserine).

3. *Mitotic spindle inhibitors* Cause mitotic arrest and include colchicine and Vinca alkaloids (vinblastine and vincristine).

Plant alkaloids form a broad group (including cocaine, morphine, quinine, atropine and Vinca alkaloids).

4. *Antitumour antibiotics* Bind with DNA to block RNA production, e.g. adriamycin, daunor-

ubicin, mithramycin, actinomycin D, mytomycin C
and bleomycin.

5. *Miscellaneous*

- Antiproliferative enzymes (L-asparaginase) act
  on protein synthesis.
- Nitrosoureas affect DNA cross-linkage.
- Inorganic platinum compounds (cis-platinum).
- Others (procarbazine, hydroxyurea).

Drug resistance and toxicity

Malignant cells may have primary (natural) or
secondary (acquired) drug resistance (the latter is
due to adaptation and/or mutation).

Toxicity occurs as a result of damage to rapidly
dividing normal tissues:

- Bone marrow: anaemia, haemorrhage and infection (most drugs).
- Gastrointestinal tract: stomatitis, vomiting,
  diarrhoea (most drugs).
- Lymphoreticular: immunosuppression and infection (most drugs).
- Hair follicles: epilation or alopecia (cyclophosphamide, vincristine and adriamycin).
- Lung: damage (chlorambucil and bleomycin)—
  dose related.
- Urinary bladder: cystitis and sterile haematuria
  (cyclophosphamide).
- Hepato- and nephrotoxicity (methotrexate).
- Skin: impaired wound healing, vesiculation and
  oedema.

- Cardiotoxicity (daunorubicin and adriamycin)
  —dose related.
- Fetus: teratogenesis and abortion.
- Tissue damage if extravasated.

Careful choice of cytotoxic combinations, strict
observance of total doses (many effects are dose-
related) and serial blood counts with symptomatic
control (e.g. antiemetics) will minimise toxicity.

Contraindications

Use of ineffective agent, availability of another
superior approach, very advanced disease (fatal
toxicity is likely), pre-existing bone marrow depression or active infection and when there are no means
of assessing the progress of treatment.

Methods of cytotoxic use (Fig. 25)

Single-agent continuous therapy

A constant blood level of a single cytotoxic drug is
maintained until unacceptable toxicity, drug resistance or cure results.

Combination therapy

Continuous

This uses a number of drugs with various actions
continuously; the cancer mass reduces only at the

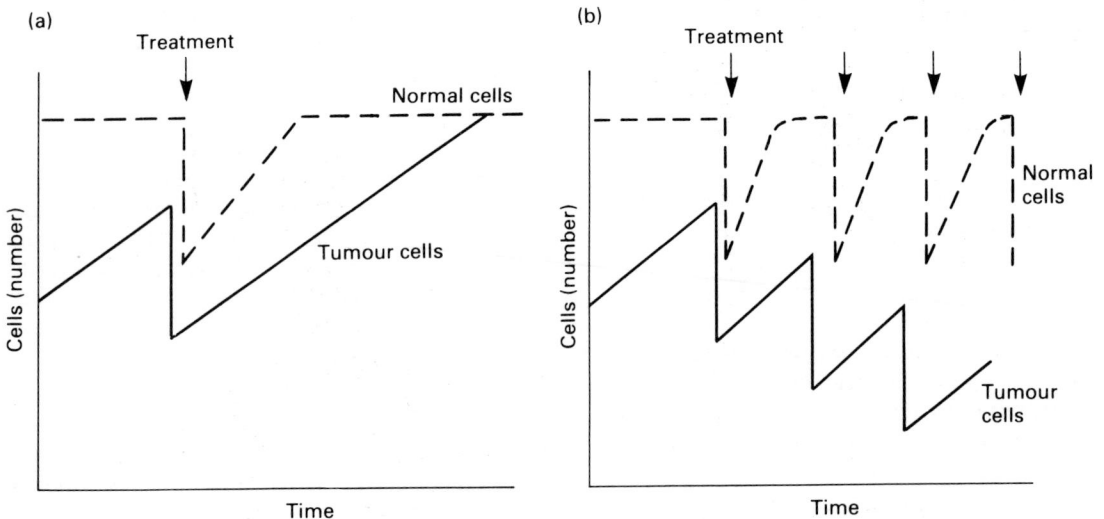

Fig. 25 Comparison of (a) single and (b) pulsed combined cytotoxic
therapies

expense of simultaneous normal tissue toxicity which necessitates a rest phase for recovery during which time the cancer will repopulate.

Pulsing combination therapy

This is the most widely used treatment. Treatment is split into short intervals each of which is referred to as a pulse. Its advantages are:
- Maximal exploitation of the differential in recovery times between normal and malignant tissues.
- Relative lack of toxicity allows therapy to continue indefinitely so increasing chance of cure.
- Allows higher doses of individual drugs to be given so that a higher proportion of cancer cells are killed.
- Recovery of normal tissues in between treatment pulses includes the restoration of the immune system which has further tumoricidal action against small cancer cell populations.

Sequential therapy

When combination chemotherapy is given in sequence it is called sequential therapy. In Hodgkin's Disease Stages IIIb and IV there is 70–80 % remission following the MOPP schedule:

Mustard (nitrogen mustard)	$6 \, mg/m^2$ i.v.	Day 1 and 8	
Oncovan (vincristine)	$1.4 \, mg/m^2$ i.v.	Day 1 and 8	
Procarbazine	$100 \, mg/m^2$ (0)	Day 1–14 (inclusive)	
Prednisolone	$40 \, mg/m^2$ (0)	Day 1–14 (inclusive)	

Prednisolone is given only during the first and fourth courses. Six courses are given with 2 weeks rest between the end of one course and the beginning of the next.

The early stages of Hodgkin's lymphoma (I, II, IIIa) are treated with radiotherapy (Fig. 26).

Cytotoxic administration

Systemic (oral and i.v.)

More toxic but drug can reach micrometastases.

Local

Similar in effect to the localised methods of treatment (i.e. surgery and radiotherapy). Includes:

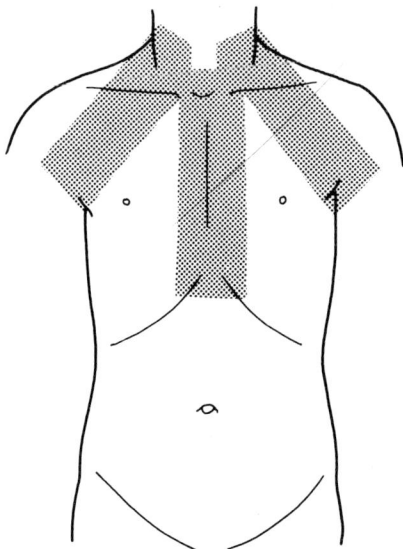

Mantle technique
above diaphragm

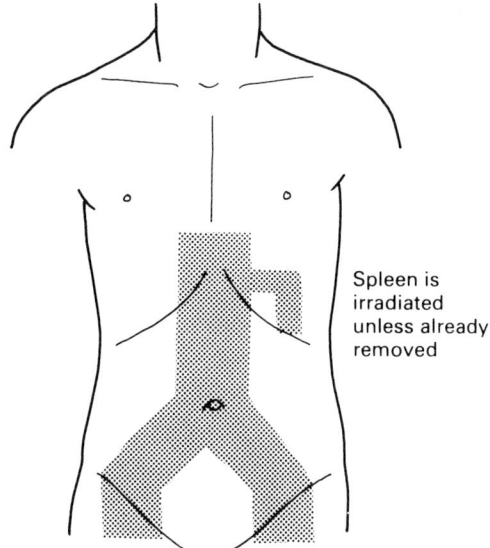

Inverted Y technique
below diaphragm

Spleen is irradiated unless already removed

Fig. 26 Radiotherapy in Hodgkin's disease

Regional cytotoxic therapy

Arterial infusion

- Malignant melanoma recurrence—phenylalanine mustard,
- Head and neck tumours—through the external carotid artery with methotrexate followed by antidote folinic acid for rapid neutralisation,
- Liver secondaries—through the hepatic artery during laparotomy with 5-fluorouracil.

Extracorporeal limb perfusion The main artery and vein to the tumour-bearing area are cannulated to maintain artificial circulation. Limb temperature can be raised (by immersing the limb in a water bath or covering it with hot towels) to cause vasodilation for increased rate of cytotoxic perfusion (also hyperthermia may be lethal to cancer cells). This method is used in malignant melanoma or soft tissue sarcoma of the limb (Fig. 27).

Intracavitary

For example:

- Pleural effusion due to secondary deposits or complicated malignancy of the breast and bronchus may lead to dyspnoea and may be treated with instillation of cyclophosphamide or thiotepa causing pleurodesis and fibrosis.
- In ascites thiotepa or cyclophosphamide instillation is used with three objectives—control of ascites, control of advanced primary disease and as adjuvant therapy at the time of resection for primary gastric, rectal and ovarian cancers.

Intrathecal

For example, subarachnoid methotrexate injection in acute lymphatic leukaemia since most cytotoxics cannot cross blood-brain barrier.

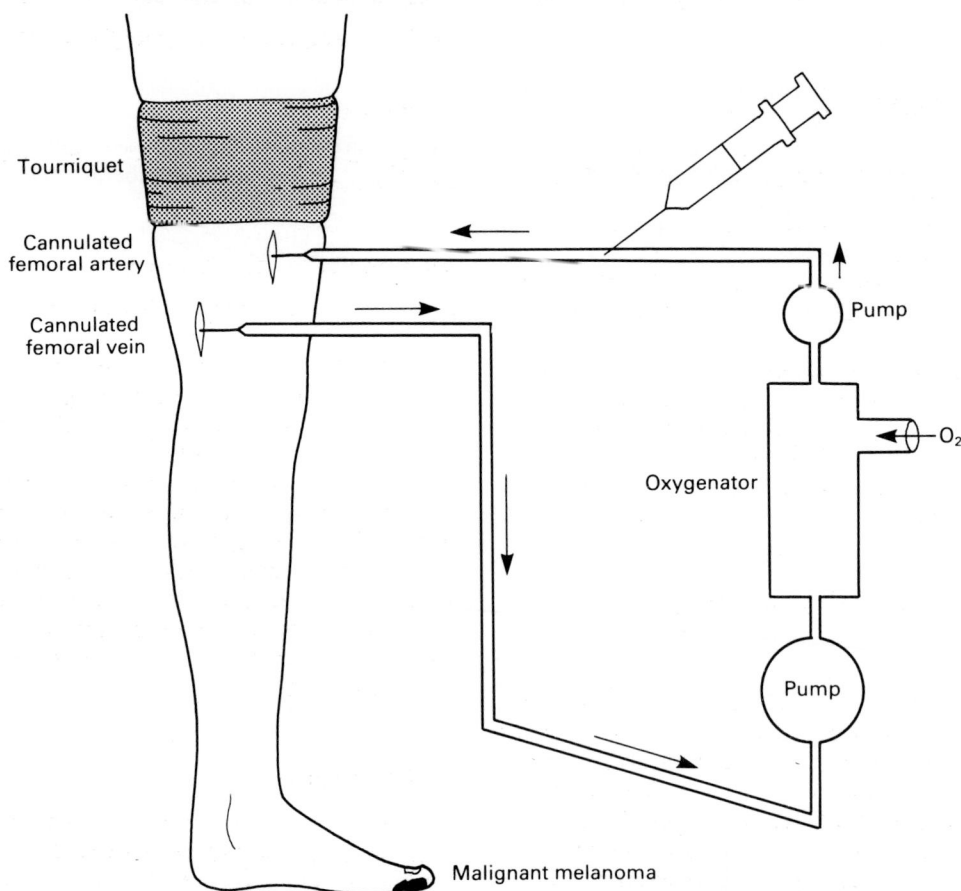

Fig. 27   Extracorporeal isolated lower limb perfusion

Topical

Creams and ointment, e.g. 5% 5-fluorouracil twice daily for 2 weeks in skin carcinoma. It causes intense local reaction and is inferior to other means.

Therapeutic potential of cytotoxic agents

Influenced by drug toxicity, tumour kinetics (the larger the G_f and the higher the cell loss coefficient, the more vulnerable the tumour to cytotoxics and vice versa), drug pharmacokinetics (drug should reach the tumour site and remain there in a sufficient concentration for sufficient time) and the method of cytotoxic use.

The cancer response to cytotoxics is therefore classified as:

Group A Striking, e.g. Burkitt's lymphoma
Group B Less effective, e.g. endometrial carcinoma
Group C Ineffective, e.g. oesophageal carcinoma

ENDOCRINE THERAPY

Therapeutic manipulation of endocrine environment is carried out either by:
- Ablative therapy (surgical removal or radiation destruction of particular endocrine organ); or
- Additive therapy (medical castration) where exogenous natural or synthetic hormones are administered.

Endocrine therapy (unlike cytotoxics) is never curative—eventually all hormone-sensitive tumours will become resistant—and offers only a form of palliation in advanced endocrine-sensitive cancer (in less than 30% of cases) with successful growth control lasting for a maximum of 2 years.

Endocrine pharmacology

Oestrogen

Has many anticancer actions: direct action on breast and prostatic tissue; pituitary-mediated effect as antiprolactin in breast carcinoma and anti-interstitial cell-stimulating hormone in prostatic carcinoma; immune stimulation in both breast and prostatic carcinoma; increases testosterone-binding globulin, thus decreasing free testosterone in prostatic carcinoma. The preparations include (with oral daily doses):

Ethinyloestradiol 0.1–0.5 mg three times daily
Stilboestrol 1–5 mg three times daily
Tripara-anisilchlorethylene (Tace) 12–24 mg

Fosfestrol tetrasodium (Honvan)

Usually inert, but under the action of acid phosphatase of prostatic carcinoma, free stilboestrol will be liberated and leads to sacral and pelvic pain rapidly following injection (daily i.v. dose 250–500 mg) in patients with metastases to these areas (thus it is diagnostic and therapeutic in these cases).

Androgens

Testosterone propionate 100 mg three times weekly (i.m.); may lead to hirsutism, hoarseness, skin changes, increased libido and baldness (in men).

Progestogens

Medroxyprogesterone acetate (Provera).

Antiprolactins

CB_{154}, L-Dopa and CG_{603}; used in advanced breast cancer.

Aminoglutethimide (Orimeten)

A steroidogenesis enzyme blocker inhibiting oestrogen synthesis by blocking desmolase, which mediates the first step in the conversion of cholesterol to androgens in the adrenal glands (medical adrenalectomy), and aromase, which mediates the conversion of androgens to oestrogens peripherally. Clinically 250 mg three times daily with hydrocortisone 20 mg twice daily (to prevent a reflex rise in ACTH, which might overcome the adrenal block) is used in postmenopausal or oöphorectomised women with metastatic breast cancers (especially oestrogen positive) producing remission in 30% with results comparable to those of surgical adrenalectomy.

Anti-oestrogens

Inhibit oestrogen by blocking receptor sites in target organs in oestrogen-dependent tumours. They have minimal side-effects, mild oestrogenicity and possible prolactin inhibition. They are (with oral daily doses):

Tamoxifen   10–20 mg twice daily (may cause thrombocytopenia)—very popular drug

Nafoxiden   60–90 mg three times daily (causes dry skin, photophobia and cataract)

Clomiphene-   50 mg twice daily
citrate

Glucocorticoids

Cancer complications such as hypercalcaemia (due to bone metastases, immobilisation with osteoporosis precipitated by oestrogen therapy), cerebral oedema, autoimmune haemolytic anaemia, general depression and anorexia are all treated with prednisolone. However, prolonged glucocorticoid therapy may cause many side-effects—suppression and atrophy of adrenal glands, Na^+ and H_2O retention, K^+ depletion, weight gain and risk of heart failure, hypertension, susceptibility to infection, cushingoid appearance with moon face and buffalo hump, gastrointestinal tract problems (e.g. dyspepsia, peptic ulcer and perforation), osteoporosis, hyperglycaemia and diabetes, psychosis with euphoria, skin changes, cataract and myopathy.

Clinical uses

Breast carcinoma

Only 30% respond to hormonal manipulation. Prediction of the response depends on laboratory tests (positive oestrogen receptors, tumour culture with different hormones and hormonal assay) and clinical factors (older age and long disease-free interval between primary treatment and appearance of first recurrence have a better response; menopausal status also counts).

Early breast carcinoma

Treated by surgery ± radiotherapy. Adjuvant prophylactic chemotherapy is now also given even if axillary lymph nodes are not involved.

Advanced breast carcinoma

Treated by (in order of procedure):
1. Palliative surgery.
2. Radiotherapy: in bone and skin metastases.
3. Premenopausal: ovarian ablation.
4. Perimenopausal (5 years after menopause): anti-oestrogens or androgens.

5. Postmenopausal: oestrogen but use prednisone in hepatic and lung infiltration. An anti-oestrogen is the drug of choice in soft tissue and pulmonary involvement. Relapses after ovarian ablation need secondary endocrine ablation (adrenalectomy or hypophysectomy). In postmenopausal relapses, stop the treatment and look for a withdrawal response and if none then perform a secondary endocrine ablation.

Cytotoxic therapy is indicated in endocrine failure or is used initially if the tumour is found to be hormone insensitive (e.g. negative oestrogen receptors) and in fairly aggressive diseases like fulminating hepatitis lymphangiosa. Either single or, usually, intermittent combination therapy is used (5-fluorouracil, cyclophosphamide and methotrexate). It is the treatment of choice in rapidly progressing breast carcinoma.

Immunotherapy (by non-specific stimulation of immune defence mechanism) and neutron therapy are still under trial.

N.B. In male breast carcinoma (1% of total breast carcinoma) bilateral surgical orchidectomy is effective in two-thirds of cases. If relapse occurs, steroid therapy is better than ablative therapy.

Prostatic carcinoma

Ninety per cent are hormone dependent. Oestrogen (stilboestrol) is the initial treatment. If thromboembolism occurs, whether induced by oestrogens or already present due to malignant infiltration of lymphatics or venous drainage of lower limbs by prostatic carcinoma, then:
- Perform bilateral subcapsular orchidectomy.
- Relapses need steroid or ablative therapy.
- Bone metastases are controlled with megavoltage radiotherapy and obstructive uropathy is controlled with prostatic transurethral resection (TUR).

Cancers of ovary, uterus (endometrial) and kidney (adenocarcinoma)

These organs are the embryological derivatives of the urogenital ridge and their cancers are all treated with progestogens.

Thyroid carcinoma

Thyroxine 0.1 mg three times daily (or alternatively T_3 20 μg three times daily) is given to suppress TSH and to prevent the growth of the primary residual tumour and its metatases (after total thyroidectomy ± block dissection in papillary carcinoma, medullary carcinoma and malignant lymphoma; after hemithyroidectomy in follicular carcinoma). However, T_4 is required as replacement therapy and careful observation for toxicity is needed. Radiotherapy, especially ^{131}I therapy, is indicated in lethal anaplastic carcinoma, for postoperative treatment of residual malignant tissues and in multiple secondaries (especially bone metastases of follicular carcinoma).

IMMUNOTHERAPY

The high incidence of cancers in kidney transplants and immune-deficient states together with the rare phenomenon of spontaneous tumour regression indicate the value of immune defences. Tumours differ antigenically from their host—this antigen difference is evident from host ability for allogenic inhibition (tumour cells lacking antigen will not grow when they are in the company of normal cells) and immunological surveillance to restrain tumour growth. Host immunoglobulins act either as:
- An agent enhancing tumour growth.
- Unblocking antibodies that reverse the enhancement (*see above*).
- Beneficial cytotoxics that activate the complement system.
Cell-mediated immunity against a specific tumour antigen (Type IV) as well as antibody-dependent cell-mediated (killer) cytotoxicity (Type VI) can be demonstrated in cancer patients.

Clinical uses

Immunotherapy in humans is capable of destroying only very small quantities of malignant cells in subclinical forms, usually after the completion of other therapies. It is either specific or non-specific.

Specific

Stimulation of the host immune exaggerated response can be:
- Active: autologous tumour, e.g. patient's own tumour cells irradiated and reinjected.
- Adoptive: e.g. transfusion of donor-sensitised or immunised cytotoxic cells as well as transfer factor.
- Passive: use of antiserum specific to a particular antigen, e.g. antilymphocyte serum in leukaemia.

Non-specific

To stimulate general immune mechanisms by injecting BCG into melanoma nodules (leads to regression) or intrapleural injection of BCG in pneumonectomy (for lung cancer). *Corynebacterium parvum* and levamisol are other boosting agents.

RETINOIDS

Non-toxic chemical modifications of preformed vitamin A (alcohol retinol). Vitamin A deficiency results in squamous metaplasia which can be converted after vitamin replenishment to actively secreting columnar epithelium; therefore, retinoids prevent squamous metaplasia and their role in differentiation may be used in cancer prevention and preneoplastic conditions. (Vitamin A is inferior to retinoids as it may cause hepatic toxicity.) Clinical regression is noticed in actinic keratosis, basal cell carcinoma and malignant melanoma after topical therapy. Specific retinoid cytoplasmic receptors as well as immunostimulation may explain their mode of action. Further clinical studies are needed.

INTERFERON

Inerferon (IF) is a protein which interferes with viral infection. If the inducing agent is a virus or double-stranded inducer it is called Type 1 IF. Type 11 IF is produced if the immunocompetent cells are stimulated by unrelated substances. IF has three actions:
- Binds to a surface receptor in the target cell and sets in motion a series of secondary messengers culminating in a change in the cell's general metabolic state (such changes inhibit virus replication using the genetic machinery of the host cell).
- Complex inhibitory effect on cell growth and division.
- Profound effect on the immune system (acting as a lymphocyte hormone).
According to heterogeneity, there are three families of IF: α (predominantly produced by leucocytes), β (produced by fibroblasts) and γ (produced by antigen- or mitogen-stimulated lymphocytes). Including subtypes there is a total of 14 different molecular species of IFs. Clinically the use of IF in myeloma, breast cancer and non-Hodgkin's lymphoma results in objective regression of these tumours. It can cause some side-effects (dose-

related) including anorexia, weight loss and central nervous system toxicity (metabolic encephalopathy). Other tumours, such as melanoma, renal cell carcinoma, lung cancer and Kaposi's sarcoma, respond to IF at a low rate (less than 20%). This anticancer potential of IF could possibly be utilised in adjuvant therapy in the early stages of solid tumours as well as in advanced disease.

SUPPORTIVE THERAPY

Consists of non-specific symptomatic measures to control the primary complications of cancer (e.g. cachexia, dysphagia, infection) or to counteract the side-effects of anticancer treatment (e.g. bleeding, infection). Includes nutrition (enteral or parenteral), blood transfusion, antibiotics, analgesics and terminal care measures.

1.44. Tumour Markers and Cancer Screening in Surgery

TUMOUR MARKERS

These are products of the metobolic acitivity of tumours and are either tumour-derived or tumour-associated, although not necessarily tumour-specific. They may be secreted (into blood, urine or other body fluids) or expressed (at the cell surface) in quantities larger than those in normal tissue. Their concentrations in body fluids are measured by radioimmunoassay or detected on the cell surface (in paraffin sections, smears or fresh biopsy tissue). They include (with their typical tumour):

Hormones with their subunits

ACTH and related	
MSH	(bronchogenic carcinoma)
ADH	(bronchogenic carcinoma)
Hypothalamic releasing factors	(bronchogenic carcinoma)
PTH	(bronchogenic carcinoma)

Calcitonin	(bronchogenic and breast carcinoma)
Prostaglandins	(colon and breast carcinoma)
HCG	(chorion carcinoma and teratoma)

Notice that these hormones are ectopic (i.e. their production is inappropriate to the tissue of origin of the tumour). Eutopic hormones (i.e. appropriate to the tissue of origin of the tumour) are also markers, e.g. calcitonin in medullary thyroid carcinoma, catecholamines and urinary vanillylmandelic acid in phaeochromocytoma, and urinary homovanillic acid in neuroblastoma.

Oncofetal products and antigens

CEA (carcinoembryonic antigen)	(gastrointestinal tract carcinoma) (Table 8)
AFP (α-feto protein)	(hepatoma and teratoma) (Table 8)
Ferritin	(many)
Cancer basic protein	(all)
Pregnancy associated proteins	(breast and teratoma)
Placental type enzymes	(many)

Table 8. Non-specific rise of AFP and CEA in various conditions in order of frequency

AFP	CEA
Neoplastic	
Liver	Colon and rectum
Biliary tract	Pancreas
Pancreas	Liver
Stomach	Bronchus
Colon and rectum	Breast
Lung	Uterus
Malignant melanoma	Ovary
Non-neoplastic	
Viral hepatitis	Ulcerative colitis
Alcoholic cirrhosis	Alcoholic liver disease
Chronic active hepatitis	Chronic bronchitis and emphysema
Ulcerative colitis	Fibroadenosis
Crohn's disease	

Enzymes and isoenzymes

Prolyl hydroxylase   (hepatoma and breast)
Sialyl transferase   (many)
Prostatic acid phosphatase

Macromolecules

Paraproteins (monoclonal
   immunoglobulins with urinary
   light chain Bence–Jones
   protein)   (myeloma)
Milk protein   (breast)
Polyamines   (many)
Nucleosides   (many)
Other tumour-associated proteins
   (acute phase reactive proteins and
   urinary hydroxyproline)

Hormone receptors   (breast carcinoma)

? Hormonally induced cancer-associated phenomena
(*see* Table 9)

Clinically useful markers

Those suitable for routine management and general screening are very limited. They include the following.

HCG

Produced by placenta (reaching maximum concentration in the eighth gestational week) and abnormal trophoblastic tissue. It is composed of α-non-specific and β-specific subunits. It increases in chorion carcinoma and can detect a tumour mass of 1 mg; it is therefore used as a screening test in all cases of hydatidiform mole after uterine evacuation to judge the progress, to monitor chemotherapy and to detect early metastases. β-HCG (above 10 i.u./l) is found in 50% of testicular teratomas and in few pure seminomas. False high levels may occur after orchidectomy and hypogonadism owing to high LH (luteinising hormone) (identical to α-HCG subunit), and retesting after testosterone administration is therefore needed. HCG also increases in carcinoma of the pancreas, stomach and bronchus.

AFP

Normal range 1–16 μg/l in adults. This is a protein synthesised by yolk sac, liver and gastrointestinal tract and is the major serum protein of the fetus.

Levels above 40 μg/l are found in 60% of teratomas and although high levels of AFP are non-specific (*see* Table 8) its assay in conjunction with β-HCG gives positive results in 75–95% of testicular teratomas and both levels are crucial in the subsequent management.

Staging   Preorchidectomy high marker levels that fall to normal postoperatively suggest Stage I while persistently high levels after orchidectomy suggest undetected Stage II (retroperitoneal lymph node) or Stage III (supradiaphragmatic node involvement). Slow falls in AFP levels may indicate a residual AFP-producing tumour.

Assessing prognosis   Levels of HCG $< 5 \times 10^4$ i.u./l and AFP < 500 μg/l are associated with 10% mortality whereas levels above 1×10^5 i.u./l and 1 mg/l respectively carry a mortality in excess of 40% (the marker level is proportional to the bulk of metastatic teratoma).

Monitoring therapy   Eighty per cent of metastatic teratomas undergo remission on combined chemotherapy, the duration of which is judged by assay of markers (if they become normal, there is no need for maintenance therapy). If marker levels fall to normal but there is static residual disease (evident on chest X-ray or CAT scan) biopsy of the residual lesions will be consistent with differentiated teratoma or necrotic tissue (further therapy is not indicated). On the other hand advancing disease with static marker levels indicates non-marker-producing tumour cells and change of therapy is indicated.

CEA

A complex glycoprotein synthesised by tumour cells and by normal colonic epithelium. It is carried on the cell surface membrane and normally shed with faeces. In cancer it is shed into surrounding serum and serous fluids. Although raised levels are non-specific (*see* Table 8) the serum levels detected in 65% of all colorectal cancers depend on:
● Tumour stage: CEA is raised in 30% of patients with Duke's Stage A tumour and in 90% of those with hepatic metastases.
● Tumour site: CEA levels are low or absent in right colonic and rectal tumours and higher in left colonic, particularly sigmoid cancer.
● Degree of differentiation.
● Functional hepatic status.

CEA therefore has no role in screening among the normal population. However, it is used as a prognostic indicator (very high preoperative levels suggest a poor prognosis) and as an indicator for second-look surgery for cure in early colonic recurrence. In monitoring therapy, falling CEA levels suggest a response to chemotherapy or radiotherapy.

Hormone receptors

Hormones are defined as chemical mediators secreted by cells to affect 'target cells' at a distance, e.g. most hormones (endocrine effect); to stimulate nearby cells to secrete other hormones, e.g. glucagon from α-cells of the pancreas stimulating β-cells to secrete insulin (paracrine effect); or to act as neurotransmitters (neurocrine effect). Each hormone binds a protein situated on the cell membrane or within the cell (receptor) with a high affinity and specificity. There are two types of receptor mechanism:

Hormone-receptor complex

Situated at the cell membrane, this complex activates adenyl cyclase enzyme, leading to the production of adenosine monophosphate (AMP) as a second messenger which in turn stimulates intracellular metabolic events. Such a mechanism can be seen in catecholamines and peptide hormones, i.e. glucagon, LH, FSH, ACTH, while protein hormones, i.e. growth hormone, insulin and prolactin, activate membrane receptors by production of a second messenger other than AMP (probably a peptide).

Steroid hormones

Diffuse through the cell membrane to bind to a specific cytoplasmic receptor protein which then undergoes a change in conformation and translocates to the cell nucleus, acting on the genome to induce transcription (RNA synthesis). Some target cells possess more than one receptor type, e.g. thyroid hormone acts via multiple receptor sites in the cell membrane, on the mitochondria, within the nucleus and in cytoplasm. The receptor assay, e.g. oestrogen receptor, is done by preparation of a particulate fraction from the tissue, incubation with radioactive hormone and separation of the hormone portion bound to the receptor from the free portion; the ratio of these two components is determined by scintillation counting. Receptor assays have considerable clinical impact:

- Development of hormone inhibitors that compete with the natural hormone for binding to receptor sites leading to no response, e.g. anti-androgen (cyproterone) used in prostatic carcinoma as well as in sexual offenders, anti-oestrogen (tamoxifen) used in breast cancer treatment, histamine H_2 receptors blocker (cimetidine), β-adrenergic receptor blocker (atenolol).
- Testicular feminisation syndrome (male genotypically but female phenotypically) represents end organ insensitivity and/or abnormal androgen receptors.

Oestrogen receptors in breast cancer

Provide a method of predicting the hormonal sensitivity of breast cancer   About 32% of breast cancers have no detectable or significant receptor activity and must be spared ineffective endocrine therapy (better treated by cytotoxic therapy). The remaining two-thirds, mainly in postmenopausal patients, must be considered for endocrine therapy with a 50% chance of response. Tumours with high receptor levels are more likely to respond. As samples of metastatic disease for assay may be difficult to obtain, receptor analysis should be an essential investigation in all primary breast cancers (since quantitative differences in the receptor concentration in primary cancers and their later metastases will not disturb the differentiation between receptor-positive and receptor-negative tumours).

Androgen and progesterone receptors have also been discovered. The latter are present in a proportion of oestrogen receptor-positive tumours which respond to hormonal treatment better than those possessing oestrogen receptors alone (70% response versus 25% respectively). Progesterone receptors are only rarely found in tumours without oestrogen receptor activity.

Tamoxifen   A potent oestrogen receptor-blocking drug which competes for binding to cytoplasmic receptor sites yielding no response. It is now the initial treatment of choice for advanced breast cancer with oestrogen receptor activity. Tamoxifen has a similar efficacy to high dose oestrogen therapy but *lacks its side-effects*; therefore, it is also the treatment of choice in those with unknown receptor status and is a suitable treatment for asymptomatic early disease (since in the majority of patients, breast cancer is already a systemic disease at the time of presentation, necessitating systemic as well as local therapy). Adjuvant tamoxifen with chemotherapy after mastectomy is therefore more effective in delaying recurrence than chemotherapy alone.

Provide a prognostic guide Recurrence is less and survival rates are better in receptor-positive cancers than in receptor-negative cancers. Oestrogen receptor activity is a sign of a biologically favourable tumour since there is a higher proportion of receptor-positive tumours in patients with well-differentiated (Grade I or II) tumours, those without axillary lymph node involvement and those in whom focal elastosis is prominent.

? Hormonally-induced cancer-associated phenomena

Hypercalcaemia

Ectopic parathormone explains a few cases but osteolytic metastases are often associated with biochemical changes not consistent with the hyperparathyroid state. Breast cancers have been found to release prostaglandins E and F which have the ability to mobilise bone calcium, a property that is inhibited by the addition of aspirin or indomethacin. These macromolecular factors (prostaglandins) can explain hypercalcaemia and can have prognostic implications. The cell source is unknown.

Cachexia

The commonest cause of cancer death. The progressive weight loss, anorexia, malabsorption and wasteful pattern of tumour metabolism have a complex underlying cause. Toxohormone and cytotoxic polypeptides have been postulated but remain questionable.

Gastrointestinal changes

The recent recognition of gastrointestinal tract hormones (Table 9) has helped significantly to explain some of the tumour manifestations. These hormones may be produced ectopically or released by endocrine tumours.

VIPomas

Also known as the Verner–Morrison or WDHA syndrome = watery diarrhoea, hypokalaemia and

Table 9. Circulating alimentary hormones

Hormone	Location	Physiological role	Pathology
Gastrin	Antrum	Stimulates acid secretion. Maintains mucosal growth. Causes gastric motor activity	High in atrophic gastritis and achlorhydria. Fasting gastrin level is normal in duodenal ulcer while high in gastrinoma in Zollinger-Ellison syndrome
Secretin	Duodenum	Stimulates pancreatic bicarbonate	Failure of secretion leads to faulty pancreatic bicarbonate mechanism for neutralising acid in duodenal ulcer
Cholecystokinin	Duodenum and jejunum	Stimulates gall bladder contraction Stimulates pancreatic enzyme secretion	High in chronic pancreatitis
Motilin	Jejunum	Causes upper alimentary motor activity	—
Glucose-dependent insulin-releasing hormone (GIP)	Jejunum	Stimulates insulin release	—
Neurotensin	Ileum	Unknown (hypotensive)	High in dumping syndrome (in partial gastrectomy or vagotomy)
Enteroglucagon	Ileum and colon	Maintains mucosal growth. Slows intestinal transit	High after bowel resection but low in massive resection
Pancreatic polypeptide	Pancreas	Anticholecystokinin	High in minor or acute pancreatitis, low in severe pancreatitis and steatorrhoea

achlorhydria. Occur in non-B-islet cell tumours of the pancreas and 15% of neural childhood tumours (ganglioneuroblastomas). A vasoactive intestinal peptide (VIP) (made up of two amino acids related to the gastrointestinal peptide group) is responsible for this syndrome which may also include diabetes mellitus, hypercalcaemia, tetany and flushing. Death occurs from renal failure. This syndrome should be distinguished from the Zollinger–Ellison syndrome (gastrin-producing islet cell tumour associated with refractory peptic ulceration). Diagnosis may be delayed, leading to metastasis; streptozotocin (cytotoxic) is effective in producing prolonged remission. The diarrhoea may be controlled with high-dose steroids. Early diagnosis is based on suspicion in any case of profuse diarrhoea and hypokalaemia in which case VIP estimation should be done. VIP is usually grossly high and treatment by localised pancreatic resection may be curative. VIP may be normal (pseudo-Verner-Morrison syndrome) and total pancreatectomy may be the only method of treatment to remove the responsible product (other than VIP).

CANCER SCREENING

The aim is to detect and treat the disease in the population at an early curable stage in order to reduce cancer mortality.

Advantages
- Improved prognosis.
- Less radical curative treatment.
- Reassurance for those with negative test results.
- Resource savings from less radical treatment.

Disadvantages
- Longer morbidity for those with unaltered prognosis.
- Overtreatment of borderline abnormalities.
- False reassurance for those with false negative results.
- Anxiety and morbidity for those with false positive results.
- Cooperation from population to accept screening and carry out repeated tests cannot be relied on.
- Hazards of screening test.
- Resource costs from screening, diagnostic investigations and overtreatment.

In the absence of effective methods of primary prevention or effective treatment of symptomatic tumours, screening offers the best hope of controlling the mortality from some cancers. Health education promoting self-examination is also a form of screening, e.g. breast cancer, skin melanoma and testicular cancer. Medical follow-up, e.g. hydatidiform mole by HCG assay for chorion epithelioma is another form of screening.

The *sensitivity* of a test is the number of positive tests per 100 patients with the disease. The *specificity* of the test is the number of negative tests per 100 patients who do not have the disease.

Mass screening tests

Uterine cervix

Cytology with 80% sensitivity and very high specificity. It has the disadvantage of overtreatment of borderline abnormalities. Colposcopic biopsy and laser excision of affected epithelium may reduce this disadvantage. The age and frequency of screening is controversial. Five-yearly repeats may miss up to 40% of invasive cancer.

Stomach

Double-contrast barium meal detects early gastric carcinoma. It carries a radiation hazard and is very non-specific with almost 25% of screened individuals requiring further investigation involving fluoroscopy, cytology and endoscopy. Mortality has been reduced by 20% since the test was introduced but the natural history of this disease is ill understood and it is argued that both incidence and mortality from gastric cancer were falling already.

Breast

This is the only cancer in which screening reduces the mortality rate (proven in randomised controlled trial). Mammography (by a single oblique view) is highly sensitive and specific with low radiation dose and low cost; 20–40% of detected cancers are preinvasive. Breast self-examination needs greater exposure in the general population. Although widely advocated, its sensitivity, specificity and effectiveness in reducing mortality require further research.

Lung

The multifocal, often bilateral, distribution of lung cancers along with their rapid growth rate make attempts to control mortality by screening disappointing. Chest X-ray and sputum cytology combined and repeated at 4-monthly intervals detect nearly 90 % of cases especially in high-risk groups. Neither is sufficiently sensitive on its own: X-rays lack specificity whereas with cytology localisation of lesions is difficult. Health education aimed at primary prevention and measures to curtail cigarette smoking seem much more profitable means of control.

Large intestine

- Identification and treatment of premalignant conditions, e.g. polyposis coli.
- Sigmoidoscopic screening (practised in USA) is hazardous and not acceptable to the general population.
- Guaiac—impregnated filter paper test for occult blood (do-it-yourself test) is a promising new screening tool. The specimen can be posted to a laboratory for analysis. The test lacks specificity (bleeding gums after toothbrushing may give false positive results which require the patient to undergo colonoscopy and barium enema both of which are unpleasant for the patient and expensive for the Health Service). Lack of acceptability by some because of distaste for taking a faecal sample is another problem.
- CEA is non-specific (discussed on p. 153).

Bladder

Workers exposed to carcinogenic chemicals in their occupation (e.g. rubber and dye industry) may be screened by urinary cytology at 6-monthly intervals. Its sensitivity, specificity and effectiveness need to be evaluated.

Thyroid

First-degree relatives of patients with medullary thyroid carcinoma can be screened by measuring calcitonin levels (20 % of these carcinomas have a familial history with an autosomal dominant inheritance).

1.45. Some Important Paediatric Problems

GASTROINTESTINAL OBSTRUCTION IN THE NEONATE

Functional ileus is a common problem. However, only organic causes will be discussed here.

Presenting features are severe vomiting, failure to pass meconium and progressive abdominal distension ending in strangulation and death (in oesophageal atresia, constant drooling of saliva with choking attacks and cyanosis during feeding occur). Other causes of death are fluid and electrolyte metabolic disturbances and inhalation of vomitus with asphyxia.

Causes and treatment

Oesophageal atresia Either as absent oesophagus (2 %) or partial absence or web but no fistula (10 %) or commonly atresia with tracheo-oesophageal fistula (85 %). Lipiodol swallow is needed to identify the type. The condition occurs within the first 48 h. Treatment is by quick metabolic correction and thoracotomy with disconnection of fistula and reconstruction of oesophageal continuity (end-to-end anastomosis).

Congenital pyloric stenosis Occurs in 4/1000 births usually in males with a familial history. It never occurs after 4 months of age. Clinical findings are non-bilious forcible and projectile vomiting ± palpable epigastric lump ± visible peristalsis. Treatment is quick metabolic correction followed by pyloromyotomy (Ramstedt's operation) under general anaesthesia via an upper abdominal incision. The hypertrophied pylorus is incised and muscle fibres are teased apart without breaching the mucosa (if accidently opened then patch with omentum just like perforated peptic ulcer). Medical treatment with atropine-like drug (e.g. Eumydrin) usually ends in failure.

Duodenal atresia Usually associated with Down's syndrome. It is usually due to web or stenosis in the region of the ampulla of Vater or rarely to annular pancreas (failure of complete rotation of the ventral segment) with a characteristic double-bubble radiological appearance. Visible peristalsis and vomiting with or without bile are the main presentations. Treatment is by duodenoduodenostomy with an intraluminal catheter passed via the anastomosis and brought out through the gastrostomy.

Jejunal and ileal stenosis   With abdominal distension within 24 h of birth—confirmed radiologically (multiple fluid levels). Treatment is by Mikulicz procedure of exteriorisation, resection and spur enterostomy.

Midgut malrotation   In the form of arrested rotation due to transduodenal band of Ladd leading to a volvulus neonatorum after clockwise rotation of the whole midgut around the axis of the superior mesenteric artery. Treatment is by division of the band and untwisting the bowel.

Meconium ileus   Is the neonatal manifestation of mucoviscidosis with characteristic soap bubble appearance of meconium in the terminal ileum (seen in right iliac fossa). Adequate preoperative preparation followed by laparotomy. The proximal ileum is anastomosed end-to-side to the collapsed colon distal to the obstruction. The distal ileal opening is formed into an ileostomy through which meconium can be removed.

Intussusception   Usually in 6–9 month old male with facial pallor, vomiting, screaming and 'red-currant jelly' stool. A sausage-shaped lump around the umbilicus is felt. Operative reduction (by milking) or resection of an irreducible or gangrenous segment (with end-to-end anastomosis).

Hirschsprung's disease   Due to a variable aganglionic rectosigmoid segment with an obstruction at the anorectal junction. Identified by rectal biopsy and radiology, including barium enema (prior to rectal washout). Constipation, abdominal distension with empty rectum gripping the examining finger are classical features. Treatment is surgical when the child is 8.2 kg in weight and thriving. Laparotomy and full mobilisation followed by anal pull-through. The anterior half of the inverted rectum is opened transversely and the proximal colon is pulled through the opening with an end-to-end coloanal anastomosis covered by a proximal temporary colostomy.

Anorectal agenesis   In the form of imperforate anus, low or high anomalies. X-ray of the infant upside down with a coin strapped to the anus can reveal the rectal gas which in turn can identify the level of agenesis. Treatment is according to the level usually with pull-through operation protected by colostomy. Any rectourethral fistula should be divided.

GASTROINTESTINAL BLEEDING IN CHILDREN

The treatment is according to the cause. The common causes are:

Haematemesis
- Swallowed maternal blood.
- Peptic oesophagitis.
- Oesophageal varices.
- Gastritis and stress ulcer.
- Haemorrhagic disease of the newborn and blood dyscrasias.
- Hiatus hernia.
- Gastric duplication.

Rectal bleeding
- Swallowed maternal blood.
- Peptic oesophagitis.
- Oesophageal varices.
- Meckel's diverticulum.
- Stress ulcer.
- Haemorrhagic disease of the newborn and blood dyscrasias.
- Necrotising enterocolitis.
- Intussusception/midgut malrotation.
- Anal fissure/constipation with impaction.
- Infectious diarrhoea.

1.46. Medical Imaging and Interventional Radiology

MEDICAL IMAGING

Ultrasonography, computerised axial tomography and isotope scintillography have changed the radiologist into a medical imager. The improvement in the accuracy of diagnoses and the delineation of disease processes by these non-invasive modalities has had a major impact on the management of surgical patients.

Ultrasound

Ultrasound is a non-invasive technique with no contraindications which allows the visualisation of internal organs. Using 1–15 MHz mechanical vibrations (above the range of human hearing), generated and detected by a transducer, an image of body structures can be obtained owing to reflection of the transmitted sound at the interface of tissues with different impedance. The returning pulse-echo information can be stored electronically or photographically. In addition, precise measurements of organ size and pathological lesions can be made with electronic calipers.

Grey-scale ultrasound

This allows the production of non-moving cross-sections (tomographs) of soft tissues by storing pulse-echo information as the ultrasound transducer is moved around the patient. The image is displayed on a black-and-white television screen.

Real-time scanning

Transducers capable of registering 20 frames/s give continuous moving (real-time) images of internal organs instead of static pictures. Real time allows imaging of moving structures and the rapid scanning of large-volume organs in an omnidirectional fashion merely by moving the transducer. This makes it ideal for examining the liver and vascular tree.

Doppler ultrasound

Using ultrasonic Doppler-shifted pulse-echo signals from moving blood it is possible to detect blood vessels and to map them out in a two-dimensional plan. Dilated vessels and aneurysms can be demonstrated and the presence or absence of difficult vessels such as foot pulses detected. The quality of blood flow through vessels can be indicated and, using more sophisticated analysis of the signals, a quantitative estimation of blood flow obtained. Doppler ultrasound is of value in the investigation of obstructive arterial and venous disease.

Therapeutic ultrasound

Using sound vibration of 1 million cycles per second (1 MHz) frequency can lead to the following effects:
- Activation of cells.
- Increased absorption of intracellular fluid.
- Stimulation of blood and lymph flow.
- Increased heat in the tissues.

- Microcellular massage—ultrasound hits cells and flattens them and the cells then return to their original shape (pressure and relaxation).
- Analgesia—only pulsed ultrasound has this effect. The rhythmical effect of sound waves numbs the nerve endings.

These effects are utilised therapeutically in:
- Traumatic and inflammatory conditions including osteoarthrosis.
- Scar softening, e.g. following haematomas, carbuncles, Dupuytren's contracture and plantar fasciitis.
- Miscellaneous, e.g. tenosynovitis, low back pain, sports injury, varicose ulcers, pressure sores, facial scars, scleroderma, carpal tunnel syndrome and renal stone disintegraton.

Therapeutic ultrasound is contraindicated (due to its thermal, shaking and cavitation effects) in:
- Tumours: since it activates benign and malignant cells.
- Areas irradiated (deep X-ray therapy) or having radioactivity or post thyroidectomy after the use of radioactive drugs (because of ultrasound thermal effect).
- Areas with localised sepsis (since the sepsis may be spread).
- Thrombosis (detachment with embolism).
- Retina (detachment).
- Pregnancy (abortion).

Recently *pulsed electromagnetic energy* (PEME) is becoming more popular and is replacing many applications of therapeutic ultrasound. The PEME spectrum ranges in frequency from as small as 27 MHz (shortwave therapy, shortwave radio) up to 2450 MHz (infrared and visible light).

The high-frequency equipment currently used is either Diapulse or Megapulse. They are used to improve wound healing postoperatively in orchidopexy and foot and recent injuries, and to aid nerve and spinal cord regeneration. PEME has no thermal effect, it improves the rate of oedema dispersion, encourages haematoma absorption, reduces inflammation, encourages collagen layering at an early stage, stimulates osteogenesis and improves healing of the peripheral and central nervous system.

Computerised axial tomography

CT scanning (Table 10) has been available for just over a decade. Utilising X-rays, three-dimensional body images can be presented as a series of two-dimensional 'slices'. CT scanning gives sensitive definition of soft tissues in a way that conventional

Table 10. Comparison between ultrasound and CT scanning

	Ultrasound	CT scanning
Image	Sectional tomographs	
	Omnidirectional	Axial
	Interpretation required	Excellent high resolution
Limitations	Operator dependent	Expensive
		Only available regionally
		Radiation hazard
	Fat patient	Thin patient
Considerations for use	Capability of answering certain clinical questions	
	Where there is an overlap in usefulness use the cheapest first	
Uses	Obstetrics	Brain
	Blood vessels	Lung
	Eye	Orbit
	Cardiac	Staging malignancy
		Deep X-ray therapy planning
	Liver, pancreas, biliary tree guided biopsy techniques	
Contraindications	None	Obstetrics

radiography cannot. The use of contrast medium can further improve the delineation of organs.

The CT system comprises four units.

The scanning frame The scanner consists of an X-ray tube and a detector system. X-rays pass through the patient and the emergent beam is stored as a 'profile'. The patient is rotated and another profile obtained. Depending on the exact type of scanner, a varying number of profiles are obtained.

The processing unit The image data of each body plane in the form of profiles are then processed by computer and 'assembled' into a form which can be displayed visually.

The viewing unit The assembled data are presented on a television screen. The picture can be manipulated in such a way that the visual information of particular organs or areas of interest can be enhanced.

The storage system In addition to the normal polaroid photographic method of storing the televi-

sion picture of the body slice, image profiles of each body plane can be committed to computer memory, floppy disc or magnetic tape for retrieval at a later date.

ISOTOPE SCANNING

In contrast to X-rays, CT scanning and ultrasound, isotope scanning (IS) depends on the administration to the patient of a radionuclide energy source which emits γ-radiation. The distribution of the radionuclide is determined by the biological properties of the vehicle to which it is attached. The γ-ray emission is detected by a scintillation crystal as light emissions which can be counted electronically. The low-resolution image can be displayed on an oscilloscope or photographic paper. The picture obtained cannot be relied on to demonstrate detailed anatomy but since IS is based on count density which can be measured against time it readily lends itself to functional or dynamic studies of the target organ. Using computer analysis, graphs and histograms can present measurements of function in a readily understandable form.

Bone scanning

^{99m}Tc attached to a radionuclide vehicle such as methylene diphosphonate is taken up by bone. In conjunction with normal X-rays it can be used to detect bony metastases from the lung and breast and prostatic primary malignancies. It is also of value in the early detection of osteomyelitis and the diagnosis of Perthes' disease and stress fractures. In these clinical situations detailed anatomical display is unnecessary.

Isotope kidney scanning

Conventional intravenous urography not only gives a suitable anatomical display of the kidney, collecting system and bladder but also provides information about renal function. IS can also give anatomical information but its particular value is in measuring differential renal function. Using technetium-labelled DPTA, perfusion images of the renal arteries can be obtained along with the transit time of the isotope through the renal parenchyma and pelvis separately. Using a computer, differential renal function can be plotted graphically. In a similar manner differential perfusion images of the cerebral hemispheres can be obtained.

Localisation of endocrine tumours

[75]Se-selenonorcholestrol has been used to differentiate bilateral adrenal hyperplasia from adrenal adenoma. Normal or hyperplastic adrenal glands take up the isotope but with unilateral adenoma the abnormal gland takes up the radionuclide but the normal side is suppressed. Technetium-thallium subtraction imaging is the most sensitive method of localising parathyroid adenomas.

INTERVENTIONAL RADIOLOGY

In parallel with non-invasive diagnostic techniques, a variety of invasive percutaneous procedures have been developed. These enable the radiologist to provide the clinician with tissue, cytological and microbiological specimens as well as to carry out a broad spectrum of therapeutic procedures.

The surgeon should familiarise himself with these recent advances and be aware of their availability within the hospital or region. The therapeutic and diagnostic techniques performed by the interventional radiologist encroach on the traditional territory of the surgeon. The most appropriate method of diagnosis and treatment of certain conditions requires close cooperation between surgeon and radiologist since they may benefit the patient by avoiding a traditional surgical procedure. Not only do the patient and surgeon benefit, but in-patient time can be minimised with subsequent benefit to the health-care budget.

Percutaneous biopsy

Percutaneous biopsy using fine-bore needles guided by ultrasound or CT imaging has enabled biopsy specimens to be obtained from areas previously only accessible to the surgeon. Percutaneous needle biopsy of lung lesions, abdominal and retroperitoneal masses and pelvic viscera is now well established. Laparotomy, laparoscopy, thoracotomy, mediastinoscopy and craniotomy may all be obviated. In the presence of coagulation disorders the radiologist can biopsy the liver by the transjugular route.

Drainage and extraction procedures

The obstructed urinary tract

The percutaneous placement of a pigtailed catheter into the obstructed pelvicalyceal system under local anaesthesia may circumvent the need for an open surgical operation in a severely ill patient with electrolyte and acid-base disturbance. Percutaneous nephrostomy is of particular benefit in cases of bilateral obstructive uropathy, the obstructed unilateral kidney or the transplanted kidney. Following percutaneous nephrostomy, microbiological and cytological specimens can be taken and antegrade pyelography carried out. The repertoire of the radiologist can extend to the removal of calculi using a steerable catheter and basket retrieval system, the dilatation of strictures using a balloon catheter and the placement of permanent ureteral stents.

Decompression of the kidney may allow the recovery of renal function and the correction of metabolic disturbances. The cause of the obstruction may have meanwhile resolved spontaneously (the passage of a stone) or may have been improved by non-surgical treatment (radiotherapy, chemotherapy or hormone manipulation) and in these cases operation may be avoided entirely. In other cases the patient may have been rendered fit for anaesthesia and an open operation.

Jaundice and gall stones

Preoperative biliary drainage

In the jaundiced patient who is seriously ill, a period of preoperative biliary drainage to allow the recovery of hepatic function prior to surgery seems theoretically advantageous. The value of percutaneous drainage is currently being evaluated (probably of no value).

The residual common bile duct stone

The retained common bile duct stone after choledochotomy, which previously could only be tackled by reoperation, can now be treated by endoscopic methods and by the interventional radiologist. Both methods are safer than surgery. If a T-tube is still *in situ* and a stone is demonstrated in the common bile duct, the tube is left for 6 weeks until a fibrous track to the skin has matured. Using a steerable catheter and basket retrieval system the stone may then be removed. In a patient without a T-tube and in whom endoscopic retrograde cholangiopancreatography is contraindicated, the radiologist can still gain access to the common bile duct by a percutaneous transhepatic approach.

Percutaneous transhepatic prosthetic insertion (*in unfit jaundiced patients*)

The removal of foreign bodies

Upper gastrointestinal foreign bodies and those in the intravascular compartment (e.g. catheter tips) have been removed successfully by the interventional radiologist.

Intraperitoneal abscess localisation and drainage

Using abdominal ultrasound guide and needle aspiration under X-ray screening.

Vascular disorders

Percutaneous transluminal balloon angioplasty

Recent advances in balloon catheter technology have allowed the relatively safe dilatation of arterial stenoses and the technique of transluminal balloon angioplasty is now firmly established in the management of peripheral ischaemia, renal artery stenosis and coronary artery disease. The restoration of circulation to ischaemic limbs may be successful in circumventing the need for endarterectomy or bypass surgery under general anaesthesia and may salvage limbs in patients unfit for anaesthesia. Angioplasty of the coronary arteries will prevent the need for thoracotomy or sternotomy.

Venous thrombosis and pulmonary embolism

In the management of the poor-risk patient with iliofemoral thrombosis and in patients where anticoagulants have failed or are contraindicated, the interruption of the inferior vena cava to prevent pulmonary embolism can be achieved by the placement of an umbrella filter proximal to the thrombus via the transjugular approach.

Massive pulmonary embolus is also amenable to treatment without recourse to surgical embolectomy. Utilising the percutaneous transjugular or femoral approach a catheter can be steered into the pulmonary artery via the right heart. The embolus can either be dislodged into more peripheral segments of the artery or extracted using a suction cup. Following embolectomy an umbrella filter can be placed in the inferior vena cava.

Acute arterial bleeding

Therapeutic embolisation of the arterial tree is a major advance in the management of the poor-risk patient with surgical bleeding. Following the selective catheterisation of the appropriate vessel, absorbable or non-absorbable emboli are injected into the artery. Bleeding from tumours, gastrointestinal and urological lesions, fractures, ruptured viscera, aneurysm and biopsy sites has been controlled successfully in this manner. Provided there is sufficient collateral circulation there is little danger to other viscera.

Bleeding oesophageal varices

In addition to balloon tamponade, injection sclerotherapy, vasopressin infusion and various surgical portasystemic disconnection procedures, the interventional radiologist has added another method of control of variceal bleeding. Via a transhepatic or jugular approach, the portal venous system can be entered and the varices occluded by embolisation.

Arteriovenous malformations

The surgery of arteriovenous malformations may be difficult because of their anatomical position and the difficulty is compounded by their vascularity. Surgery may also be impermanent because of subsequent enlargement of collateral vessels. Embolisation of arteriovenous malformations has been used both as a definitive method of treatment and as a method of reducing vascularity prior to definitive surgery.

In neurosurgical practice a variety of lesions have been treated by this method. Previously, flow-guided embolisation of vessels was the only method of therapy but more recent advances have improved the accuracy of the procedure. The introduction of fine flexible catheters now allows the selective catheterisation of cortical vessels and the more accurate placement of emboli. Sophisticated balloon catheters have also been developed which facilitate hyperselective catheterisation of vessels and make flow-guided embolisation less hazardous by preventing aberrant embolisation.

The management of tumours

Preoperative embolisation

Embolisation of certain tumours preoperatively may be of benefit. Not only is the vascularity of the neoplasm reduced, helping to prevent operative blood loss, but the chance of tumour emboli being thrown off by operative handling may be reduced. Some authors maintain there is a theoretical advantage of provoking an immune response against the tumour cells as a result of tumour cell necrosis and the release of their specific antigens.

Palliation of neoplasms

The benefit of pain relief and reduction of haemorrhage from inoperable neoplasms has ensured therapeutic embolisation a place in the palliation of malignant disease. Embolisation of hormone-producing tumours is of value in that the distressing endocrine effects, e.g. sweats, palpitations and diarrhoea in the carcinoid syndrome, can be reduced.

Endocrine ablation

It is now possible to infarct the adrenal gland by the occlusion of adrenal veins using percutaneous embolisation. This has proved to be useful in the management of Cushing's syndrome. It may acquire a place in the management of advanced breast cancer in preference to medical adrenalectomy using aminoglutethimide which is toxic or surgical adrenalectomy which is a major surgical procedure.

Conclusions

Interventional radiological techniques have become firmly established in the management of surgical patients. Their scope will increase as radiologists with the necessary technical expertise are trained. This brief account of just some of the exciting developments in the field will it is hoped spur the Fellowship candidate on to investigate the subject more thoroughly and to become aware of the benefits that are likely for the patient and the surgeon. An account of catheter technology and precise accounts of the procedures can be found in the further reading list.

1.47. Clinical Implications of Contraceptive Pills in Surgery

The contraceptive pill is not free from major side-effects. These include the following.

- Thromboembolism is four times more likely to occur than in non-pill takers. This may be:
  —Venous thrombosis (unrelated to the period of pill use)—in superficial veins (proportional to age and parity), in deep veins and in pulmonary embolism.
  —Arterial thrombosis in both coronary and cerebral arteries. The predisposing factors are: oestrogen dose in the pill; age; cigarette smoking; obesity; other conditions such as diabetes, hypertention and familial hyperlipidaemia.
- Cardiovascular complications such as myocardial infarction—hypertension due to salt and water retention—obesity and cardiac failure.
- Gastrointestinal side-effects: abdominal bloating, persistent nausea, vomiting and weight gain. Breakthrough or withdrawal bleeding may sometimes mimic acute abdomen.
- Cholestatic jaundice with lithogenic bile. Gall bladder disease is common in postpartum primiparas who were prepregnancy pill takers.
- The hepatobiliary lesions attributed to anabolic steroids and/or the contraceptive pill are:
  —Cholestasis—both
  —Gall bladder disease—contraceptive pill
  —Liver tumours and nodules—both
  —Budd–Chiari syndrome—contraceptive pill
  —Peliosis hepatis (blood-filled cysts in the liver parenchyma)—anabolic steroids
  —Sinusoidal dilatation—contraceptive pill
- Breast pains and stimulation of fibroadenosis of the breast. The contraceptive pill may activate breast carcinoma and provokes galactorrhoea in females and gynaecomastia in males.
- Special medical problems, e.g. benign intracranial hypertension and erythema nodosum.
- Special surgical problems:
  —Carpal tunnel syndrome
  —Budd–Chiari syndrome (thrombosis of hepatic veins and portal hypertension)
  —Acute pancreatitis
  —Cholangiocarcinoma (no statistical support)
  —Acceleration of fibroid enlargement
  —Swollen painful legs
- Central nervous system side-effects such as stroke, severe migraine/headache and exacerbation of epilepsy. Anxiety and depression can also occur.
- Increased susceptibility to infections—vaginal candidiasis and even cervical erosions, and various skin conditions, e.g. pigmentation, eczema.
- Interferes with diagnostic tests for hydrocortisone assay, thyroxine level and serum iron

because it increases the plasma binding proteins, giving false results.

- Drug interference, e.g. antituberculous drugs, ampicillin and tetracyclines, and hypoglycaemic agents.

1.48. Malignant Melanoma

The incidence of cutaneous malignant melanoma in white-skinned people is increasing on a world-wide basis. It is estimated that both the incidence and the mortality are doubling every 10 years. While malignant melanoma is a potentially curable disease in its early stage, it is fatal in the late disseminated stage.

Malignant melanoma arises *de novo* or in a pre-existing benign naevus. The benign melanotic hamartoma (or naevocellular naevus or mole) is derived from a neural crest and may be junctional, compound, intradermal or blue naevus. These naevi may be small or large, pedunculated, sessile or flat, with or without hair. They are benign and usually remain so, or they may undergo spontaneous regression, leaving a halo (or Sutton's naevus) representing an autoimmune phenomenon (which may also occur in malignant melanoma). However, 10–40% of benign naevi undergo malignant change and this should be suspected if there is an increase in size, a change in colour (whether darker, lighter or mottled), bleeding, ulceration, crusting, itching or the formation of satellite spots.

Aetiology

- Exposure of fair-skinned people, particularly the Celts, to excessive sunlight. The ultraviolet irradiation causes nuclear damage and collagen disruption. The incidence of malignant melanoma is strongly influenced by the amount of ultraviolet light and duration of exposure.
- Familial or hereditary melanoma with 20% incidence of multiple lesions.
- Precancerous lesions (i.e. the giant bathing-trunk naevus) and *in situ* melanoma (i.e. conjunctival melanosis and lentigo maligna or Hutchinson's freckle).
- Trauma and hormonal changes (e.g. pregnancy) are doubtful.

CLINICAL PATHOLOGICAL ASPECTS

Clinical classification and staging

There are three main clinical types:

Lentigo maligna malignant melanoma develops slowly at the site of a previous Hutchinson's freckle on the faces of elderly people. It is regarded as a pre-invasive *in situ* melanoma with a relatively good prognosis.

Superficial spreading malignant melanoma represents a flat junctional activity anywhere on the skin with late dermal invasion and nodular transformation (the latter is associated with lymph node metastasis).

Nodular malignant melanoma with early dermal invasion and lymph node metastasis. The prognosis is poor.

There are three clinical stages in the spread of malignant melanoma:

Stage I   No evidence of regional spread.

Stage II   Clinical involvement of lymph nodes by embolism or regional spread by lymphatic permeation producing local satellite nodules and/or 'in-transit' deposits between the primary tumour and the regional lymph nodes. However, there is no evidence of distant spread.

Stage III   Distant spread: bloodborne metastases are seen in lungs, liver, brain, bones and skin. Secondary black deposits may involve unusual sites, e.g. small intestine, heart and breasts, and may cause melanuria.

Prognostic Factors in order of importance are:
1. Tumour thickness.
2. Infiltration level.
3. Presence of ulceration.
4. Mitotic activity.
5. Location.

Factors which on multivariate analysis do not appear to influence prognosis are: sex, age, histogenetic type of tumour, vascular invasion and lymphocytic infiltration.

Histological microtomal prognostic evaluation (or classification)

Tumour thickness (Breslow, 1970) Simple vertical measurement through the tumour centre is a reliable, accurate, objective and important determinant of the therapy and prognosis, since there is a close correlation between tumour thickness and prognosis. Tumours less than 0.75 mm are very unlikely to metastasise and rarely, if ever, recur if a margin of at least 2 mm clearance is achieved; thus excisional biopsy with 2 mm clearance is recommended generally for diagnosis and may be therapeutic if the tumour thickness is less than 0.75 mm.

Tumour infiltration or penetration level (Clark-McGovern level classification, 1976) Although important, this was proved to be highly subjective with up to 30% variation in the estimate of levels by different pathologists, and the system is replaced by the Breslow tumour thickness measurement. In the Clark-McGovern system the tumour is stated to be (Fig. 28).

Level 1   (*in situ* malignant melanoma). Confined to basal epidermis.
Level 2   Invasion of the papillary dermis (subepidermal connective tissue).
Level 3   Invasion to the junction level between the papillary and reticular dermis.
Level 4   Invasion of the reticular dermis.
Level 5   Invasion of the subcutaneous tissues.

This system is well correlated with patient survival.

MANAGEMENT

Surgery remains the mainstay in Stages I and II. Radiotherapy has no place and chemotherapy is only considered in Stage III. The clinical-histological work-up consists of excision biopsy (with 2 mm clearance margin) to measure the tumour thickness. Incisional, needle and scrape biopsies are contraindicated owing to the risk of tumour spread. Surgical treatment follows in the form of adequate excision of the primary tumour, with or without lymph node block dissection. Troublesome metastatic lesions are occasionally removed.

Stage I

Wide excision (5 cm clearance) of skin and subcutaneous tissue down to deep fascia (rarely including deep fascia) with split skin graft taken from the unaffected limb is the ideal approach (since the incidence of local recurrence is very low). The exceptions are:
● Lesions less than 0.75 mm thick and invasion level II: treated by local excision and closure without grafting (same as excisional biopsy with 2 mm margin clearance).
● Malignant melanoma of the face: treated by wide excision and rotational flap.
● Subungual malignant melanoma: treated by amputation via the neck of the proximal phalanx (no need for complete disarticulation of the finger).
● Malignant melanoma of the choroid of the eye necessitates eyeball enucleation or removal.
Prophylactic lymph node block dissection is indicated in tumours within the territory of the

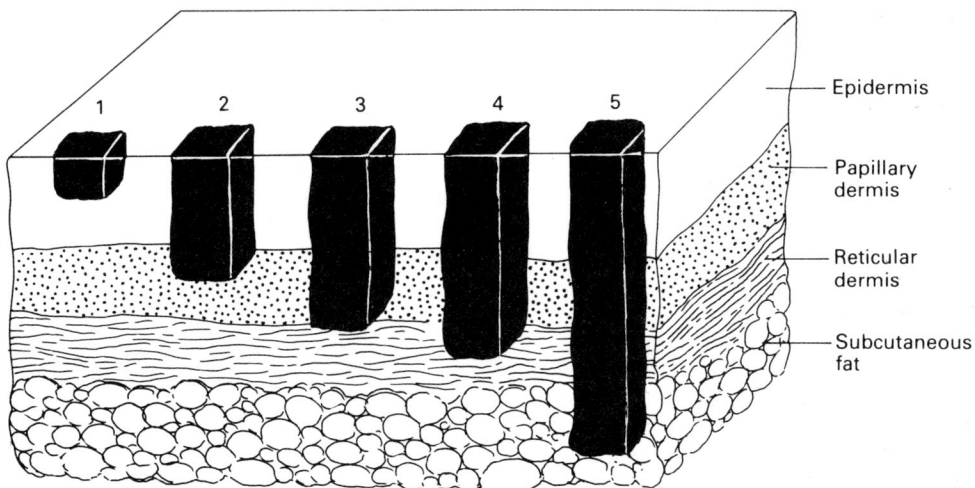

Fig. 28   Clark–McGovern level classification of malignant melanoma

lymphatic drainage (e.g. groin malignant melanoma) and for tumours of 2–5 mm thickness because of documented increase in 5 year survival. In tumours greater than 5 mm, the survival is so poor that node dissection may be postponed since blood-borne spread will probably appear before lymph nodes reveal evidence of recurrence. For these thick tumours node dissection represents a form of prophylactic palliative surgery for future troublesome locally fungating lesions.

Stage II

For 'in-transit' metastases, it is necessary to perform an in-continuity dissection and remove all potentially contaminated tissue between (and together with) the primary malignant melanoma and the draining lymph nodes, i.e. prophylactic and therapeutic dissection.

Clinically palpable lymph nodes necessitate careful therapeutic lymph node block dissection (inadequate node-picking operations should be abandoned because of the risk of tumour spillage— local wound recurrence is almost invariably fatal). Such a radical clearance of inguinal lymph nodes (in leg malignant melanoma) or axillary lymph nodes (unilateral in arm malignant melanoma and bilateral in midline back malignant melanoma) is invariably followed by lymphoedema and requires elastic stockings. Axillary dissection must be more radical than that used in breast cancer. Theoretically, a central midline back malignant melanoma should be excised with combined bilateral axillary and bilateral inguinal lymph node block dissection. Practically however, in view of the high associated morbidity, some surgeons prefer to excise the melanoma alone and to monitor the patient, performing block dissection only in clinically palpable lymphodenopathy (staged operation).

Stage III

- Palliative surgery is often worthwhile as a debulking procedure and to remove the painful, ulcerated lesions.
- Chemotherapy either i.v. or intralesionally using dimethyltriazinoimidazole-carboxamide (DTIC) in subcutaneous and pulmonary recurrences. Visceral metastases are difficult to treat.
- Isolated limb perfusion with phenylalanine mustard (in limb recurrences), with or without hyperthermia, remains a useful treatment and is occasionally curative for localised metastatic

disease (the treatment of Stage II in-transit metastases).
- Immunotherapy using BCG intralesionally.
- Heavy neutron radiotherapy is used for recurrences.

1.49. Solitary Thyroid Nodule

Discrete nodule formation in an otherwise normal thyroid gland is not uncommon. Clinically diagnosed solitary thyroid nodule (STN) may prove to be multinodular on the operating table or at subsequent histological examination. True STN is known for its malignant potential (especially in younger patients). Differentiated thyroid carcinoma may present itself clinically in one of the following forms:

1. STN.
2. STN + lymph node in neck.
3. STN + skeletal metastases.
4. STN + pulmonary metastases.
5. STN + cross-over combination 2, 3, 4.

Management

Management of STN is based on examination, both local and general, which allows assessment of thyroid status and of possible sites of metastases. Five specific investigations are: thyroid function tests (T3, T4, FTI, TSH); fine needle aspiration cytology (requiring special expertise); ultrasound scan; radioactive isotope ^{127}I scanning; surgical exploration with frozen section facilities.

The most common presentation is the euthyroid patient with an apparently simple STN; the basic problem is to define whether the nodule is cystic or solid, single or multifocal.

Aspiration

In the absence of ultrasound facilities immediate needle aspiration will establish the physical nature of the nodule. Needle aspiration of a simple cyst is usually perfectly adequate. Aspiration biopsy cytology by fine needle technique for a solid lesion does not exclude malignancy with certainty and also relies on considerable cytological expertise.

Ultrasound and radioactive isotope scanning

Ultrasound examination will establish whether a nodule is solid/cystic, single/multifocal, with irregularity of a cyst wall; or refractory and solid suggesting malignancy.

Radioactive isotope scanning, complementary to ultrasound, divides STN into:

- Hot (high uptake) with overactive hyperthyroid function.
- Warm (normal uptake) with active euthyroid function.
- Cold (subnormal uptake) with inactive function.

Hot STN is *usually* not malignant. It represents a toxic follicular adenoma requiring treatment by excision or radioiodine therapy.

Warm STN is a functioning adenoma without endocrine disturbance (histologically follicular adenoma, Hurthle cell adenoma, embryonal adenoma and fetal adenoma). Rarely well-differentiated carcinoma occurs and warm STN may develop into hot STN. Surgical excision is necessary.

Cold STN is malignant in about 12% of cases (either follicular, papillary or medullary) and should be excised. Other causes of cold STN include degenerative cyst, haemorrhage, calcification, abscess and hydatid parasitic cyst. Degenerative adenoma (i.e. hyperplasia in multinodular goitre) and occasionally autoimmune Hashimoto's thyroiditis can present as cold STN.

Surgical exploration and treatment

The foregoing methods may help in planning surgical treatment, but surgical exploration with the help of frozen section remains the end-point of assessment with a view to treatment and it should be preceded by independent inspection of the vocal cords. Local resection of a simple lesion, subtotal resection of a lobe or subtotal removal of the whole gland will suffice for the innocent disorder depending on its single or multifocal nature.

For differentiated carcinoma presenting as STN treatment is as follows.

Papillary carcinoma (metastasises to lymph nodes) Total lobectomy with subtotal lobectomy on the contralateral side, ensuring protection of parathyroid and recurrent laryngeal nerve function. Lymph node enlargement should be diagnosed by frozen section as being due to reactive hyperplasia or secondary deposits. In the latter case a modified neck dissection is carried out (by removing adjacent lymph nodes only, avoiding excision of the sternomastoid and cervical vessels).

Follicular carcinoma (skeletal metastases via bloodstream) Total thyroidectomy removes the lesion and any residual tissue which may compete for radioactive iodine when skeletal deposits may demand treatment at a later date.

Medullary carcinoma Best treated by total thyroidectomy with positive nodes removed by regional resection.

In all these situations thyroxine replacement is required and ideally it is used to suppress TSH in the case of papillary and follicular carcinomas (hormone dependence).

Aetiology of malignant thyroid tumours

- Familial or genetic (medullary thyroid carcinoma).
- Radiotherapy in childhood with radioactive iodine (papillary thyroid carcinoma). *N. B.* Radiotherapy with radioactive iodine should never be given to patients under 45 years of age nor to pregnant women.
- Iodine deficiency goitre or goitrogenic drugs (e.g. thiouracil).
- Autoimmune thyroiditis (malignant lymphoma of thyroid).
- Rarely, benign adenoma changed into malignant.

1.50. Hypercalcaemia and Primary Hyperparathyroidism

The blood level of calcium is influenced by various interacting factors. However, abnormal calcium levels can be caused by a variety of conditions (Table 11). Primary hyperparathyroidism and malignant disease are the two most common causes.

Differential diagnosis of hypercalcaemia

- Primary hyperparathyroidism.
- Sarcoidosis.
- Myelomatosis.
- Hyperthyroidism.
- Milk-alkali syndrome.
- Vitamin D intoxication.
- Immobilisation with Paget's disease.

Table 11.   Disturbed calcium metabolism (modified from Walter and Israel, 1974)

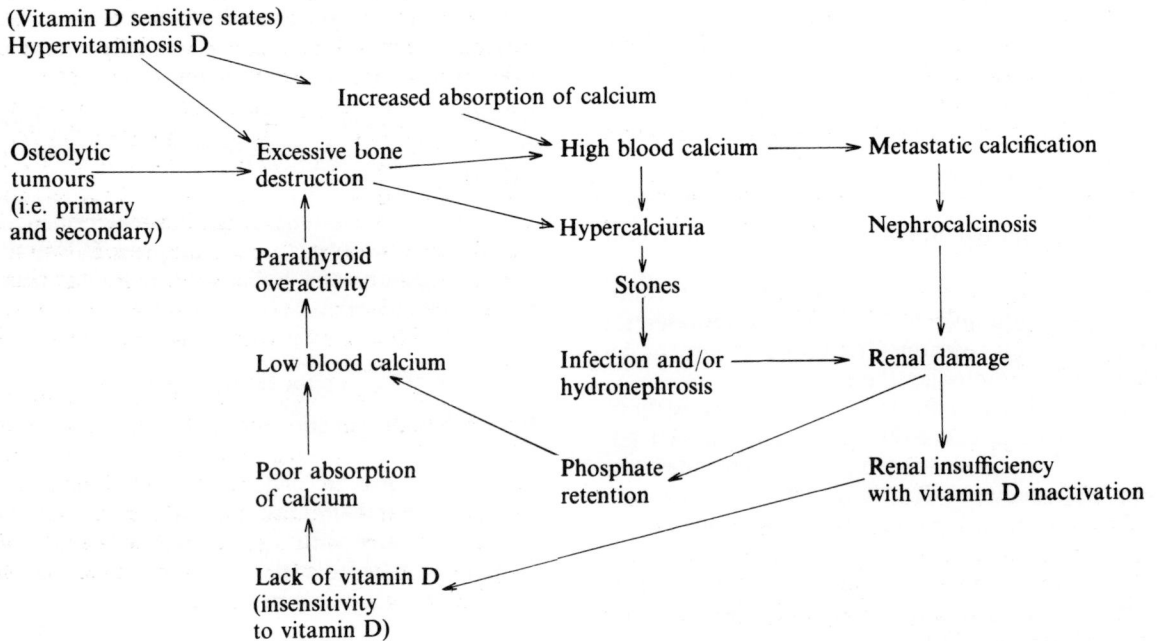

```
(Vitamin D sensitive states)
Hypervitaminosis D
                              Increased absorption of calcium

Osteolytic            Excessive bone        High blood calcium  ───→  Metastatic calcification
tumours               destruction
(i.e. primary                                                         Nephrocalcinosis
and secondary)                              Hypercalciuria
                      Parathyroid
                      overactivity          Stones

                      Low blood calcium     Infection and/or  ───→  Renal damage
                                            hydronephrosis

                      Poor absorption       Phosphate             Renal insufficiency
                      of calcium            retention             with vitamin D inactivation

                      Lack of vitamin D
                      (insensitivity
                      to vitamin D)
```

• Malignant disease with endocrine function (e.g. carcinoma of bronchus or kidney); or skeletal metastases in breast, prostate, bronchus, kidney and thyroid cancer.

Clinically, hypercalcaemia leads to anorexia, nausea, vomiting, constipation, muscle weakness and decreased reflexes, thirst, polyuria, nocturia and corneal calcification.

Preoperative diagnosis of primary hyperparathyroidism

Clinically it is the disease of bones (osteitis fibrosa cystica, cyst formation and generalised osteoporosis), stones (renal tract stones and nephrocalcinosis), abdominal groans (due to acute pancreatitis and peptic ulcer) and psychic moans. Laboratory investigations reveal hypercalcaemia, hypercalciuria, hypophosphataemia, hyperphosphaturia and elevated serum alkaline phosphatase. Blood samples for serum calcium estimation should be taken from a fasting patient without application of an arm tourniquet. X-rays show subperiosteal bone resorption in the hands with generalised cystic bone disease and renal stones and/or nephrocalcinosis.

The steroid (cortisone) suppression test is used to exclude hypercalcaemia of sarcoidosis, vitamin D intoxication or metastatic bone disease. Cortisone

150 mg is given daily for 10 days. The calcium level before the injection as well as on the 5th, 8th and 10th day of the test is estimated. It will be reduced in these conditions but hypercalcaemia will persist in primary hyperparathyroidism. Other laboratory tests are full blood count, liver function tests, urea and electrolytes, serum proteins (for serum calcium correction) and protein chromatography with Bence–Jones protein in urine (to exclude multiple myeloma), and uric acid estimation.

Preoperative parathyroid localisation tests

Identification of all parathyroid glands is necessary for successful surgery. Failure rate due to incomplete intitial exploration is 5 % and most undetected adenomas are in the neck or upper thymus.

Isotope scan using *technetium* and *thallium subtraction imaging* is extremely sensitive in accurately locating adenomas, particularly when there has been previous neck surgery or previous failed parathyroid explorations. The technique principle is first to outline the thyroid with ^{99m}Tc and then to give ^{201}Tl isotope which is taken up by both the thyroid and the parathyroid; the computerised subtraction of the two captured images (by gamma camera) will then show the parathyroid as a 'hot spot'. The other localising tests are rarely used now because of their insensitivity. Surgical exploration is required for persistent hypercalcaemia even if all the tests are negative. They include:

- Cine oesophagography (barium swallow showing indentations).
- Ultrasound scan.
- Arteriography and digital subtraction angiography.
- Retrograde venography and venous sampling of parathormone levels performed by radiologist via the femoral vein.
- CT scan.
- Nuclear medical radiography.
- Thermography.
- Lymphography.

Operative localising tests

Careful thorough exploration of the neck is essential. Parathyroids are small and tongue-shaped, dull orange in colour, and, when pinched with forceps, demonstrate a typical subcapsular blush. The following tests facilitate parathyroid identification at operation:

Staining with methylene blue Methylene blue 5–7.5 mg/kg in 500 ml of 5% dextrose commenced 1 h preoperatively and allowed to flow so that there are about 150 ml in the bottle still to run at the time of induction of anaesthesia. This last amount is run through after induction and while the neck is being opened at operation. Some surgeons believe that this test stains the cervical lymph nodes as well as giving false positive results; others find it helpful especially in localising ectopic parathyroids (e.g. in the thymus) which stain blue.

Flotation density test in 20% mannitol Adenoma or hyperplasia sink (no fat) while normal tissue floats (due to fat). The test is not widely practised.

Biopsy and frozen section This is helpful but may lead to infarction of the remaining biopsied glands. Many surgeons doubt the value of frozen section and prefer to wait for paraffin section.

Selective venous sampling Performed by the surgeon to identify the level of the hyperfunctioning gland.

Parathyroidectomy

The aim is to remove the diseased gland or glands and leave the patient normocalcaemic. The approach is similar to thyroidectomy with only middle thyroid vein disconnection to allow for thorough mobilisation and exploration. A lower collar incision and a stitch applied to the lateral border of the thyroid to pull it forwards and medially are useful. Meticulous care is taken to ensure an absolutely bloodless field—once bleeding occurs on any scale it becomes exceedingly difficult to recognise the subtle features of the small (and occasionally oddly located) parathyroids. There is no need for superior or inferior thyroid vessel ligation–division under usual circumstances. Adenoma is usually solitary, and once it is found excision without further search is adequate. In hyperplasia, however, full exploration of all four glands with excision of three and a half is recommended.

Postoperative evaluation of tetany clinically and of hypocalcaemia chemically is important. Prolonged i.v. calcium infusion may be required for 2 days in hypocalcaemia. Regular life-long follow-up is important—missed hypocalcaemia may lead to serious problems, e.g. cataract. Indefinite oral calcium replacement 2.5 g four times a day ± vitamin D therapy are needed.

Treatment of hypercalcaemia in general

In order of importance:

1. *Treatment of hypercalcaemia itself.* Because of its dangerous renal, gastrointestinal, neuropsychiatric and musculoskeletal effects, hypercalcaemia should be treated until the underlying cause is diagnosed and treated. The following measures are helpful:

- Rehydration: 4–6 litres in the first 24 h.
- Diuresis: with saline or even frusemide to decrease tubular reabsorption of calcium.
- Calcitonin: reduces bone resorption and causes calciuresis.
- Corticosteroids: reduce bone resorption (are both diagnostic and therapeutic).
- Mithramycin: is a cytotoxic antibiotic with specific toxic action against osteoclasts (single i.v. dose of 25 µg/kg).
- Diphosphonate: is an inhibitor of calcification.
- Low-calcium diet.

2. *Treatment of the underlying cause*, e.g. parathyroidectomy, tumour removal, bone radiotherapy, chemotherapy (for myeloma and bronchial small-cell carcinoma) and endocrine therapy (in metastatic breast carcinoma).

3. *Treatment of complications*, e.g. nephrocalcinosis and/or renal stones are treated finally on their merit. Surgery is indicated only in obstruction, pain and infection; otherwise treatment is expectant and conservative.

1.51. Terminal Care in Surgery

The terminal stage of any illness can be defined as beginning at the moment when the clinician says 'There is nothing more to be done' and then begins to withdraw from his patient. At this stage the patient can be managed in hospital, home or hospice. The aims of the palliation are:
- To restore the quality of living (symptom control).
- To take the fear out of dying (spiritual support).

Pain

Terminal cases due to cancer form the majority and about 87% of these patients have pain as the main complaint. Malignancy can produce pain by many mechanisms:
- Nerve compression by tumour or pathological fracture caused by the tumour bony metastases (sharp well-localised pain).
- Infiltration of nerve or blood vessel or their perineural or perivascular lymphatics or lymphoedema (diffuse burning, sympathetic).
- Gastrointestinal or genitourinary tract involvement and obstruction (either dull diffuse colicky or burning, as in cystitis).
- Vascular obstruction by tumour (ischaemic or venous engorgement).
- Tension and distension pain due to tumour infiltration of bones and closely investing fascia, and periosteum (pain-sensitive structures).
- Central necrosis and infection.
- Headache due to raised intracranial pressure.

Pain in advanced cancer is constant, and analgesics should be given at 4 h intervals on a regular basis and not *pro re nate*. Prescriptions are illogical and lead to inadequate pain control and possible consequent tolerance. Opiate addiction does not occur in chronic severe pain and would be immaterial in dying patients. Dose increase, however, indicates a change in the underlying pathology and not the development of tolerance. The oral route is preferred and injections should only be necessary during the last few days of life.

Analgesics

Peripherally acting non-narcotic analgesics

The effectiveness of aspirin (300–600 mg after food) or paracetamol (500–1000 mg tablets 4-hourly) should not be underestimated. However, osseous deposits (in carcinoma of the breast, bronchus, thyroid and multiple myeloma) produce severe bone pain through release of prostaglandins. Since non-steroidal anti-inflammatory drugs (NSAIDs) are potent prostaglandin synthetase inhibitors, they are effective in bone pain relief, e.g. diflunisal (Dolobid) 250 mg 12-hourly, salsalate (Disalcid) 500 mg 8-hourly or indomethacin sustained release (Indocid) 75 mg 24-hourly. Corticosteroids, although they modulate the inflammatory process by preventing prostaglandin release (stabilise cell membranes), are effective in relieving pain caused by nerve compression but not in relieving bony pain.

Centrally acting drugs

The following drugs, given in 4-hourly oral regular doses, can be extremely effective:

Non-narcotics
- Buprenorphine
- Nefopam

Weak narcotics
- Dihydrocodeine (DF 118) 10 mg
- Dihydrocodeine combined with paracetomol (Paramol 118)—contraindicated in asthma and liver dysfunction
- Dextropropoxyphene (Doloxene) 100 mg—causes drowsiness
- Dextropropoxyphene combined with paracetamol (Distalgesic)
- Aspirin and papaveretum

Strong narcotics may, however, be needed:
- Phenazocine 10 mg sublingually 6-hourly
- Morphine slow-release tablet (MST Continus) 10 mg 12-hourly
- Diamorphine i.m. or orally in chloroform water 4-hourly

When dysphagia, intestinal obstruction and persistent vomiting present, one of three *suppositories* is the choice:
- Morphine hydrochloride 10, 30 or 60 mg
- Oxycodone pectinate 30 mg
- Dextromoramide 10 mg

Morphine and diamorphine are probably the best *injectable analgesics.*

Sublingual analgesics include:
- Dextromoramide 5 or 10 mg
- Phenazocine 5 mg
- Buprenorphine 0.2 mg
- Diamorphine hypodermic tablet 10 mg

Note that a syringe driver can give continuous i.v. infusion in chronic pain. The patient can keep the syringe in his pocket and move around without pain. It is becoming an increasingly popular method since it:
- Maintains plasma level of narcotics, antiemetics and phenothiazine.
- Reduces injections to once daily or on alternate days.
- Reloads 12- or 24-hourly.
- Dosage as for i.m./subcutaneous injection.

Terminal cases in children
Should be given oral weak narcotic analgesics. Diamorphine can result in excessive sedation and problems in withdrawal should the child go into remission. They should be nursed at home with supportive care from the family and general practitioner. Hospital can provide advice when necessary.

Analgesics to be avoided

Too short effect
- Dextromoramide
- Pethidine (any route)

Too many side-effects
- Pethidine
- Pentazocine (unacceptable dysphoria)
- Levorphanol

Unpredictable analgesics (no place in chronic pain)
- Pethidine
- Pentazocine

Bad mixtures
- Diconal (dipipanone + cyclizine) (profound sedation)
- Nepenthe and aspirin
- Brompton cocktail (contains cocaine and chlorpromazine—a pharmacological nonsense)

Inappropriate use (inadequate dose/inappropriate drug)
- Partial antagonist used with agonist (partial antagonists are pentazocine, phenazocine and buprenorphine).

- Not given according to duration of action.
- Prostaglandin inhibitors not given for bone metastases.
- Inadequate use of narcotic potentiators.

Non-drug methods

May need sophisticated equipment and technical expertise. Such facilities (discussed in Section 1.2, 'General principles') are available in pain clinics (found in special directory).
- Secondary deposits can be treated with radiation or short or single doses of chemotherapy.
- Pathological fractures are a common source of pain and are best treated by fixation (plaster of Paris or preferably internal).
- Visceral upper abdominal pain (intra-abdominal cancer) can be relieved by coeliac plexus destructive block (alcohol or phenol).
- Unilateral pain below C6 level can be treated by contralateral cordotomy.
- Bilateral or midline pain is relieved by pituitary ablation.

Nausea and vomiting

Have different causes and are therefore treated differently (careful history is essential).

Drug-induced (by narcotics)

Treated with prochloperazine mesylate (Stemetil) 12.5 mg i.m. 4-hourly (produces moderate sedation while Largactil 25 mg i.m. 8-hourly is the most sedative but least effective antiemetic of the phenothiazines). The antiemetic of choice is haloperidol (Serenace) 2.5 mg i.m. 8-hourly (minimal sedation).

Hypercalcaemia

Can cause vomiting and anorexia. Occurs in carcinoma with bone secondaries or excess parathormone secretion, e.g. bronchial carcinoma. It is relieved rapidly by prednisolone 5 mg four times a day reducing to 5 mg daily or dexamethasone 4 mg i.m. 6-hourly for 48 h. Calcitonin can also be used.

Primary or secondary cerebral tumour (raised intracranial pressure)

Can cause vomiting, headache, blurred vision and mental confusion. Dexamethasone 4 mg should be given 6-hourly for 48 h by which time there should be a response (in this case a low maintenance dose of

2–4 mg/24 h should continue). If there is no response after 7 days, the patient should be reassessed.

Intestinal obstruction

Treated with i.v. infusion and nasogastric suction if obstruction is complete. If obstruction is incomplete a stool softener should be used, e.g. Dioctyl Forte two tablets twice daily. Analgesics and antiemetics should be given rectally (Stemetil or thiethylperazine malate (Torecan) suppositories). Metoclopramide may be used to increase gastric emptying in gastric stasis (can cause extrapyramidal symptoms as do phenothiazines).

Radiation or cytotoxic-induced vomiting

Is almost impossible to control; however, tetrahydrocannabinol can be effective.

Uraemia

Due to advanced obstructive uropathy.

Constipation

Due to inactivity, anorexia, low-residue diet and analgesic drugs (occupying opioid gut receptors). Treated by combined faecal softener and peristalsis-inducing (stimulant) laxative, e.g. Dorbanex 10 ml twice daily. Suppositories, enemas or manual disimpaction may also be required. (Senokot or Dulcolax are also useful stimulant laxatives. Lactulose 15 ml twice daily is an osmotic stimulant—an expensive alternative.)

Diarrhoea

Has many causes. It may be due to constipation with overflow (spurious diarrhoea) and treated as above. In subacute intestinal obstruction antiperistaltics can be used, e.g. loperamide (Imodium) or diphenoxylate with atropine (Lomotil). In malabsorption, usually due to pancreatic insufficiency, two tablets of pancreatin with each meal provide replacement. In rectal carcinoma (with mucus discharge) prednisolone retension enema or suppository is used.

Dyspnoea

Should be treated according to the cause, e.g. diuretics in cardiac failure and bronchodilators (salbutamol and aminophylline) in bronchospasm. In superior vena cava obstruction, dexamethasone 12 mg is given daily prior to radiotherapy. The same is used for lymphangitis carcinomatosa. Treat with antibiotics (in chest infection), drainage and possibly bleomycin instillation (in malignant effusion), opiates to relieve the sensation of dyspnoea (although they cause respiratory centre depression) and hyoscine (Scopolamine) 0.4–0.6 mg to dry up the accumulated secretions (death rattle). Oxygen may also be used. Corticosteroids in patients with short prognosis are the drugs of choice. The patient should be propped up in left ventricular failure, placed semiprone in bronchogenic carcinoma and on one side in pleural effusion.

Depression

Treated by *tender loving care* along with mood-elevating prednisolone 5 mg twice daily. Amitriptyline 25–75 mg daily is a useful antidepressant. It potentiates the analgesic effects of opiates in addition to its inherent analgesic activity. When giving amitriptyline oral hygiene is important as it causes a dry mouth. For anxiety diazepam (Valium) 5 mg three times a day is adequate. Largactil 25 mg three times a day can be given in the very last days. Emotional and spiritual support is important.

Muscle spasm

Due to tumour pressing on or irritating a nerve. It is treated with diazepam or dantrolene (Dantrium) 25 mg daily.

Anorexia

Small amounts of the patient's favourite food attractively presented can work wonders. Periactin (an appetite stimulant) is disappointing. Steroids are the drugs of choice (marked effect).

Pruritus

Due to bile acid accumulation in the skin as a result of obstructive jaundice. Treated with cholestyramine 4 g three times a day, Betnovate skin ointment or trimeprazine (Vallergan—a phenothiazine with marked antihistamine action).

Fits and convulsions

Due to primary or secondary brain deposits. Treated with diazepam 10 mg three times a day, phenytoin 100 mg three times a day or sodium valproate (Epilim) 200 mg three times a day. However, dexamethasone may reduce or eliminate the need for anticonvulsants.

Insomnia

Treated with short-acting benzodiazepines (Temazepam 10 mg at night). However chlormethiazole (Heminevrin) 1 g is a useful hypnotic for the elderly.

Miscellaneous

Urinary frequency and incontinence
- Emepronium bromide (Cetiprin) 200 mg at night
- Condom
- Indwelling catheter

Fungating growths
- Radiotherapy, cytotoxic, hormonal manipulation

- Betadine with liquid paraffin (1/4) cleansing Antibiotics
- Desloughing agents (natural yoghurt is good)

Oesophageal carcinoma
- Radiotherapy
- Insertion of oesophageal tubes

Nerve compression
- Strong analgesic
- Steroids, e.g. dexamethasone 4 mg/24 h
- Nerve block (intercostal/intrathecal/epidural 5–7.5% phenol glycerine + lactic acid)
- Tricyclic antidepressant, occasionally

Stretched liver capsule
- Paravertebral nerve block, occasionally
- Strong analgesic
- Methyl prednisolone 125–250 mg/24 h × 7 (i.m.)

Note: The following natural agents could be made use of:
- Yoghurt is a good skin desloughing cleansing agent.
- Honey is an excellent surgical dressing for bed sores and ulcers.
- Pineapple juice is a good solution for oral hygiene.

SECTION 2
Clinical Surgery

Introduction

The clinical part of the examination takes place in a hospital atmosphere (except in England where it is held in an examination hall). The clinical part is *the most essential* section. You have to pass it clearly in order to pass the Final FRCS. In the Irish Fellowship you may compensate for a written section but you have to score a clear double pass mark in the clinical section (120 out of 360). In other Colleges you have to pass clearly both the clinical and written sections *individually* as a prerequisite for passing the Final FRCS.

Clinical assessment is composed of two components—a few 'short cases' and one 'long case'—which are examined together and usually scored as a double mark. Clinical examination is the biggest hurdle since the examiner and examinee meet face to face and the examinee examines the patient under the dissecting microscope of the College examiners. The candidate's method of examining the patient and his presentation of the case are extremely important. Candidates should bring with them their own surgical instruments, i.e. stethoscope, torch and measuring tape.

The following areas are worth considering.

Examinee–patient relationship

BE:
- Smart. Good appearance is essential. Have your hair cut and dress professionally (for men, three piece dark suit with conservative tie) and wear clean shoes. Avoid school motifs and club dress. Smell should be acceptable and hands should be clean and warm (i.e. *appear, talk and behave like a doctor*).
- Polite and courteous. Introduce yourself, ask patients' permission for examination, thank them at the end, help them with their night clothes and tuck in the sheets. Seeing a semi-naked patient left uncovered after physical examination gives the examiner a very bad impression.
- Gentle. Ask the patient if he or she is suffering from pain; examine gently, looking at the face from time to time for any painful facial expression. Never examine patients as if you are manipulating experimental animals and remember that if the patient shouts 'ouch' you have failed your final FRCS!
- A shrewd observer. A surgeon should have a lion's heart (for courage), a lady's hand (gentle fine touch) and an eagle's eyes. You should try to spot as many abnormal physical signs as you can (even if not relevant to patient's main complaint) and therefore must examine the patient as a whole and not just the part related to his or her complaint. Abdominal examination is never complete without examining external genitalia and performing rectal examination (the foreskin should be inspected for phimosis and, if normal, retracted to inspect possible external urethral meatal stricture. Testicles are abdominal organs and should be palpated routinely especially for tumours since this may explain a vague abdominal mass such as a para-aortic lymph node). Rectal examination should be performed unless you are specifically requested not to. Do not forget to examine the patient's back and both legs, and examine the peripheral pulses carefully. Patient should be examined in the lying and standing position as well as walking since you may discover limping, scoliosis or paraplegia. However, you must be quick and comprehensive in your examination.
- Methodical. Many able candidates fail their examination, not because of ignorance of facts but because they examine the patients haphazardly, illogically or incompletely. Diagnosis is not very important—even the layman can diagnose hernia or varicose veins. The doctor should go through his patient methodically step by step according to a well practised routine, which has become instinctive, before reaching his final conclusion. Stress the importance of inspection and observation before embarking on palpation (e.g. ask the patient to lie flat and to lift his head

against your hand resistance. Ask him to cough while you look at hernial sites, then ask him to cough again and feel the impulse or the thrill at hernial or varicose vein sites). Make sure that you are being seen by the examiners (like a driving test where you have not only to follow the rule of mirror, signal, manoeuvre but also to be seen while you are doing it). Some candidates prefer to do a running commentary of their findings, others prefer to sum up at the end; both approaches are acceptable but the latter is preferable to avoid disturbing the patient with your commentary.

- Careful. When forced to discuss the causes of a patient's swelling at his bedside, avoid the word 'malignancy' or 'tumour' but use 'mitotic lesion' or 'neoplasia' instead. Always mention the common causes first before thinking of rarities. Do not be clever, be careful.
- Friendly. Especially in the long case, since this may guarantee the diagnosis, either volunteered by the patient himself or easily concluded after asking indirect leading questions (e.g. What investigations were performed? What did the doctor tell you?)

    If the examiner asks you later on 'Did you ask the patient about diagnosis?,' answer diplomatically, 'I asked him as a part of my routine systematic enquiry.' (Do not say 'No' since the examiner may take you to the patient to find out the truth).

Examinee–examiner relationship

DO:
- Appear professional (*see above*).
- Talk clearly, slowly and concisely (to the point), presenting a well-planned precise answer.
- Praise the patient (in the long case) by saying 'he is a good cooperative gentleman' or 'she is a nice lady and quite a good historian'. Avoid the negative aspects of patients.
- Keep it simple. Basic principles should always be mentioned first, emphasising the importance of history, examination and investigation and mentioning the simplest, most relevant investigation first. In emergencies always discuss under the plan of 'resuscitation, review then repair'. Common sense should be stressed, e.g. do not mention the fetus as a cause of an abdominal swelling in a male or prostatic enlargement as a cause of urinary retention in a female.
- Look confident. Give the impression that you know exactly what you are talking about and

know quite well how to substantiate your answers. The examiner may take a contrary view just to test your knowledge. You are expected to discuss the advantages and disadvantages of opposing views without emotion and to be sufficiently flexible to allow another opinion but at the same time to be firm in your own beliefs.
- Sound interesting and listen to the examiner's point of view especially when he wants to tell you his approach. Never ever tell him that his technique is old-fashioned.
- Lead the examiner to areas of the discussed topic which you know very well.
- Thank the examiner at the end.

DO NOT:
- Argue with the examiner even though you know that you are correct.
- Repeat his question while thinking of an answer and do not ask him to repeat his question since this indicates either that you did not listen to him carefully or that he was not able to phrase his question in an understandable way. However, if uncertain as to your instructions, do not hesitate to ask the examiner for clarification and hopefully he will rephrase the question better.
- Produce bizarre facial expressions when asked a question and do not smile too much when you are answering. This is an irritating habit. Do not make unnecessary hand or body movements and do not lean on the examiner's table.
- Become aphasic because of the shocking stress of the examination since examiners think that you should function properly under the stress of surgical emergencies and major operations, which is similar if not greater than examination stress, i.e. you are not suitable to be a surgeon. Relax and impress the examiner with your quiet confident ability.
- Be too friendly with the examiner or be tempted to crack jokes. Be reserved, smile a little with confidence and keep the discussion smooth, comfortable and to the point.
- Ask the examiner to help you while conducting your physical examination (e.g. do not ask him to support the patient while she bends forward for inspection of the breasts). Hopefully he will volunteer to help you.
- Spoil the examiner's X-rays when shown films on the viewing box by touching them or marking them with biro since these films may be treasured by him.
- Be clever. Do be careful. Always try and talk from the general to the specific and from the

common to the rare. Do not bring up rarities or syndromes unless you are prepared to talk about them and do not mention them first before common diseases. You are being tested on clinical surgery and not on the latest breakthrough in an obscure subspeciality with which you happen to be conversant.

- Be overconfident and authoritative toward the examiners, especially in controversial issues, e.g. breast cancer or peptic ulcer treatment. Never express your instructions to the patient dogmatically, e.g. in Buerger's disease do not say: 'Either you stop smoking or I amputate your legs', but 'I *advise* you to stop smoking since you cannot both smoke and keep your leg.' Careful phrasing in such situations is important.
- Abbreviate or use vague terms. PR may mean pulse rate or per rectum or pityrasis rubra. MI may mean myocardial infarction or mitral incompetence. Also avoid words such as minimal, slight, tinge, minor since physical signs are either normal or abnormal, black or white (even in grey cases you have to give your impression and a provisional diagnosis and not list a long differential diagnosis). Do not use meaningless phrases. Your ability to communicate as well as your surgical knowledge and judgement is being assessed.
- Answer irrelevantly. Listen carefully, plan your answer and then answer the particular question asked. At the bedside do not jump to conclusions but examine the findings, then plan and think of the possible causes that support the conclusion (use your eyes and hands, then your brain, then open your mouth).
- Assume that the examiner always knows the answer or that he knows more than you.

A. Short Cases

These cases are chosen (by the Consultant and his deputy organiser, e.g. Registrar or Senior Registrar) from surgical out-patient clinics and they will be admitted to hospital for operation at the end of the clinical examination. Some of them are in-patients with obvious physical signs that merit discussion. However, in the English Fellowship these cases are brought into an examination hall

(for which they are paid) for the clinical examination. Such cases must be transportable, not acutely ill, elective not emergency and able to appear for consecutive examinations. They may not even need an operation, e.g. pectoral lipoma, large sebaceous cyst, Dercum's disease. (Remember to ask the patient: 'When did you have this swelling?' 'Does it give you any problem?' If it is asymptomatic say there is no need for operation.)

Diagnosis is usually no problem in short cases as they can be spot diagnosed. Listen carefully to the examiner's wording and his phrasing of the questions. Approach each case in three stages:

1. Examine your patient: elicit physical signs in a methodical way, be accurate and comprehensive and make sure the examiner knows what you are doing. (Do not be hesitant or clumsy in your steps of examination.) Make a point of inspection because although you may have noticed the signs to be seen on inspection, it is important that you are seen to be. Every action should be clear, simple and look well practised. Be very gentle and polite with patients.

2. Give your physical findings at the conclusion of the examination (this is preferred to a running commentary).

3. Discuss the diagnosis.

Pay special attention to the examiner–examinee and examinee–patient relationships.

A1. ABDOMINAL MASSES
('*examine this patient's abdomen*')

1. Ask patient to lie flat with the abdomen completely exposed from the xiphisternum down to and including the external genitalia—from nipples to knees. (*N.B.* testicles are abdominal organs.)

2. Make a point of inspection, paying particular attention to hernial sites, general abdominal distension (fat, fluid, flatus, faeces, fetus or tumour), epigastric pulsation (normal in a thin patient; otherwise indicates gastric carcinoma overlying the aorta, right ventricular failure). If the pulsation is expansile, it indicates aortic aneurysm. Visible peristalsis indicates intestinal obstruction or pyloric obstruction (with a succession splash heard on gentle shaking of patient). Notice abdominal striae, umbilicus, distended veins (inferior vena cava obstruction, portal obstruction with caput medusae) and pigmentation.

3. Make an effort to search for a hernia or post-operative incisional herniation by asking patient to lift his head against your hand resistance applied on forehead while you are looking at his abdomen. Ask

patient to cough twice—once so that you can locate the hernial site and the second time to enable you to confirm it by palpation for impulse on coughing.
4. Warm your hand, kneel by the patient's bedside and gently palpate his abdomen using your flat hand, palpating mainly through the metacarpophalangeal joints. Palpate the whole abdomen first to feel whether it is soft or rigid, painless or tender (always look at the patient's face). Then palpate for any localised organomegaly and LUMPS (*see below*).
N.B. Organomegaly—tumours connected with the liver, spleen and stomach move freely with respiration; those of the kidney and other abdominal organs do not.

Hepatomegaly

Palpate from the right iliac fossa upwards towards the right hypochondrium. It is confirmed by percussion for hepatic dullness from the chest towards the abdomen for the upper border and *vice versa* for the lower border. Auscultate for hepatic haemangioma. The gall bladder is impalpable unless distended in which case it is a pyriform swelling opposite the ninth costal cartilage and moves freely with respiration. Right hydronephrosis is differentiated from enlarged gall bladder by bimanual palpation, which is possible only in kidney cases.

Splenomegaly and renal tumour

Palpate from the right iliac fossa upwards towards the left hypochondrium. Splenomegaly may be mistaken for left renal tumour. The following points will help in differentiation:
- A renal tumour is bimanually palpable moving backwards and forwards between one hand on the loin behind and the other on the anterior abdominal wall. Splenomegaly is not palpable bimanually.
- Fingers can usually be passed between the kidney and the ribs but not between the ribs and splenomegaly.
- The spleen has a sharp edge with a notch. The kidney edge is always rounded and has no notch. An enlarged kidney tends to bulge forwards. Perinephric abscesses bulge backwards.
- Because of overlying colonic splenic flexure percussion on splenomegaly may be resonant.
N.B. With any abdominal tumour, examine for LUMPS:

- Liver enlargement.
- Umbilicus secondary malignant deposits from gut primary tumour, especially stomach (Sister Joseph's nodule).
- Moving (or shifting) dullness for ascites confirmed also by transmitted fluid thrill. Ascites causes lateral abdominal bulging with flank dullness (shifting) and bulging transverse umbilicus. Ovarian tumour causes anteroposterior abdominal bulging with central (non-shifting) dullness and a vertical umbilicus that is drawn upwards.
- Per rectal or vaginal examination for ovarian or pelvic deposits, prostatic enlargement and secondary anal conditions, e.g. piles, abscesses and fistulae.
- Supraclavicular lymph node enlargement (e.g. testicular and gastric tumours).

Causes of right iliac fossa mass

Consider the following in order of frequency:
1. Appendicular mass or abscess.
2. Carcinoma of the caecum: the mass is not tender in an anaemic elderly patient over a long period; occult blood in stool and barium enema are positive.
3. Crohn's disease: diarrhoea, weight loss, occult blood in the stool, high ESR, and barium follow-through showing 'string sign' of Kantor (US gastroenterologist) in long-standing Crohn's disease.
4. Gynaecological masses: parametritis, twisted ovarian cyst, uterine fibroid.
5. Pelvic kidney: congenital or history of kidney transplantation; IVU is essential.
6. Iliac lymphadenitis.
7. Rare conditions: ileocaecal tuberculosis, actinomycosis, haematoma, carcinoid tumour, intussusception and appendicular tumours.

A2. LEG ULCER
('*examine this patient's leg*')

The three commonest causes of leg ulcers are venous, arterial and traumatic. However, an arterial ulcer due to peripheral vascular insufficiency may be associated with varicose veins. Therefore careful methodical examination is essential. A quick preliminary history is sometimes necessary. Ask about the ulcer duration and any past history of deep venous thrombosis, postoperative leg swelling and history of tuberculosis or syphilis.

1. Kneel by patient's leg and inspect closely and carefully, observing:
- Skin colour
- Hair
- Nails
- Muscle wasting
- Inflammation and oedema
- Ulcer
- Gangrenous toe
- State of veins and their filling
- Any obvious pulsation

2. Palpate for:
- Ulcer base
- Periulcer induration and liposclerosis
- Fascial defects (sites of venous perforators)
- Temperature
- Capillary filling
- Sensation

3. Palpate all peripheral pulses bilaterally:
- Femoral artery in midinguinal point between the anterior superior iliac spine and symphysis pubis (patient is supine).
- Popliteal artery deeply in the midline of the popliteal fossa (knee flexed to a right angle and patient lying supine or prone). Palpation should be very deep, commencing medially and bringing the fingertips transversely across the line of the artery.
- Posterior tibial artery: midway between the back of the medial malleolus and the medial border of the tendo Achillis (foot is dorsiflexed and inverted).
- Dorsalis pedis artery: in the groove between the first and second metatarsal bones upwards towards the ankle (foot is steadied by left hand and right hand finger pulps are directed slightly towards the first metatarsal bone).

4. Auscultate the femoral artery and adductor hiatus for any bruit (atherosclerosis).

5. If the pulses are absent or poor do Buerger's postural test (skin pallor on leg elevation and skin rubor on leg dependency). If pulses are present and normal consider a venous origin and examine for varicose veins of the leg.

6. Do culture and sensitivity tests of the discharge in infected ulcer and do biopsy if the ulcer edge is irregular or elevated (in a suspected malignant ulcer).

REMEMBER
- Microscopic death of cells is called 'necrosis'.
- Macroscopic dead soft tissue is called 'slough', e.g. skin, fascia or tendon.
- Macroscopic dead bone is called 'sequestrum', e.g. in chronic osteomyelitis.
- Macroscopic death with putrefaction is 'gangrene' (including both soft tissues and bone as in lower limbs or organs, e.g. appendix, gall bladder, small intestine). Gangrene is either dry (atherosclerosis or Buerger's disease) or wet with infection and swelling (embolism and diabetes).

Causes of ulcer

Ulcers and wounds are both breaches in the epithelial surface but the former are due to internal causes while the latter are due to external causes. Self-inflicted ulcer is a combination of both. You should define the ulcer in terms of site, size, shape, edge (margin), floor (the visible part within the ulcer margin), base (the tissue on which the ulcer is situated—examined by palpation), regional lymph nodes and ulcer discharge.

1. *Venous*: in varicose veins or post-phlebitic syndrome. The ulcer is on the lower medial third of the leg, irregularly shaped with terraced margin and pink granulated floor sitting on a bony base.

2. *Arterial*: with signs of ischaemia and absent pulses. Gangrenous toe may be seen (atherosclerosis and Buerger's disease).

3. *Traumatic*: can be caused by adhesive bandages, plaster-of-Paris, but more commonly by patient lying in one position for too long (decubitus pressure sore). The latter is prevented by frequent changing of the patient's position and rubbing the bony prominences with spirit and talcum powder. Common in comatose and hemiplegic geriatric patients and is difficult to heal (may need excision and skin graft).

The above three causes are the commonest, followed by:

4. *Infective*:
- Pyogenic ulcer: acute infection commonly with staphylococci and healed with antibiotics.
- Tuberculous ulcer: chronic after rupture of a cold abscess. It has an undermined margin, a soft base covered with thin serous discharge and bluish surrounding skin. An example is erythema induratum of Bazin, which produces purple nodules on the calves of the legs in adolescent females. It is due to *Mycobacterium tuberculosis* and treated with antituberculous drugs.
- Syphilitic gummatous ulcer: usually on upper third of the leg with punched out edge, dirty sloughed floor and hard base (due to *Treponema pallidum*).

- Oriental sore (Baghdad boil): due to *Leishmania tropica*.
- Meleney's ulcer: leads to progressive skin gangrene (synergistic bacteria) (*see* Section 6).

5. *Neuropathic (trophic sore) ulcer*: skin anaesthesia caused by diabetes mellitus (with vascular insufficiency and repeated infection) may lead to perforating ulcers of the sole of the foot which practically never heal. Other causes of neuropathic ulcers are spina bifida, tabes dorsalis, leprosy, peripheral nerve injury, syringomyelia and alcoholic polyneuritis.

6. *Malignant ulcer*: with its premalignant Marjolin's (French surgeon) ulcer. Premalignant ulcers include chronic scar (due to burn), chronic varicose ulcer and sinus of chronic osteomyelitis.

7. *Vasculitic ulcer*: frequently occurs on the lateral aspect of the leg in collagen diseases, such as rheumatoid arthritis, and in ulcerative colitis.

8. *Cryopathic ulcer*: in chilblains and cold injury.

9. *Hypertensive ulcer (Martorell's ulcer)*.

10. *Haematological ulcer*: in leukaemia, sickle cell and haemolytic anaemia and polycythaemia.

11. *Self-inflicted ulcer*.

Causes of gangrene

1. Secondary to RESTED (Raynaud's disease, Ergot, Senile atherosclerosis, Thrombosis, Embolism and Diabetes).
2. Infective, e.g. gas gangrene.
3. Traumatic, e.g. pressure sores, supracondylar fracture of femur pressing on popliteal artery.
4. Physical, e.g. burns, frostbite, chemicals.
5. Venous gangrene due to idiopathic or visceral neoplasm (Trousseau's sign) and in polycythaemia vera.

Pathogenesis and treatment of varicose ulcer

Venous ulceration does not appear to result from blood stasis within dilated tortuous veins of the lower limb with local deoxygenation (Homans theory, 1916) nor to be caused by arteriovenous shunting (Pratt theory, 1948). The current and widely accepted theory of its pathophysiology is that of venous pressure. Normally the pressure of foot veins is 100 mmHg at rest. This falls to 30 mmHg during exercise due to sucking action of the calf muscle squeezing blood out of the soleal sinusoids and deep veins towards the heart (this calf muscle pump is sometimes known as the peripheral heart.) When the valves in the deep venous system have been destroyed, e.g. post-thrombotic, or rendered incompetent by venous dilatation, blood oscillates up and down the deep veins and venous pressure recorded from the superficial veins during exercise remains constant.

Such venous hypertension results in local capillary bed dilatation which leads to increased permeability owing to stretching of the intraendothelial pores. Fibrinogen leaks in great amounts and polymerises within the tissues to form insoluble fibrin clots in the interstitial fluid around capillaries within the skin and subcutaneous tissues of the calf (pericapillary fibrin cuff). Owing to an associated deficient fibrinolytic activity, the fibrin breakdown is reduced and a greater amount of interstitial thrombosis occurs (liposclerosis). Liposclerosis blocks oxygen and nutrients from reaching the overlying dermal cells (microcirculation diffusion block) leading to tissue anoxia and cellular death which is seen clinically as ulceration. The usual location of this ulcer on the medial lower third of leg is due to constant ankle perforators with maximal venous hypertension at that site. Thus prolonged elastic support (to prevent venous stasis and hypertension) supplemented by fibrinolytic enhancement is the best method of prophylaxis (and treatment) in patients with phlebographic evidence of severely damaged veins.

Varicose ulcer requires daily antiseptic cleansing (Chlorhexidine, EUSol or H_2O_2) and elastic compression bandaging. Once the ulcer is dry, absorbent dressing is applied to promote drying and scaling. Calaband or Viscopaste may be advocated with fibrinolytic enhancement using a course of *stanozolol*. Up to 90% of venous ulcers will heal with the above measures.

Operative indications

- No response to medical measures.
- Multiple or large ulcer (over 2.5 cm in diameter) with liposclerotic area of 5 cm or more.
- Associated saphenofemoral incompetence or obvious perforators should be treated prior to ulcer treatment (deep venous system should be normal).

Contraindications to operation

1. Severe ulceration with diffuse oedematous skin (operation will lead to necrosis).
2. Infected ulcer or infected eczematous skin.
3. An obstructed deep venous system.

Operative procedures

Dodd's operation involves subfascial dissection and ligation of perforators via a midline posterior incision curved towards the medial malleolus while Cockett's operation involves suprafascial ligation of perforators (above the deep fascia). Linton's operation is directed towards excision of the ulcer, including its deep fascia (followed by split skin grafting), together with removal of superficial varicose veins and flush ligation and disconnection of the saphenofemoral junction. Combined subfascial perforator ligation, ulcer excision (and split skin grafting) and treatment of varicose veins is the procedure currently used.

A3. VARICOSE VEINS
('examine this patient's leg')

These enlarged elongated dilated veins may be present with leg ulcer (proceed as described above then continue for varicose vein examination) or without, in which case follow the procedure outlined below:
1. Ask the patient, uncovered from the umbilicus downward, to stand up on a stool.
2. Inspect in good daylight and carefully scrutinise the front (long saphenous vein) and the back (short saphenous vein) of the lower limbs.
3. Palpate over the course of the short and long saphenous veins, as well as the groin (saphina varix) and above possible ulcers to feel vaguely visible varicosities and to detect deep fascial defects or gaps (sites of perforators) which are felt as venous blown-out areas.
4. The cough impulse test is performed by applying the right hand to the groin just below the saphenous opening and asking the patient to cough. A fluid thrill is felt in the middle finger if the valve at the saphenofemoral junction is incompetent.
5. The percussion (tap) sign is elicited by placing the left-hand fingers just below the saphenous opening and tapping the main bunch of varicosities once with the right middle finger. If the valves are incompetent within that examined segment, there will be an upward wave, producing an impulse felt by the left hand overlying the long saphenous vein above.
6. Perform the Brodie–Trendelenburg test: ask the patient to lie down on the couch; elevate her lower limb, keeping it straight, and milk the veins to drain the blood out. Place a thumb firmly over the saphenous opening, lower the limb and instruct the patient to stand. Remove the thumb suddenly, and

if the veins fill immediately this proves saphenofemoral junction valve incompetence.

The triple tourniquet test (Oschner and Mahorney) is a modification of the above, using three successive applications of one tourniquet or three tourniquets applied at once around the upper thigh, above the knee and below the knee then releasing them in order (from above downward) to demonstrate the level of communication between the deep and superficial systems (through the incompetent valve).
7. To demonstrate patency of the deep venous system, occlude the superficial venous system (but not the deep veins) by applying a rubber tourniquet around the thigh (Perthes' bandage walking test) with the patient in a standing position. The patient is then allowed to walk for 5 min: severe pain is experienced with more pronounced varicosities in the lower limb.
8. Finally examine the lower abdomen in the lying position (if time permits) to differentiate secondary from primary varicose veins. The causes of secondary varicose veins are:
- Pregnancy.
- Intrapelvic neoplasm (uterus, ovary, prostate, rectum) obstructing deep venous return leading to superficial varicosities.
- Compensatory varicose veins complicating iliofemoral phlebothrombosis.
- Arteriovenous fistula, often associated with superficial varicosities. The primary cause should be treated.

Treatment

Current methods of treating varicose veins are:
- Triple saphenectomy procedure, i.e.
  —Saphenofemoral junction flush ligation-disconnection (mistakenly called Trendelenburg's operation, which referred originally to high mid-thigh varicose vein ligation).
  —Varicose vein stripping. (This should be confined to the femoropopliteal segment of the great saphenous vein to avoid saphenous nerve neuritis, interruption of lymphatics and pain produced by extirpation of the low segment between the ankle and knee joints. Furthermore, extirpation of below-knee segment does not remove ankle perforators which communicate with the posteromedial branch of long saphenous vein.)
  —Multiple varicose vein avulsions (mainly below knee).

- Injection-compression technique. Indicated in:
  —Postoperative recurrence especially below the knee.
  —Primary varicose veins, especially when confined to below the knee, as an alternative to surgery.
  —Troublesome vulval varicosities.
- It is contraindicated in deep venous thrombosis or in contraceptive pill takers, and in the presence of saphenofemoral junction incompetence.
- The sclerosing material used is 5 % ethanolamine oleate (Ethamolin) or 3 % sodium tetradecyl sulphate (STD). Each varicosity is injected with 0.5–1 ml not exceeding a total of 10 ml per session (otherwise haemolysis occurs). Injections must always be intravascular (otherwise skin ulceration may occur). The varicosities are marked in the standing position and injection is done in the lying position with the leg elevated. Each injection is maintained temporarily by supporting the needle with a dental roll until all injections are finished. Then all injection sites are compressed by Sorbo-rubber pads maintained in position by a crêpe bandage and a full-length elastic stocking for 6 weeks. The recurrence rate is higher than with surgery.

A4. SWOLLEN LEG
('examine this leg')

A swollen lower limb is due either to medical central (often bilateral) or surgical peripheral (often unilateral) local disease.

1. Exclude the medical causes (cardiac, renal, hepatic and hypoproteinaemia) by history and physical examination, e.g. increased jugular venous pressure, puffiness of face, ascites. The swelling is often bilateral, indicating a systemic cause.

2. Unilateral leg swelling has either a venous or a lymphatic origin (rarely it is caused by arteriovenous fistula).

- Venous origin is suggested by: history of deep venous thrombosis after pregnancy, operation or immobility; presence of pain, varicose veins or complications such as ulcers or dermatitis usually with pitting oedema. The contraceptive pill in females and stilboestrol in males are predisposing factors.
- Lymphatic origin is suggested by absence of pain, healthy skin (no ulceration or pigmentation) and non-pitting oedema (primary lymphoedema is bilateral in 50 %).

3. Arteriovenous fistula is rarely present and is either congenital or acquired (after stab or gunshot trauma). Hot leg ulcer, varicose veins with port-wine skin discoloration. local gigantism, warmth, machinery murmur or bruit as well as collapsing arterial pulse (due to high pulse pressure) and cardiac enlargement and failure are all indicative of congenital or acquired fistula. (The latter is diagnosed on the basis of history and lacks gigantism if it occurs after completion of epiphyseal fusion of the limb bones.)

REMEMBER
Difficult cases can be investigated by;
- Ascending deep functional venography.
- Lymphangiography.
- Arteriography (valuable in arteriovenous fistula).

Treatment of lymphoedema is mainly conservative (limb elevation, bed rest with antibiotics for cellulitis attacks, elastic bandages, intermittent diuresis, pneumatic intermittent external compression and massage). In severe cases surgery can be tried (flaying operation, swiss roll operation, Kandoleon's operation, lymphovenous microsurgery). In resistant cases limb amputation may be indicated.

Peripheral causes of leg swelling

Venous origin
- Post-phlebitic syndrome.
- Deep venous thrombosis.

Lymphatic origin
- Primary lymphoedema manifested at birth (lymphoedema congenita; when familial, called Milroy's disease), at adolescence (lymphoedema praecox) or after age 35 years (lymphoedema tarda).
- Secondary lymphoedema after
  — Radical surgical excision of lymph nodes.
  — Radiotherapy.
  — Malignant infiltration, e.g. breast carcinoma.
  — Inflammation.
  — Parasitic infestation (filariasis).

Secondary lymphoedema differs from primary in being of rapid onset, unilateral in distribution and always having an obvious known cause.

Miscellaneous
- Arteriovenous fistula.
- Lipoedema.
- Erythrocyanosis frigida.
- Tight bandage or plaster.
- Injuries, e.g. muscle contusion or fracture.
- Infection, e.g. cellulitis.

A5. LOCALISED INTEGUMENTAL SWELLINGS
('*examine this lesion*')

Inspect and palpate the lesion thoroughly. You can ask the patient how long he has had the swelling and whether it causes him any problems (if the lesion is benign, asymptomatic and present for a long period, leave alone). Describe the lesion in terms of number (solitary or multiple), site, size, shape, overlying skin colour, contour (smooth or irregular surface), consistency (jelly-like, soft, firm, hard or stony hard), tenderness, tethering (mobility) and transillumination.

Sebaceous cyst

Small intracutaneous firm smooth spherical swelling (moves with skin), usually associated with a punctum (can be revealed by gently squeezing or pulling the lesion under tension). It commonly occurs on the scalp, postauricular area, scrotum and face as a retention cyst (due to blocked sebaceous gland duct). Treatment is by excision for cosmetic reasons and to prevent complications (infection, ulceration in Cock's peculiar tumour, calcification and sebaceous horn formation).

Lipoma

Soft multilobulated, commonly subcutaneous (skin moves over it) with no punctum. It has positive fluctuation (fat is fluid at body temperature) and slipping sign (if the lump edge is pressed, it slips from beneath finger). If the lipoma is subfascial or submuscular ask the patient to contract that particular muscle and the lipoma will decrease in size or disappear with no more lobulation. Lipoma is best left alone unless it is:
- Large and unsightly (cosmetic).
- Symptomatic, i.e. painful or tender in adiposis-dolorosa or Dercum's disease (multiple subcutaneous lipomas with one or more tender or painful). Only the painful lipomas should be removed.
- In the thigh or retroperitoneally located as these are more likely to progress to liposarcoma.
The treatment is surgical excision.

Dermoid cyst

Sequestration dermoid occurs at sites of closure of embryonic fissures in the midline of the neck, abdomen, mediastinum and scalp and at the inner or outer angles of the orbit. It is a firm tense subcutaneous mobile cyst (skin moves over it). It differs from an implantation dermoid in that its wall contains hair, hair follicles, sweat and sebaceous glands. Implantation dermoid is associated with a scar from a precipitating injury (thus its wall is stratified squamous epithelium) and commonly affects the hand, palm or fingers, usually of gardeners.

Treatment is excision to prevent infection and for cosmetic reasons. Both dermoid and sebaceous cysts contain pultaceous material that can be moulded; therefore such large cysts give an indentation sign.

Cavernous haemangioma (as well as lymphangioma and meningocele)

Give emptying sign when compressed and refill again when pressure is released. De Morgan's spots, though vascular cutaneous lesions, do not give emptying sign. Treatment of cavernous haemangioma is conservative.

Papilloma

Common benign, sessile or pedunculated, pigmented or non-pigmented, single or multiple squamous cell lesion. When on the sole of the foot it may be difficult to differentiate from a corn (localised horny plug of epithelial cells in the epidermis). Treatment is by surgical excision or chemical application (silver nitrate).

Ganglion cyst

A tense cyst that communicates with a synovial membrane of a joint or a paratenon (tendon sheath) and contains gelatinous fluid. It usually occurs on the dorsum of the wrist or foot, but it may be related to flexor tendons in the palm or to peroneal tendons at the ankle. It represents a herniation of synovial membrane and may cause pain or interfere with tendon function. Treatment is by rupturing it with external pressure or by excision under anaesthesia (local, Bier's block or general) with a bloodless field. The recurrence rate is high.

Muscle tumour

When the muscle is relaxed, the lump can be moved freely across the long axis of the muscle; when the muscle is contracted, the movement becomes abruptly limited. Treatment is surgical excision.

Pulsating lesion

The pulsation may be transmitted from a nearby artery or the swelling itself may be pulsating. These are differentiated by the 'expansile impulse', placing the index and middle fingers over the swelling; if the pulsation is transmitted, the fingers move up and down, but if the swelling is expansile the fingers move apart. Auscultation can reveal a systolic murmur in pulsating lesions while arteriovenous fistulae emit a continuous murmur. A pulsating swelling can be an aneurysm or a sarcoma.

Toenails

Ingrowing toenail

Caused by pressure necrosis. Treated initially by conservative means (correct trimming, clean socks and foot baths, antibiotic course for infection). If these means fail, try simple avulsion and if this fails then radical ablation of the germinal matrix surgically (either partial by unilateral or bilateral wedge excision or total by Zadik's operation) or chemically (80% phenol solution applied for 3 min to the germinal matrix after simple nail avulsion).

Onychogryphosis

Overgrown toenail—treated by Zadik's operation as conservative means do not succeed.

Nail bed lesions

* Subungual haematoma: due to trauma; treated by nail trephine and evacuation of clot.
* Subungual melanoma: treated by excisional biopsy followed by amputation of the digit through the distal interphalangeal joint.
* Glomus tumour: composed of encapsulated arteriovenous plexuses concerned with heat regulation. It is a very painful tiny benign tumour which needs excision (with simple nail avulsion if subungual) leading to dramatic lasting relief.

A6. HERNIA
('examine the groin')

Hernia (protrusion of a viscus or part of a viscus through a normal or abnormal opening) is either internal (e.g. hiatus hernia) or external (e.g. inguinal, incisional or femoral, in this order of frequency). It is the latter which are often presented in examinations. The three common scrotal swellings are hydrocele, epididymal cyst and varicocele.

1. The patient, stripped below the waist, should be examined lying and standing (hernia reduces itself in the first position and becomes obvious in the second position). Initially you should never touch the patient but ask him to cough and look for the visible cough impulse to locate the hernial site.

2. Ask him to cough again and confirm the presence of hernia by feeling the palpable impulse preferably by employing the hand corresponding to the side to be examined (e.g. right hand to right groin), placing the index, middle and ring fingers over the indirect inguinal, direct inguinal and femoral hernial sites respectively while the patient is coughing (Zieman's tests—surgeon from Alabama). Inguinal hernia usually bulges above and medial to the pubic tubercle while femoral hernia bulges below and lateral to it. Incisional hernia is diagnosed on the basis of history of abdominal incision with a hernia, and protrusion through the abdominal musculature is easily confirmed when the patient lies down and coughs or lifts his head against resistance. Femoral hernia is diagnosed by its location, and when the invagination test demonstrates that the inguinal canal is empty. It is difficult to reduce, and taxis is contraindicated. It is common in females (because of wide broad pelvis).

3. Academic differentiation of direct from indirect inguinal hernia. Follow four steps:

(a) On inspection, direct hernia emerges straight through Hesselbach's triangle and not obliquely along the inguinal canal.

(b) *Invagination test*: employ the hand corresponding to the side to be examined and invaginate the scrotum *gently* with the little finger; direct hernia is suggested if it passes directly backwards into the abdomen instead of obliquely upwards and outwards or if the cough impulse is felt hitting the pulp rather than the fingertip.

(c) *Occlusion test*: after reducing the hernia (e.g. by the patient lying down) and then occluding the internal inguinal ring 1 cm above the midpoint of the inguinal ligament (stretched between the anterior superior iliac spine and the pubic tubercle which is different from the midinguinal point stretched between the anterior superior iliac spine and the symphysis pubis—a landmark of the common femoral artery) ask the patient to cough. Any bulging is strongly indicative of direct hernia coming forwards since indirect hernia is prevented from coming down medially through the canal and external inguinal ring.

(d) On lying down, a direct hernia reduces itself instantly and the bulge reappears with equal suddenness when the patient strains.

4. Assess whether the hernia is reducible or complicated (i.e. irreducibility, inflammation, incarceration and strangulation) and determine its contents (if possible). On lying down, the small intestine is reduced with a gurgle; the omentum is doughy on palpation and difficult to reduce due to adhesions. Both femoral hernia and saphina varix have a cough impulse but saphina varix is faintly blue, softer on palpation and usually associated with pronounced varicosity of the long saphenous vein and a positive 'tap sign'. Enlarged lymph node of Cloquet is very difficult to differentiate from irreducible femoral hernia and if no possible focus of infection is found, surgical exploration will be the final answer. Irreducible inguinal hernia in females is difficult to differentiate from hydrocele of the canal of Nuck (Anatomist from Holland) (the hydrocele is smooth, fixed, fluctuant and brilliantly translucent) and from cyst of Bartholin's gland (not translucent and confined to labium majus; it is easy to get above it).

5. In the presence of an obvious lump try to get above the swelling by grasping it between the finger and thumb; if this is not possible it is an inguinal hernia but otherwise consider intrascrotal lesions.

Indirect (oblique) inguinal hernia

● The most common hernia.
● Due to congenital preformed sac (partially or completely patent processus vaginalis).
● More common on the right side in young males owing to later descent of right testicle, but after the second decade left inguinal hernias are as frequent as those on the right.
● Unilateral usually (bilateral in 30%).
● Common in men.
● Treated by herniotomy; repair of the stretched internal ring with lateral displacement of the cord; and reconstruction of the weak posterior wall of the inguinal canal (darning usually).

Direct inguinal hernia

● Represent 15% of inguinal hernias.
● Always acquired.
● Usually bilateral.
● Only in men (never females or children).
● Associated with Malgaigne's bulges.
● Presence of predisposing factors, e.g. chronic bronchitis, ascites, obesity, obstructive prostatic uropathy, elderly man with constipation or chronic intestinal obstruction, and postoperative injury to iliohypogastric or ilioinguinal nerves (in appendicectomy).
● Rarely large, rarely descends into the scrotum and rarely strangulates because of wide neck.
● Treated by reduction and inversion of sac (not herniotomy), repair of fascia transversalis in front of it, and reconstruction of the posterior wall of the inguinal canal.

Femoral hernia

● Third most common (incisional hernia is second).
● Common in females (because of wide broad pelvis).
● Difficult to reduce and the most likely to strangulate.
● Truss is contraindicated (it can be used in inguinal hernia whenever operation is contraindicated).
● Treated by low or high approach.

Incisional hernia
(*see* Abdominal wound dehiscence, p. 31)

A7. SCROTAL SWELLING
(*'examine the scrotum'*)

If you can get above the swelling then:

1. Palpate the intrascrotal swelling. If its bulk lies in front of and to a variable degree above the body of the testis but it cannot be felt distinctly from the testis it is vaginal hydrocele which is usually bilateral. If the swelling is tense, somewhat lobulated above and behind the body of the testis and felt distinctly from the testicle it is an epididymal cyst, spermatocele or encysted hydrocele of the cord.

2. Do transillumination test by applying a torch behind the cyst and looking from the front of the scrotum through a piece of paper made into a tube and applied directly to the scrotum to prevent scattering of light. Brilliantly translucent swellings are vaginal hydroceles or encysted hydroceles of the cord. Epididymal cysts look tessellated. Remember that:

● All scrotal inguinal hernias are non-translucent except for those of an infant or young child which contain the small intestine (translucent).
● All vaginal hydroceles are translucent except those of many years' duration and those which have been aspirated many times (because of

deposition of fibrin and blood pigments on their walls). Aspiration reveals a straw-coloured fluid (urine-like) from vaginal hydroceles, milky (like barley water) from spermatoceles and crystal clear (like water) from epididymal cysts.

3. If the palpation reveals a thickened enlarged epididymis with tenderness and a thickened vas it is epididymo-orchitis. If the scrotal swelling (often left-sided) gives a soft feeling like a 'bag of worms' in the standing position, and when the patient is asked to lie down the veins empty and the swelling disappears on testicular elevation, it is a varicocele. In this case the testicle size should be assessed as it is often smaller than on the other side (due to atrophy).

A testicle located at the superficial inguinal ring usually indicates maldescended testicle in children and torsion in adults. The former is usually associated with congenital indirect inguinal hernia. Unilateral hard heavy enlarged testicle (same shape but larger size) usually indicates a testicular tumour.

Small testicle (due to atrophy)

If unilateral, consider:
- Infarction consequent upon torsion.
- Epididymo-orchitis of mumps.
- Postoperative following spermatic artery damage, inguinal hernia, varicocele and orchidopexy.
- Varicocele.

Bilateral atrophy is caused by leprosy, hepatic cirrhosis and oestrogen therapy for carcinoma of the prostate.

Hydrocele

Collection of fluid in the tunica vaginalis and is either congenital or acquired. The latter is either primary (idiopathic) or secondary to trauma, tumours or infection. Vaginal hydrocele is treated by tapping, Lord's operation (multiple radial gathering stitches using catgut—without delivery of the hydrocele), or subtotal excision which entails complete delivery of the hydrocele through a large incision. The tunica vaginalis can be inverted (Jaboulay's method).

Testicular torsion (see also p. 236)

Usually occurs within the first 20 years of life.

Aetiology (the underlying abnormality(ies)):
- High investment of tunica vaginalis (common).
- Extreme motility of scrotal contents (neonates).
- Separation of testis and epididymis (very rare).
- May be no underlying abnormality.

Predisposing factors:
- Spiral attachment of cremaster.
- Unusual body movements.
- Trauma.
- Cycling.
- Cold.
- Pubertal growth spurt.

Testicular viability depends on:
- Testicular descent.
- Possibility of spontaneous reduction.
- Interval before operative reduction.
- Degree of twisting of the cord.

Physical examination (testicular torsion should be differentiated from acute epididymo-orchitis):
- Elevation test of testicle increases twisting and is therefore painful while elevation relieves epididymo-orchitis.
- Degree of funiculitis (tender spermatic cord in the inguinal region) and prostatitis (tender rectal examination) with fever in epididymo-orchitis but not in torsion.
- Presence of mid-stream urine pus cells and/or high WBC in epididymo-orchitis and their absence in torsion.
- Patients with epididymo-orchitis are more than 25 years of age.

Investigations:
- Ultrasound doppler.
- Radionucleotide testicular scanning.

There is evidence now that once torsion occurs the endocrine function remains normal but the exocrine function becomes disturbed, i.e. sterility results even if the testis was salvaged possibly due to a sympathetic orchidopathia in the normal testicle. Treatment is by operative untwisting of the torted testis and bilateral orchiopexy.

A8. BREAST MASS
('*examine the breasts*')

Never ever touch the breast before careful inspection:
1. Ask the patient to undress down to the waist and from a distance ask her to sit up so that you can compare the level of the breasts.

2. Ask her to lean forward and then lift her arms, and then ask her to put them against her waist and contract her pectoral muscles.

3. Palpate the normal breast in quadrants, then examine the axilla for axillary lymph nodes (hold the patient's left hand with your left hand and examine the left axilla with your right hand and *vice versa*).

4. Palpate the supraclavicular lymph nodes by approaching the patient from behind, moving the patient's head gently towards the examined side and asking her to shrug her shoulders while you examine them.

5. Palpate (in supine position) the pathological breast carefully looking for the 10 breast cancer signs including: breast elevation, four nipple changes—retraction, eccentric nipple, ulceration (Paget's disease) or blood discharging—and five skin changes—skin dimpling due to pull of the ligaments of Copper (the fibrous bands anchoring the mammary gland to the dermis), peau d'orange due to subcutaneous lymphatic obstructions, direct skin infiltration or fungation, malignant ringworm due to multiple skin nodules secondary to centrifugal lymphatic permeation, and finally confluent skin nodules ('cancer *en cuirasse*'). *Do not forget to examine the normal breast.*

6. When palpating the breast mass, describe its site, size, shape, number, consistency, borders, mobility and then the state of the axillary lymph nodes on the side of the lesion.

7. Ask the patient to lie back and examine her liver (for visceral metastases) and her arm for possible lymphoedema (non-pitting).

N.B. In the mastectomy patient ask about haemoptysis (pulmonary metastasis), bony pain (skeletal metastasis) and weight gain (ascites—visceral metastasis) and whether radiotherapy, endocrine therapy or chemotherapy had been given. Examine as above and also look for any evidence of local recurrence (in mastectomy scar) and radiation effects.

A9. CERVICAL SWELLING
('*examine the neck*')

Midline swelling should suggest the possibility of a thyroid nodule of the isthmus, thyroglossal cyst, subhyoid bursa or dermoid cyst. Lateral swelling has many causes: commonly the cause is either lymphadenopathy (commonly inflammatory in nature due to infection or tuberculosis in Asians but can also be due to primary Hodgkin's lymphoma or secondary carcinoma from a primary tumour elsewhere) or thyroid nodule. Less common causes are salivary masses, neurogenic tumours, vascular swellings, pharyngeal pouch, skin tumours, and congenital masses such as branchial cyst and cavernous haemangioma. You are allowed to ask the patient 'How long have you had this swelling?' and 'Does it cause you any problems?' Quickly look at the ear, nose and throat (ENT). Look at the scalp in suspected thyroglossal cyst asking the patient to protrude her tongue (thyroglossal cyst will move up while isthmic nodule will not).

Thyroid swelling

1. Inspect the eyes, and thyroidectomy scar or telangiectasia following radiotherapy. Look at the swelling while the patient is swallowing. It is wise to let the examiner know that you would examine the thyroid while the patient is swallowing a mouthful of water (it is more humane), even if a glass of water is not available. During swallowing you may palpate the radial pulse quickly (for rhythm and rate) and feel the palm (sweaty hot hand with tremor in thyrotoxicosis and dry skin in hypothyroidism).

2. Palpate the neck bimanually from in front and behind (again while patient is swallowing water) to determine size, symmetry, consistency and tenderness.

3. From behind, palpate the regional lymph nodes especially the supraclavicular nodes in the supraclavicular hollows (after patient shrugs his shoulders or bends his head towards the side under examination).

4. Percuss the manubrium to detect any dullness indicating retrosternal extension.

5. Auscultate for bruits.

6. If you are given time, then confirm the state of thyroid functioning by examining for three thyrotoxic eye signs (exophthalmos, lid lag and ophthalmoplegia). Examine the legs for pertibial myxoedema and the limbs for proximal myopathy—both occur in thyrotoxicosis. Myxoedema is suggested by characteristic facies, hoarseness of voice and dry skin. For thyroid assessment *see* Section 1.49.

Lymph nodes

Pyogenic lymph nodes are tender and hot, with evidence of infection (of the respiratory tract and mouth). Cold matted lymph nodes are tuberculous. Fixed stony hard lymph nodes are metastatic in origin. However, in lateral swellings that do not

move with swallowing and have a rubbery consistency, suspect Hodgkin's lymphoma (in adults) and non-Hodgkin's lymphoma (in the elderly)
Then:
1. After examining the cervical lymph nodes bilaterally, palpate for axillary and inguinal lymph nodes on both sides.
2. Palpate the abdomen for para-aortic lymph nodes, spleen and liver enlargement.
3. The next important step is to biopsy the cervical lymph nodes. If lymphoma is found to be present, staging laparotomy will be considered (splenectomy, liver biopsy and para-aortic lymph node biopsy). CT scanning, IVU and lymphangiography are done later.

Note on Hodgkin's disease classification

Based on histological grading or clinical staging.

1. Histological grading

Lukes, 1963	Rye, 1966 (currently used)
Lymphocyte and/or histiocyte (L & H) nodular diffuse	Lymphocyte predominance (young)
Nodular sclerosis	Nodular sclerosis (young)
Mixed cellularity	Mixed cellularity
Diffuse fibrosis	Lymphocyte depletion
Reticular	(elderly)

2. Clinical staging (Peters et al., 1966)

Stage I   Disease limited to one anatomical region.
Stage II Disease limited to two contiguous anatomical regions on same side of diaphragm; or
Disease in more than two anatomical regions or in two non-contiguous regions on same side of diaphragm.
Stage III Disease on both sides of diaphragm but limited to involvement of lymph nodes, Waldeyer ring and spleen.
Stage IV Extralymphatic involvement of bone marrow, lung parenchyma, pleura, liver, bone, skin, kidneys and gastrointestinal tract.

All stages are subclassified as A or B to indicate the absence or presence, respectively, of systemic symptoms. Treatment is radiotherapy (Stages I and IIA) or chemotherapy (Stages IIB, III and IV).

Branchial cyst

This is a unilateral cystic swelling at the anterior border of the sternomastoid at the junction of the upper third and lower two-thirds. It is common in young females, and usually arises from the second branchial cleft (first branchial cleft cysts are suprahyoidal and juxta-auricular with possible communication to the auditory meatus). The treatment is surgical excision.

A10. PAROTID SWELLING
('examine this patient's neck')

1. Inspect carefully for unilateral enlargement, facial symmetry and any incision.
2. Ask the patient to blow or whistle, close his eyes against resistance (signs of facial nerve paralysis). Then ask him to open his mouth as far as he can (difficulty in moving the jaw—ankylosis).
3. Feel the overlying skin (while the patient closes his eyes) and test for loss of touch sensation.
4. Palpate the tumour, describing its exact site, shape, size, consistency, mobility and overlying skin fixation.
5. Palpate the cervical lymph nodes (pre- and postauricular and supraclavicular groups).
6. Ask the patient to open his mouth. Use a wooden spatula and torch to see Stensen's duct and massage the parotid gland from outside to express any pus (superimposed parotitis).

Causes of parotid swelling

Inflammatory (acute parotitis)

Due to viral or pyogenic infections, actinomycosis, tuberculosis. This may follow major operation, debilitating disease (e.g. typhoid fever and cholera), radiotherapy.

Suppurative sialoadenitis

Secondary to obstruction of a salivary duct by a stone or stricture.

Neoplastic

Either primary or secondary (to nasopharyngeal carcinoma, bronchial cancer or lymphoma).
Primary epithelial tumours include pleomorphic adenoma (benign circumscribed firm lobulated encapsulated tumour with no sex predilection with potential for recurrence after enucleation and

developemt of carcinoma), monomorphic adenoma such as adenolymphoma (Warthin's tumour is a less common benign tumour—a slowly enlarging soft cystic fluctuant tumour in middle-aged or elderly males which can be bilateral; unlike pleomorphic adenoma it produces a hot spot in ^{99m}Tc pertechnetate scan) and mucoepidermoid tumours.

Primary non-epithelial tumours include acinic cell tumour and carcinoma (with fixation, bone resorption and ankylosis, skin and mucous membrane anaesthesia, muscle paralysis, facial nerve paralysis and pain).

These tumours are assessed clinically (*not* biopsied), then excised by suprafacial or superficial partial parotidectomy. In suspected malignancy, an outpatient fine-needle aspiration cytology biopsy or operative frozen-section may be used to confirm its nature (postoperative radiotherapy may be required to avoid radical parotidectomy for residual deep tumour).

REMEMBER

- *Fascial slings* (from fascia lata) may be used to support facial tissues and mask the deformity of facial nerve palsy (could be shown as a short case).
- *Frey's syndrome* is facial flushing and sweating on gustatory stimulation due to auriculotemporal nerve injury. It is either postoperative after parotid or temporomandibular joint surgery, traumatic or congenital (birth trauma). The cause is union of postganglionic parasympathetic fibres from the otic ganglion with sympathetic nerves from the superior cervical ganglion. In severe cases division of the lesser superficial petrosal nerve within the skull is the treatment.

Autoimmune

Sjögren's syndrome (dry eyes — keratoconjunctivitis sicca; dry mouth — xerostomia; and rheumatoid arthritis) causes enlargement of the salivary and lacrimal glands. Mikulicz disease (symmetrical enlargement of all salivary glands, narrowing of the palpebral fissures due to enlarged lacrimal glands and dry mouth) is a variant.

Cysts

As in sarcoidosis with Heerfordt's syndrome (uveitis, salivary and lacrimal gland enlargement).

Metabolic

Includes diabetes, acromegaly, liver cirrhosis and reaction to drugs (e.g. antithyroid drugs and atrophy).

A11. MALIGNANT SKIN TUMOURS
('*examine the skin*')

Usually presented in the form of malignant ulcers. The order of frequency is basal cell carcinoma, squamous cell carcinoma, malignant melanoma. Inspect carefully for site, size, shape, edge, floor and discharge. Palpate for ulcer base (soft or hard, or indurated) and enlargement of adjacent lymph nodes.

Basal cell carcinoma

Rodent cell ulcer is a misnomer since there may only be a nodule. However if ulcer is present it is usually circular and commonly confined to the face (the area between a line joining the upper and lower borders of the ear with the outer canthus of the eye and the outer angle of the mouth respectively) but may occur anywhere in the body except the soles and palms. It has a raised rolled-out beaded edge, a network of blood vessels and a temporary healing crusty floor covered with serous discharge. The base is slightly indurated. It spreads slowly by local invasion. Blood or lymphatic spread does not occur. The diagnosis is confirmed by excisional biopsy (therapeutic) or elliptical biopsy from the lesion and normal surrounding skin. Treatment is by surgical excision, radiotherapy or cryosugery.

Squamous cell carcinoma

The ulcer is irregular in shape with an everted or raised edge. The base is hard and indurated with blood-stained discharge. The regional lymph nodes may be enlarged due to secondary infection (painful) or actual involvement (painless hard). The ulcer is rapidly growing and may have superadded infection. The diagnosis is confirmed by elliptical biopsy (from lesion and normal skin). Treatment is by wide surgical excision or radiotherapy.

Comment on treatment of basal and squamous cell carcinomas

Surgical excision is the quickest and safest approach, especially for recurrent lesions. Radiotherapy is recommended when the surgical reconstruction after excision is a problem, e.g. lesions of the eyelids, in which case radiotherapy can be delivered more precisely. Radiotherapy, however, is contraindicated for lesions in cartilaginous areas (i.e. earlobe and nose) because of the risk of radionecrosis, and surgery is preferred, e.g. wedge excision with modified 'L' shape in carcinoma of the earlobe to prevent helical stricture. Cryosurgery is indicated for multiple small lesions.

Malignant melanoma (see also p. 164)

A pigmented naevus with possible signs of malignancy raises suspicions. The diagnosis is confirmed histologically on the basis of frozen or rapid paraffin sections taken after local excisional biopsy with a narrow margin of clearance (0.2 cm). This is safely performed provided the supplementary wide surgical clearance (3–5 cm) is performed within 48 h of biopsy, depending on the degree of vertical invasion. Treatment is wide excision and split skin grafting ($\pm$ block dissection).

A12. MISCELLANEOUS CASES

Any patient, whether operated on or not, may be presented as a short case provided it serves as spot diagnosis case.

Dupuytren's contracture

Localised thickening of palmar fascia, puckering the overlying skin and flexing the ring and little finger—affects the metacarpophalangeal and proximal interphalangeal joints. It is familial and occurs more often in cirrhotics and epileptics on Epanutin.

Treatment Early cases (uncomplicated puckering) need night splintage and gentle stretching of the fingers by the patient. In advanced cases treatment is either single limited or multiple palmar fasciotomy but more commonly partial palmar fasciectomy (removing the affected fascia only). Radical total palmar fasciectomy (excising the affected and normal fascia) is an extensive operation and is indicated in patients with high Dupuytren's diathesis (young patient, rapid progressive disease, strong family history, history of epilepsy and/or alcoholism and the presence of ectopic deposits such as knuckle pads, plantar and penile lesions). Excision of the skin and replacement with skin grafts is indicated only in recurrent cases. (Figs 29 and 30).

Amputation is used for chronic severe cases with irreversible flexion-contracture deformities.

Hallux valgus

Either congenital (metatarsus primum varus) or acquired in women who wear tight narrow shoes.

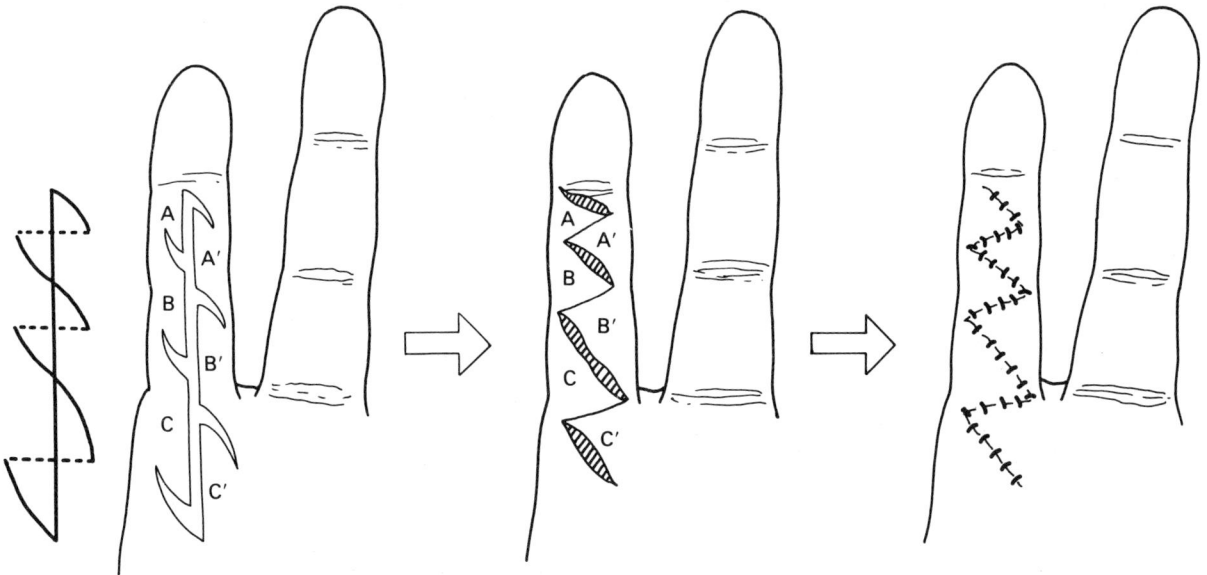

Fig. 29 A continuous multiple Z-plasty used in Dupuytren's contracture of the little finger

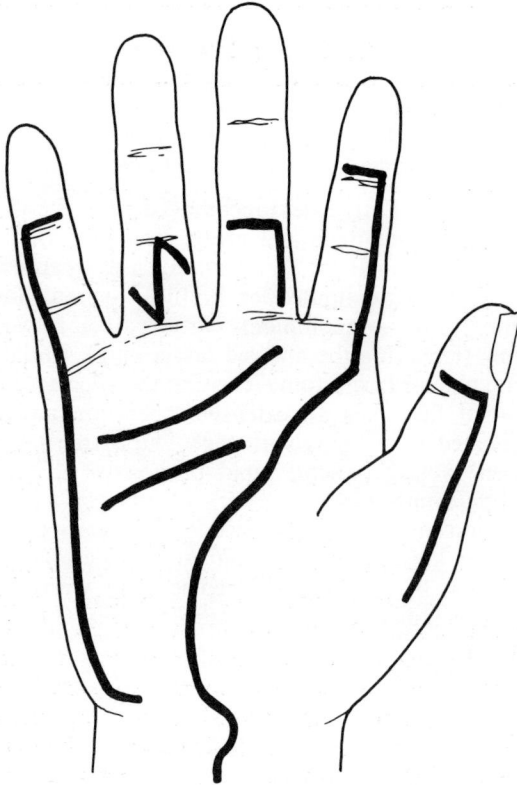

Fig. 30 Commonly used incisions in hand surgery

Consists of four elements: bony exostosis of the first metatarsal head; an adventitious bursa — first metatarsal bunion with or without fifth metatarsal bunionette; osteoarthrosis of the first metatarsophalangeal joint; and overriding or underriding of the second toe by the first. Treatment is by Keller's operation (American surgeon) which is an excision arthroplasty of the base of the proximal phalanx, being careful of the flexor tendon, with excision of the exostosis and final reconstruction of the medial collateral ligament. (The excised base of the proximal phalanx can be replaced with an implant.)

Hallux rigidus

This is simply monoarticular osteoarthrosis of the first metatarsophalangeal joint, producing a stiff painful joint. Treatment is by Keller's operation.

Chronic bursitis

In the prepatellar bursa (housemaid's knee), olecranon bursa (student's or miner's elbow) or syn-ovial cysts in the popliteal fossa (Baker's cysts). Baker's cysts arise from semimembranous bursa or, in rheumatoid arthritis of the knee, from posterior rupture of the joint capsule. They are either aspirated or left alone to disappear spontaneously. Bursa elsewhere can be excised.

Ruptured Achilles tendon

Represents the commonest tendon rupture in middle-aged men after games or even after a trivial stumble. The case is diagnosed by history and by examination for a palpable and even visible gap (at the rupture site), free dorsiflexion and reduced plantar flexion (but never abolished due to action of the long flexors of the toes and tibialis posterior). The patient usually cannot stand on tiptoe. Treatment is by early suture and ankle immobilisation in a plaster for 6 weeks. Late suture is disappointing because of retracted ruptured ends; instead, the gastrocnemius and soleus muscles are relaxed.

Pyogenic granuloma

Ranula

Submandibular salivary calculus

Long lower limb incision over course of long saphenous vein (to be used for coronary bypass)

Look for a median sternotomy incision immediately.

Cushing's syndrome or Cushing's disease

Cushing's syndrome is due to steroid therapy or adrenal cortical hyperplasia, adenoma or malignancy while *Cushing's disease* is due to secretion of ACTH by basophilic tumour of the anterior pituitary.

Perianal abscess or fistula

Remember Goodsall's rule (*see* p. 365).

T-tube

This will be shown in a patient.

Continuous irrigation

Mounted on a three-way Foley urinary catheter after open prostatectomy (in the presence of an abdominal incision with a suprapubic drain) or transurethral resection of prostate or bladder tumour (no abdominal incision or drain).

Abdominal faecal fistula

Caecostomy, ileostomy or colostomy

In caecostomy there is a Foley catheter in the right iliac fossa. Notice the spout in ileostomy but not colostomy. You may be asked about the complications after ileostomy or colostomy and why they were constructed. (See also p. 43 and p. 269.)

Subclavian set

For parenteral nutrition (notice the intralipid milky solutions covered with black bags because of photosensitivity) and/or CVP monitoring (notice the manometer and absence of intralipid parenteral solution). You may be asked about the indications for parenteral nutrition or CVP monitoring.

Appendicectomy

You may be asked *what to look for*. If you are seeing an appendicectomy patient on the third postoperative day, ask him about bowel action, examine his wound locally for infection or surrounding tenderness and look at his temperature chart since postoperative pyrexia may indicate wound infection or chest infection (X-ray), urinary infection (midstream urine), thrombophlebitis (see if he has an i.v. line), deep venous thrombosis, rectal pelvic abscess or subphrenic abscess ('pus nowhere, pus somewhere else, pus under diaphragm').

Male gynaecomastia

Causes are:
- Idiopathic—unilateral or bilateral.
- Hormonal, e.g. stilboestrol therapy in prostatic cancer and testicular teratoma; anorchism; rarely, ectopic hormones from bronchogenic carcinoma; and adrenal or pituitary disease.
- Liver failure in cirrhosis.
- Klinefelter's syndrome.
- Drugs, e.g. digitalis, spironolactone, isoniazid.
- Leprosy.

B. Long Cases

Time allowed is 20–30 min with one patient. You are required to take a history, perform a physical examination and interpret your findings to reach *one* diagnosis. You have to prepare yourself for possible relevant investigations and work out a differential diagnosis (to be presented only when you are asked). Enlarge on the chief complaint and its present history, mention all *positive* clinical findings and ask for the simplest relevant tests. Be friendly with the patient, while following the general points above. One useful tip is to ask the patient, 'Did you come here specially today, or are you a patient in this hospital?'. Also obtain the name of the consultant the patient is under since you may well find yourself being examined by him. Ask the patient about the investigations performed and what he was told as a result of them. Examine the patient methodically and comprehensively, and elicit the physical signs related to his complaint as well as other signs. Most patients know the diagnosis and it is worth telling the patient what you think the diagnosis is as he will usually agree with you if you are right.

Leave 5 min for reorganising your presentation. Underline the important points in the history and stress the positive findings in the physical examination. Give your provisional diagnosis and support it with the most relevant investigations, starting with the simplest and cheapest, since the more sophisticated the test or investigation the more delay there is for the patient. For example, in surgical anaemia, contrast radiology (in the form of a barium study) and endoscopy should head your list since the commonest causes of anaemia are malignancy (i.e. gastric and caecum carcinomas) and peptic ulcer; other possible causes, e.g. ulcerative colitis, Crohn's disease and the malabsorption syndrome, would be investigated later. In a jaundiced patient, urine examination for bilirubin and urobilinogen, plain abdominal X-ray and abdominal ultrasound come before transhepatic cholangiography, ERCP and liver biopsy. In colorectal diseases, rectal examination, sigmoidoscopy (or colonoscopy) and biopsy come before carcinoembryonic antigen test and barium enema since the latter may precipitate an intestinal obstruction in annular carcinoma of the rectosigmoid junction. In upper abdominal pain of unknown origin, barium swallow (in Trendelenburg's position) and meal will exclude hiatus hernia and peptic ulcer respectively. Abdominal ultrasound will exclude biliary stone and possibly pancreatic and renal swelling (oral cholecystography can be done if ultrasound is inconclusive). Intravenous urography will exclude any urinary system pathology.

The examination organisers may leave X-ray films beside the patient purposely to help you, so have a good look at them. The films will most probably show abnormal radiological findings such as a stone or an ulcer (normal films will usually not be included).

A well-planned presentation of the case history and positive physical findings is the most important part of this test. The examiner will tell you to present the case as if he knows nothing about the patient. Intermittent interruptions by the examiner with mutual discussion of the findings, diagnosis, investigation and possible operative treatment will reveal your capability for reasonable argument, mature clinical judgement and accuracy in requesting relevant investigations and interpreting data.

Case-taking

The following scheme is recommended.
Patient: name, age, occupation, married or single, address, date of admission.
Chief complaint (one, rarely two) and *duration*.
History of present illness: e.g. if the presenting complaint is pain enquire about: similar attacks in the past; pain severity and character; location; radiation and direction (epigastric pain radiating to the back by penetration is consistent with pancreatitis and by encirclement around the right side is consistent with cholecystitis); duration since the first attack; intermission and intervals of freedom (for how long?); relation to meals; does it wake him at night (nocturnal pain); aggravating factors and relieving factors; associated features such as vomiting (amount, colour, does it look like coffee grounds, taste and food residue); bowel habits, appetite, weight loss, heartburn and dysphagia (if any). In biliary pain it is very important to ask about associated fever and rigor (in cholangitis), jaundice, itching and coloured urine, pale stool.
Past history:
● Of hospital admissions in chronological order, with hospital names, causes of admission and names of operations performed.
● Of allergies whether atopic, e.g. asthma, or to drugs (especially penicillin, iodine contrast media and zincplast—Elastoplast).

● Of drug intake, especially:
—Oral hypoglycaemic agents in diabetes mellitus (should be stopped 24–48 h prior to surgery and insulin given instead).
—Anticoagulants for valve replacements (should be stopped 48 h prior to surgery and heparin given instead as well as vitamin K injection and prophylactic antibiotics to prevent subacute bacterial endocarditis).
—Contraceptive pill in females and stilboestrol in males, e.g. for prostatic carcinoma (contraceptive pill should be stopped 1 month prior to surgery and if impossible Dextran 70 should be used during operation to prevent possible deep venous thrombosis).
—Other drug intake such as anti-epileptic and antiheart failure measures can continue during the immediate perioperative period.
● Of previous illnesses (e.g. rheumatic heart disease) and accidents (e.g. road traffic accident).
Quick family history: cause of death of parents, children, brothers or sisters; and familial disease, e.g. haemophilia, gall stones, hypertension and diabetes mellitus.
Quick social history: habits as regards alcohol, tobacco, food and exercise.
Systemic inquiry: only the positive symptoms in each system, e.g. alimentary, respiratory, cardiovascular, urinary, nervous and musculoskeletal systems.
Impression should now be made based on the history alone to be confirmed by physical examination.

Physical examination

Vital signs: temperature, pulse rate, blood pressure and respiratory rate.
General appearance (e.g. lying in bed in agony, doubled up with pain, cooperative) as well as JACCOL (jaundice, anaemia, cyanosis, clubbing, oedema, lymphadenopathy).
Head and neck: scalp swelling, exophthalmos, pupils' size and reaction, mouth—tongue, jugular venous pressure, central trachea, goitre, carotid bruit).
Chest: quick examination, except if patient is female look for breast carcinoma. Otherwise inspection, palpation, percussion and auscultation. Examine the back of the chest (e.g. for possible pulsating collaterals in coarctation of the aorta).
Abdomen (in detail):
● Inspection for generalised or localised swelling,

hernial sites (ask patient to cough), visible peristalsis, pulsation, dilated vessels, scars and umbilicus.

- General palpation for soft or rigid abdomen and special palpation for tenderness or rebound tenderness, for impulse on coughing in hernias as well as for organomegaly, fluid thrill and splashing.
- Percussion to confirm the upper limit of hepatomegaly, the dull nature of enlarged urinary bladder in retention and shifting dullness in ascites.
- Auscultation for bowel sounds at the McBurney point (borborygmi and tingling sound in intestinal obstruction and quiet in paralytic ileus). Also for vascular lesions, e.g. hepatic haemangioma and aortic aneurysm.
- Abdominal examination is not complete without examining the genitalia (phimosis, hypospadias in penis and since testicles are abdominal organs a discovered seminoma may explain huge abdominal para-aortic lymph nodes which may be misdiagnosed initially as intestinal masses). The rectum should also be examined (essential in rectal carcinoma or villous adenoma and prostatic carcinoma).

Limbs: especially lower limbs for pitting oedema, ulcers and pulses.

Provisional diagnosis should be single. Differential diagnosis is only acceptable in a vague unexplained symptomatology with few or no physical signs.

At this point, reorganise yourself once again, underlining the *positive* physical findings, and present your clinical data in a logical format. Think of the most simple relevant investigation (and why) and prepare yourself psychologically for discussion face-to-face with the examiners.

The following are common often repeated long cases.

B1. DUODENAL ULCER

History is essential since there may be slight epigastric tenderness or absolutely no physical signs. The case may have been complicated before by perforation (notice the abdominal scar), bleeding or pyloric stenosis. Give *one* personally recommended operation that you would perform and substantiate your approach. Do not say it could be managed *either* by partial gastrectomy or vagotomy and pyloroplasty.

B2. CHOLECYSTITIS ± HISTORY OF PANCREATITIS ± JAUNDICE

It is essential to distinguish between pain due to gall stone cholecystitis (sudden dull continuous pain in the right hypochondrium radiating to the interscapular area and back by encirclement; associated with retching and vomiting together with tachycardia and pyrexia and usually comes at night after a fatty meal, e.g. fish and chips), and pain due to biliary colic from a common bile duct stone or, rarely, a cystic duct stone with ball-valve mechanism (pain is on and off, associated with ascending cholangitis, which is manifested by rigor, fever and even septicaemia, and with the fluctuating jaundice of Charcot's triad). Remember that fluctuating jaundice can also be due to periampullary carcinoma (high ESR and positive occult blood in stool with palpable gall bladder).

In acute pancreatitis pain is usually very severe and constant, radiating from the upper abdomen to the back by penetration; it is associated with vomiting and relieved by leaning forward. Ask for history of gall stones and alcoholism. Rarely, acute pancreatitis is presented on its own (in examinations), but commonly it is presented as a gall stone cholecystitis (electively admitted for cholecystectomy) with past history of pancreatitis. Notice here the type of patient (e.g. fertile, fatty, flatulent, 50-year-old female). On physical examination, a palpable gall bladder should make you consider the following:

- Acute cholecystitis: wrapped in protective greater omentum (just like appendicular mass).
- Mucocele: painless swelling with no jaundice.
- Empyema of gall bladder: with pyrexia and tachycardia.
- If the patient is jaundiced then carcinoma of the head of the pancreas is likely (Courvoisier's sign or statement).
- Very hard swelling indicates gall bladder carcinoma or liver tumour (metastatic or primary).

Courvoisier's statement (not law): 'If in a jaundiced patient the gall bladder is palpably enlarged, it is *probably* NOT a case of stone impacted in the common bile duct, because in that case previous cholecystitis has already made the gall bladder fibrotic.' This is a negative statement and not a law. Courvoisier only made a statement of probability (approximately 75% of cases); therefore double stone impaction in the cystic and common bile ducts and oriental chlonorchiasis (although regarded as exceptions to Courvoisier's law) are actually included within the 25% of his correct statement.

B3. RECTAL CARCINOMA

Rectal examination is the vital step. Once you feel the hard rectal cancer (whether ulcerative, cauliflower or annular) you *have* to proceed wth proctoscopy. (Proctoscopy or sigmoidoscopy *with* biopsy is the key investigation. Barium enema is not recommended in *low* rectal lesion and may be dangerous since it may cause obstruction in annular rectosigmoid carcinoma. Enema is indicated in high colonic lesions beyond the reach of the rigid sigmoidoscope and in order to reveal the possible double colonic primary tumours in 5 % of colonic cancers). In villous adenoma the tumour is soft and covered with mucus and not blood (make sure you have asked the patient about mucus discharge and symptoms of hypokalaemia; also stress that you will send the patient's serum for potassium estimation). You have to make up your mind whether you are planning to excise the tumour by anterior restorative resection or by abdominoperineal excision with permanent left iliac colostomy (and why) or whether you leave this decision until after laparotomy (and assessment of spread).

B4. CHRONIC URINARY RETENTION

Commonly due to prostatic carcinoma: it is important to reveal a history of prostatism. On physical examination of the abdomen, an enlarged urinary bladder is confirmed by:
- Palpation: one cannot get a hand under it since it is an intrapelvic organ.
- Percussion: dul and one can define upper border easily.
- Palpation and pressure may squeeze some urine out. Ask the patient about his desire to micturate when you press.

Remember that the size of the prostate cannot be assessed while the patient is in retention (only rectal examination after catheterisation is correct). Stress the characteristics of prostatic carcinoma that can be revealed by rectal examination:
- Obliteration of median prostatic sulcus.
- Hard prostate ⎫ and whether
- Fixed prostate ⎭ flat or bulging.

Benign prostatic enlargement is generally bigger than malignant enlargement.

You may discover a swollen leg or legs which may be caused by:
- Deep venous thrombosis due to disseminated intravascular coagulation.

- Metastatic obstruction of lymphatic drainage of the lower limbs.
- Metastatic obstruction of venous drainage of the lower limbs.
- Thromboembolic effect of stilboestrol treatment; hormonal therapy should be stopped and operative treatment—subcapsular orchidectomy—carried out. (Low-dose stilboestrol is recommended as 2 or 3 mg daily initially for 10 days, to be continued as 1 mg/day indefinitely).

Catheterisation

May be discussed with its complications. Remember that it should be done under aseptic conditions with a Silastic self-retaining Foley catheter (preferable to irritant rubber catheter). Complications include false passage, traumatic bleeding, infection and bacteraemia as well as catheter bladder tumour (oedematous mucosa with central pit due to irritating catheter tip). The two most important complications (which the examiners are after) are inflation of the balloon inside the urethra, causing urethral rupture, and induced paraphimosis. Therefore, make absolutely sure that you inflate the catheter balloon *only* if you see the urine running first and do not forget to pull back the foreskin after you finish catheterisation. Make a note of drained urine—whether clear or infected (murky), blood-stained or with clots—since you may need a Simplastic (harder material) catheter with a large draining tip (whistle tip). In stricture, a catheter with a Tiemann tip is useful. If it is impossible to negotiate the urethra and the bladder is quite distended then suprapubic catheterisation may be indicated.

The number on the catheter, e.g. 18 Fr, indicates the circumference (circumference = diameter × 22/7); thus, an 18 Fr catheter has a diameter of 18 divided by 22/7 (or approximately 3) = 6 mm. French gauge is also applied to urethral sounds, T-tubes and drains. In urethral dilators or bougies there are two figures, e.g. 24/28, which indicate the smallest and largest circumferences respectively (or diameters of 8 mm and 9.3 mm respectively). Ureteric catheter figures should be divided by 6, not 3; thus size 6 means 1 mm diameter.

Investigations and treatment

Investigations include haemoglobin (Hb), white cell count (WCC), erythrocyte sedimentation rate (ESR), prostatic acid and alkaline phosphatases (false acid phosphatase increase after admission is possibly due to repeated rectal examination or diurnal variation). Also mid-stream urine (MSU) or catheter stream urine (CSU), with plain X-ray of kidney, ureter, bladder (KUB), of intravenous urography (IVU), and abdominal ultrasound followed by diagnostic cystoscopy (prostatic biopsy). Treatment is by transurethral resection ± radiotherapy. (Hormonal therapy is usually reserved for skeletal metastases and recurrent prostatic obstructive uropathy.)

B5. VASCULAR CASE

As patients with peripheral vascular disease spend many weeks in hospital, you may well be asked to examine one of these patients. Those who have had inverted Y side-to-end aortofemoral bypass in Leriche's syndrome or iliofemoral or femoropopliteal bypass in lower limb ischaemia may be presented. Other suitable candidates for long cases are recently recovered embolectomy patients (with mitral stenosis, atrial fibrillation or past history of myocardial infarction) or patients who have had carotid endarterectomy or bypass in transient ischaemic attack. Unoperated vascular cases such as lower limb ischaemia may also be shown; gangrene, however, is shown as a short case.

B6. MISCELLANEOUS CASES

You may be shown any practically available patient in the ward with a detailed history such as:
- Recurrent goitre whether colloid or malignant.
- Unilateral or bilateral renal stones (whether operated on or not).
- Carcinoid syndrome.
- Inflammatory bowel disease such as ulcerative colitis or Crohn's disease.
- Unoperated colonic lesion such as carcinoma or polyposis coli.
- Hip osteoarthritis.
- Complicated gastrectomy.

SECTION 3
Operative Surgery

Introduction

An operation does not start with skin incision nor does it finish with skin closure. There are various preoperative preparations to be undertaken (routine and special)—anaesthesia, positioning, skin preparation and draping under completely antiseptic conditions—before the actual operative procedure begins. This is followed by postoperative care and instructions (to avoid postoperative morbidity and mortality). The preoperative and postoperative periods are as important as the operative procedure itself.

1. *Routine preoperative preparations*

A. Obtain permission for operation (signed consent form) and inform relatives.

B. Explain operation to patient.

C. Preparation of patient.

(i) Articles which should be *removed*:
Artificial eye
Contact lenses
Hearing aid
Artificial limbs
Dentures
Wig, toupée and hair grips
Jewellery
Pants/trousers (pyjamas) (except for dental patients).

(ii) Check for pacemaker.

(iii) Shave operative site and bathe.

(iv) Test urine (routinely).

(v) Nil by mouth—4 h prior to surgery.

(vi) Mark operative site, e.g. varicose veins, ileostomy or colostomy site, and breast mass. The side should also be marked with an arrow, e.g. right or left inguinal hernia, nephrectomy and limb amputation.

(vii) Check identiband with case sheet and X-rays.

(viii) Give premedication.

The essential points in preoperative preparation can be summarised as follows: well-prepared patient, consent obtained and operation explained.

2. *Special preoperative preparations*

According to the type of surgery, e.g. urinary catheterisation and bowel preparation in colorectal surgery; nasogastric suction, i.v. infusion in gastric surgery; antithyroid drugs, cervical X-ray and direct laryngoscopy in thyroid surgery.

3. *Anaesthesia*

4. *Positioning*

For example Lloyd–Davis (combined lithotomy-Trendelenburg position) in rectal carcinoma; supine in gastric and biliary operations; hyperextended neck with head supported by a ring and the shoulders by a sandbag in thyroidectomy.

5. *Skin preparation in antiseptic theatre and draping of the operative site*

6. *Surgical procedure*

Irrespective of its nature, usually involves the following stages

I Exposure and exploration.
II Mobilisation.
III Vascular dissection, ligation and division.
IV Excision.
V Reconstruction.
VI Closure with or without drainage.

Therefore, if you are asked the technical details of any operation you can discuss it safely and correctly according to the above six stages. Think of the above stages in thyroidectomy, gastrectomy, mastectomy, nephrectomy or any other major operation and you will find a striking similarity in their technical principles.

7. *Postoperative instructions*

For example, to continue antibiotics in bowel surgery if indicated, T-tube cholangiography on the 10th day in common bile duct exploration, nasogastric suction until there are bowel sounds or bowel action (flatus or faeces), urinary catheterisation if indicated. Removal of tube drain when dry (usually 3 days) or after creation of a fistulous track when requested (usually 7 days). Removal of stitches in 4 days (neck), 5 days (head), 7 days (limbs) or 10 days (abdomen) approximately.

Note: If the operation is performed as an emergency (life-threatening conditions, e.g. perforated viscus, appendicitis or strangulated hernia) there is insufficient time for full investigations and adequate preparations due to the urgency of the situation; the diagnosis should therefore be mainly clinical (which may sometimes prove wrong after operation). If the operation is elective (no immediate threat to the patient's life), there will usually be sufficient time for full investigations and adequate preparations. Morbidity and mortality are therefore less than in emergency operations.

EMERGENCY OPERATIONS

3.1. Emergency Laparotomy for Generalised Peritonitis

Indicated in perforated viscus, i.e. acute appendicitis (majority), peptic ulcer (5–8% of emergency laparotomies), colonic diverticular rupture and rarely gall bladder perforation. Quick assessment and preoperative preparation in the form of nasogastric suction, i.v. drip, CVP line and urinary catheterisation as well as prophylactic antibiotic may be required.

1. Under general anaesthesia with patient in supine position.
2. Right central paramedian incision (in uncertain diagnosis) or incision according to the suspected pathology from history and examination (grid iron in appendicitis, upper midline in peptic ulcer and gall bladder perforation and lower midline or left paramedian in diverticular perforation).
3. Aspirate any free fluid and sample it for bacteria then perform a quick exploration to identify the source of perforation and deal with it accordingly.

Appendicitis (Fig. 31)

1. Appendix base is identified by tracing taeniae coli of caecum; deliver the caecum through the incision and then deal with the appendix.
2. Apply Babcock's tissue forceps around the tip and base of appendix. Viewing the mesoappendix against light, make a window near its base then clamp the appendicular vessels (branches of ileocolic branch of superior mesenteric artery) and divide close to the appendix.

3. Insert 2/0 chromic catgut purse-string seromuscular stitch 1 cm from appendix base and leave untied.
4. Crush the appendix base, then recrush it and apply forceps 0.5 cm higher. Ligate the lower crushed part then cut off the appendix flush to the lower border of the crushing forceps and discard the contaminated knife, appendix and forceps in a dish (bowel is opened here). Now tie the purse-string suture to invaginate the ligated stump after application of forceps.
5. Check haemostasis then replace the caecum. Using a swab on sponge forceps, mop pus from the paracolic gutter and pelvis. Remember that peritoneal lavage with warm normal saline, Noxyflex or antibiotic solution is indicated *only* in generalised faecal peritonitis. Such peritoneal toilet may be harmful in spreading a localised peritonitis and is therefore contraindicated.
6. Drain the area (if necessary) with a wide-bore tube drain (closed system), then close in layers with or without interparietal povidone-iodine spray.

Special points

- In difficult high retrocaecal or deep pelvic appendix do not hesitate to enlarge the incision laterally or medially with generous muscle cutting. Good exposure and dissection under direct vision are essential.
- Retrograde or base-first appendicectomy is sometimes helpful.
- Oedematous appendix base does not need to be crushed before ligation and if it is impossible to invaginate the stump then diathermise its lumen and direct the drain mouth to it.
- Drainage of pus alone without appendicectomy is acceptable *only* in difficult cases when one cannot find the appendix.
- If an appendicular mass is felt it can be removed after careful dissection. If carcinoma of the

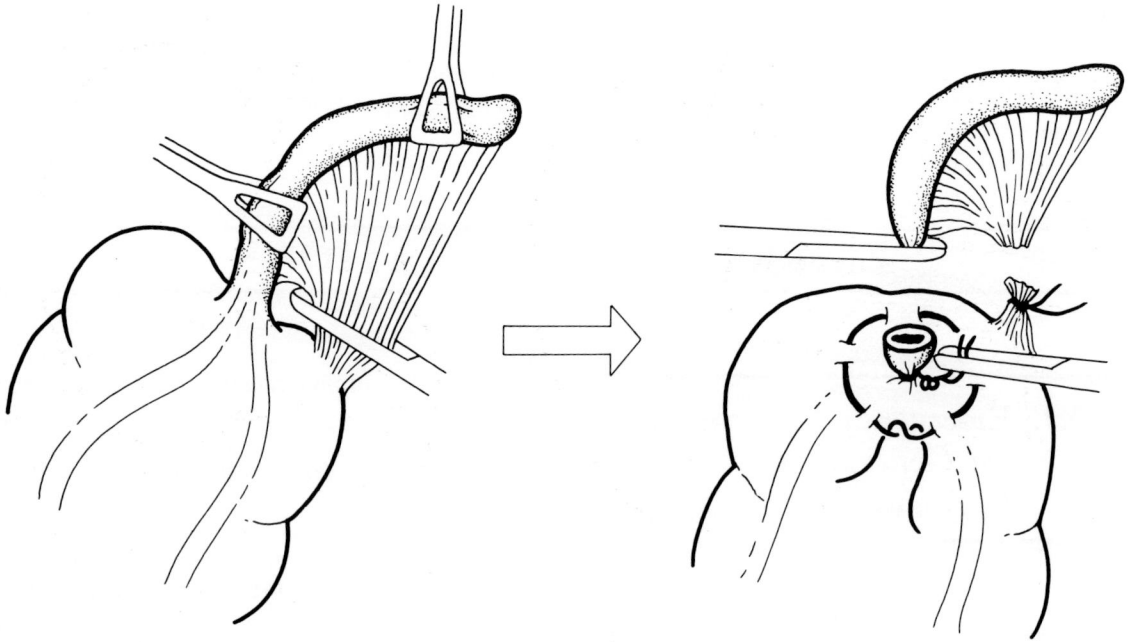

Fig. 31   Standard appendicectomy

caecum with secondary appendicitis is suspected, or can't be excluded, right hemicolectomy can be performed even if the pathology report reveals a benign appendicular mass later on.

- If after abdominal closure the histology report reveals carcinoid tumour of the appendix, no further action is required, only regular follow-up for life. However, if adenocarcinoma is reported then right hemicolectomy must be performed.

- If the appendix was normal, check the terminal ileum (for Crohn's disease), Meckel's diverticulum, the ovaries (for ruptured Graafian follicles) and lymph nodes (mesenteric lymphadenitis). Appendicectomy should be avoided in caecal Crohn's disease since this may trigger external fistula formation. However, the appendix can be removed in ileal Crohn's disease if it is inflamed. Meckel's diverticulum should be removed only if involved; otherwise leave alone and label the case clearly for future action.

Peptic ulcer (Fig. 32)

1. Ask the assistant to pull the pyloric antrum.
2. Carefully close the duodenal perforation with three interrupted 2/0 chromic catgut sutures inserted 1 cm from the proximal edge, passing through the perforation and emerging 1 cm from the distal edge. This two-stage biting avoids inadvertent stitching of the posterior to the anterior pyloric wall. The closure is done in a transverse fashion as longitudinal suture causes stenosis at the site of closure.
3. Mobilise a fold of omentum and patch it over the perforation, then tie the sutures to close the perforation.
4. Peritoneal toilet and wide-bore tube drainage (closed system) are carried out.

Special points

- In gastric perforation, ulcer cancer is present in 5–10% of cases so take four angle biopsies then perform simple closure, limited wedge gastric resection and suturing, or formal partial gastrectomy (Billroth I). Substantiate your decision in examination.
- Associated bleeding ulcer should be underrun (duodenal) or excised (if in stomach).
- If there is bile peritonitis but no anterior perforation, open the gastrocolic ligament to look for posterior gastric or pyloroduodenal ulcer and treat as above.
- Simple closure is the safest treatment because of its low mortality and the patient's poor health. An experienced surgeon (and expert anaesthe-

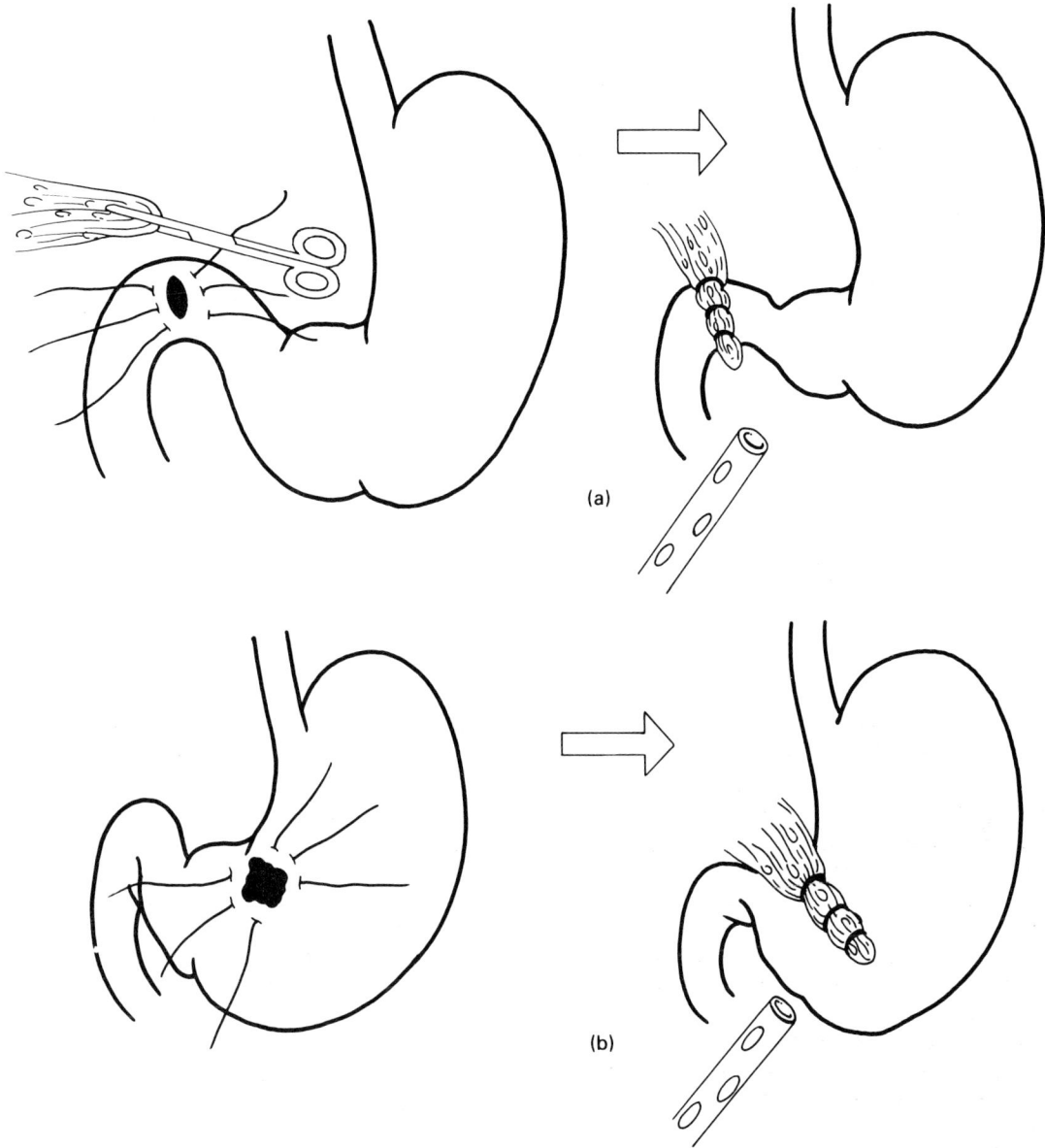

Fig. 32   Closure of perforated peptic ulcer with omental tag and peritoneal drainage. (a) Perforated duodenal ulcer. (b) Perforated gastric ulcer. Biopsy should be taken from the edge of the perforated gastric ulcer.

tist) can undertake definitive treatment if there is a chronic history of peptic ulcer, gastric ulcer from the start, or combined bleeding and perforation.

- Patients with simple closure of the perforation should be advised to have definitive elective operation and should be followed up regularly (roughly one-third are cured, another one-third remain symptomatic and the last third suffer complications).

Colonic diverticulum

Patch with greater omental tag using 2/0 chromic catgut stitches with or without temporary transverse loop colostomy.

After full recovery perform sigmoidoscopy and barium enema to examine the distal colon and to test the sutured area for leakage. Six weeks later resect the diseased segment with anastomosis and follow by closure of the colostomy at a third stage. Alternatively resect the diseased colonic segment from the start and perform Hartmann's procedure by bringing up a proximal end colostomy and closing the distal colonic end and dropping it into the pelvis (this option eliminates the toxic focus of infection). This will be followed by a second stage— restoration of continuity. (The distal colonic end is sometimes brought up as a mucocutaneous fistula to prevent its retraction into the pelvis. However, in difficult identification Foley's balloon catheter inserted rectally can be used to facilitate its dissection.)

Special points

In concomitant colonic perforated carcinoma biopsy should be taken and followed as above. Alternatively, a primary resection and anastomosis protected by colostomy to be closed later on can be performed. However, in examination the *safest* procedure should always be mentioned as the first choice, i.e. A staging procedure (temporary colostomy, resection with anastomosis, then closure of colostomy).

Gall bladder

Cholecystectomy, preferably in the antegrade (fundus first) fashion. If impossible to perform, because of obscured anatomy and friable inflamed tissue, then try partial cholecystectomy and/or cholecystostomy with Foley's catheter left in for 7–10 days to create a fibrous external fistula together with drainage of the subhepatic area. The common bile duct should be examined and an operative cholangiogram should be considered (if feasible) since exploration of the duct may be required.

3.2. Intestinal Obstruction

Surgical relief is carried out electively after routine gastroduodenal nasogastric suction coupled with fluid replacement and correction of electrolyte imbalance. The three indications for emergency operation after suction and i.v. fluid replacement are:

External hernial obstruction or strangulation Obstruction (irreducible hernia containing an intestine with obstructed lumen but good blood supply) often culminates in strangulation (serious impairment of blood supply of hernial content with imminent gangrene). Clinical distinction is difficult and it is better to assume that the case is strangulation and treat accordingly. Classically, femoral hernia strangulates in women and inguinal hernia strangulates in men while incisional hernia strangulates in both sexes. External hernia is the commonest cause of intestinal obstruction in developing countries while adhesion band is the commonest cause of intestinal obstruction in developed countries (owing to the great number of laparotomies performed).

Internal intestinal strangulation Is the most urgent condition since gangrene follows quickly. Clinically there is intestinal obstruction with shock in an ill toxic patient. Pain may fluctuate up and down but is never absent, and persistence of pain for 2 h in spite of gastroduodenal aspiration is diagnostic of strangulation. There is always tenderness and rebound tenderness (peritonism) over an intra-abdominal strangulated coil (in obstruction, only tenderness presents). Strangulated intestine in external hernia presents as a tense, tender, irreducible lump with no expansile cough impulse and which has recently increased in size. Late internal strangulation leads to generalised tenderness and rigidity.

Acute or acute-on-chronic intestinal obstruction Usually involves the upper gastrointestinal tract. Sudden intestinal colicky pain and vomiting are the first symptoms. Distension is usually absent (but borborygmi and high-pitched bowel sounds may be present on auscultation). Absolute constipation is late, as there is natural action of the bowels after onset, yielding some faeces below the site of intestinal obstruction even if it is complete.

There is no constipation in acute intestinal obstruction due to:

Richter's hernia (partial enterocoele).
Gall stone ileus.
Mesenteric vascular occlusion.
Intestinal obstruction associated with pelvic abscess.

(Chronic intestinal obstruction usually involves the lower gastrointestinal tract. It starts first with constipation that becomes absolute as a result of completely obstructing colonic carcinoma or diverticular disease. Abdominal distension then follows, leading to a fully blown caecum and pain. Vomiting is late).

Obstructed or strangulated inguinal hernia

Approach and repair is similar to that in elective cases. Differences in treatment depend on the site of intestinal obstruction and whether the bowel is viable or dead.
1. Make a suprainguinal incision parallel and 2 cm above the medial two-thirds of the inguinal ligament cutting through skin, subcutaneous tissue and Scarpa's fascia down to the external oblique aponeurosis after proper haemostasis.
2. Identify the external inguinal ring and split the external oblique ring in the line of the inguinal canal to reveal the spermatic cord (male) or the round ligament of the uterus (female).
3. Isolate the hernial sac by sharp dissection in the line of the cord (through cremasteric and internal spermatic fascias) and expose fully the internal inguinal ring, safeguarding spermatic vessels and vas deferens.
4. Pick up the sac with two or three artery forceps and open. Identify its contents and see whether it is viable. Gently draw up the bowel and never let it slip back into the abdomen. If it is viable replace and pass a finger to check for the presence of femoral hernia from inside the peritoneal cavity (if present can be repaired simultaneously). If viability is suspect then cover it with warm moist packs for 5–10 min (asking the anaesthetist to give a higher percentage of oxygen), then re-examine for sheen, colour, peristalsis and mesenteric pulsation. A black segment of small intestine with no sheen, no peristalsis or pulsation should be resected with end-to-end anastomosis (2/0 chromic catgut in two layers—mucosal continuous and seromuscular continuous) then replaced intraperitoneally. If the large bowel is resected it should be protected proximally with a temporary loop colostomy via a separate left iliac muscle cutting (or appendectomy-like) incision to be closed 6 weeks later when barium enema (done at least 2 weeks postoperatively) shows no anastomotic leak in the suture line. Again, the large bowel (usually sigmoid colon in left inguinal hernia) is closed in one or two layers—using mainly interrupted seromuscular 2/0 silk and mucosal continuous 2/0 chromic catgut (*optional* gas-tight barrier). Take care not to exert tension or cause strangulation during suturing. Replace the bowel intra-

peritoneally with paracolic drainage.
5. Resect the hernial sac and close its neck after transfixion ligature or purse-string suture (herniotomy).
6. Repair is carried out by suturing the inguinal ligament to the conjoined tendon, using non-absorbable nylon or Prolene, from the pubic tubercle medially to the internal inguinal ring, displacing the cord laterally.
7. Close in layers—chromic catgut to external oblique aponeurosis refashioning the external inguinal ring so that it permits entry of the little finger. If Halsted repair is required in an elderly patient (over 60 years) to strengthen repair then close the external oblique aponeurosis posterior to the cord which will be subcutaneous. In women the ligament is excised and in orchidectomy done in the elderly (consent should be obtained preoperatively) the repair is made easier by complete closure of the external oblique aponeurosis. Closure of subcutaneous tissue (plain catgut) and skin (Prolene or clips) follows.

Internal intestinal strangulation

1. Laparotomy via right paramedian incision usually.
2. If the caecum is collapsed it is small bowel intestinal obstruction and if distended then it is large bowel intestinal obstruction. Expose the site of obstruction clearly after withdrawal of intestinal coils using moist warm packs.
3. Decompress the intestinal obstruction by Savage's intestinal decompressor (or similar decompressor) via a stab in the bowel, using a purse-string suture to control any spillage. Higher small bowel intestinal obstruction may be milked upward towards the nasogastric suction controlled by the anaesthetist.
4. Assess viability (as above) and act accordingly. In small bowel intestinal obstruction adhesion bands can be divided and bowel released, volvulus is dismantled and fixed. In acute large bowel intestinal obstruction due to carcinoma involving:
- Ascending colon up to proximal part of the transverse colon, emergency right hemicolectomy is advocated *but* if the tumour is irremovable or the patient is elderly and extremely ill then ileotransverse enterostomy is indicated. Impending or actual caecal perforation may necessitate caecostomy (alone or in addition to above procedure).
- Splenic flexure down to rectum, temporary transverse loop colostomy is performed, fol-

lowed 4 weeks later by resection of the obstructing tumour (when the condition of the patient has stabilised) with closure of colostomy simultaneously (two stages) or 6 weeks later (three stages).

However, with an irremovable tumour or in elderly patients, transverse sigmoid colocolic bypass (side-to-side anastomosis) is recommended. In massive pelvic infiltration, loop transverse proximal colostomy is constructed permanently. In diverticular sigmoid disease perform Hartmann's operation—resecting the area, establishing proximal left iliac end colostomy, and closing the distal rectal end to be resutured later on (rectal or distal end can be brought out to skin level as a mucocutaneous fistula to facilitate later anastomosis).

Colostomy

Either end colostomy (usually permanent as in abdominoperineal excision of rectal carcinoma but can be temporary as in Hartmann's operation for diverticular disease) or loop colostomy (usually temporary but can be used permanently). The colostomy can be iliac or in the transverse colon.

Left iliac end colostomy

The site is marked, a disc of skin is removed and an appendectomy-like (but muscle-cutting) incision is made in the left iliac fossa. The proximal colonic end (clamped with either an intestinal or Zachary-Cope clamp) is delivered through the incision. Then colonic serosa is stitched to the abdominal wall muscle using 2/0 chromic catgut and mucosa is sutured to the skin with eight interrupted stitches. This is followed by application of a colostomy bag over the functioning colostomy. The laparotomy wound should be closed and covered before the colostomy is constructed to avoid faecal contamination.

Transverse loop colostomy (Fig. 33)

The most widely used temporary colostomy. General anaesthesia is important since traction on the mesentery causes pain and nausea.
1. Transverse incision (8–10 cm long) in the right upper abdomen midway between the umbilicus and xiphisternum over the rectus abdominis muscle and extending laterally to the lateral border of the rectus muscle.
2. Cut down all layers including the rectus muscle, which is divided transversely (ligating and dividing the epigastric artery).

3. The most *proximal* loop of transverse colon is prepared by cleaning omentum from its anterior surface; then a small hole is made in the transverse mesocolon through which a rubber tube is passed to facilitate delivery of the colon through the incision (in sigmoid colostomy a left iliac muscle-cutting incision is made—sigmoid colon has no omentum). Close the laparotomy wound at this stage.
4. The colonic loop is held by an underlying glass rod (or by a colostomy bar or skin bridge incised initially). Open the colostomy on its antimesocolic border longitudinally (along taenia coli) or transversely.
5. Insert mucocutaneous sutures (2/0 chromic catgut) and close the skin so that the colonic loop fits snugly, allowing one finger to pass down each side. The colostomy appliance should be constructed immediately (the colon should be opened at operation and not later).

Complications of colostomy

- Loss of viability (blood supply is interfered with).
- Separation of colostomy and retraction (due to tension and infection).
- Infection—cellulitis (due to haematoma); scarring and stenosis. Stenosis occurs at the mucocutaneous junction. The colostomy should be refashioned with excision of skin disc.
- Paracolostomy hernia especially in end terminal colostomy. Colostomy should be resited and the hernial defect closed.
- Prolapse in transverse colostomy is not important (since it is usually temporary) but in end colostomy it leads to dysfunction; treated by reconstruction or resiting.

Colostomy closure

1. Apply stay (silk) sutures to the mucocutaneous junction under general anaesthesia and mobilise the colostomy.
2. Separate the colostomy from the anterior abdominal wall, removing the skin edge with it.
3. Perform simple two-layer closure: 2/0 chromic catgut using continuous Connell stitch (loop on mucosa to invert it) taking in all layers followed by fine silk seromuscular Lambert (interrupted) layer.
4. Conduct the anastomosis outside and replace it intraperitoneally since an extraperitoneal location is associated with inadequate mobilisation and unsatisfactory anastomosis under tension.
5. Close the abdominal wall ($\pm$ drainage).

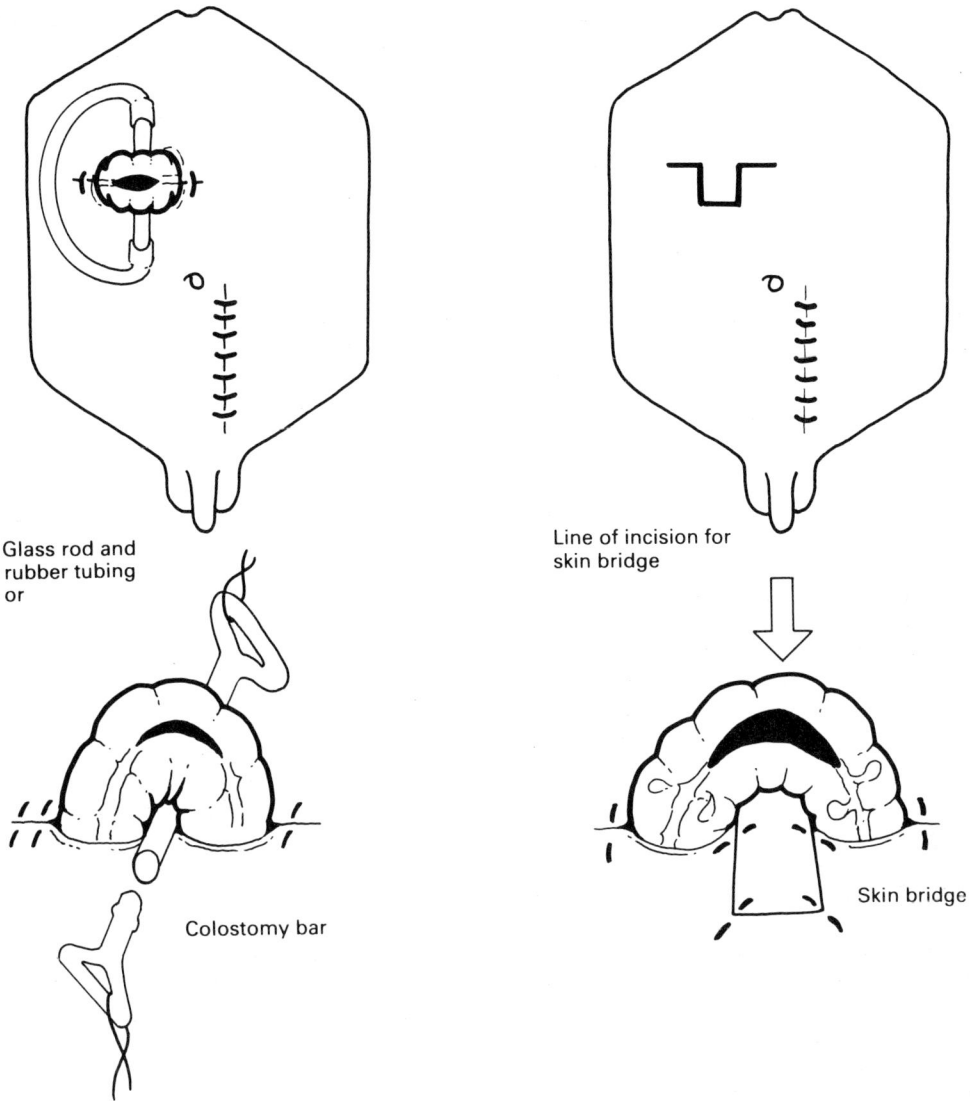

Fig. 33 Loop colostomy

Glass rod and
rubber tubing
or

Colostomy bar

Line of incision for
skin bridge

Skin bridge

3.3. Femoral Hernia Repair

Indications

Uncomplicated femoral hernia Because of the constant risk of strangulation and the highly un-

satisfactory result of femoral truss (urgent operation).

Strangulated femoral hernia Occurs when blood supply of its contents is impaired (gangrene occurs 6 h later). The intestine is obstructed already and its blood supply is constricted impeding venous return and leading to congestion and fluid exudation within the hernial sac. Later, the arterial supply is compromised leading to blood effusion into the lumen and wall of the intestine (the sac becomes blood-stained with transmigration of bacteria followed by haemorrhage and thrombosis of vessels, subserosal blood decomposition, perforation and gangrene). Clinically the findings are those of intestinal obstruction (generalised abdominal pain following its initial localisation over hernia, vomiting, abdominal distension and constipation) combined with local signs of a tense tender irreducible hernia which has recently increased in size with no expansile impulse on coughing. Rebound tenderness is often present. When gangrene starts, peristaltic pain paroxysms cease (grave sign) due to peritonitis or paralytic ileus and the patient passes into septic shock.

Approaches to femoral hernia repair (Fig. 34)

Low approach (Lockwood, Surgeon, St Bartholomew's Hospital, London)

A 10 cm skin crease incision over the hernia, a finger's breadth below the medial half of the inguinal ligament. Deepen the incision, expose the preperitoneal fat-covered sac and incise the sac on its *lower lateral aspect* to avoid bladder injury, dilate

the neck digitally, examine bowel viability, and reduce the bowel if possible. Close the femoral canal with interrupted non-absorbable 2/0 suture (monofilament nylon or silk mounted on a fish-hook J-shaped needle) approximating the inguinal ligament to the pectineal ligament and making sure not to constrict the femoral vein laterally (place your index finger on it).

Inguinal approach (Lotheissen, Surgeon, Kaiser Josef Hospital, Vienna)

The incision is as for inguinal hernia—2 cm above and parallel to the medial two-thirds of the inguinal ligament. Deepen the incision medial to the inferior epigastric vessels after cord mobilisation and external oblique division. Intraperitoneally expose the obstructed contents and retract the lower end of the wound to manipulate and reduce the contents (hernia repair is as above). This approach is condemned since it weakens the inguinal area and predisposes to inguinal hernia formation.

High approach (McEvedy, Surgeon, Ancoats Hospital, Manchester)

A 10 cm vertical incision centred on the inguinal ligament (over the femoral canal through the lower 5 cm). The sac is dissected as above. If strangulated or the contents cannot be reduced then cut through the upper 5 cm; incise the rectus sheath parallel to the lateral border of the rectus muscle and dissect between transversalis fascia and peritoneum (no posterior rectus sheath behind the lower one-third of the rectus muscle below the arcuate line). Reduce the contents, manipulating from above and below, then repair from above (in order to visualise the accessory obturator artery and avoid its injury).

Henry's approach (Henry, British surgeon, found this approach accidentally while performing it on bladder bilharziasis in Egypt)

A 10 cm midline infraumbilical extraperitoneal incision deepened between the peritoneum and transversalis fascia. Repair from above. This approach is very good for bilateral femoral hernias.

Preperitoneal approach (Nyhus, USA)

A transverse anterior abdominal wall incision (modified from Henry) is used to repair femoral hernia from behind. The transversalis fascia is closed, assisted by external direct manual reduction from

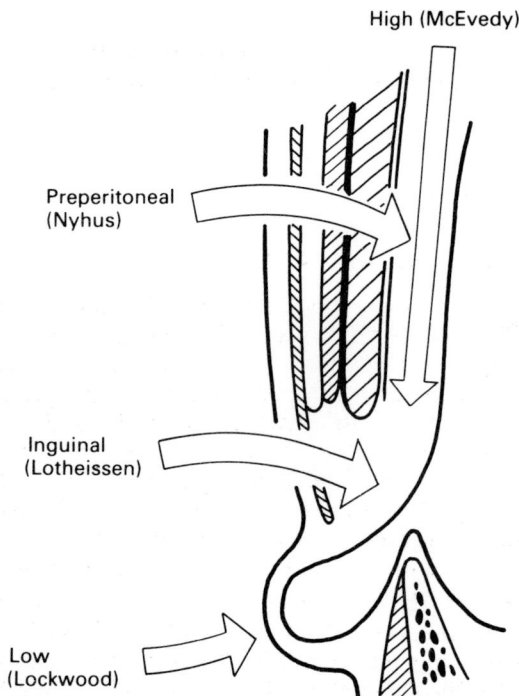

Fig. 34 Approaches in femoral hernia repair

below. This approach also allows repair of direct, indirect and recurrent inguinal hernias through one incision. (Not practised in the UK.)

Inguinal ligament multipartial division
(Ellis, Westminster Hospital, London)

Via low approach (to allow ample room for reduction and/or resection); is not widely practised.

The commonest approaches for strangulated femoral hernia are:
- Lockwood approach (with or without paramedian laparotomy).
- McEvedy approach: probably the most widely practised.
- Nyhus approach: very good approach practised widely in the USA (not UK).

Technical points

- Ascertain bowel viability from:
   Sheen and colour.
   Arterial mesenteric pulsation.
   Bowel peristalsis.
   If good, replace. If doubtful, cover with warm moist packs and give 100 % oxygen for 5–10 min by the clock and re-examine. If by the above criteria it is judged viable, replace. If not, resect and do end-to-end primary anastomosis for small bowel (in two layers—2/0 chromic catgut to the mucosa and a seromuscular layer).
- Avoid *taxis* in femoral hernia since dislodgement of gangrenous bowel requires laparotomy. If such a gangrenous segment slips back into the abdomen during hernia repair, perform laparotomy (paramedian incision is essential) to resect it and restore bowel continuity.
- A grooved director may be used to cut the lacunar medial ligament (the theoretical possibility of injury to accessory obturator artery is often exaggerated) in order to enlarge the hernial neck.
- Omentocele should be excised rather than replaced since adhesions are vascular and difficult to reduce. Richter's hernia (partial enterocele) is treated either by wedge excision and anastomosis (in transverse fashion in two layers) or by inversion within the bowel lumen with two layers.

3.4. Arterial Embolectomy

Indications

Major acute interruption to the circulation of a limb thought to be due to embolism requires embolectomy provided that the limb is still potentially viable and that the patient is not in circulatory failure.

Preoperative preparation

Intravenous heparin 10 000 units as soon as diagnosis of embolism is made. Measures to improve cardiac state if necessary. Aortography unnecessary initially, as diagnosis is made by clinical findings, particularly loss of pulses.

Position of patient

Supine. For lower limb, leg externally rotated at hip and flexed at knee, permitting access to femoral and distal popliteal arteries. For upper limb, arm abducted on arm board.

Anaesthesia

Local infiltration anaesthesia may be used in the critically ill patient; otherwise general anaesthesia is preferred.

Procedure

Femoral embolus (Fig. 35)

The common and superficial femoral arteries are the commonest peripheral sites. The common femoral artery and its bifurcation is exposed through vertical incision; tapes or silicone slings are placed round the common femoral, superficial and profunda arteries. Open the common femoral artery with a transverse incision opposite the profunda opening. Remove wire from a No. 3 or 4 Fogarty catheter, and test balloon. No more than the correct amount of fluid for inflation should be drawn into the syringe. Pass the catheter gently down the profunda as far as possible. Then inflate the balloon (the surgeon does this himself) until resistance is felt and gently withdraw the catheter while adjusting inflation by feel to keep the balloon in contact with the arterial wall. Clot emerges from the arteriotomy

Common
femoral
artery

Fogarty catheter

Profunda
femoris

Superficial femoral
artery

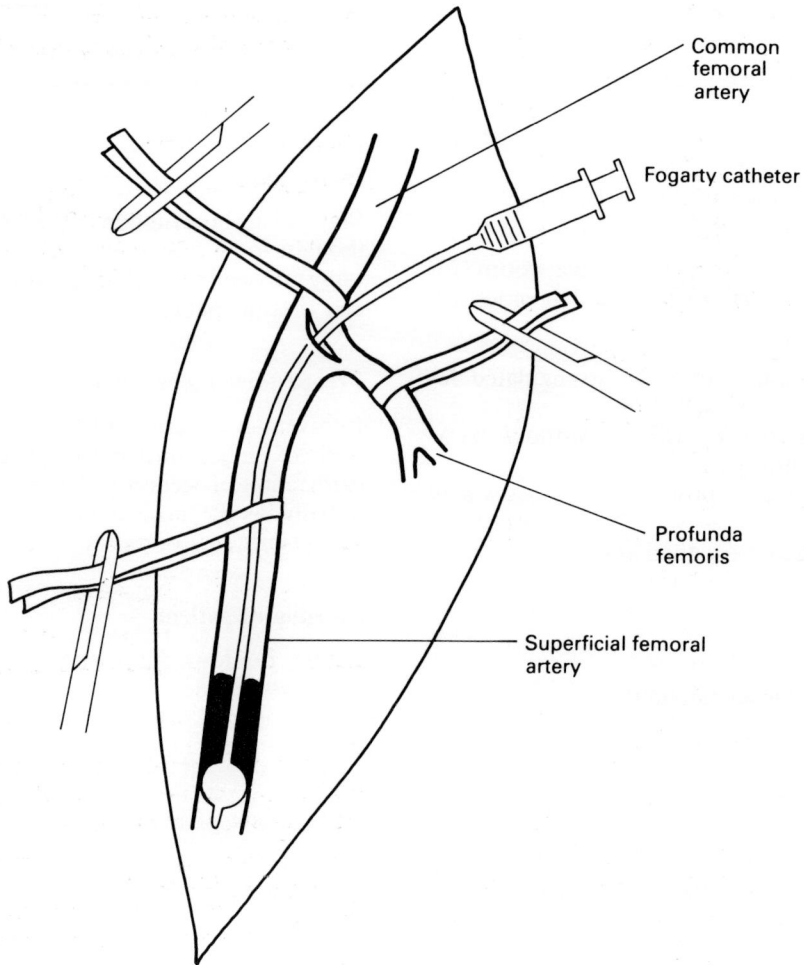

Fig. 35   Femoral embolectomy

in front of the balloon. Repeat the pass into the profunda until no further clot is obtained. Apply bulldog clamp to the profunda. A catheter is then passed down the superficial femoral artery as far as possible. In favourable cases it reaches the ankle. Withdraw clot and repeat until no further clot is obtained. If the embolus does not shoot out with the initial arteriotomy, a No. 4 or 5 size Fogarty should be passed upwards and withdrawn with the balloon inflated as before, until a good forward flow is obtained. Clamp the common femoral artery and close the arteriotomy with 5/0 Prolene.

Popliteal embolus

These may often be removed through the common femoral artery. If unsuccessful, the distal popliteal artery should be exposed by a vertical incision a finger's breadth behind the medial border of the tibia, division of the deep fascia and backward retraction of gastrocnemius, and division of the medial hamstrings near the tibia. The popliteal bifurcation can be displayed by this approach.

Aortic saddle embolus (Fig. 36)

This can usually be removed with Fogarty catheters via a bilateral femoral approach. One side is clamped while as much embolus as possible is withdrawn from the other. The process is then reversed. The superficial femoral and profunda arteries should also be 'catheterised' to remove clot that may have migrated distally.

theter to be passed upwards and into each forearm vessel, both of which should be cleared.

Failed embolectomy

This usually means coexisting occlusive disease, or that occlusion was thrombotic not embolic. Emergency arteriography is indicated so that arterial reconstruction may be undertaken if feasible.

3.5. Leaking Aortic Aneurysm

In patients reaching hospital alive with a leaking abdominal aneurysm, survival depends very much on prompt action by the surgical and anaesthetic team, the aim being to secure control of the aorta proximal to the aneurysm with the least possible delay; resuscitation can then proceed and the remainder of the operation is carried out much as in an elective case.

Preoperative preparation

Even if the patient arrives in a stable and satisfactory condition, arrangements for operation should be put in hand immediately. Twelve units of blood should be crossmatched, two i.v. drips set up, and a urethral catheter and a nasogastric tube should be passed. In theatre, the patient is placed straight on the operating table; the surgical team are ready scrubbed and gowned and the patient is draped before anaesthesia is started (in case sudden catastrophic bleeding occurs when the abdominal wall relaxes). Patients in shock should ideally be taken straight from the ambulance to the theatre; little time should be wasted on attempts at resuscitation, and for patients *in extremis* immediate laparotomy and aortic control may offer the only chance of survival.

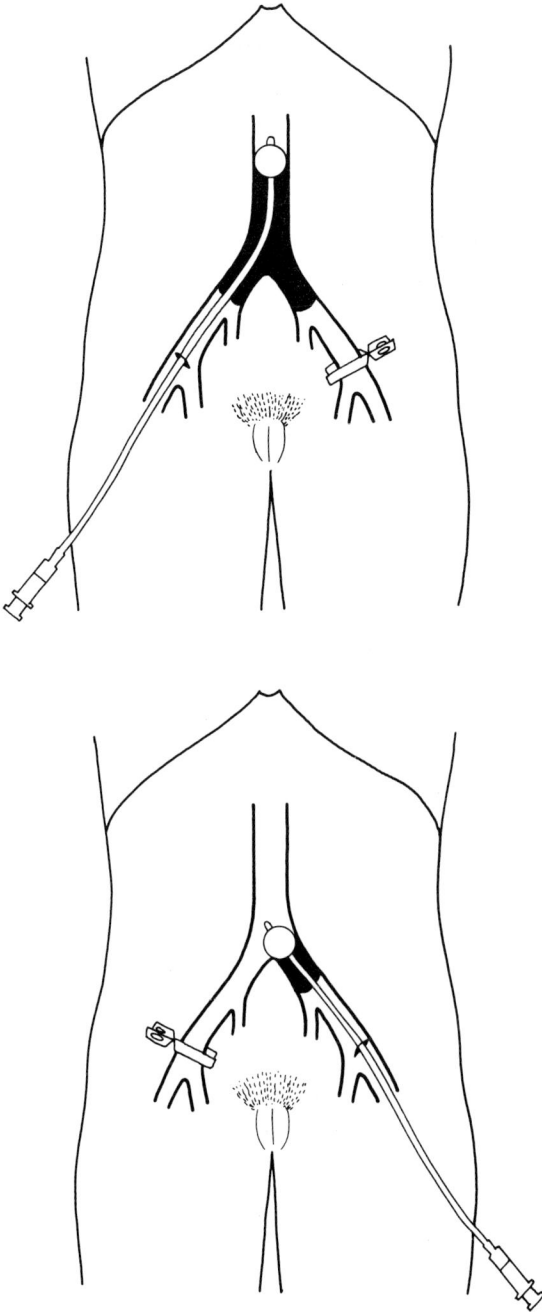

Fig. 36 Bilateral embolectomy for aortic saddle embolism

Brachial embolus

Expose brachial bifurcation via an S-shaped incision, the proximal limb being medial. Transverse arteriotomy above the bifurcation allows the ca-

Procedure

If the patient's condition is still stable after anaesthesia and opening the abdomen through a long midline incision, the duodenum can be quickly mobilised and the neck of the aneurysm looked for through the haematoma; after giving i.v. heparin, it is clamped as in the elective procedure. If this proves difficult or the patient is deteriorating or *in extremis*, the upper abdominal aorta should be compressed. This can be done by backward pressure against the spine with the end of a suitably shaped wooden spoon, or the blade of a weighted vaginal speculum pointing upwards parallel with the aorta and pressed backwards in the midline. Alternatively, with the left lobe of the liver retracted the supra-coeliac aorta can be exposed by dissection through the upper part of the lesser omentum and partial division of the right crus, and clamped at this level. At the lower end the common iliac arteries are clamped, and time can then be taken to dissect the neck of the aneurysm for clamping the aorta below the renal arteries.

If necessary, the aneurysm can be opened and a finger pushed up through its neck as a guide for the application of the clamp at this point. A Foley catheter passed up into the aorta, and then inflated, is another possibility; and if difficulty is experienced in clamping the common iliac arteries, they can be controlled in a similar manner.

Once the clamps are in place, the operation proceeds as for an elective aneurysm. A woven graft should always be selected to minimise blood loss through the graft wall. Before completing the distal anastomosis a Fogarty catheter should be passed down the lower limb arteries to withdraw any clots.

3.6. Compound Fracture

Procedure (Figs 37–39)

Should be managed urgently with prophylactic antibiotics, tetanus prophylaxis, preoperative immobilisation (splintage), careful X-ray assessment (to decide whether closed or open reduction is required). Then:

1. Under general anaesthesia with X-ray screening control try to assess the pulses. Try closed manipulation and feel pulses again. Check for swelling and haematoma under tension.

2. Clean the skin thoroughly, shave the wound margins and remove all foreign bodies and dirt. Irrigate the wound generously and remove blood clots.

3. Extend the incision (after debridement of devitalised margin) to visualise clearly all dead muscles and damaged fascia in order to remove them. Decompress the enclosing fascia if necessary. Identify and safeguard main arteries and nerves. Remove small spiky bone chips but do not remove big pieces, otherwise bone shortening may result.

4. Reduce the fracture under screening usually by closed manipulation; rarely open reduction is required (primary internal fixation is better avoided because of high rate of infection).

5. Once the fracture is reduced, it is usually stable and the limb is suitable for padded plaster cast immobilisation which can be split to allow for oedema development. If the fracture is unstable

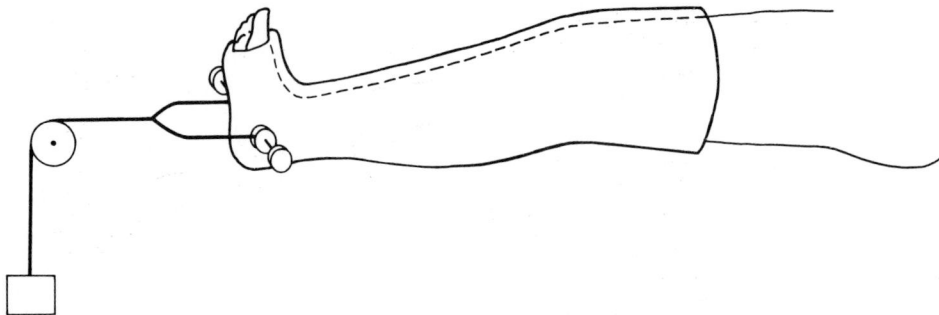

Fig. 37   Calcaneal skeletal traction, closed reduction of compound fracture of tibia and fibula, and plaster-of-Paris immobilisation

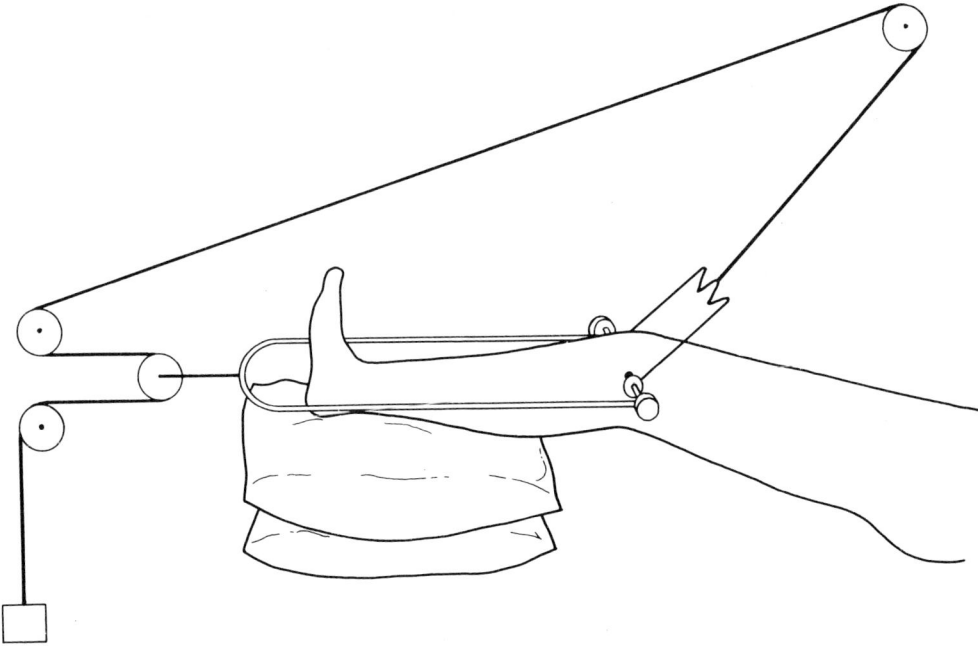

Fig. 38 Hamilton–Russell skeletal traction for fractures around the hip

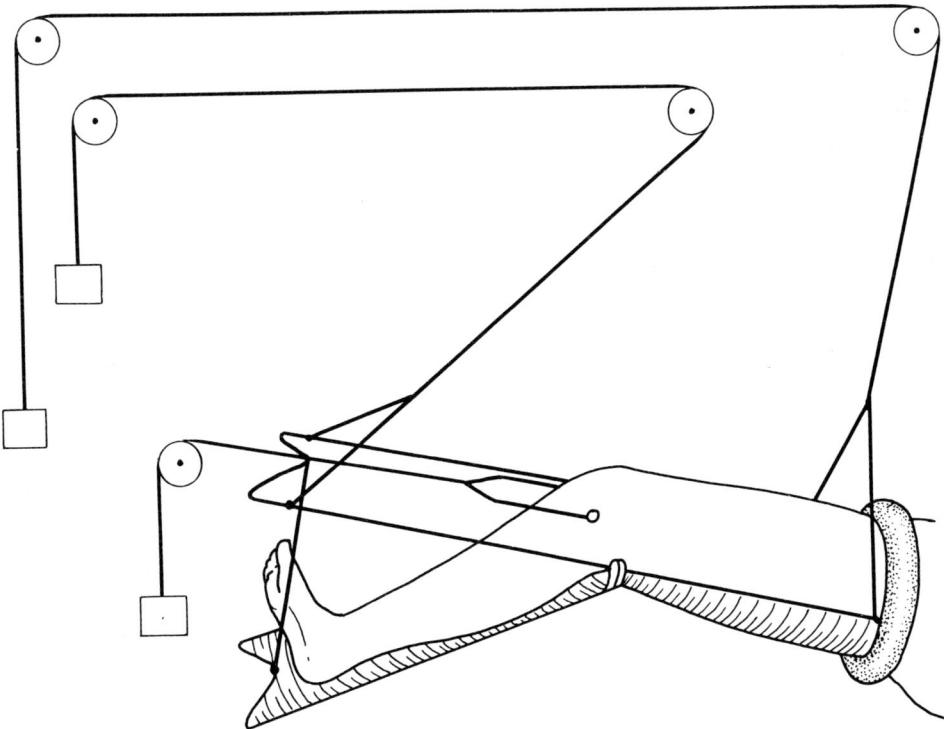

Fig. 39 Sliding skeletal traction with a Thomas' splint for shaft and supracondylar fractures of the femur

after reduction *skeletal traction* should be added. In compound femoral fracture, after nicking the skin (always under general anaesthesia), insert upper tibial Steinmann pin or Denham pin mounted on a T-handled introducer from the lateral to the medial aspect 2.5 cm posterior-inferior to the tibial tuberosity. In compound fractures of tibia and fibula (ignore fibula and reduce tibial fracture) introduce a calcaneal pin 2.5 cm posterior inferior to the lateral malleolus. Attach a traction stirrup to the pin (e.g. Bohler stirrup) and set sliding skeletal traction on a Thomas' splint (in femoral fracture) or use calcaneal skeletal traction with a Bohler–Braun frame (in compound tibial and fibular fracture).

6. Remember to close the skin without tension, using a relief incision if necessary. If impossible to close then delayed primary suture 5 days later or split skin grafts are needed.

3.7. Head Injury and Burr Hole Procedure

Indications

1. Closed head injury when one of the following signs, suggestive of intracranial haemorrhage (mainly extradural), is present:
- Sudden deterioration in the level of consciousness.
- Dissociation of vital signs due to increased intracranial pressure, i.e. systemic hypertension and bradycardia (opposite to internal haemorrhage signs of hypotension and tachycardia). Such hypertension (due to hypoxia induced by intracranial haematoma and increased intracranial pressure) leads to reflex bradycardia (via baroreceptors) and the combination is termed Cushing's reflex.
- Focal neurological signs, i.e. sluggish dilating unilateral pupil and contralateral hemiparesis.

2. Open head trauma if it is depressed compound fracture. Burr hole should be performed in the vicinity of the fracture over an intact bone to lift the depressed fragment for proper decompression. Close dural tear if present to prevent development of epileptogenic focus.

3. Intracranial pressure monitoring with an extradural or subdural transducer, subdural bolt or intraventricular cannula (carries risk of infection in 1–5% of cases). Such investigation provides baseline pressure and gives warning of complications (intracranial haematoma) before there are clinical signs in conscious and stable head injuries so that the decision whether to operate can be made.

4. Ventricular access for relief of increased intracranial pressure, air or contrast ventriculography, drug administration and external ventricular drainage (burr hole here is elective and not an emergency as in the above three indications).

Preparations

Under local anaesthesia preferably with endotracheal intubation to ensure an adequate airway; or under general anaesthesia. Position the head over a horse-shoe head rest or between sandbags, shave and cleanse the whole head with an antiseptic solution (e.g. Disadine). Mark the surface for proposed burr hole(s) under strict sterile circumstances and infiltrate the scalp beneath these markings with 1% lignocaine and 1:200 000 adrenaline. The site of the burr hole is determined by:
- The side of bruising in the temporal muscle.
- The side of skull fracture (seen on skull X-ray).
- The side of initial dilatation of pupil.

Use a sterile ruler to delineate the midline of the scalp in the sagittal plane; then mark two 4 cm incisions, each 3 cm from the sagittal plane at a point 13 cm from the nasal root (frontal burr holes). Two more incisions are marked—one 3 cm above the midzygomatic point (temporal burr hole) and one 8 cm posterior to the temporal burr hole (parietal)— along an imaginary half circle (Fig. 40).

Procedure

1. Incise and deepen the skin down to bone (at proposed sites, preferably starting with the temporal site first). Use finger tips to press and stop the bleeding vessels, applying artery forceps to the galea aponeurotica to arrest bleeding. Insert a self-retaining retractor.

2. Strip back pericranium with a rugine or periosteal elevator. Use a Hudson brace with perforator to penetrate the outer and inner tables of the skull and then use a burr to complete the skull hole. Stop bleeding from diploë with bone wax.

3. If extradural haematoma is seen, enlarge or extend the burr hole (craniectomy) by bone nibbling forceps (bone rongeur). Remove the blood clot. Irrigation with saline and gentle suction is applied. Middle meningeal arterial bleeding can be con-

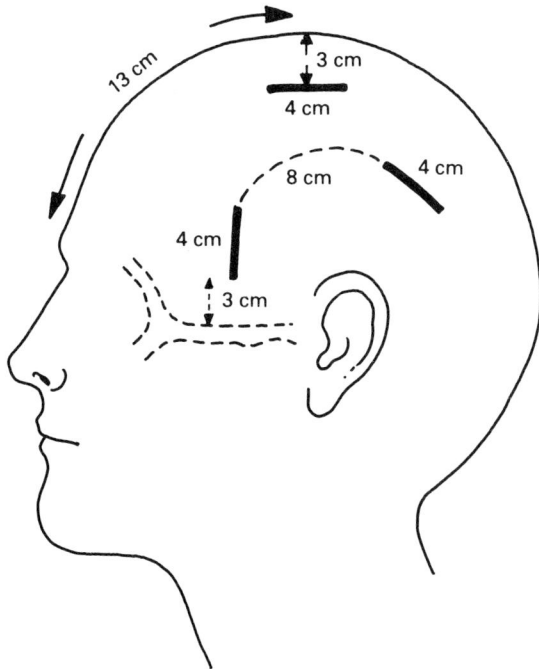

Fig. 40 Sites of burr holes

trolled by coagulation and/or underrunning or transfixing the artery with 3/0 silk. Secure haemostasis. Oxycel may be used for this purpose. To prevent recurrence of bleeding, stitch dura over the bone edge to pericranium using interrupted silk suture.

4. If no extradural haematoma is found, open the dura with a sharp hook and blade No. 15 to locate subdural haematoma. If no haematoma is seen but the brain bulges then make further burr holes until haematoma is located; it is then drained and the brain decompressed.

5. Leave burr hole open, with a Redivac drain for the next 24 h, and close in layers.

6. Flat position is adopted postoperatively to encourage the brain to expand.

3.8. Tracheostomy

Objectives and rationale

- To relieve upper respiratory tract obstruction.
- To decrease respiratory work by bypassing oropharynx and reducing dead space.

- To afford direct access to tracheobronchial tree for aspiration of secretions and bronchial lavage.
- To allow intermittent positive pressure ventilation in case prolonged ventilation is required.
- To stabilise the thoracic cage in chest injuries where it decreases paradoxical respiration and reduces the traumatic chest wall deformity.

Indications

Obstructed upper respiratory tract

- Acute infections, e.g. acute laryngotracheobronchitis in children, acute epiglottitis, laryngeal diphtheria.
- Oedema of glottis (whether traumatic, infective or allergic), e.g. Ludwig's angina.
- Facial burns.
- Head and neck injuries, e.g. faciomaxillary fractures and cut throat.
- Tumours, e.g. carcinoma of larynx and thyroid.
- Bilateral abductor paralysis of vocal cords following recurrent laryngeal nerve injury in thyroidectomy.
- Foreign body.
- Stenoses and atresias, e.g. congenital web or atresia and chronic stenosis following tuberculosis or scalding.

Impaired respiratory function

In obstructive and restrictive airway diseases, aims to reduce the anatomical dead space and improve the physiological dead space due to retained secretions.
- Fulminating bronchopneumonia.
- Chronic bronchitis with severe emphysema.
- Chest injuries, e.g. flail chest.
- Lower respiratory tract obstructed by secretions, e.g. post-thoracotomy or upper abdominal operations or prolonged coma.

Respiratory paralysis

- Unconscious patients with head, maxillofacial or spinal cord injuries.
- Prolonged coma, e.g. drug overdose, poisoning (such as barbiturate).
- Bulbar type of poliomyelitis, polyneuritis and myasthenia gravis.
- Tetanus.
- Vocal cord paralysis.

Operative necessity

- Laryngectomy and laryngopharyngectomy (always).
- Following total thyroidectomy, and/or bilateral block dissection of the neck (sometimes).

Options

Crash or emergency tracheostomy (vertical incision from cricoid cartilage down to suprasternal notch with or without local anaesthesia and oxygen administered via face mask) is not recommended since endotracheal intubation or emergency laryngotomy are better and quicker alternatives (Widebore needle or tube inserted and directed backwards through cricothyroid membrane via a puncture or small horizontal stab respectively until air begins to hiss in and out; an oxygen source is then attached to the needle or tube). Prophylactic elective tracheostomy, planned at leisure under ideal circumstances in an operating theatre, is best.

Elective tracheostomy (Fig. 41)

1. Search for the correct size of tracheostomy tube before starting (e.g. 28 Fr in adults).
2. Under general anaesthesia with endotracheal intubation.

3. Horizontal skin crease incision midway between the cricoid and suprasternal notch.
4. Confine the deep dissection to the midline, separating pretracheal muscles and dividing the thyroid isthmus between clamps, oversewing the cut ends. Arrest any bleeding vessels (transverse branches of anterior jugular veins).
5. In a bloodless field with good exposure, retraction of wound edges and cricoid hook in place perform the tracheal cut in the 2nd, 3rd and 4th tracheal rings. An inverted U-shaped tracheal incision hinging the flap downwards and forwards and stitching it temporarily to the lower edge of the skin incision is the commonest form of tracheostomy. It facilitates postoperative tube changing, reinsertion in case of accidental tube displacement and prevents stenosis. Other variations are a vertical tracheal cut or resection of a circular disc.
6. Suck out the blood entering the trachea and insert the tracheostomy tube (after asking the anaesthetist to pull the endotracheal tube up to the level of the cricoid cartilage under your supervision).
7. Tie the tracheostomy tube with tapes around the neck. Close the skin. An inflatable rubber or polyethylene cuff-tube is preferred to a metallic outer and inner tube combination for sealing the air passage and preventing aspiration pneumonia after vomiting.

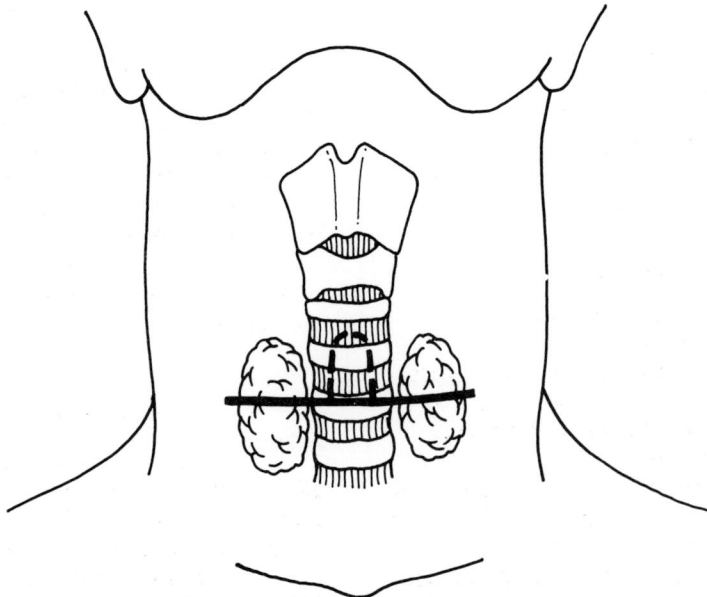

Fig. 41 Tracheostomy

In children beware:

- Laryngotomy is impracticable since the crico-thyroid space or membrane is too small.
- In performing tracheostomy remember the five possible pretracheal structures that must be dealt with properly:
  1. Innominate vein.
  2. Anterior jugular vein.
  3. Thymus.
  4. Inferior thyroid plexus of veins.
  5. Thyroidea ima inconstant artery.

Postoperative (nursing) care

1. Maintain patent airways
- Frequent atraumatic suction.
- Humidification.
- Mucolytic agent.
- Encourage coughing and physiotherapy.
- Occasional bronchial lavage.
2. Prevent infection and other complications
- Aseptic suction, handling and tube changing.
- Antibiotics: remember that *Pseudomonas aeroginosa* (the main microorganism of intensive therapy units) is often found here.

- Avoid tube impinging on posterior tracheal wall (pressure necrosis).
- Deflate cuffed tubes for 5 min every hour (to prevent pressure necrosis).
- Repeated daily clinical and radiological assessments.
3. Final removal of tracheostomy tube (weaning) depends on the status of blood gases before and after removal.

Complications of tracheostomy

- Operative haemorrhage (venous or arterial).
- Encrustation due to tracheal trauma and dry or inadequate humidified inhaled air.
- Tracheal ulceration and tracheo-oesophageal fistulation.
- Tracheal pressure necrosis and stenosis.
- Surgical emphysema.
- Mediastinal emphysema and pneumothorax (due to intermittent positive pressure venti-lation).
- Infection of wound, lung or passages especially by *Pseudomonas aeruginosa*.
- Accidental tube displacement and blockage.

ELECTIVE OPERATIONS

3.9. Vagotomy, Oesophageal and Gastric Operations

Truncal vagotomy

Nasogastric tube in the stomach helps to drain it and to define the oesophagus.

1. A midline incision. Explore and assess whether there are extensive subphrenic adhesions (if found, may make the operation difficult or unwise).
2. Mobilise the left lobe of the liver by dividing its coronary ligament and pack it off to the right; introduce retractors on the right and left. Stretch the stomach downwards.
3. Divide the peritoneum over the oesophagus transversely and retract the oesophagophrenic ligament upward.

4. Mobilise the oesophagus and encircle it with a finger then a rubber tube. By exerting traction on the tube, dissection of the surface is facilitated. Locate the anterior nerve and strip it up and down, freeing 5 cm. Resect 2.5 cm (vagectomy). Similarly deal with the posterior vagus nerve which lies away from the oesophagus and to the right (LARP = left vagus anterior and right vagus posterior). Dissect off and divide every suspicious nerve structure on the oesophagus.

Pyloroplasty (Fig. 42)

The pyloric muscle only may be divided longitudin-ally or the full thickness of the wall may be transected longitudinally and the opening closed transversely (to avoid stenosis) in two layers, or in one layer and covered with omentum (Heineke–Mikulicz). Judd as well as Holt and Lythgoe advocated prior excision of any anterior ulcer

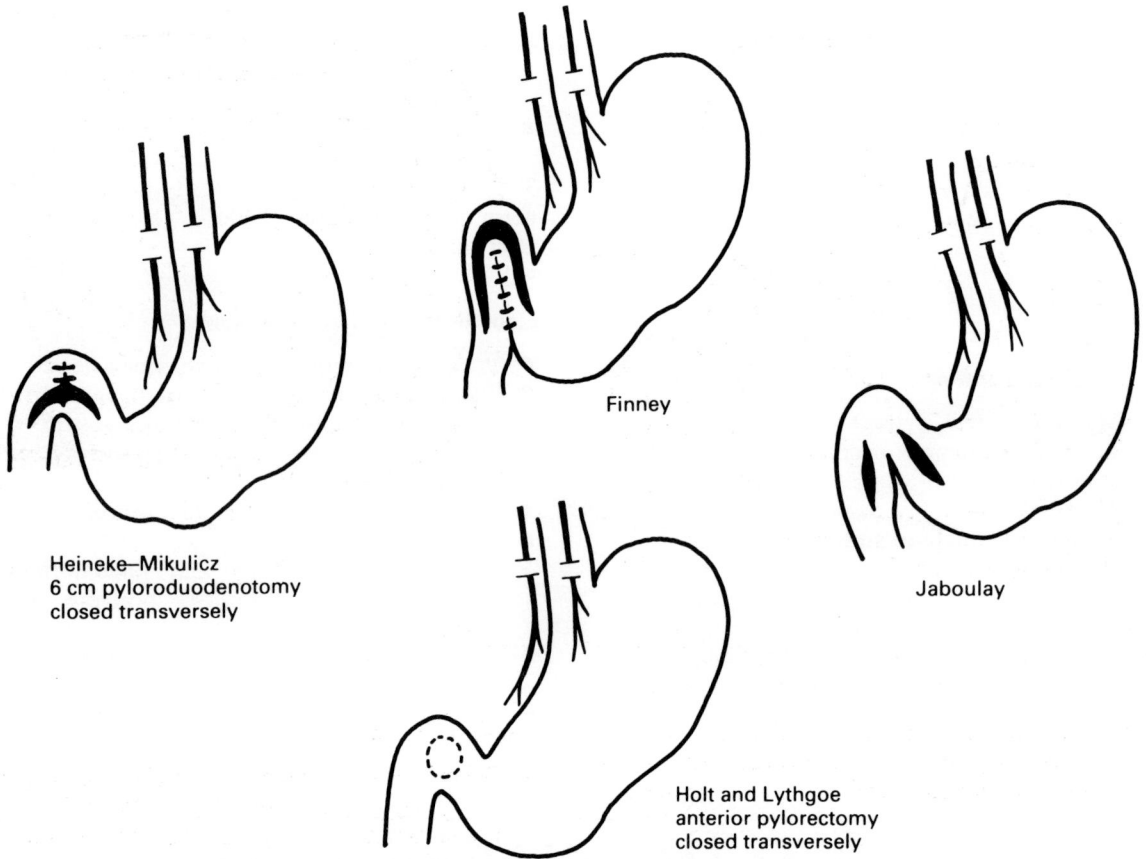

Fig. 42 Types of pyloroplasty accompanying truncal vagotomy

present, excision of a portion of the sphincter and pyloric antrum longitudinally, and suturing of the gap transversely. Pyloroduodenostomy (Japoulay) or continuous U-shaped pyloroplasty (Finney) are other alternatives.

Gastrojejunostomy (Fig. 43)

1. Draw the great omentum upwards to display the transverse mesocolon and decide whether posterior retrocolic or anterior high antecolic anastomosis is required. Retrocolic is preferred unless the distal gastric outlet is obstructed by malignant tumour.
2. Identify the middle colic artery and open the mesocolon on the left of the main artery.
3. Seize the greater and lesser curvatures of the stomach with Babcock tissue forceps and draw the most dependent part (posteroinferior) of the stomach through the hole.

4. Rotate the forceps anticlockwise—the greater curvature then moves to the right.
5. Bring up a short loop of jejunum, apply intestinal clamps and establish a 7 cm long isoperistaltic anastomosis in two layers (haemostatic and seromuscular—both by continuous 2/0 chromic catgut).
6. Approximate the edges of the hole in the mesocolon to the stomach.
7. Check that the afferent loop is not under tension. Make certain there are no peritoneal holes left, then close.

Operations for oesophageal carcinoma

The oesophagus is subdivided into:
Upper third: from cricopharyngeus to aortic arch; includes the cervical segment and supra-aortic segment.
Middle third: from aortic arch to inferior pulmonary vein.

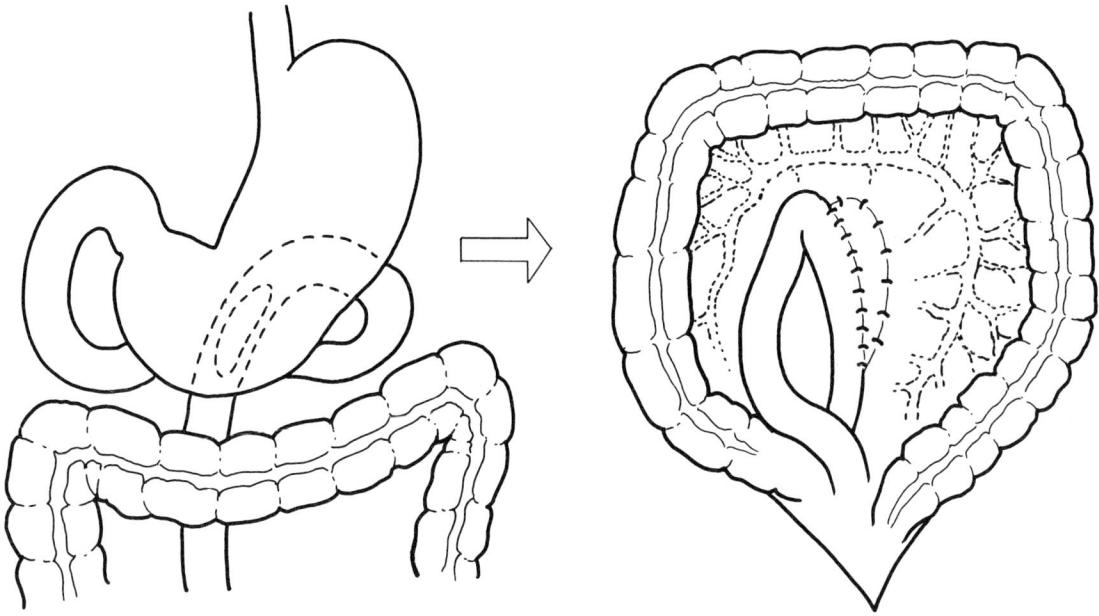

Fig. 43 Posterior retrocolic gastrojejunostomy

Lower third: from inferior pulmonary vein to gastro-oesophageal junction; includes the supra-diaphragmatic segment and abdominal segment.

Operative principles

Upper third carcinoma

Is treated by either:
- Radiotherapy; or
- Three-stage total oesophagectomy (McKeown).

Middle third carcinoma

- In the lower half: needs Lewis–Tanner (two-stage procedure).
- In the upper half: is removed by the two-stage procedure followed by a third stage (McKeown) consisting of clearance and mobilisation of the cervical oesophagus through a right supraclavicular incision (left supraclavicular approach may damage thoracic duct); delivery of the oesophagus into the neck wound; oesophagectomy with closure at the oesophagogastric junction; and restoration of continuity by anastomosing the cervical oesophagus to the gastric fundus. This will avoid anastomotic leak into the mediastinum (fatal). Any leak will be onto the skin cervical incision (external).

Lower third carcinoma

- Below the diaphragm (in the absence of peritoneal or visceral spread): needs radical left abdominothoracic approach (Garlock), excising the tumour-bearing area with the stomach, spleen, pancreatic tail, greater and lesser omenta, and the regional lymphatic field and restoring continuity by oesophagojejunal anastomosis (Roux-en-Y) or oesophagogastrostomy.
- Above the diaphragm: is better excised by Lewis–Tanner operation (the two-stage procedure). Via a laparotomy, the stomach is mobilised on the right gastric and gastroepiploic arteries with Kocherisation of the second part of the duodenum and pyloromyotomy (vagotomy is done with tumour excision). After the abdominal closure, the second stage is performed, consisting of right thoracotomy through which the tumour and the lower oesophagus are mobilised and the stomach is drawn into the chest. The tumour, with adequate clearance of normal oesophagus, and the proximal stomach are resected and continuity is restored by oesophagogastric anastomosis.

The anastomosis is of two layers interrupted with non-absorbable sutures (mucosa is the toughest coat). The gastric fundus is anchored posteriorly by stitching it to the mediastinal pleura and anteriorly it is folded over the anastomosis to reinforce the suture line.

Nasogastric tube suction (although it splints the anastomosis) may have the disadvantages of:
- Introducing infection to the suture line.
- The swallowed saliva and secretions may become stuck to the suture line because of the tube.
- Trauma from the tube in the form of pressure necrosis or accidental suction. The patient is therefore better managed without nasogastric tube suction.

Preoperative preparations are like those for total gastrectomy. Postoperative i.v. fluids (and nothing orally) with small Gastrografin swallow on the 5–7th day when the chest drain may be removed if there is no anastomotic leak.

Billroth I partial gastrectomy (Fig. 44)

1. Mobilise the greater curvature and divide the left gastric vessels.
2. Dissect out the first and second parts of the duodenum (Kocherisation).
3. Divide the duodenum and keep it closed with a non-crushing clamp.
4. Divide the stomach, leaving approximately one-fifth. Close the upper part of it, leaving an aperture the size of the duodenum adjacent to the greater curvature, and approximate it to the duodenum with two layers of sutures.
5. Close the dangerous superior duodenogastric angle of Sorrow with a triple stitch, i.e. take a bite first of the anterior wall of the stomach, then the posterior wall, and finally the superior aspect of the duodenum. If possible, this suture may be repeated at a higher level as a reinforcement.
6. Drain the anastomosis and close the abdomen.

Polya partial gastrectomy (Fig. 45)

1. Nasogastric tube and i.v. drip. General anaesthesia and supine position.
2. The incision is usually midline, but may be on the left for gastric ulcer or on the right for duodenal ulcer. Quick peritoneal exploration is then done.
3. Mobilise the greater curvature of the stomach and preserve the middle colic vessels and mesocolon. Excise three-quarters of the stomach and ligate and divide the left gastric vessels.
4. Mobilise all aspects of the first portion of the duodenum, ligating the right gastric artery. When dissecting the duodenum, keep close to it.
5. Apply two occluding and two crushing clamps and carefully clear the stomach at the proposed site for anastomosis. Divide and close the duodenum with two layers of sutures.
6. Bring up a short loop of the first part of the jejunum and anastomose it to the divided stomach, usually afferent to the lesser curve.
7. The results with antecolic or retrocolic anastomoses are similar; antecolic are easier to dismantle and are therefore preferred.
8. The afferent loop of jejunum is kept as short as possible. It may be fixed to the colon with a suture to prevent internal strangulation.

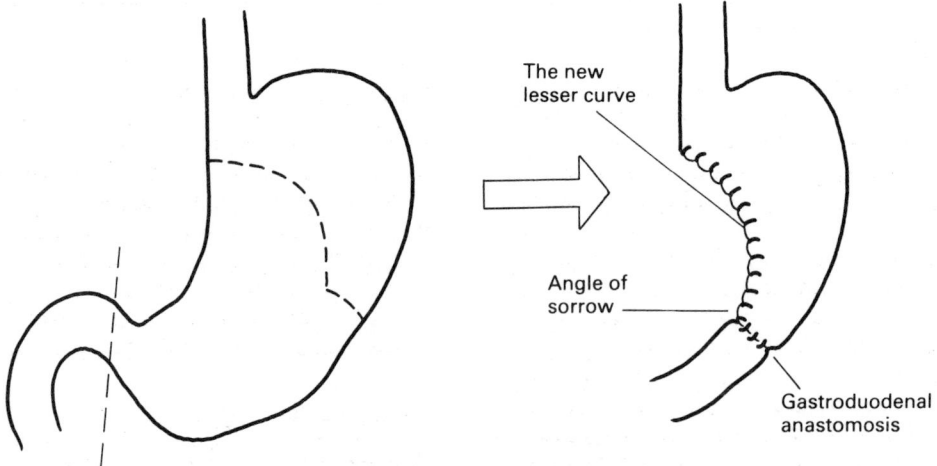

The new lesser curve

Angle of sorrow

Gastroduodenal anastomosis

Fig. 44   Billroth I partial gastrectomy

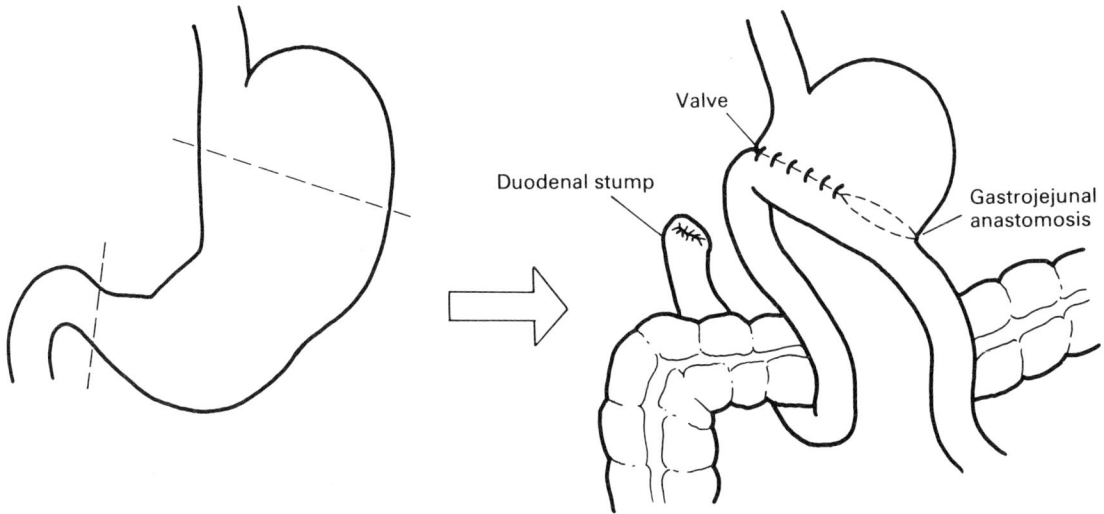

Fig. 45 Polya partial gastrectomy

Notes.
- An adherent gastric ulcer may be pinched off the pancreas with the fingers or, if this is impossible, excluded by excision.
- The upper part of the divided stomach may be closed to form a Hofmeister valve.
- Difficult duodenal ulcer may require Nissen's procedure, i.e. closure of the duodenum by suturing the anterior duodenal wall onto the ulcer.

Total gastrectomy

1 A drip and nasogastric tube are *in situ*. A long left paramedian incision followed by quick peritoneal exploration.

2. Mobilise the greater curvature up to the oesophagus. Divide the left gastric vessels and extend the division of the lesser omentum as far as the oesophagus. This manoeuvre is aided by mobilising the left lobe of the liver by dividing the coronary ligament.

3. Mobilise all aspects of the first part of the duodenum, divide and close it.

4. A loop of jejunum is brought up either in front of, or behind, the colon and anastomosed to the oesophagus in two layers behind the stomach, which is amputated only when the anastomosis is nearly completed. The mucosa is the strong layer in the oesophagus. To avoid 'drag', suture the anastomosis to its surroundings. Great care should be employed in forming this anastomosis as it leaks easily. It is performed in two layers with non-absorbable material. Alternatively, a Roux-en-Y procedure may be used. A side-to-side anastomosis is made in the jejunal loop (Braun). The Ryle's tube may be left in, either with its tip just above the anastomosis, or through it (*see* 'Operations for oesophageal carcinoma').

3.10. Splenectomy

Indications

- Traumatic splenic rupture.
- Shunt operations in portal hypertension except for distal splenorenal shunt.
- Haemolytic anaemia in congenital spherocytosis and thrombocytopenic purpura.
- Staging laparotomy in Hodgkin's lymphoma.
- Part of proximal and total gastrectomy, lower oesophagectomy and distal pancreatectomy.

Procedure (Fig. 46)

Preoperatively a nasogastric tube is passed (to facilitate the operation and prevent postoperative

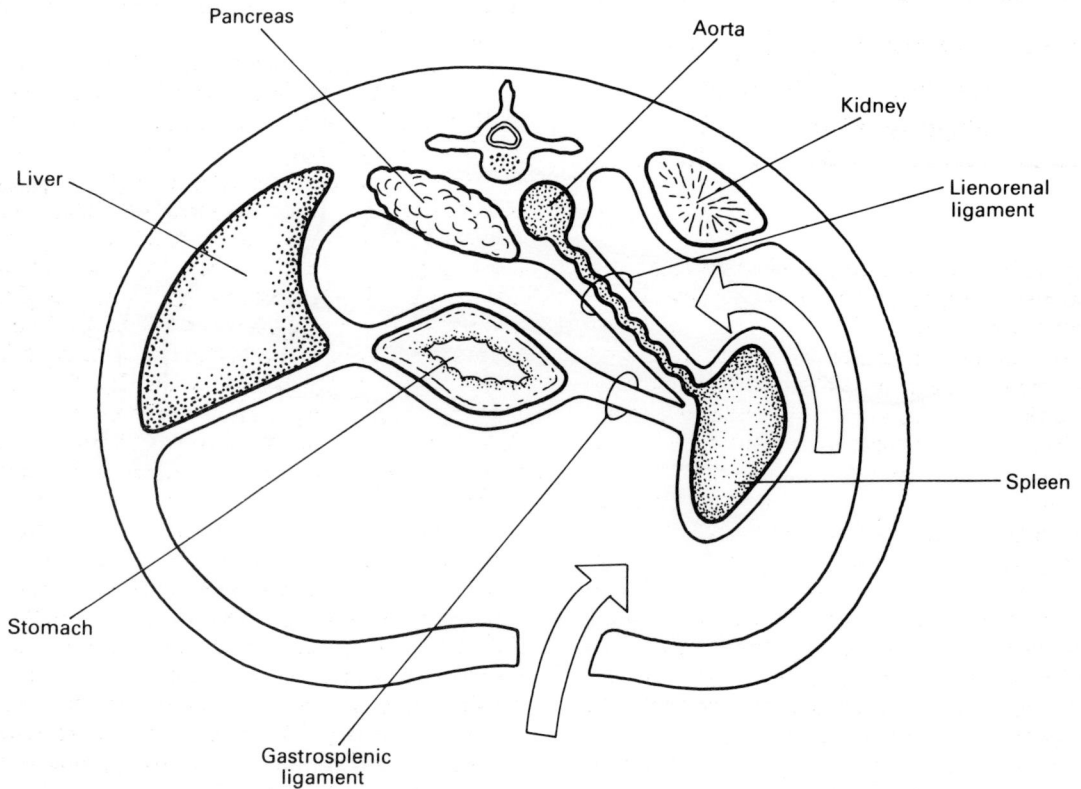

Fig. 46 Splenectomy—surgical approach

gastric distension and paralytic ileus), with intravenous drip and possible blood transfusion (in trauma) or platelet solution (in thrombocytopenia).

1. Under general anaesthesia and supine position.
2. Left upper paramedian or left subcostal incision.
3. Once in the peritoneal cavity, quick exploration.
4. The surgeon (standing to the right of the patient), passes his left hand round the spleen while the assistant retracts the skin for good exposure. The surgeon uses his right hand to cut the posterior layer of the lienorenal ligament by sharp and blunt dissection.
5. Spleen is rotated medially and delivered through the incision while a large pack is inserted.
6. Gastrosplenic ligament containing the vasa brevia and part of the left gastroepiploic blood vessel is ligated and divided without traumatising the stomach's greater curvature.
7. Careful separation of the pancreatic tail from splenic hilum followed by double ligation of splenic blood vessels, individually if possible, with a non-absorbable suture, e.g. silk.
8. Search for spleniculi and then insert sump drain (in case of unrecognised damage to pancreatic tail).
9. Closure in layers.

Complications

Unexplained postoperative abdominal pain with fever may herald portal vein thrombosis (when anticoagulants and antibiotics must be given). Other possible complications include acute gastric distension, paralytic ileus, left basal atelectasis, haematemesis (due to gastric mucosal congestion after vasa brevia ligation), pancreatic leak and possible abdominal wound dehiscence or persistent hiccup due to left subphrenic irritation by blood collection or an abscess.

3.11. Cholecystectomy and Common Bile Duct Exploration

Prophylactic antibiotics (cefuroxime 750 mg. i.m. three times a day) to prevent postoperative infection, 500 ml mannitol 10% infusion pre- and peroperatively to prevent hepatorenal shut-down and failure, low-dose heparin (5000 i.u. subcutaneously daily) with premedication until mobilisation postoperatively with stockings to prevent deep venous thrombosis are all recommended especially in *jaundiced* patients with recent biliary obstruction. Preoperative reduction of weight and cessation of smoking with postoperative physiotherapy are essential to reduce pulmonary atelactasis. (Nasogastric suction, used peroperatively to decompress the stomach for the benefit of the surgeon and anaesthetist, should be avoided postoperatively since there is no anastomosis to rest and the transnasal tube makes coughing difficult, dries inspired air and results in higher incidence of pulmonary atelactasis. Postoperatively acute gastric dilatation is rare and when nausea or vomiting starts postoperatively then only suction is required.)

1. Under general anaesthesia and supine position (with right arm extended) on special radiolucent operating table. Surgeon is better operating on right side of the patient in cholecystectomy and should change his position to the left side when he attempts exploration of the common bile duct.

2. Via right upper paramedian in narrow costal margin, subcostal Kocher's (wide costal margin) or upper midline incision. Quick exploration for associated hiatus hernia and diverticular colonic diverticula (Saint's triad), and of stomach, duodenum (e.g. ulcers), pancreas (e.g. chronic pancreatitis with enlarged head and foci of fat necrosis) and liver (e.g. cirrhosis or cancer). Insert a finger into the foramen of Winslow (epiploic foramen) to palpate the bile duct for stone. Insert the right hand above the liver to allow air to pass behind it and to help drop it for easy operation on the gall bladder. Decide whether it is necessary to preserve the gall bladder for bypass (e.g. in carcinoma of pancreatic head).

3. The assistant's help is required in packing off the lesser curvature of the stomach to the left, and the duodenum and colon downwards (insert retractors). A third retractor on the liver exposes the cystic duct area.

4. To aid dissection apply sponge-holding forceps to the fundus of the gall bladder and Moynihan forceps to Hartmann's pouch to manipulate the cystic duct.

5. Nick and strip off the peritoneum over the ducts. With further dissection using a swab on sponge forceps and/or Lahey's swab (baby dab) identify the cystic artery by tracing it to the gall bladder. It runs inside the Calot triangle formed by the cystic duct, bile duct and lower hepatic edge. Free, clamp and divide it followed by application of ligatures (linen).

6. Dissect further to show clearly the termination of the cystic duct—ligate proximally. Operative cholangiography may now be carried out using 25% Hypaque through a Stoke-on-Trent cannula fixed in place by ligature after being introduced into the cystic duct. The proximal end of the cystic duct may then be divided. Two films are taken after an injection of 5 ml (to delineate small impacted stones) and 10 ml (to reveal the biliary flow into the duodenum) of Hypaque respectively. Look at the diameter of the common bile duct (should not be more than 12 mm), filling defect, dye flow to duodenum and lower narrow intramural biliary segment (Fig. 47). The cystic duct stump is then ligated (00 linen or silk) 3 mm from common bile duct as flush ligation may cause stenosis.

7. Remove the gall bladder by dividing its attachments to the liver and its peritoneal reflection. Gall bladder bed haemostasis is established by coagulation with no need for suturing the bed. A drain is left in the gall bladder area and brought out through a separate opening in the flank.

8. The classical indications for opening the common bile duct if operative cholangiogram is not available are:

● History of jaundice, abnormal liver functions, Charcot's triad (fever, pain and jaundice); oral cholecystogram showing multiple small stones in the gall bladder with patent or dilated cystic duct.

● Operative finding of dilated common bile duct more than 12 mm, palpation of stone (or aspiration of biliary mud), periductal fibrosis and pancreatitis (indurated), thickened gall bladder with no stone or with single-faceted stone.

9. To open the common bile duct free a part of its anterior wall *above the duodenum*, then insert two stay sutures through the wall. If identification of the duct is uncertain, aspirate the contents with a needle. Before opening the common bile duct, pack off the area and have a sucker in readiness. The stay sutures are held taut and a small longitudinal cut is made in the common bile duct *as close to the*

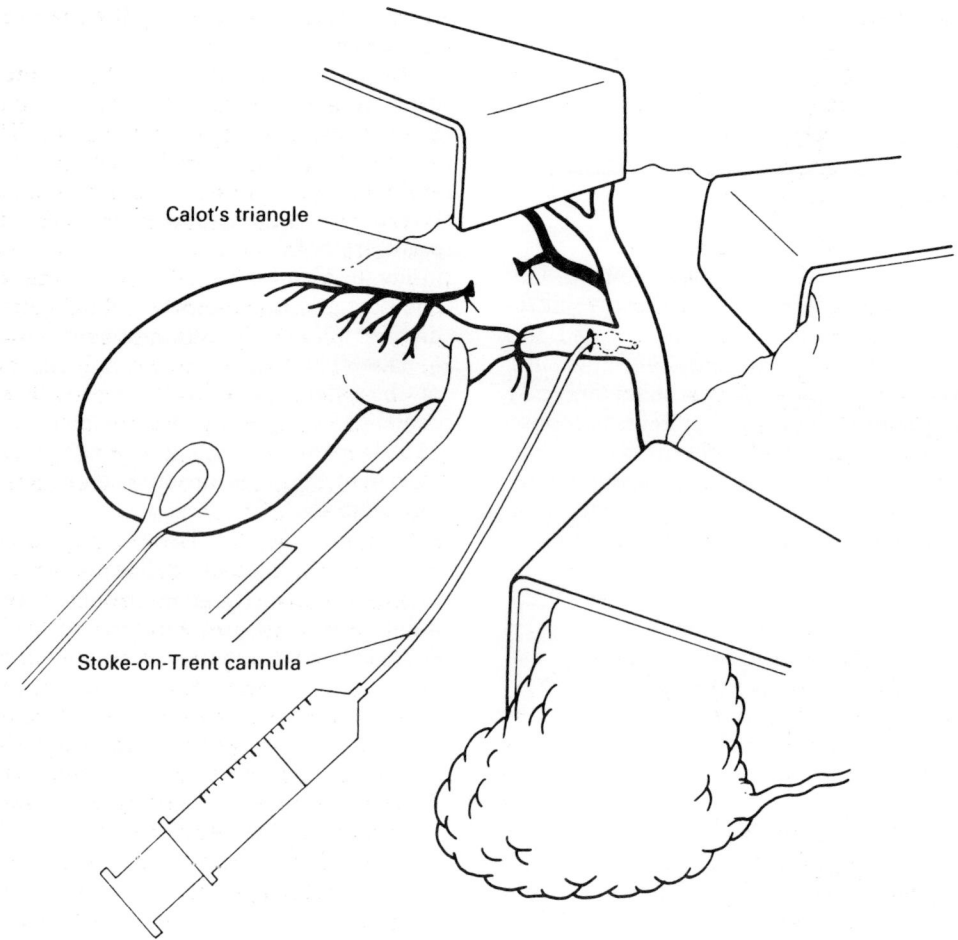

Fig. 47 Cholecystectomy and peroperative cholangiogram

duodenum as possible to leave a good upper portion as a safeguard in case further surgery is required.

10. The duct is explored. A variety of instruments are available, for example, Bakes' dilators, Lister's bougies, gum elastic bougies, Desjardin's forceps, Jack's catheter and Fogarty's biliary catheter. The duct is thin-walled and stones usually stick at the lower end causing ball-valve obstruction and poor visualisation of the terminal distal narrow part of the common bile duct on cholangiography. Exploration should be atraumatic; the use of a Fogarty catheter is usually successful and clearly demonstrates the site and patency of the sphincter of Oddi. Rigid metallic instruments such as bougies and Desjardin's forceps can cause damage to the duct wall and false passages and should be used carefully. After removal of any stones and debris, the duct is washed out with saline (Fig. 48a).

11. An attempt is now made to dilate the sphincter of Oddi by the passage of bougies. These instruments must be passed through the sphincter.

12. If unsuccessful because of stricture or impacted stone at the lower end of the common bile duct then the second part of the duodenum is mobilised (Kocherisation), opened vertically, and the sphincter of Oddi is divided under vision. Find the site of the sphincteric opening by palpating the tip of the Fogarty catheter or probe passed down the common bile duct from above. Divide the sphincter at 12 o'clock (sphincterotomy), or sphincteroplasty may be carried out.

13. Close the duodenum with two layers transversely.

14. In the elderly, unfit patient with difficult anatomy, e.g. gross obesity, and if there is concern about residual stone or biliary mud, choledo-

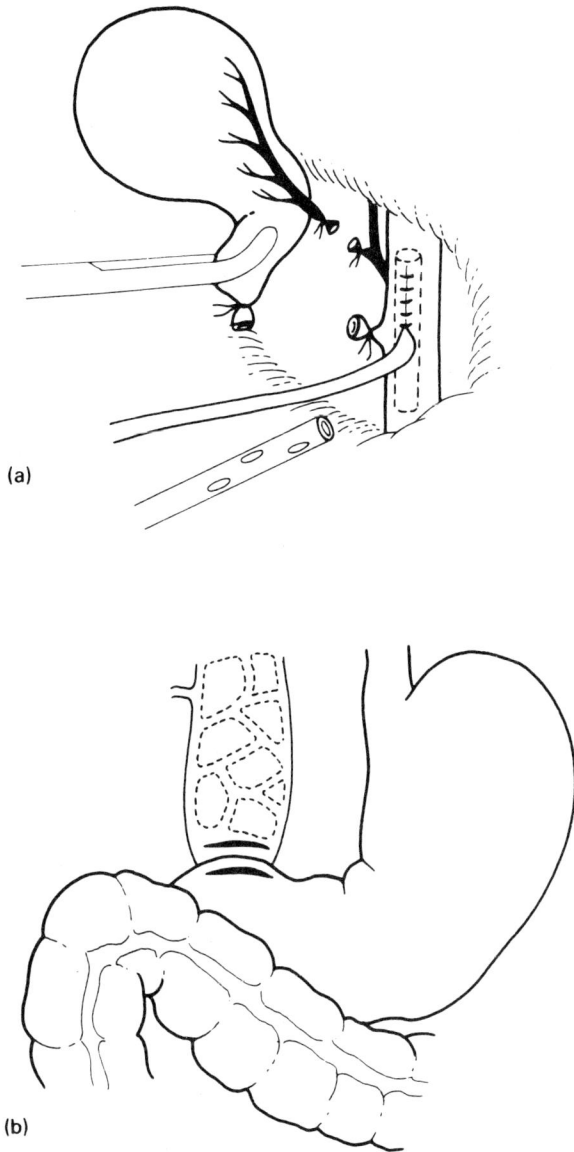

(a)

(b)

Fig. 48 Common bile duct exploration (temporary and permanent drainage). (a) Supraduodenal common bile duct exploration with T-tube insertion. (b) Choledochoduodenostomy

choduodenostomy is recommended (Fig. 48b)—a transverse low incision in the common bile duct is sutured to a longitudinal parallel duodenal incision after Kocherisation to construct a stoma as wide as the duct calibre permits. There is little evidence to support the claim that there is a higher incidence of ascending cholangitis with such a bypass operation.

Sphincteroplasty is necessary if there is a concomitant stricture.

15. Insert a T-tube into the supraduodenal common duct opening. Close the opening around the tube with 2/0 catgut (interrupted). The duct is not closed until it is established that there is no residual pathology as this leads to immediate and late complications. Any rise in pressure in the duct is associated with increased leakage around the T-tube into the peritoneal cavity, and continued obstruction makes ascending cholangitis and septicaemia more likely. Although such pathology can be dealt with postoperatively by retrieval under radiographic control via T-tube track and retrograde cannulation of the sphincter and papillotomy, this does not avoid prolonged hospitalisation, patient suffering and further anaesthetics. The available alternatives are:

- T-tube postexploratory cholangiography (with or without contact cholangiography). Has the disadvantage of leakage around T-tube during injection of dye preventing adequate filling of the distal end where spasm may have occurred as a result of manipulation of the sphincter area. Serial films can reduce this problem. Contact cholangiography by inserting a dental film below the second part of the duodenum after Kocherisation can improve visualisation of the distal part of the duct, revealing small impacted stones. However, it is not widely used.
- Foley cholangiography requires practise to ensure adequate obstruction of the lumen of the duct to prevent backflow.
- Choledochoscopy is expensive as regards purchase of the instrument, requires practise, is impossible in narrow ducts and does not permit examination of the smaller proximal ducts.

16. Add a tube drain to drain the gall bladder bed. Place Surgicel into the gall bladder bed if oozing.

17. Bring out drainage tubes carefully through separate openings.

Postoperative points

- If the T-tube is pulled out by accident, open the abdomen and replace it immediately.
- Clamp T-tube from the fifth day.
- Remove the tube drain on the fifth day.
- T-tube choledochogram is taken on the 10th day.
- Remove the T-tube if X-ray is satisfactory.

Postoperative excessive biliary leak

From the abdominal drain or as a persistent fistula is due to:

- Accidental damage of a duct during the operation.
- Residual impacted stone in the lower part of the common bile duct causing obstruction, increased intrabiliary pressure and bursting of cystic duct ligature.
- Distal stricture especially in chronic pancreatitis.
- Slipped cystic duct ligature (technical).
- Leak from gall bladder bed due to congenital cholecystohepatic duct. Accumulation of bile subhepatically or subphrenically may lead to upper abdominal or chest pain, tachycardia, hypotension and is often mistaken for coronary thrombosis. The condition needs immediate re-exploration and bile drainage, which produces dramatic relief. The condition is termed the *Waltman–Walters syndrome*.

3.12. Restorative Rectal Resection and Abdominoperineal Excision of Rectum

Restorative rectal resection

Requirements

- The growth should be early cancer, i.e. stage A or B, maximum C1.
- On biopsy the histological differentiation should be good or moderate (but never undifferentiated = anaplastic).
- The growth should be at least 10 cm above the anal verge since 5 cm is needed for macroscopic tumour clearance to prevent future recurrence and another 5 cm is needed for intact sensation and to prevent incontinence. Owing to the tortuous course of the rectum the growth felt by a finger in rectal examination at a level of 7.5 cm from the anal verge could be telescoped; after operative mobilisation it may be found to be 10 cm from the anal verge.
- Colon should be normal, i.e. free from ulcerative colitis, Crohn's disease, diverticular disease and polyposis coli. Pelvic mesocolon is preferably long for anastomosis.
- The patient should not be too fat.

- The patient's pelvis should be normal or wide, i.e. shallow wide female pelvis is preferred to the male pelvis which is deep and narrow.
- When hepatic secondaries are present this operation is preferred if other requirements are fulfilled.

Thorough preoperative bowel preparation is essential (*see Section 1.21*).

Procedure

1. A nasogastric tube, an i.v. drip and urethral catheter are placed *in situ*. General anaesthesia and Trendelenburg's position, with the surgeon standing on the left side of the patient.

2. A long left paramedian incision is made. The abdomen is opened and explored for another primary colonic cancer and hepatic secondaries. After examining the blood supply of the mesocolon and the growth, the sites for division of the colon and rectum are decided upon.

3. The pelvic colon is held and the rest of the bowel packed away; a self-retaining retractor is placed in the wound. In females the uterus with adnexae can be sutured and retracted anteriorly (Fig. 49).

4. The pelvic colon is partly freed by dividing the congenital adhesions on its lateral aspect and the peritoneum of the pelvic floor is then demarcated by dividing it with scissors; the incision runs from the colon at the proposed site of division laterally over the mesocolon, anteriorly across the base of the bladder or region of the cervix 12 mm in front of the lowest point of the peritoneal floor, then upwards on the medial side of the mesocolon, returning to the original level. The peritoneum of the pelvis is then raised by sharp and blunt dissection safeguarding the ureters and genital vessels.

5. Commencing at the proposed site for division of the colon (Fig. 50a), the mesocolon is divided down to its root. The main pedicle containing the superior haemorrhoidal vessels is dissected free and (after ensuring that both ureters are safe) ligated and divided.

6. Good mobilisation then follows and the rectosigmoid mesentery is freed from the sacrum by a few cuts with the scissors; by digital dissection posteriorly, the fascia of Waldeyer may be reached posterior to the rectum. The dissection anterior to the rectum is then commenced and the seminal vesicles or vaginal wall identified. By division of bands behind the seminal vesicles or vaginal wall, the fascia of Denonvilliers is opened and a plane of dissection found leading down to the apex of the prostate or the perineal body. The lateral ligaments

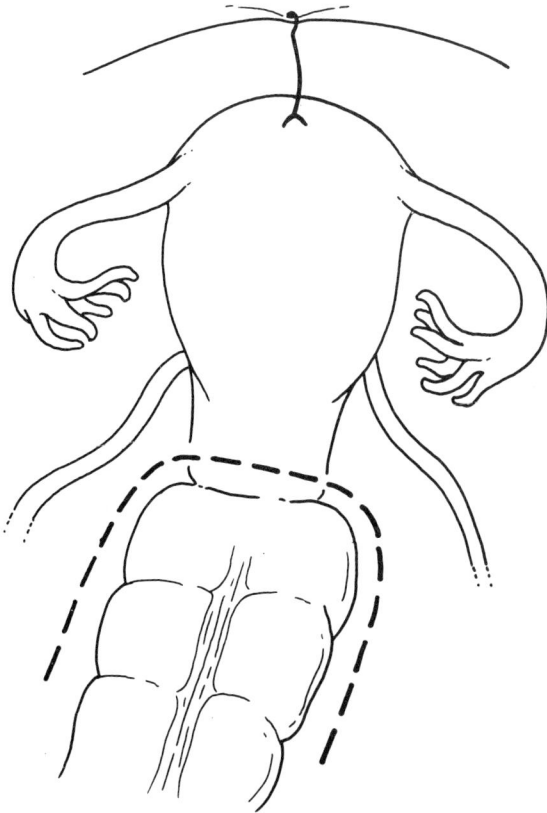

Fig. 49 Division of pelvic peritoneum prior to rectal mobilisation in the female

containing the middle haemorrhoidal vessels are ligated and divided. Mesorectum is also divided.

7. Proposed sites for division are cleared of fat. A right-angled clamp is placed over the rectum, and the rectum may be washed out, e.g. with Noxyflex solution (Fig. 50b), after a gentle anal stretch. Crushing clamps are now placed above and below, and the diseased bowel and its mesentery removed. For clearing faecal contents of the upper bowel end perform an intraoperative washout. Foley's catheter is inserted into the caecum through a purse-string in the terminal ileum (Fig. 50c) and fluid is let out through a corrugated tube fitted to the proximal end. This end is then recut and prepared for anastomosis.

8. The end of the colon is anastomosed to the upper end of the rectum using single interrupted seroso-submucosal (2/0 silk), or double-layer seromuscular interrupted (2/0 silk) and continuous mucosal (chromic catgut) sutures. Horizontal mattress sutures of non-absorbable material are recommended.

9. The floor of the peritoneum is closed (con-troversial) with paracolic tube drainage, then the wound is closed.

Abdominoperineal excision of rectum

Abdominal dissection

The dissection proceeds as described in 'Restorative rectal resection'. However here the patient is in the lithotomy-Trendelenburg position, using a Lloyd–Davies' apparatus. A sandbag or 'rest' under the sacrum facilitates the approach to the coccyx.

Perineal dissection

1. The anus is closed with two purse-string sutures. An elliptical incision is made around the anus and is deepened through the perineal space and fascia into the ischiorectal fossa.

2. This incision is extended on both sides so that a finger may be introduced around the ileococcygeus to facilitate its division, and the inferior rectal vessels are ligated.

3. A self-retaining retractor may be inserted.

4. Mobilisation: the fascia of Waldeyer posterior to the rectum is divided, and the tissues are divided anterior to the rectum, keeping behind the transverse perineal muscles. Anteriorly the pubococcygeus muscle is divided. The prostate and urethra with catheter are identified and by further careful division, the plane of Denonvilliers is entered, lying behind the prostate. The bowel turns sharply backwards at the anorectal junction and the dissection must follow this line to avoid urethral damage. The abdominal surgeon assists in defining the tissue planes (until both surgeons shake hands inside the pelvis). The lateral ligaments are ligated and divided. With anterior growths (in females), the whole posterior portion of the vagina is excised.

5. The perineal wound is closed with drainage (either Redivac or wide tube inserted via ischiorectal fat). The vaginal orifice is re-formed.

3.13. Thyroidectomy

Indications for operation

● Solitary thyroid nodule.

● Pressure symptoms, e.g. on trachea (dyspnoea),

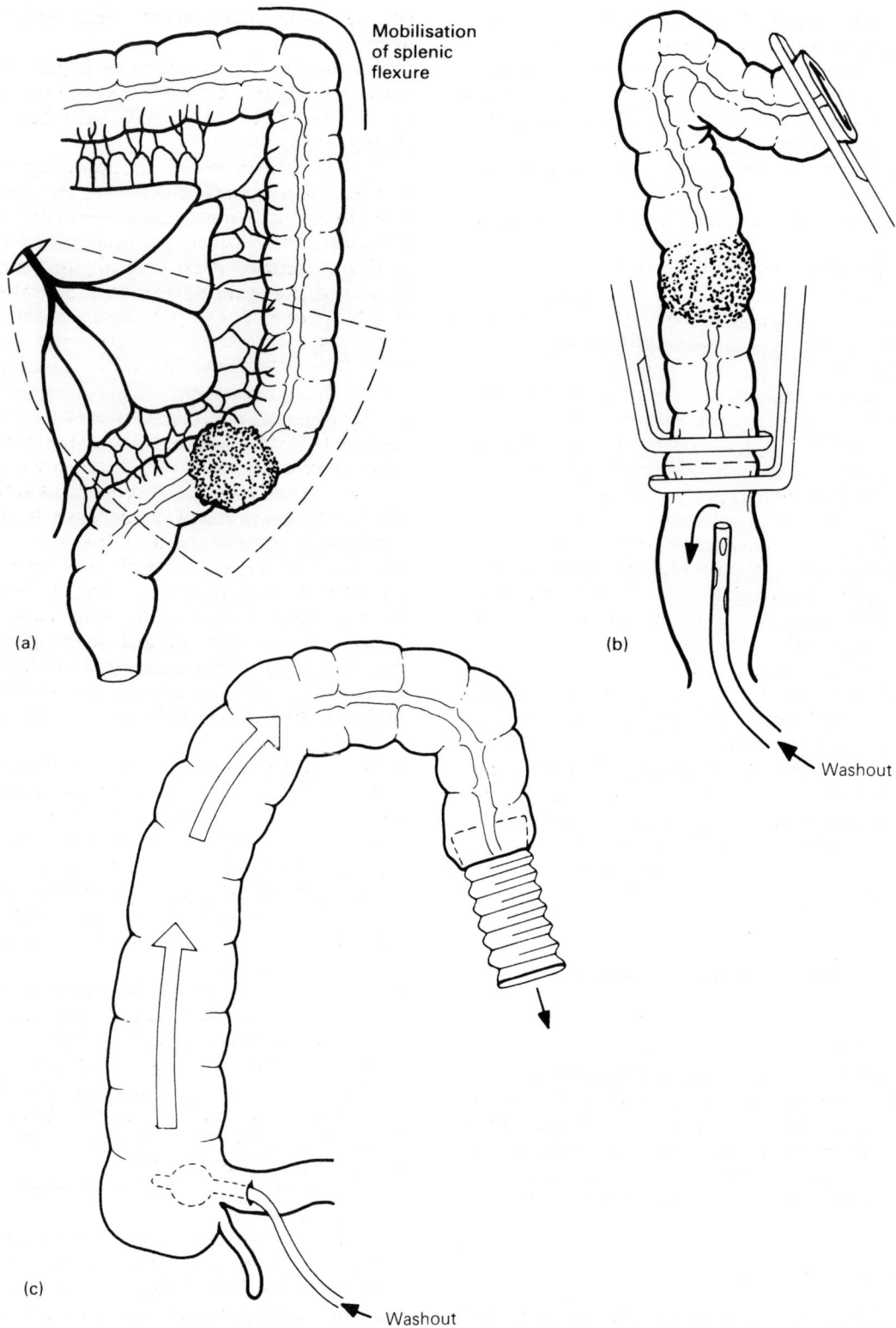

Mobilisation of splenic flexure

(a)

(b)

Washout

(c)

Washout

Fig. 50 Restorative rectal (anterior) resection

on oesophagus (dysphagia) and on recurrent laryngeal nerve (hoarseness).

- Ectopic thyroid, e.g. lingual or retrosternal goitre due to dysphagia and dyspnoea respectively with possible future mitotic (malignancy) changes and bleeding.
- Secondary thyrotoxicosis in multinodular goitre.
- Primary thyrotoxicosis (this is medically treated) only if:
  —Ineffective medical treatment.
  —Recurrence after medical treatment.
  —Allergy or side-effects of drugs.
  —Economic consideration (drug price).
- Cosmetic.
- Malignant thyroid disease (treated by total thyroidectomy); suspected when there is:
  —A rapidly enlarging solitary thyroid nodule or recent change in a long-standing goitre.
  —Hard swelling in part or whole.
  —No mobility of gland with swallowing.
  —Berry's sign: absent carotid pulsation because of surrounding infiltrating tumour. Classically goitre displaces the carotid artery backward and outward, so the pulsation is felt behind the posterior edge of the goite.
  —Tracheal obstruction.
  —Local spread suggested by hoarseness and Horner's syndrome (meiosis, enophthalmus, ptosis and anhidrosis).
  —Lymph node enlargement usually unilaterally. Biopsy is essential. The so-called ectopic thyroid is in fact thyroid metastatic disease in the lymph node which may be the only manifestation of an occult primary impalpable thyroid carcinoma.

Partial (subtotal) thyroidectomy

Preoperative

Cervical X-ray to show any calcification or tortuous trachea (important for anaesthetist). Indirect laryngoscopy to detect any recurrent laryngeal nerve paralysis and treatment of thyrotoxicosis (e.g. propranolol (Inderal) 40 mg tablet three times daily until sleeping pulse rate is below 100 per min.

Procedure (Fig. 51a–c)

1. Endotracheal general anaesthesia with neck hyperextension. A sandbag between the shoulders and horse-shoe ring below head and special draping.
2. A collar incision is made one finger's breadth above the suprasternal notch. Deepen the incision through the platysma on both sides beyond the sternomastoid borders.
3. By sharp dissection raise the upper flap until the thyroid notch is reached and raise the lower flap down to the suprasternal notch. Joll's self-retaining retractor is then applied.
4. Divide the deep fascia vertically in the midline until the thyroid isthmus is exposed. Raise the strap muscles on one side to expose the lateral lobe, insert retractors and continue the dissection until the entire lobe is clearly visible. Divide and ligate the middle thyroid vein.
5. Full mobilisation using sharp scissors and blunt dissection (Lahey's swab); dislocate the lateral lobe into the wound. If necessary, to improve exposure, divide the strap muscles between forceps at the level of the cricoid cartilage, to preserve their nerve supply (from ansa cervicalis below).
6. Dissect in the middle, laterally and posteriorly to the lobe of the thyroid and identify the inferior thyroid artery, recurrent laryngeal nerve (in the groove between the trachea and oesophagus close to the terminal branches of the inferior thyroid artery) and parathyroids. Ligate the artery in continuity *well away from the gland* to avoid recurrent laryngeal nerve injury.
7. Mobilise the upper pole, insert Kocher's director behind it and doubly ligate the superior thyroid vessels. Apply artery forceps and divide *close to the gland* to avoid injuring the external branch of the superior laryngeal nerve (supplies cricothyroid muscle and its damage causes hoarseness of voice).
8. Expose the front of the trachea by dividing the inferior thyroid *plexus of veins* and free the pyramidal lobe, if present.
9. Change to the opposite side of the patient; free the other lobe and deal similarly with its vessels.
10. Apply a series of forceps (markers) around the gland and divide it. Continue dividing the gland by applying forceps to the gland substance until the trachea is reached and the gland is shaved from it. Most of the lateral lobes, the whole of the isthmus and pyramidal lobe are removed. Two small posterior portions (4 g) of gland are left on either side of the trachea.
11. Suture the remaining part of the gland, if it is bleeding, to the side of the trachea (reconstruction). Insert two Redivac drains so that they emerge through the deep fascia at the lateral aspects of the wound or through individual stab wounds. Close

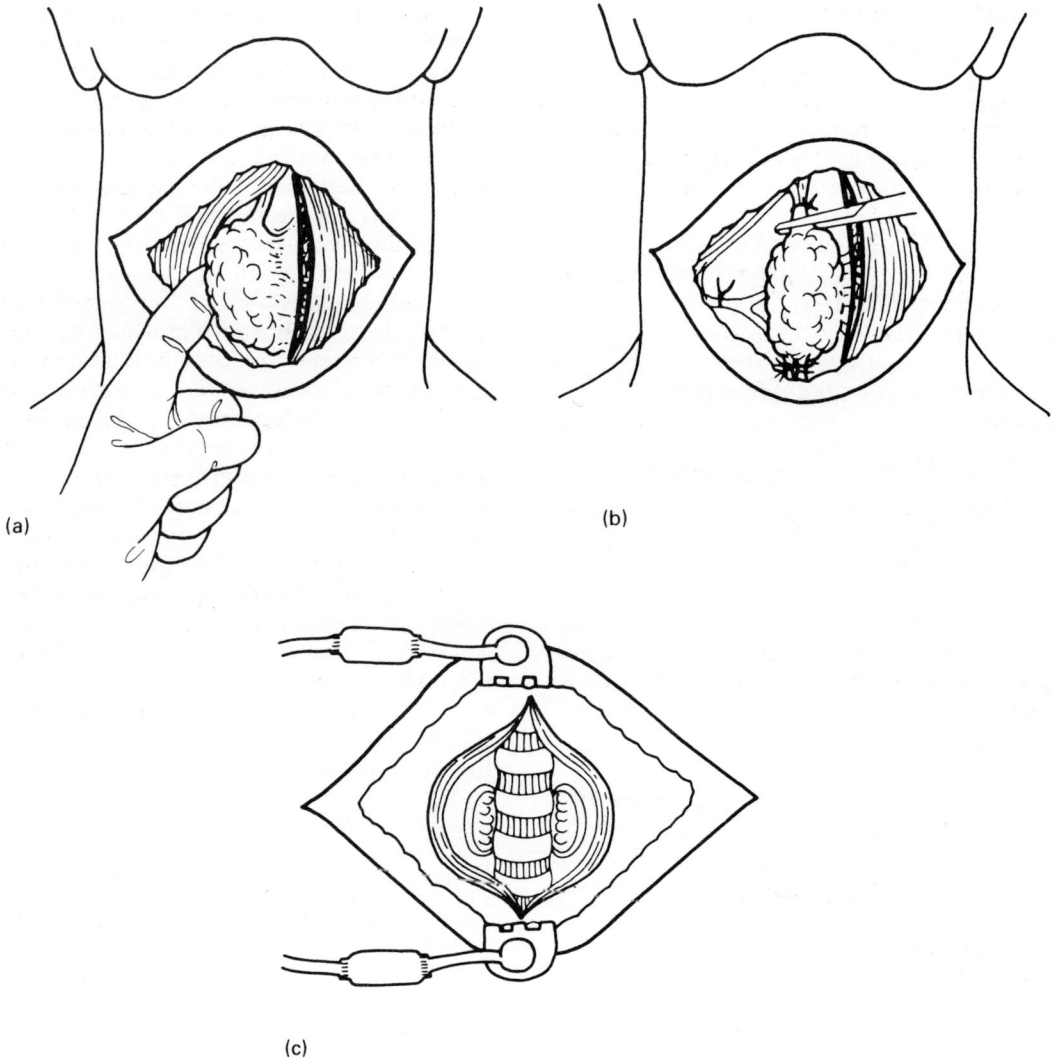

Fig. 51 Partial thyroidectomy. (a) Exposure and mobilisation. (b) Vascular ligation and division. Joll's retraction in (a) and (b) is not shown. (c) Reconstruction after excision

the deep fascia (interrupted 2/0 chromic catgut). Remove the sandbag from beneath the shoulders and approximate the platysma with fine plain catgut (interrupted). Suture drainage tubes to the skin, then close the wound with clips.

Postoperative complications

Early

- Tension haematoma—needs immediate evacuation or aspiration.

- Respiratory obstruction due to tension haematoma, laryngeal spasm, unilateral or bilateral recurrent nerve paralysis, or rarely to collapse or kinking of the trachea—needs endotracheal intubation, steroids for several days and, rarely, tracheostomy.

- Recurrent laryngeal nerve paralysis (unilateral or bilateral, complete or partial, transient or permanent). Superior laryngeal nerve paralysis lead to hoarseness of voice only.

- Thyrotoxic crisis occurs rarely in thyrotoxic patients with inadequate preparation—treated by hydration, antipyretics, steroids and propranolol 20 mg 6 hourly.

Intermediate
Include parathyroid insufficiency after 2–5 days, occasionally delayed for 3 weeks. Treated by calcium therapy.

Late
Include wound infection, keloid scar and thyroid insufficiency (occurs within 2 years) or recurrent thyrotoxicosis.

3.14. Superficial (Suprafacial) Parotidectomy

Procedure (Fig. 52)

Warn the patient of possible damage to the facial nerve, or even of its deliberate removal if found necessary.

1. General anaesthesia with hypotension, if necessary. The table head is tilted upwards to collapse the external jugular veins and the patient's head is extended and turned away from the surgeon.
2. Make a cervicomastoid-facial S-shaped incision which runs vertically down just in front of the pinna and curves backwards below it; the pinna may be sutured and retracted.
3. The skin flaps are widely mobilised and held back by stay sutures to reveal all aspects of the gland. The great auricular nerve may be preserved or sacrificed (a piece of the nerve may be saved in saline to be used as a nerve graft in case of inadvertent facial nerve injury during operation).
4. Identify and safeguard the facial nerve and its two major subdivisions, the upper temporofacial and lower cervicofacial nerves (joined in a goose-foot fashion—*pes anserinus*), by identifying the junction of the cartilaginous and bony meatus behind the gland and following the nerve up above the posterior belly of the digastric and as it emerges from below the mastoid process. Pinching the nerve elicits facial twitching, and a nerve stimulator is sometimes useful.
5. Fine mosquito forceps are thrust with blades

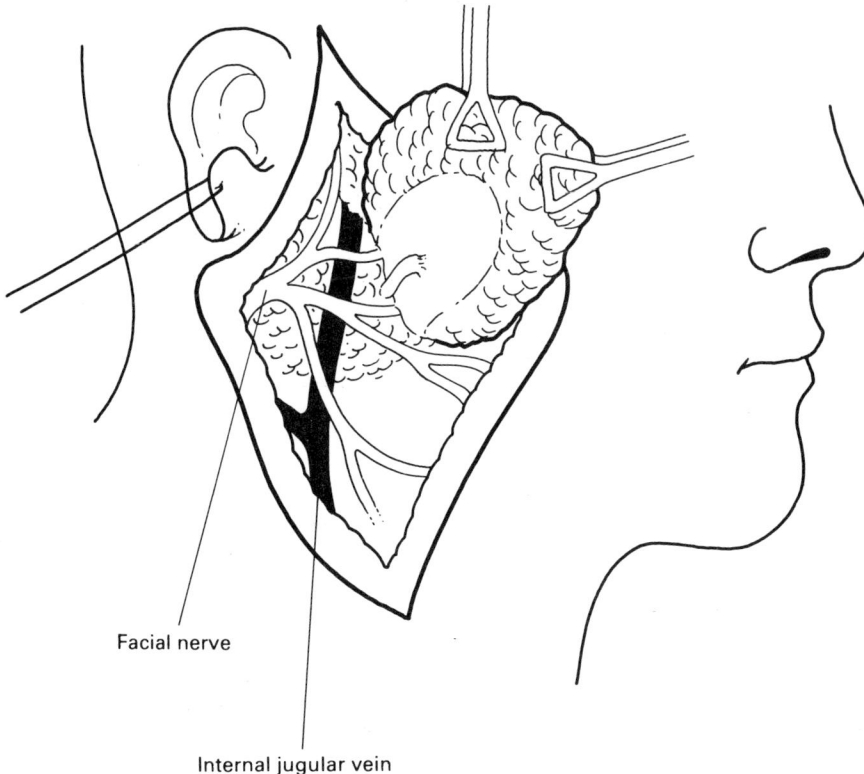

Facial nerve

Internal jugular vein

Fig. 52 Superficial (suprafacial) parotidectomy

closed along the facial nerve branch then opened and lifted and the overlying tissue cut with scissors. This manoeuvre can be repeated for full exposure of facial nerve branches.

6. The superficial lobe is removed with the duct after division near the masseter, preserving the facial nerve (remember that the facial nerve is sandwiched between the superficial and the deep part of the gland, which are connected by the isthmus).

7. Close the skin with or without a Redivac drain.

3.15. Block Dissection

This is a radical wide excision of the lymphatic field (including lymph nodes and intervening lymphatic pathways). It is done either *prophylactically* if the lymphatic field is adjacent to but not involving the primary tumour (e.g. face and neck, axilla in breast cancer, or back melanoma and groin) or *therapeutically* if the lymph nodes are enlarged because of infiltration by an operable curable adjacent primary growth. Preferably no prophylactic block dissection is carried out if the primary tumour is remote from the lymphatic field, e.g. in melanoma of the sole of the foot there is no need for groin block dissection *unless* the inguinal lymph nodes are enlarged. No block dissection is performed:

- If the primary growth is not curable or is inoperable.
- When there are distant metastases.

Sites

Cervical block dissection

Crile's complete block dissection Performed unilaterally (when bilateral block dissection is required it must be undertaken consecutively with an interval of 3 weeks, and never simultaneously. Removal of both internal jugular veins is not associated with much obstructed cerebral circulation as was previously conjectured). It is indicated for primary growths involving:

- Oral cavity (tongue, mouth floor, mandible tumours).
- Larynx (glottic, subglottic, supraglottic).

- Facial area (melanoma, lip squamous cell carcinoma).
- Neck (thyroid papillary carcinoma, malignant parotid and submandibular salivary glands).

Suprahyoid block dissection Indicated in carcinoma of the lower lip, early carcinoma of the tip of the tongue and early carcinoma of the mouth floor. Bilateral block dissection is possible at one operation. Unilateral suprahyoid block dissection can be combined with Crile's block dissection of the opposite side.

Axillary block dissection

In breast carcinoma (radical and Patey's modified radical mastectomies) and in melanoma of the back (usually unilateral block dissection is performed on the side nearest to the melanoma but bilateral block dissection is done in upper midline back melanoma).

Groin block dissection

In melanoma of lower limb. Occasionally in penile, scrotal and vulval carcinomas.

Retroperitoneal block dissection

In testicular malignancy (not practised now).

Procedure of cervical block dissection (Fig. 53)

This major operation is now safe and the 5 year survival rate is 35 % with an operative mortality of less than 3 %. Surprisingly little deformity follows block dissection but the neck is stiff and there may be drooping of the mouth corner (as a result of injury to the cervical branch of the facial nerve).

1. Blood transfusion, prophylactic antibiotic; tracheostomy may be required (rarely in suprahyoid block dissection). Endotracheal anaesthesia is employed, a sandbag is placed between the shoulders and the head turned to the opposite side.

2. The incision commences behind the mastoid process, curves downwards and forwards 3 cm below the angle of the jaw, and then upwards to terminate on the chin just the other side of the midline. A vertical incision is made from the middle of this incision down to the middle of the clavicle. The skin flaps are reflected back.

3. Two veins are divided, one in front and one behind the sternomastoid. Divide the sternomastoid just above the clavicle, dividing the external

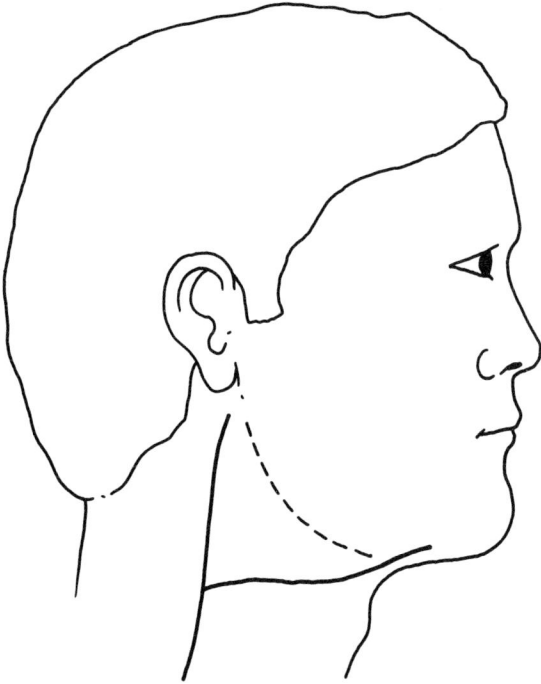

Fig. 53 Incision in cervical block dissection

jugular vein posteriorly. Dissect out the internal jugular vein anteriorly from the carotid sheath and divide it. It is dangerous to divide the internal jugular vein if it has been recently resected on the opposite side.

4. Clearance of supraclavicular fossa and division of omohyoid. The brachial nerves are seen covered by a thin layer of prevertebral fascia. Branches of the subclavian vessels are ligated. The thoracic duct on the left side is preserved. The accessory nerve and ansa cervicalis are divided.

5. Continuation of dissection to hyoid level. The tributaries of the internal jugular, middle and superior thyroid and inferior thyroid vessels, and later the common facial vein and artery, are divided. The thyroid isthmus is divided and hemithyroidectomy performed with removal of the strap muscles. Preserve the recurrent laryngeal nerve unless a laryngectomy has already been done. Identify and preserve the hypoglossal nerve, then divide the central tendon of the digastric muscle to open up the dissection. At this stage the common facial vein is divided. Identify the facial and occipital arteries arising from the external carotid, and divide them between ligatures.

6. Dissect and dislocate the submandibular gland, including its deep portion, divide the duct close to

the gland and turn it upwards. Preserve the lingual nerve.

7. Dissect out the internal jugular vein carefully and doubly ligate and divide it at the base of the skull.

8. Division of mass. Commencing posteriorly divide the sternomastoid and digastric, remove the tail of the parotid if necessary, then cut along the lower border of the jaw, ligating the facial vessels, until the opposite side of the midline is reached and the mass removed.

9. Close the skin and drain the wound with a Redivac suction drain.

3.16. Modified Patey's Radical Mastectomy

Procedure (Fig. 54)

1. Under general anaesthesia and in the supine position. The arm is held at right angles to the body on an arm board or suspended from a drip stand by a sling around the wrist. Care is taken to avoid traction injuries of the brachial plexus.

2. Define the margins of the growth. Make an elliptical semitransverse incision including the nipple, the skin over the growth, and 5 cm of normal skin beyond its margin. Avoid placing the upper part of the incision along the inferior margin of the anterior axillary fold, as a 'bridle-scar' develops.

3. Deepen the skin incision and reflect the lateral and medial flaps including a small amount of subcutaneous fat. Approximately half the subcutaneous fat is left on the skin, and the thinner the patient, the greater the care required to avoid cutting into the breast tissue (recognised by its white colour). Mobilise the lateral flap as far back as the anterior border of latissimus dorsi. Mobilise the upper half of the medial flap to the medial end of the clavicle. Confine your dissection to the lateral flap. The medial side of the mass is usually disconnected towards the end of the operation.

4. Preserve pectoralis major and the area below it. Divide the pectoralis minor tendon immediately below its coracoid insertion and the fascia on either side. The axillary vessels and nerves together with their covering fascial sheath are exposed.

5. The axilla is then dissected from the side of the

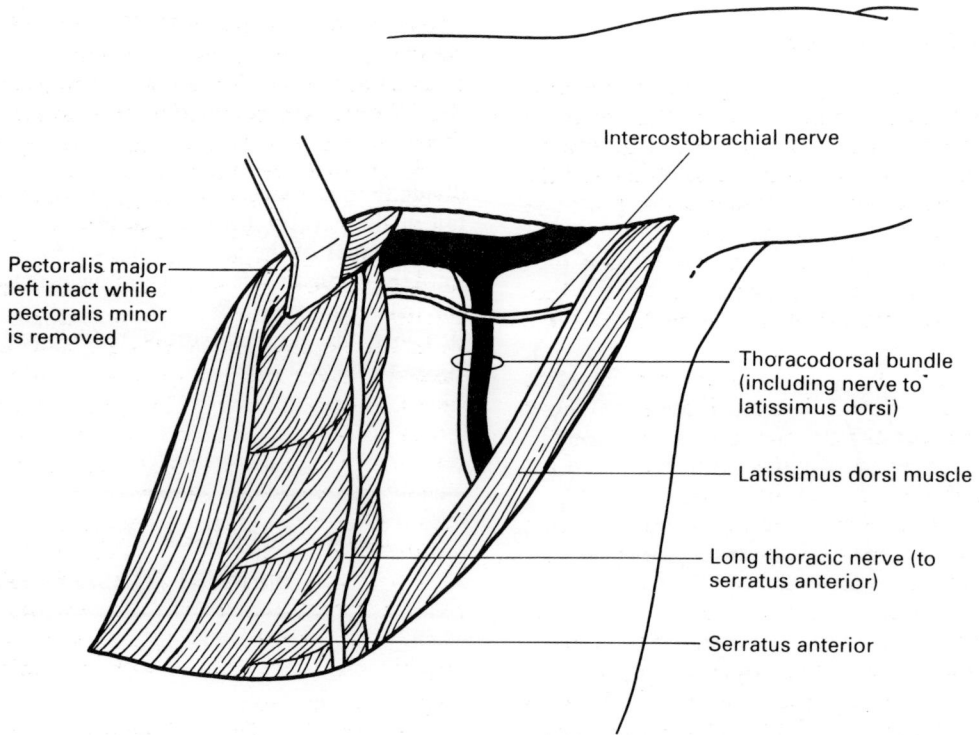

Fig. 54 Patey's modified radical mastectomy

axillary vein, proceeding medially, and from the apex of the axilla passing downwards by a combination of sharp and blunt dissection. The small vein tributaries of the axillary vein are cleared and divided 6 mm from the main vein. These veins are ligated carefully to avoid air embolus.

6. The intercostobrachial nerve and the nerves of latissimus dorsi and serratus anterior are preserved. (Note that the nerve to latissimus is found superficially near the subscapular vessels.) The nerves may rarely be sacrificed if involved glands are found to be adherent to them.

7. The breast is excised from the chest wall, clipping the lateral and anterior perforating branches before division. Excision of the mass of tissue is carried to the opposite side of the midline.

8. The rest of the medial flap still attached is mobilised to complete excision.

9. Careful haemostasis is obtained (and an immediate or late skin graft is applied, if necessary, to avoid suturing under tension).

10. Two Redivac drains are left in (axillary and subcutaneous) for 5 and 3 days respectively. The axillary tube drains lymph from axillary disturbed lymphatics (lymphorrhoea). Interrupted or subcuticular skin closure is used.

3.17. Vascular Bypass and Abdominal Aortic Aneurysm Surgery

AORTOFEMORAL BYPASS
(in Leriche syndrome)

Indications

This procedure is used in patients with severely disabling claudication or with ischaemic rest pain or gangrene in whom there is occlusive disease of the distal aorta and iliac arteries.

Preoperative preparation

Routine blood investigations, chest X-ray, ECG, 4 units of blood cross-matched; nasogastric tube, urethral catheter, preoperative wide-spectrum antibiotic.

Procedure (Fig. 55a and b)

1. Incision, laparotomy and exposure of the aortoiliac system as described below in the operation for elective aortic aneurysm grafting. The femoral arteries are exposed by vertical groin incisions; the common femoral, superficial femoral and profunda origin should be dissected and slings passed round them. If the profunda origin is diseased it should be dissected distally until a healthy portion is reached. The superficial femoral is often occluded in these patients.

2. On each side the inguinal ligament is retracted forwards, and using gentle blunt dissection a tunnel is made between the external iliac artery and the inguinal ligament, up into the retroperitoneum. On the left side the base of the pelvic mesocolon is mobilised and the tunnelling continued up behind this, taking care not to damage the ureter.

3. At the aortic end a tape should be placed round the inferior mesenteric artery and the aorta carefully examined. Disease is often found to be more extensive than shown on aortogram. The graft may be joined end-to-side to the aorta, usually between the renal vein level and the inferior mesenteric origin, or the aorta may be divided at a similar level, the distal end oversewn and the graft joined on end-to-end. The latter method is preferred provided that the distribution of occlusion is such that retrograde perfusion of the inferior mesenteric artery through the iliacs is possible.

4. A suitable Dacron graft, preferably knitted and usually 19 mm in diameter at the aortic end, is selected. Careful preclotting is done, and the graft checked for effectiveness of the preclotting before giving the patient 8000–10 000 units of heparin i.v.

5. For an end-to-side graft, a lateral clamp may be used on the aorta, but this does not permit a good view of the interior of the aorta and should only be used if the aorta is healthy at and above the level of the proposed anastomosis. If not, it should be cross-clamped below the renals and again above the bifurcation. A 3 cm vertical elliptical incision is then made between the upper clamp and the inferior mesenteric artery. For end-to-end reconstruction, the aorta is divided transversely at a similar level, and the distal end oversewn after removing loose debris with a sponge holder or gentle 'milking'. The proximal aorta between the renal arteries and the aortotomy should be carefully cleared out using squeezing, sponge holders and irrigation. An unobstructed flow into the graft is essential.

6. The aortic limb of the graft is trimmed to length so that when stretched the new bifurcation will lie above the level of the old. The upper end is cut obliquely or transversely according to the type of anastomosis, which is then made using continuous 3/0 Prolene. On completion, the anastomosis is tested by clamping the graft and releasing the aortic clamp for one beat. Further sutures are inserted if required. The graft is sucked out, and the limbs carefully drawn down through the retroperitoneal tunnels into the groin wounds.

7. With bulldog clamps on the common, superficial femoral and profunda on the first side, a longitudinal arteriotomy is made in the common femoral, if necessary extending down into the profunda until healthy artery is reached. The graft limb is placed under moderate tension and cut obliquely to the correct length. It is anastomosed to the arteriotomy with continuous 4/0 Prolene, backbleeding the clamped vessels prior to completion.

8. With the completed limb clamped near the bifurcation, one beat from the aortic end can be flushed through the free limb, which is then clamped close to the bifurcation and sucked clean. The heparin should be reversed with protamine at this stage.

9. The distal clamps are managed so that the first few beats from above are directed upwards to the iliac artery, thus avoiding the danger of *trash foot*. The aortic clamp is removed gradually over a period of some 5 min to minimise the risk of sudden hypotension. The remaining femoral anastomosis is constructed on similar lines to the first, using heparinised saline in the clamped groin vessels.

10. The posterior peritoneum is closed making sure that the whole graft is covered. Omentum may be used to aid this, if necessary. The abdominal and groin incisions are then closed, usually without drainage, but if drains are thought to be advisable they should be of the closed suction variety.

ELECTIVE GRAFTING OF ABDOMINAL AORTIC ANEURYSM

Indication

Graft replacement is advised for all infrarenal abdominal aortic aneurysms except for asymptomatic aneurysms less than 4 cm diameter, and in patients considered unfit to withstand major surgery.

Dissection proximal and distal to the aneurysm is kept to the minimum necessary for safe clamping. This saves time and avoids the danger of injury to the inferior vena cava, iliac veins and lumbar veins.

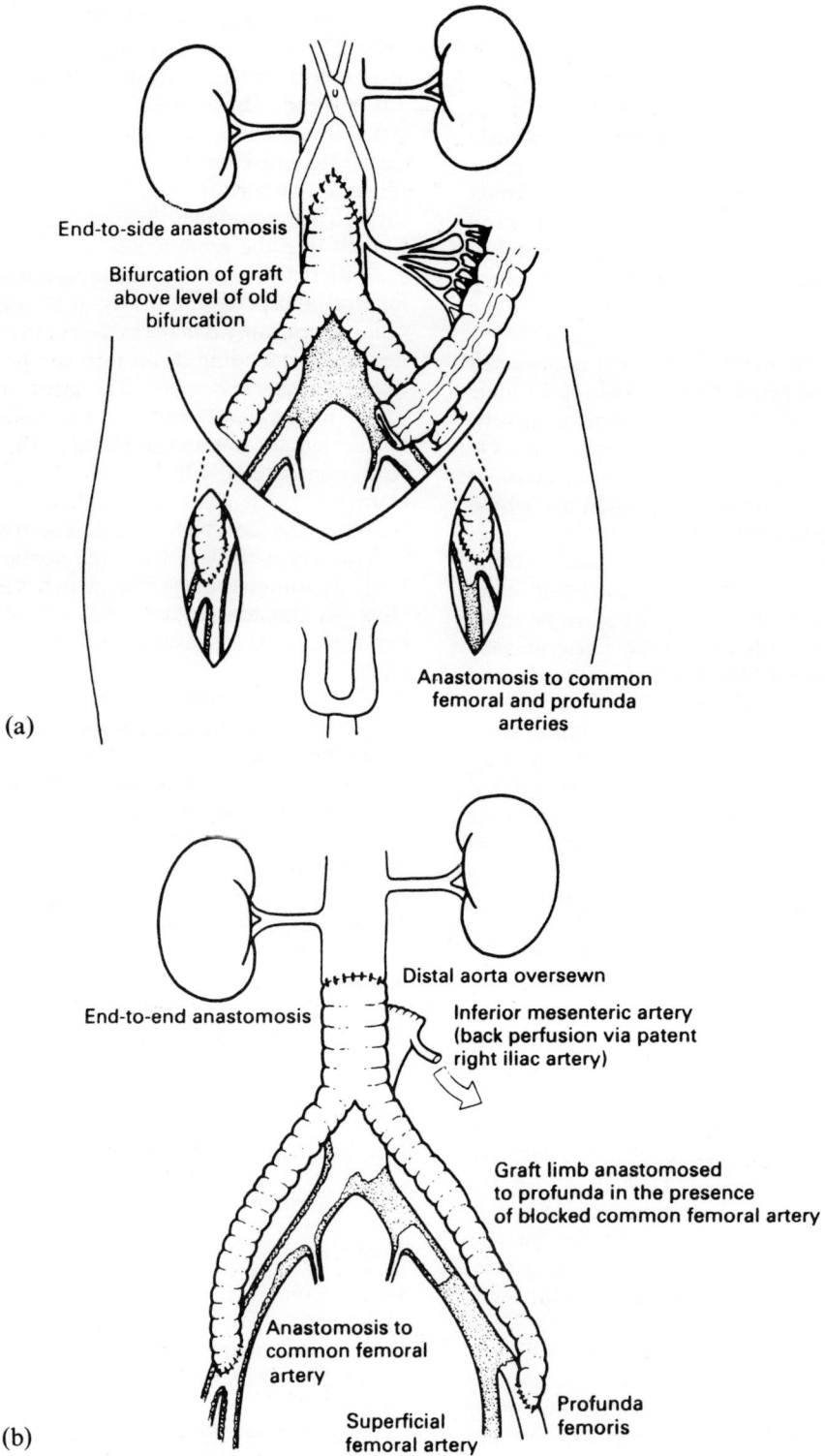

Fig. 55 Two alternative arrangements of graft and anastomoses (sites of obstruction are indicated by stippled areas)

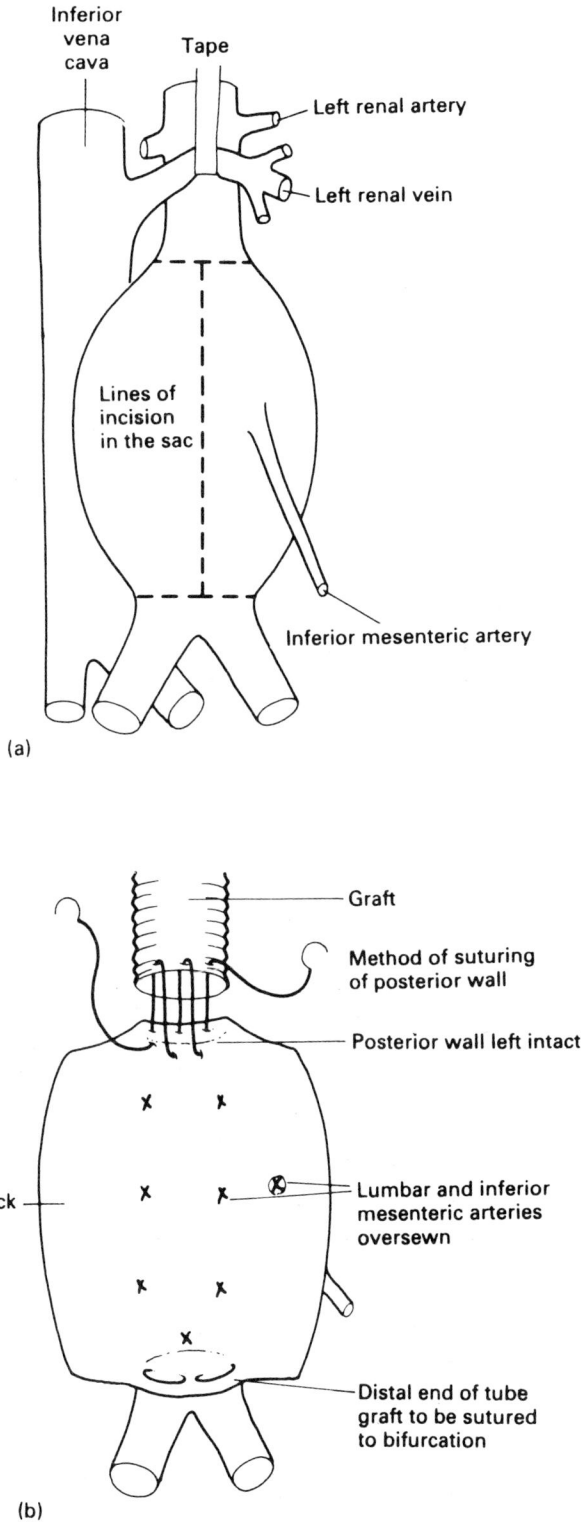

Fig. 56   Abdominal aortic aneurysm repair, using tube graft

Preoperative preparation

Routine blood, ESR, ECG, chest X-ray and ultrasound of aorta. Aortography only if associated occlusive disease. Six units of blood cross-matched. Prophylactic wide-spectrum antibiotic. Indwelling urethral catheter, nasogastric tube and CVP line are needed.

Procedure (Figs 56 and 57)

1. Supine position. Whole abdomen and upper thighs are prepared. Inflatable leggings are used to prevent deep vein thrombosis. Steridrape is used.
2. Full length midline or paramedian incision.
3. Full laparotomy to exclude other pathology. Confirm aneurysm is below renals. Examine condition of the iliac vessels—are they dilated or severely atheromatous?
4. Insert a large self-retaining retractor. Place the small bowel in a plastic gut bag outside the abdomen on the right side (or pack it off inside).
5. Mobilise the duodenojejunal flexure and duodenum off the front of the aorta and retract it to the right. Safeguard the inferior mesenteric vein. Dissect the front and sides of the neck of the aneurysm.
6. Mobilise the left renal vein if necessary by dividing its branches and retract upwards with tape.
7. Identify the space between the infrarenal aorta and inferior vena cava.
8. Divide the posterior peritoneum vertically to the right of the inferior mesenteric artery, continuing down to the bifurcation and along the line of the right common iliac artery.
9. Mobilise the peritoneum to expose the left common iliac artery (look out for the ureters). If the iliac arteries are fairly healthy a tube graft can usually be sutured to the aortic bifurcation. Assuming this is possible, proceed as follows.
10. Select a woven dacron tube graft of diameter equal to or slightly smaller than the neck of the aneurysm. Give i.v. heparin 8000–10 000 units. Clamp the aorta in the sagittal plane below the renals. The assistant holds it pressed back towards the spine.
11. Clamp the common iliac arteries, incise the anterior wall of the aneurysm from the neck down to the bifurcation and rapidly clear out clot with a finger.
12. Oversew backbleeding inferior mesenteric and lumbar arteries with 2/0 thread. At the upper and lower ends of the aneurysm extend the incision transversely on each side, but leave the posterior wall intact.

13. Anastomose the proximal end of the graft to the neck of the aneurysm, using 2/0 double-ended Prolene suture. Start posterolaterally on the left, holding the graft vertically. First insert the needle through the graft, then take a wide bite of the aorta from above down. Insert the whole row of posterior continuous suture in this manner before approximating the graft to the aorta. This makes placement of sutures much easier, and it is simple to snug down the Prolene at the end of the posterior wall. Continue around the sides and front to complete the anastomosis.
14. Clamp the graft and release the aortic clamp for one beat to test for major leaks in the suture line. Unclamp the graft and suck out.
15. Stretch the graft and trim to reach the bifurcation comfortably. Perform distal anastomosis; again posterior-layer sutures should be placed before pulling the stitch tight. The iliac arteries should be backbled prior to completion of the anastomosis. Give protamine. Allow the graft to fill from below by releasing the iliac clamps first. Manually compress the external iliac arteries and slowly release the aortic clamp; the first few beats should go into the internal iliac arteries to prevent trash foot. Then release the pressure on the external iliac arteries. Full release of the aortic clamp should be spread over some 5 min to prevent sudden dangerous hypotension. Press on the anastomosis with a finger or swab until dry. Check for bleeding from the wall of the aneurysm. Trim wall and suture sac over graft.
16. Close the posterior peritoneum; it is vital to make certain that graft material is not in contact with the bowel. Close the abdomen.
17. If a bifurcated graft is needed because of aneurysmal or diseased iliac arteries, the limbs will have to be sutured to the distal end of the common iliac arteries or to the common femoral arteries. In the latter case the distal common iliac arteries should be oversewn after dissecting and controlling the external and internal iliac arteries. It is important to maintain flow to at least one internal iliac artery.

3.18. Sympathectomy

Lumbar (Fig. 58, p. 236)

1. Under general anaesthesia. Patient is supine with the flank tilted towards the opposite side, and a

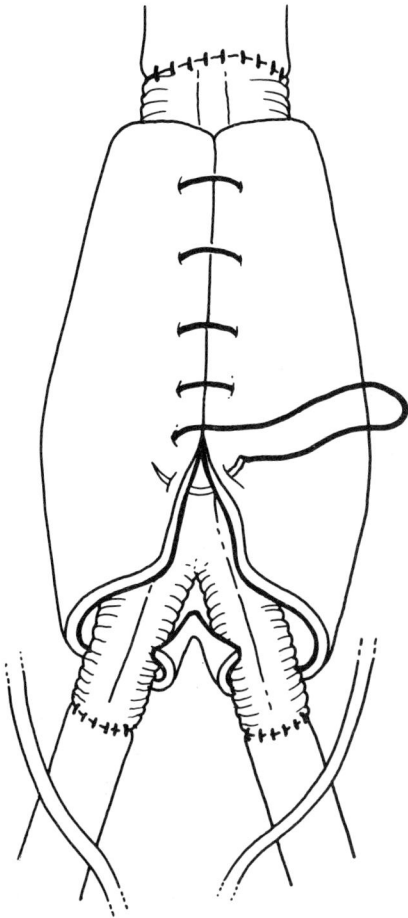

Fig. 57 Inverted Y-graft is occasionally used instead of tube graft in abdominal aortic aneurysm repair. Notice closure of the sac over the graft

sandbag placed behind the shoulder and buttock.
2. An oblique or transverse incision is made midway between the anterior superior iliac spine and costal margin towards and ending 4 cm lateral to the umbilicus. The muscles are split or divided to expose the extraperitoneal fat.
3. The peritoneal sac is raised by blunt dissection from the lateral and posterior abdominal walls to uncover the medial margin of the psoas muscle and the aorta or inferior vena cava (IVC), depending on the side (left or right respectively). The following structures may be seen: ureters, genitofemoral nerve and duodenum. Identify the ureter and place the retractors over the peritoneum and ureter. The genitofemoral nerve has no ganglia and is easily identified as it emerges through the psoas fibres.

4. The sympathetic chain and ganglia, lying anterior to the psoas muscle, are more easily felt than seen. The chain is exposed by dissecting through the overlying fascia. The chain is picked up with forceps and dissected upwards and downwards, exposing the second and third lumbar ganglia. The first right lumbar ganglion lies deep to the duodenum. The fourth lies behind the common iliac vessels.
5. Divide the chain, removing approximately 5–7 cm containing two to four ganglia. Removal of Lumbar 1 bilaterally makes the sympathectomy more certain, but may result in loss of ejaculation.
6. Lumbar veins may cross the chain and are clipped with Cushing's silver clips. Pack the area for 5 min if accidental tearing occurs.
7. The muscles are sutured in layers and the skin is closed.

Cervical (Fig. 59)

1. General anaesthesia with supine position. A sandbag is placed between the shoulders, and the head is turned to the opposite side with the table foot tilted down.
2. A skin crease incision is made 1 cm above and parallel to the medial half of the clavicle. The incision is deepened through the platysma to expose the deep fascia.
3. Dissect out and divide the external jugular vein, then divide the clavicular head of the sternomastoid. The muscle may consist of two layers. The next landmark is the omohyoid muscle and its fascia; this muscle is divided.
4. Next identify the transverse cervical vessels and trace the artery medially. It will lead to the phrenic nerve, which it crosses.
5. Mobilise the phrenic nerve from beneath the prevertebral fascia and draw it aside on a tape. The phrenic nerve is on the anterior surface of the scalenus anterior which is felt with the finger as a tight band deep to the sternomastoid and running downwards laterally to be inserted into the first rib. If in the way, the thyrocervical trunk may be mobilised and divided. Note that collateral vessels may require saving. Mobilise the scalenus anterior down to the first rib, and divide it at its insertion, preserving the medial part of it on the left side to avoid damaging the thoracic duct.
6. The subclavian artery is in the next layer, and this mobilises very easily by blunt dissection. A tape is introduced round it to act as a sling. Identify the inner border of the first rib, and detach the suprapleural membrane from it with the finger or Lahey swabs, pushing the pleura downwards. Expose the

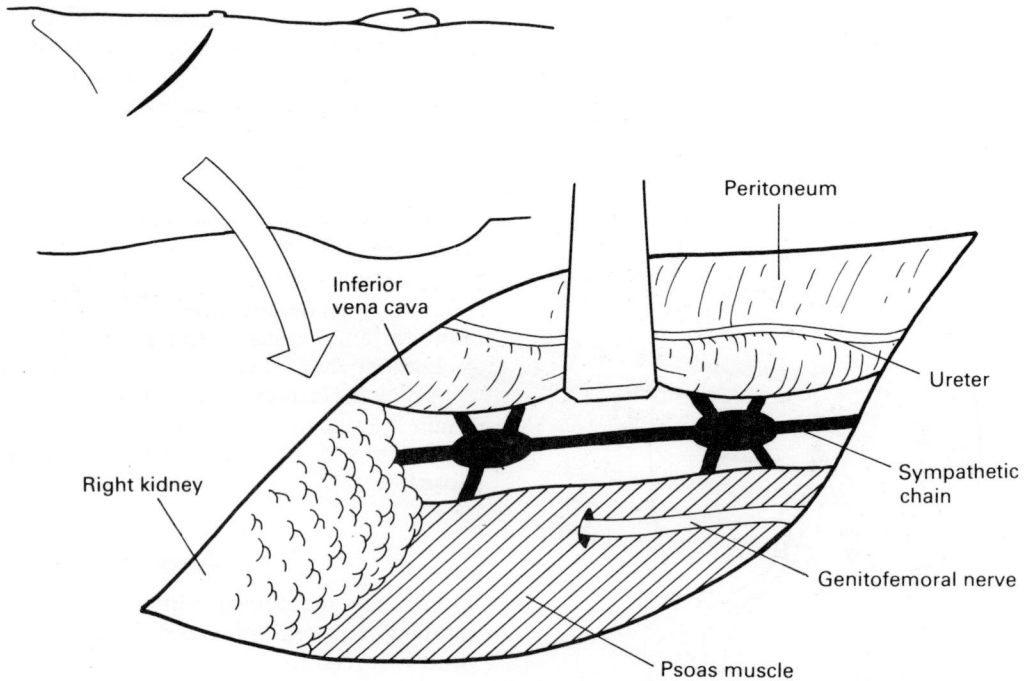

Fig. 58 Lumbar sympathectomy

necks of the first three ribs by Lahey swab dissection. A special flexible torch is used to visualise the deep area.

7. Identify the sympathetic chain with the index finger and clear off the overlying fascia. Small deep retractors are inserted and the chain is seen. At the neck of the first rib there are three structures present from medial to lateral—the sympathetic nerve, the superior intercostal vessels and the first thoracic nerve.

8. The chain is divided below the third ganglion, and dissected up by dividing its communication as far as the first thoracic and stellate ganglion, which is left with its rami communicantes to avoid Horner's syndrome.

9. Ask the anaesthetist to inflate the lungs to push the pleura back.

10. The sternomastoid and platysma are repaired and the skin approximated with clips.

N.B. In thoracic outlet syndrome pull the subclavian artery downwards and retract the brachial plexus upwards to search for the cervical rib or band. Excise the band or remove the rib with bone-nibbling forceps until no projection is left behind above the first rib.

3.19. Orchidopexy for Maldescended Testes

Badly or imperfectly descended testes are classified as:

1. *Arrested* (undescended) along the normal line of descent at the intra-abdominal, intracanalicular, emergent or high scrotal site.

2. *Deviated* from the normal line of descent (ectopic) commonly at the inguinal pouch or rarely at odd sites (e.g. perineal, pubic, penile, femoral and crossed ectopic). If a superficial inguinal pouch testis can be coaxed into the scrotum it is *tethered*, if not it is *obstructed*.

3. *Retractile*—normally descended but felt at a high scrotal site. Normal embryology includes three intrauterine phases: abdominal (1–7 months), canalicular (7–8 months) and scrotal (8–9 months). The presence or absence of a hernia is not a criterion in classification.

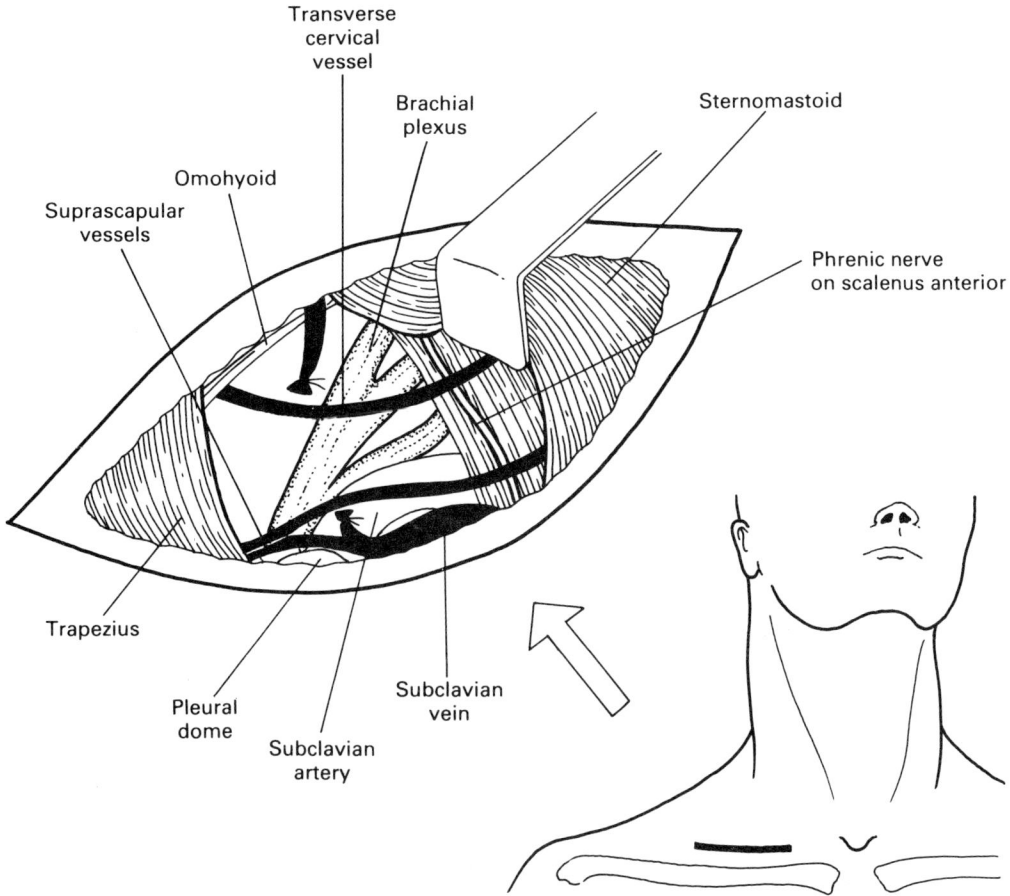

Fig. 59 Cervical sympathectomy (sympathetic chain is just under the scalenus anterior which should be cut to expose it)

Complications

- Impaired testicular function due to high temperature (affecting the normal maturation and spermatogenesis) secondary to high position. The scrotal dartos muscle and cremaster act as a thermoregulator keeping the testis 2°C cooler than body temperature.
- Malignancy.
- Hernia is an associated condition.
- Torsion occurs in 2% of maldescended testes especially testes in hernial sacs.
- Vulnerability to trauma especially inguinal testes.
- Anomalies of the epididymis and vas deferens.
- Psychological factors.

Clinical examination

- Marked variation from the norm for height, weight and fat distribution may suggest *anorchia* due to possible intersex or pituitary deficiency (require chromosomal and endocrine assessment, e.g. high LH levels or the lack of androgen response to gonadotrophin stimulation may be diagnostic).
- Penile size and scrotal development and fullness.
- Gentle palpation and milking of the groin with the boy recumbent or relaxed in warm surroundings—if testis is not found the boy should tense his abdominal muscles by straight leg raising to 45°.
- Older boy should be examined standing for evidence of hernia.

- The testis which descends fully when the boy squats is retractile.
- If no testis is found in the normal line of descent or in the superficial inguinal pouch, then perineal, pubopenile and femoral areas should be palpated and milked carefully.

Types of treatment

Gonadotrophin therapy mainly effective in retractile testes since other types are mechanically anchored. However, it is only worth considering for bilateral arrested testes, if palpable (emerged), in boys up to 5 years of age who have no hernia.

   Orchidopexy should be carried out before 5 years of age in order to:
- Enhance spermatogenesis.
- Reduce the risks of malignancy, traumatic orchitis and torsion and allow correction of any associated hernia.
- Improve appearance and so reduce anxiety in parents and child.

Procedure (Fig. 60)

1. Under general anaesthesia, using inguinal incision and exploration.
2. Mobilisation, in the following order (once sufficient length of cord has been obtained the successive steps are omitted):

(a) Inguinal mobilisation freeing the cord to the internal ring by peeling off the cremaster and incising the tunica vaginalis. A tented peritoneum or true hernia is freed initially at this stage. Gubernaculum testis is ligated and divided.
(b) Retroperitoneal dissection by dividing the lateral suspensory fascia and digital retroperitoneal dissection.
(c) Reduction of triangulation of the course of the testicular vessels by dividing the fibrous medial crus of the internal ring or blunt dissection with the finger. The inferior epigastric vessels seldom need dividing.
(d) Internal spermatic fasciectomy teasing off fascia which is then picked up, incised longitudinally and rolled off with fine dissecting forceps leaving the vessels and vas only.

3. Scrotal fixation without undue tension in an extradartos pouch (preferred to window septopexy). The scrotum is well stretched digitally; then a vertical incision is made low down near the median raphe. A chromic catgut purse-string suture is inserted before opening the dartos. Artery forceps are passed from below (guided by finger tip from above) to grasp the gubernacular remnant and pull the testis down; then the purse-string suture is tied. The skin wound is closed with absorbable sutures picking up the tunica albuginea for correct testicular orientation.

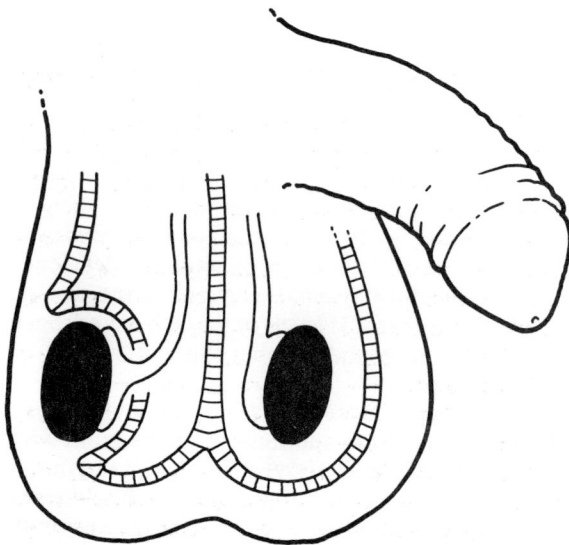

Fig. 60 Orchidopexy—scrotal fixation in extradartos pouch

3.20. Nephrectomy and Adrenalectomy

Nephrectomy

Extraperitoneal approach. Check the function of the other kidney and examine the IVU on the viewing box. The bladder is emptied.

1. Under general anaesthesia the patient lies on the sound side in a well flexed position. The opposite arm is held forward by placing it on a rest. The table may be split to widen the area between the ribs and iliac crest, or a loin rest may be used. A wide strap around the patient's pelvis and the table helps stability.

2. An oblique incision is made, commencing over the neck of the 12th rib (check the site of this rib by

X-ray). The incision runs forward over the 12th rib and may be extended up to the lateral margin of the rectus sheath.

3. The wound is deepened with cutting diathermy down to the rib. Using a periosteal elevator, periosteum is stripped first from the upper border from the back forwards then from the lower border carefully (to avoid injury to the subcostal neurovascular bundle) from the front backwards opposite to the direction of the intercostal muscles; a raspatory is then applied to the upper border, stripping periosteum backwards and forwards, followed by excision of the rib through its neck whth bone-cutting forceps.

4. Access is improved posteriorly by removing the 12th rib subperiosteally. The following structures are preserved: pleura, subcostal nerve, colon and peritoneum. The incision is deepened to expose the latissimus dorsi, serratus posterior inferior, lumbar fascia and the external oblique, and these muscles are divided and split respectively. The internal oblique and transversus muscles and transversalis fascia are divided to expose the extraperitoneal fat (Fig. 61a). The peritoneum is mobilised forwards by blunt dissection to expose the perinephric fascia of Zuckerkandl. The fascia of Gerota is opened and the kidney seen.

5. If possible, it is brought out of the wound; if not, a self-retaining retractor is inserted to aid further dissection. Two long swabs or tapes can be applied around the hilum of the kidney to aid retraction (Fig. 61b)

6. The ureter is identified and transected (in hypernephroma). In papillary tumour of the renal pelvis the lower end of the ureter is mobilised for full excision of the ureter; sleeve resection of the bladder wall is performed through a separate suprapubic incision.

7. The renal vessels are triple ligated and divided between the middle and distal ligature.

8. The wound is drained. The muscles are sutured together with interrupted sutures that are tied after removing the kidney rest or straightening the table. Lumbar fascia is sutured continuously to permit free skin movement over muscles.

The operation may be extremely difficult if the inflammation and subsequent fibrosis have spread outside the kidney. The most difficult part is the mobilisation of the kidney, so this should be performed first. The following structures may need to be separated from the right kidney—liver, diaphragm and suprarenal artery, duodenum and colon; and on the left side—stomach, spleen and colon.

Right abdominal intraperitoneal nephrectomy and right adrenalectomy (Figs 62, p. 241, and 63a, p. 242)

1. Under general anaesthesia the abdomen is opened through a right paramedian incision and explored.

2. The hepatic flexure is mobilised by dividing its attachments, and packed off downwards and medially along with the small intestine.

3. The second part of the duodenum is mobilised by dividing the peritoneum along its right border. By this procedure the duodenum and head of the pancreas can be mobilised as far as the inferior vena cava (Kocher's manoeuvre).

4. The fascia of the kidney is then exposed, picked up and divided. The hilar vessels and ureter are divided and ligated and the kidney is mobilised and removed.

For adrenalectomy exposure as above then:

5. Traction on the kidney brings down the adrenal gland.

6. Its exposure is facilitated by extending the incision in the posterior parietal peritoneum upwards and retracting the right lobe of the liver.

7. The adrenal veins (draining into the inferior vena cava) are clipped with Cushing silver clips and divided.

8. Blunt dissection mobilises the gland for its removal.

9. Accessory glands may require removal.

Left abdominal nephrectomy and left adrenalectomy (Figs 62, p. 241, and 63b, p. 242)

1. Under general anaesthesia the abdomen is opened through a long left paramedian incision and explored. The incision may be extended transversely if the patient is deep and broad (fatty).

2. The spleen is held over to the left and the posterior leaf of the lienorenal ligament divided. The hand can then be inserted behind the spleen and tail of the pancreas, and these structures can be mobilised forwards off the posterior abdominal wall. The gastrocolic ligament is also divided.

3. The kidney fascia (Zuckerkandl) is exposed, picked up and opened.

4. The kidney is mobilised manually, and the vessels of the hilum and the ureter, together with any extrapolar vessels, can be seen and dealt with. If this approach is used for the adrenal gland, this structure is seen on the upper pole of the kidney and is mobilised gently with blunt dissection. The large

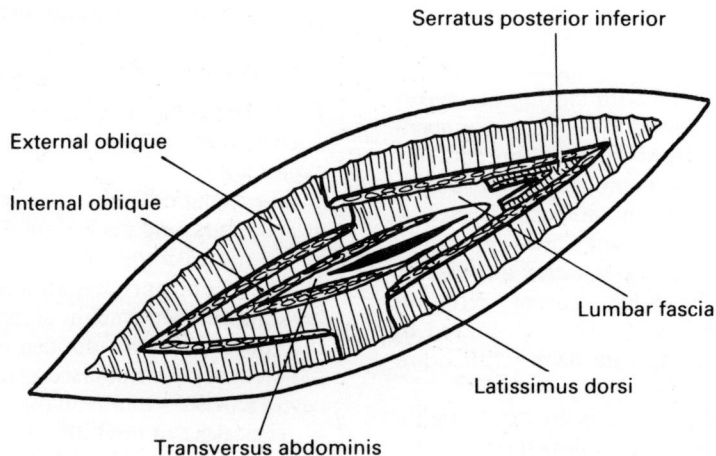

External oblique

Internal oblique

Serratus posterior inferior

Lumbar fascia

Latissimus dorsi

Transversus abdominis

(a)

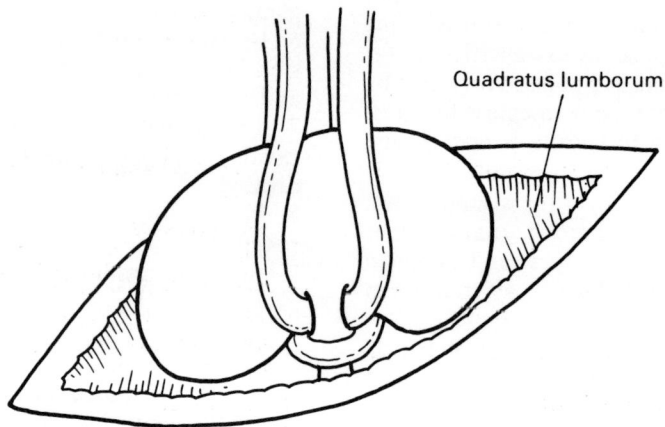

Quadratus lumborum

(b)

Fig. 61 Nephrectomy—surgical approach. (a) Muscles have been divided and split. (b) Method of handling the kidney after mobilisation and also prior to contact renogram

adrenal vein emptying into the left renal veins is clipped with silver Cushing clips and divided. Other vessels are similarly treated and the gland removed.

Partial nephrectomy

1. The kidney is exposed as above. It is secured by a tape encircling the pedicle. The vessels at the hilum are gently dissected, and if a distinct blood supply is found to the part to be removed, it is ligated and divided.
2. The segment (wedge) is removed with its calyces and associated part of the renal pelvis, leaving a fringe of healthy capsule to cover the raw area.
3. Medullary vessels are ligated, or underrun. The pelvis is repaired with plain catgut. Gauze pressure is applied for the standard 5 min.
4. The edges of the kidney are approximated with catgut over an omental graft or crushed muscle.

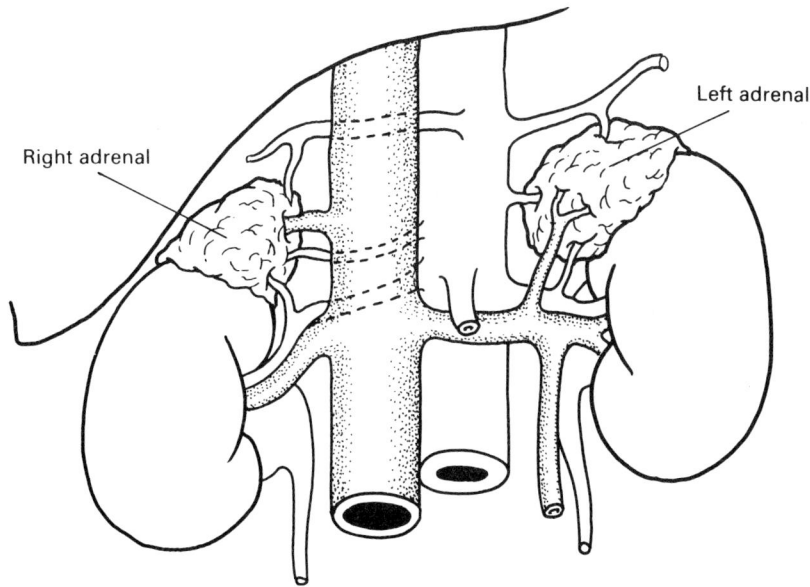

Fig. 62   Blood supply of adrenals

5. The kidney is replaced, the area drained and the wound closed.

3.21. Prostatectomy

Retropubic prostatectomy (Fig. 64, p. 243)

Preliminary bimanual examination and cystoscopy to assess the prostatic size and associated intra-vesical pathology, e.g. stone or bladder tumour. Bilateral vasectomy may be performed to prevent postoperative acute epididymitis.

1. Under general anaesthesia and with patient in Trendelenburg position.

2. Suprapubic Pfannenstiel (transverse) incision or lower midline incision. The recti are separated and the bladder separated from the pubis to expose the prostatic capsule extraperitoneally by dissection of the retropubic cave of Retzius. A self-retaining retractor is inserted.

3. The veins running over the prostate are ligated or diathermied and the bladder wall is depressed by a sponge.

4. A transverse (or vertical vesicocapsular) cut is made through the capsule (and bladder wall).

5. The cut capsule edges are held and the adenoma dissected out with a finger pressing against the pubis; the prostatic lobes are enucleated (shelled out). The urethra is divided under vision. The adenomatous tissue is thus removed.

6. A generous (V-shaped) wedge is removed from the posterior lip of the bladder (trigonectomy). Two fingers may be inserted through the bladder neck. Tags are removed and haemostasis achieved.

7. A catheter, whistle-tipped or a three-way Foley catheter size 24 Fr, is passed into the bladder, which is washed through. Continuous irrigation is then started.

8. The prostatic capsule is closed with continuous size 1 chromic catgut. The capsular repair should be watertight when tested by washing through the bladder.

9. The packs are removed and the rectus and skin closed with a Redivac drain in the space of Retzius. The urinary catheter tip can be held with a stay-suture brought out through the bladder and abdominal wall and fixed with a gauze on the abdomen to prevent its displacement and/or disruption of the capsular repair.

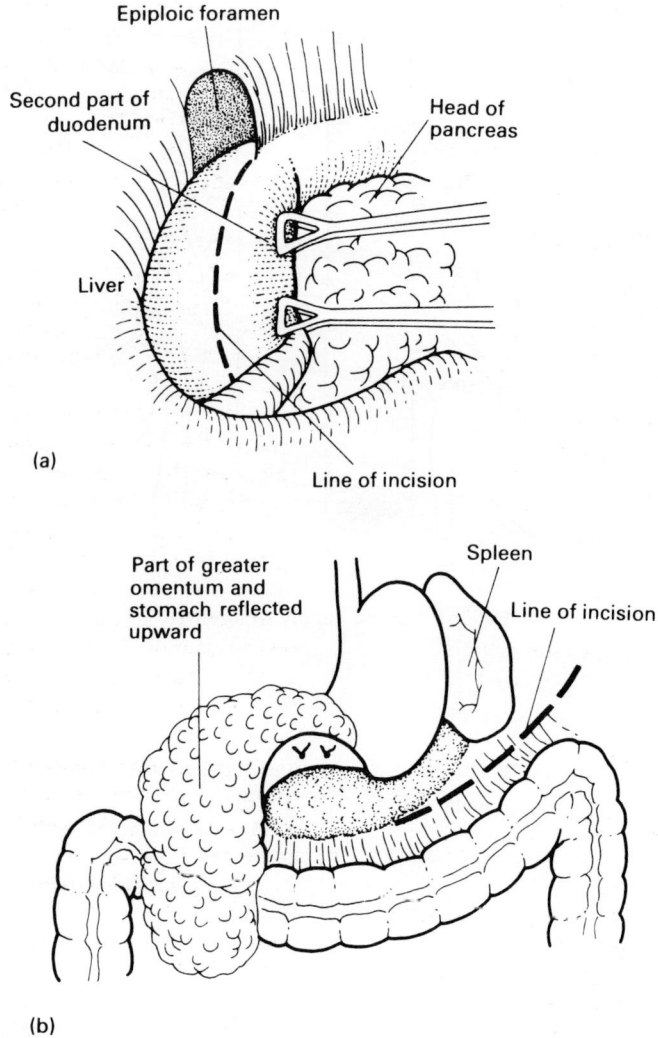

(a)

(b)

Fig. 63 Adrenalectomy. (a) Right adrenalectomy approach.
(b) Left adrenalectomy approach

3.22. Cystectomy and Ureterosigmoidostomy

CYSTECTOMY WITH ILEAL CONDUIT

This operation involves removal of the urinary bladder, with prostate and seminal vesicles in the male, and drainage of urine via an ileal loop to an external ileostomy. In the female, the uterus and adnexae are removed. May be curative or palliative.

Indications

- Invasive bladder tumour.
- Contracted bladder—tuberculosis, bilharziasis.

Associated therapy

Patients with infiltrating tumours are often given a preliminary irradiation of 4000–4500 rad.

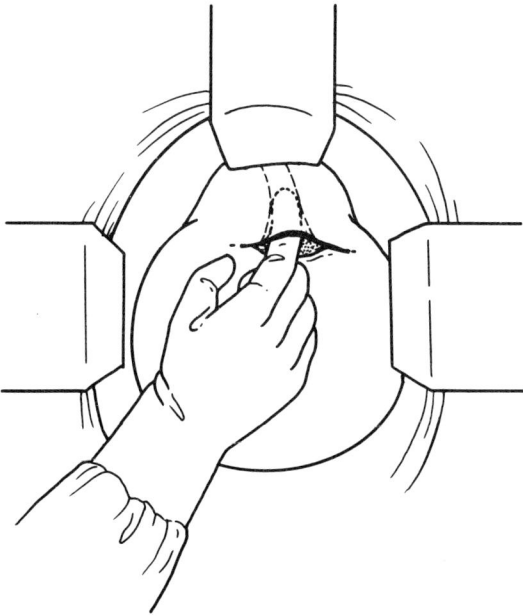

Fig. 64   Retropubic prostatectomy

Special preoperative preparation

- Intestinal tract sterilised by oral antibiotics begun 48 h before surgery.
- High-calorie, low-residue feeding over similar period.
- Restoration of haemoglobin level or correction of electrolyte levels if required.
- Advice from a previous cystectomy patient.
- Site of ileostomy marked on skin of right abdomen to accommodate comfortable siting of urine collection appliance.

Procedure (Fig. 65)

1. Patient supine catheterised, and in Trendelenburg position.
2. Lower midline incision.
3. Laparotomy and assessment of the fixity of the tumour in the pelvis. Post irradiation changes may be present.
4. If resectable, proceed to mobilise and divide the ureters—divide peritoneum over each common iliac artery bifurcation. Mobilise each ureter as it passes in front of the origin of the external iliac artery. Dissect a further 4 cm down, then divide. Hold the proximal end in light tissue forceps and ligate the lower end with non-absorbable guide ligature. The ureters may be dilated, sometimes considerably.

Draw the left ureter to the right through a convenient point in the descending mesocolon.
5. Expose and tie the internal iliac artery on each side in continuity using an aneurysm needle and non-absorbable ligature.
6. Proceed to dissect the lymph nodes on each side after exposing the anterior and lateral bladder walls and fatty tissue overlying the pelvic fascia by blunt dissection.
7. While dissecting nodes in the obturator fossa, preserve the obturator nerve and vessels. Cut and tie the vas deferens and use the proximal tied end as a later guide to the plane between the seminal vesicles and rectum.
8. As the bladder is mobilised in front, laterally and posteriorly, two lateral vascular pedicles have to be secured—lifting the bladder forwards and to the opposite side allows the superior and inferior vesical vessel pedicles to be defined, narrowed, and divided between clamps and tied. Use chromic catgut.
9. As the rectovesical fascial layer is mobilised, the bladder is dissected off the rectum. The seminal vesicles and prostate are mobilised from behind and below. The stumps of the ureters are also seen. Inferior pedicles may have to be secured in several steps.
10. Puboprostatic ligaments are now diathermised. Pelvic fascia lateral to the prostate is divided in the convexity of the retropubic area by sharp dissection. The prostate and vesicles now narrow to an apex at the urethra which is divided with scissors; remaining deep lateral connections are finally divided. Check for significant bleeding; if none, leave the pack in the pelvis and proceed to make an ileal conduit.
11. Use a length of distal ileum at least 20 cm proximal to the ileocaecal junction. The length must be adequate to extend from the ureters to the external ileostomy. Mark the selected length and prepare the mesenteric vascular pedicle with the use of transillumination. Distal mesenteric division is longer than proximal as this end passes through the abdominal wall.
12. Hold the conduit loop between light intestinal clamps. Place to the left (inframesenteric) and restore ileal continuity using 2/0 chromic catgut in a two-layer anastomosis.
13. Trim and spatulate the ureters. Suture the V of one to the apex of the spatulated length of the other with 3/0 chromic catgut. Insert the trimmed arms of a 10 Fr biliary T-tube into each ureter, wash out the ileal loop with an irrigating syringe, and draw the stem of the T-tube through it to the outer end. Complete anastomosis of the ureters to the inner

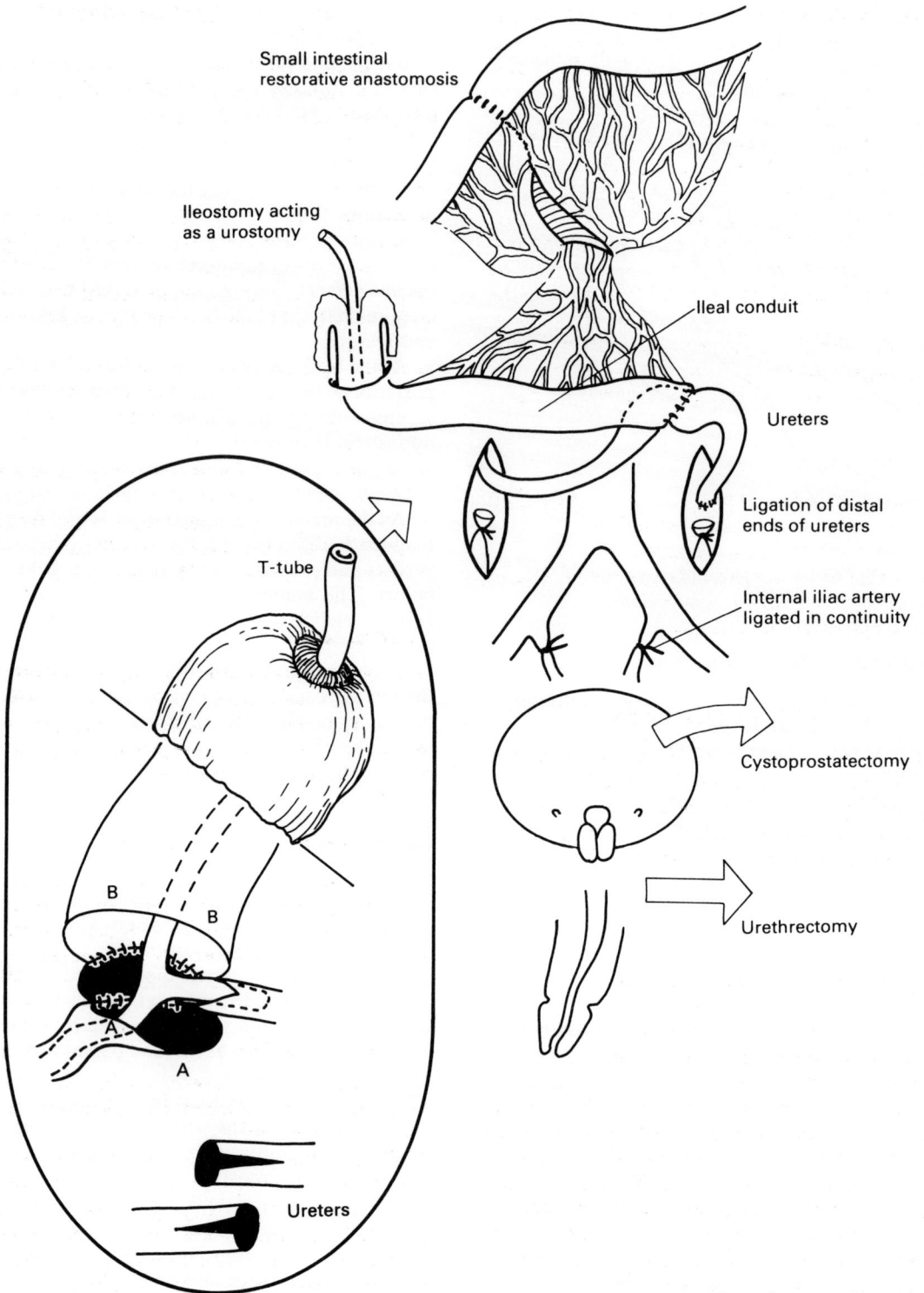

Fig. 65 Cystectomy and ileal conduit. (In the inset sides A and B will be sutured together)

ileal end with 3/0 chromic interrupted catgut stitches. T-tube splint dose *not* require suture fixation—if this were pulled out accidentally later it might disrupt the anastomosis.

14. Suture the peritoneal mesenteric incision around the ureteroileal anastomosis to make it retroperitoneal. Finally make a spouting ileostomy in the usual way through a previously marked skin circle. The stem of the T-tube can be cut suitably short and left within an immediately applied urinary appliance, where it will remain for 10 days. The abdomen is closed with tube or suction drain to the pelvis.

15. In the female, hysterectomy with bilateral salpingo-oöphorectomy is carried out after initial ureter division and internal iliac artery ligature.

Special postoperative care

1. Maintain nasogastric suction and i.v. fluid until return of adequate intestinal peristalsis.
2. Continue antibiotics as required.
3. Remove T-tube usually in 7–10 days, later than 10 days if anastomotic leak suspected.
4. Early mobilisation is useful.

URETHRECTOMY

This procedure is used for patients known to have unstable epithelium in the urethra in addition to an invasive bladder lesion. It is added to the end of a total cystectomy to prevent possible further invasive tumour appearing in the urethra.

Procedure

1. At the end of a total cystoprostatectomy, the patient is placed in the classical lithotomy position.
2. A curved incision, convex forwards, some 8 cm long, is made about 2 cm behind the scrotum.
3. The cut urethra is secured in the midline at the penile bulb as it enters the perineum through the perineal membrane and is dissected out of the whole length of the penis. The urethral dissection continues to the level of the glans. The surrounding corpus spongiosum bleeds little, as the scissors or knife are kept close to the outer wall of the urethra.
4. The perineal skin incision is closed with drainage, and a firm dressing applied.
5. In the female, the short urethra is easily dissected out via a short incision in the anterior vaginal wall behind its external opening.

URETEROSIGMOIDOSTOMY

This operation involves implantation of the ureters into the sigmoid (pelvic) colon. It is now less commonly used than ileal conduit.

Indications

- Non-malignant conditions of the lower urinary tract including congenital anomalies, e.g. exstrophy of the bladder.
- Irremediable trauma to the urethra.
- Invasive bladder tumour as an alternative to ileal conduit.
- Contracted bladder.

Advantages

- No abdominal stoma or artificial collecting device.
- Children, or individuals whose other congenital handicaps make urostomy management difficult, can accept this form of diversion.

Disadvantages

- Greater risk of ascending urinary infection.
- Hypokalaemic hyperchloraemic acidosis from absorption of urine by colonic mucosa.
- Loss of anal sphincter control, for any reason, will produce incontinence.

Special preoperative preparation

- Colon must be empty as well as sterilised.
- Oral antibiotic, high-calorie low-residue diet, and repeated enemas for 72 h before operation.
- Restoration of haemoglobin level and correction of any electrolyte imbalance.

Procedure (Fig. 66)

1. Supine position. Lower midline or transverse suprapubic incision. Insert wide rectal tube extending to rectosigmoid.
2. Pack off the small bowel and identify the ureters where they cross the origin of the external iliac arteries. Divide the overlying peritoneum and mobilise the ureters down towards the bladder; cut and tie the lower ends. The lateral leaf of the pelvic mesocolon may have to be mobilised.
3. The ureters are now inserted into the pelvic colon, the right ureter at a lower level than the left. Stay sutures hold both upper cut ends of the ureters

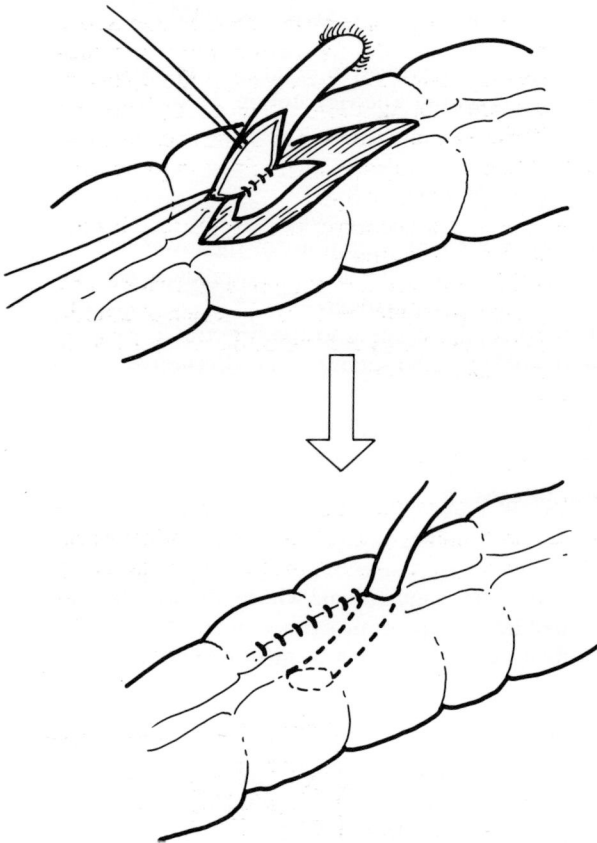

Fig. 66 Ureterosigmoidostomy

and two stay sutures are inserted about 4 cm apart in the taeni coli. The seromuscular layer of the colon is incised longitudinally between stay sutures.

4. Dissect back the seromuscular layer; open the mucosa at the distal end of the trough being formed. Lay the ureter into the trough and suture the open end to the mucosal opening with 3/0 chromic catgut.

5. After completing the posterior layer, a fine splint catheter can be passed from the ureter into the colon and thence into the rectal tube to the exterior. The anastomosis is now complete.

6. Seromuscular layers of colon are now closed over the ureter from distal to proximal with fine interrupted silk (3/0), and the lateral margin of the posterior peritoneal incision is sutured over to extraperitonealise the whole anastomosis.

7. Repeat on the left ureter at a slightly higher level to avoid tension or angulation of the ureters. This allows the pelvic colon to revert to its normal curve.

8. Secure the ureteric splints to a rectal tube at the anus. These plus the rectal tube will be passed with the first bowel motion in 4–5 days. Close the abdomen, with Penrose drainage.

Special postoperative care

1. Intravenous fluid maintains good output of urine.
2. Continue antibiotics.
3. Check electrolytes and blood urea.
4. Bicarbonate required to control acidosis.
5. Check intravenous urography in 3 months.

3.23. Pneumonectomy

Indications

Extensive lung cancer or severely damaged lung, e.g. bronchiectasis.

Surgical considerations in lung cancer

Lung cancer is the commonest cause of death among all cancers. Of 100 patients presenting with lung cancer, 70 proved to have metastatic disease already (after thorough investigations with chest X-ray—posteroanterior and lateral, sputum cytology, bronchoscopy, mediastinoscopy, radioactive scan and CT imaging, respiratory functions, percutaneous biopsy in peripheral lung cancer or scalene node biopsy, thoracoscopy and exploratory thoracotomy in this order) and die within 5 years. Only 30 had apparently localised lesions suitable for resection and of those only 8 survived 5 years.

Pulmonary resections required, in the order of frequency, are lobectomy, pneumonectomy, segmental resection and sleeve resection (with appropriate tracheobronchial reconstruction).

Operative mortality is determined by the extent of resection (lobectomy carries 5%, pneumonectomy 10% and thoracotomy without resection 10%), the presence of ischaemic heart disease, chronic bronchitis or emphysema, and the patient's age.

Postoperative prognosis depends on histological typing and cancer staging. Histologically there are four types (according to WHO): squamous carcinoma (50% of cases with 5 year survival in 28%), adenocarcinoma (including alveolar cell carcinoma; 20% of cases with 5 year survival in 17%), large-cell carcinoma (10% of cases with 5 year survival in 15%), and small-cell carcinoma (20% of cases with no 5-year survival; this is the most lethal cancer and rarely presents as a localised lesion).

Squamous, large-cell and adenocarcinoma are best treated by resection. Small-cell carcinoma is best treated by multiagent chemotherapy, i.e. cyclophosphamide, methotrexate and cyclohexyl-chlorethyl-nitrosourea (CCNU), or radiotherapy if it is localised.

There are three stages in lung cancers using the TNM classification (small-cell carcinoma is considered inoperable and is excluded):

Stage I: $T_1 (< 3 \text{ cm}) \, N_0 M_0$
$T_1 N_1$ (ipsilateral hilar node) M_0
$T_2 (> 3 \text{ cm}$ with partial lung atelectasis) $N_0 M_0$

Stage II: $T_2 N_1 M_0$
Both Stage I and II are small cancers without extrapulmonary spread.

Stage III: are large cancers which extend into nearby structures or into the proximal main bronchus or which have extrapulmonary metastases.

Stage I squamous carcinoma has the best survival of all.

Contraindications to resection

- Evidence of haematogenous metastases, e.g. in the contralateral lung, liver, brain and bones in this order.
- Lymphatic spread beyond the ipsilateral superior mediastinal nodes, e.g. scalene, posterior mediastinal and coeliac nodes.
- Direct extrapulmonary invasion: need not always preclude resection. However the following are contraindications:
  —Extensive fixed chest wall invasion.
  —Invasion of trachea or first 1.5 cm of the main bronchus.
  —Brachial plexus invasion with Horner's syndrome in Pancoast's tumour (and peripheral apical lung cancer).
  —Phrenic nerve palsy with paradoxical motion of the hemidiaphragm at fluoroscopy.
  —Intrapericardial invasion with malignant pericardial effusion and/or cardiac arrhythmias.

—Superior vena cava obstruction by metastatic mediastinal nodes (necessitates urgent radiotherapy for decompression). Oesophageal compression may also occur as indicated by barium swallow but rarely leads to dysphagia.

- Unfitness for operation especially in patients:
  —Over 70 years of age.
  —With ischaemic heart disease, chronic bronchitis or emphysema.
  —With poor respiratory reserve as indicated by pulmonary function tests. As a rule of thumb, pneumonectomy is contraindicated if FEV_1 is less than 1.2 litres.

Procedure (Fig. 67)

1. Under intermittent positive pressure, general anaesthesia with a double-lumen endotracheal tube. The lateral or, rarely, the prone position may be used.

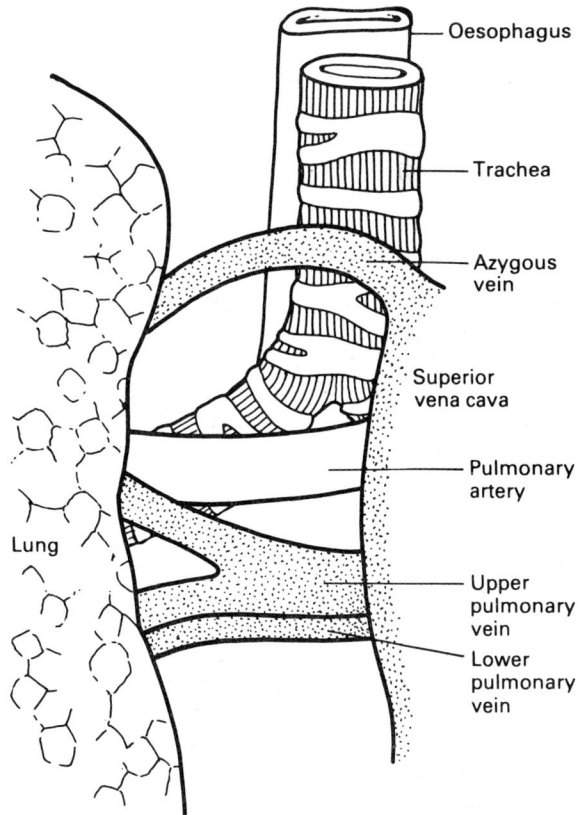

Fig. 67 Pneumonectomy—surgical approach

2. The chest is opened via a posterolateral thoracotomy incision running from the submammary crease inferior to the inferior angle of the scapula and then to the scapulovertebral interval through the fifth rib after subperiosteal rib excision. Any adhesions are divided with scissors. Areas of densely adherent pleura may have to be removed with the lung rather than risk opening a diseased lung. *En bloc* resection may be extended to include invaded chest wall and diaphragm. The subcarinal and ipsilateral tracheobronchial nodes can be removed for accurate staging.

3. The perihilar pleura and the pulmonary ligament are divided and reflected to expose the hilum. The pericardium may be opened to help in assessment of resectability.

4. The pulmonary veins are dissected and individually ligated and divided. Veins are ligated before arteries in cancer and vice versa in non-cancer cases, e.g. bronchiectasis. If necessary the left atrial wall may be secured in a vascular clamp and the veins divided flush. The atrial wall is oversewn and the clamp removed. The pulmonary artery is cleared then ligated and divided.

5. The bronchus is clamped distally and divided close to the carina. The open stump, which should be short, is closed with interrupted figure-of-8 using non-absorbable sutures, e.g. 3/0 Prolene. Alternatively the bronchus may be divided between clamps, using a non-crushing clamp proximally. Sutures are placed behind the clamp and are not tied until the clamp is removed. The hemithorax is filled with saline and the anaesthetist asked to inflate the lungs to detect any air leak from the sutured bronchus stump.

6. The chest is closed in layers without drainage or with an underwater drain but with *no suction*—the opposite lung and heart are shifted by suction with possible fatal cardiorespiratory embarrassment. Intercostal nerves are blocked or cryoprobed to reduce postoperative pain and prevent chest infection.

Postoperative complications

- Bronchopulmonary infection.
- Thoracic empyema.
- Bronchopleural fistula.
- Cardiac complications, e.g. atrial fibrillation, myocardial infarction and cardiac herniation through the resected pericardium.
- Pulmonary embolism.
- Chronic thoracotomy wound pain.

3.24. Right Hepatic Resection (Lobectomy)

The liver has remarkable powers of regeneration and resection is therefore well tolerated.

Indications

- Trauma in severe shattering liver injury.
- Tumours—primary hepatocellular carcinoma and solitary hepatic secondary carcinoma.
- High biliary tract obstruction due to cholangiocarcinoma or benign biliary stricture.
- Congenital defect—very rarely in large hepatic haemangioma.

Contraindications

- Undoubted involvement of the inferior vena cava.
- Histologically proven extrahepatic disease.
- Tumour nodules in both anatomical lobes of the liver.
- Involvement of both main branches of portal vein.

Surgical anatomy

The liver is divided into two anatomical lobes by an imaginary line between the gall bladder fossa and inferior vena cava. The left lobe is subdivided into medial (quadrate lobe) and lateral segments by ligamentum teres in the umbilical fissure. The right lobe is subdivided into anterior, posterior, superior and inferior segments. The left lobe can be subdivided into anterior, posterior, superior and inferior segments, making eight segments altogether.

Preoperative preparation

Prophylactic antibiotics (gentamicin 80 mg and lincomycin 600 mg three times a day) are given with the premedication and continued for 5 days postoperatively. Blood preparation (about 8 units) is carried out and good perioperative hydration is important.

Procedure

1. The patient is anaesthetised in the supine position. Tilting the table may help the procedure.
2. The approach depends on the underlying cause. A right paramedian exploratory incision can be extended into a right thoracoabdominal incision if, for instance, the tumour is operable or the liver is extensively injured (the diaphragm is divided, the lung is collapsed and a tape is passed around the inferior vena cava). Otherwise a bilateral subcostal oblique 'roof-top' incision using a Goligher substernal retractor with possible median sternotomy (inverted T if necessary) gives excellent exposure.
3. Ligamentum teres is sectioned and clamped for retraction. The hepatoduodenal ligament and hepatic colonic flexure are dissected and the right adrenal gland is then dissected down. The duodenum and head of pancreas are mobilised to expose the inferior vena cava and a tape is placed around this vessel above the renal veins.
4. The right lobe is mobilised, dividing the right triangular and posterior layers of the coronary ligament. The small hepatic veins are divided after ligating with metal clips or preferably transfixion with 3/0 Prolene. Then retract the liver to the left and transfix, ligate and divide the main hepatic veins.
5. At the porta hepatis the cystic duct and artery (leave the gall bladder *in situ* for the time being), then the right hepatic duct, artery and right branch of the portal vein are individually doubly ligated with non-absorbable 2/0 linen or silk and divided. A tape may be passed around the common bile duct for retraction. Notice the ischaemic line of demarcation in the floppy liver. (Step 5 may be done before Steps 3 and 4.)
6. Apply a Longmire hepatic clamp either to the right (in trauma and congenital lesions) or to the left (in tumours) of the gall bladder, then cut the liver substance and finger fracture along the ischaemic line, ligating and dividing individual vessels and bile duct inside the liver substance using 2/0 linen or silk. Then take the clamp off, watch for and ligate any more bleeding vessels.
7. Take the gall bladder out by dissection (if not already removed with the right lobe). Thorough haemostasis is required, especially at the site of the right adrenal and in the rest of the space occupied by the removed lobe.
8. Leave a silicone drain *in situ* and close the anterior abdominal wall. T-tube drainage for biliary decompression is controversial and it is probably better not to leave a T-tube in the common bile duct.

Postoperative complications

Bleeding Due to liver trauma, operative trauma, temporary liver dysfunction (liver is the factory of vitamin K dependent clotting factors II, V, VII, IX, X) or blood transfusion (with possible thrombocytopenia and coagulation factor deficiency)—may all lead to haemorrhagic shock. Massive haematemesis may also occur in the 2nd–3rd postoperative week due to intra-abdominal sepsis (stress ulcer). Routine fresh blood transfusion, vitamin K injection and selective cimetidine are required.

Infection Leaked bile and blood beneath an immobile diaphragm may become infected and lead to subphrenic abscess. Prophylactic antibiotics can be extended into therapeutic treatment. Surgical drainage may be required.

Biliary fistula Needs to be assessed by T-tube cholangiography (if a T-tube is present), ERCP or fistulogram. If there is no biliary obstruction, then parenteral nutrition and drainage of the fistula should be instituted. The presence of a stricture without fistula formation usually necessitates reoperation.

Metabolic consequences Hypoproteinaemia necessitates i.v. albumin administration, hypoglycaemia necessitates i.v. dextrose 5% infusion within the first 48 h. Mild hyperbilirubinaemia with some degree of jaundice may occur as a result of hepatocellular damage.

3.25. Amputations

Indications

- Vascular disease.
- Tumours.
- Trauma.
- Deformities whether congenital or neurological or due to chronic sepsis, pressure sores or huge lymphoedema.

Sites of election

In the upper arm, leave 20 cm measured from tuberosities, but if this is impossible, try to divide the bone 4 cm below the anterior axillary fold.

Below the elbow, 17 cm of bone are preserved as measured from the olecranon, but if this is impossible, the insertion of the biceps should be preserved. In the thigh cut 13 cm above the knee joint line. Below the knee leave 13 cm measured from the tibial tubercle.

It is important to preserve a length of stump because:

- The joint above the prosthesis should flex without interference, and the stump should retain its prosthesis.
- Muscles should be left to work the stump.
- The longer the stump, the better the muscle control and leverage.

Technical points

The use of tourniquets is avoided if the ischaemia is caused by arteriosclerosis. Equal anterior and posterior flaps are usually fashioned except in below-knee amputation. Prophylactic antibiotic is required with a properly applied bandage to protect the stump from faecal contamination.

Above-knee myoplastic flap (Fig. 68)

1. The patient lies supine under general anaesthesia. Mark the leg at the site of election. The diameter of the limb is equal to one-third the circumference (which can be measured by tape), thus giving the length of the flap from the site of election.

2. Fashion equal anterior and posterior flaps including the deep fascia and reflect them to a point 2.5 cm above the proposed line of bone section. Ligate and divide the long saphenous vein.

3. Mark the muscle groups, arbitrarily divided into four quadrants, by four stay sutures at the level of the proposed bone section.

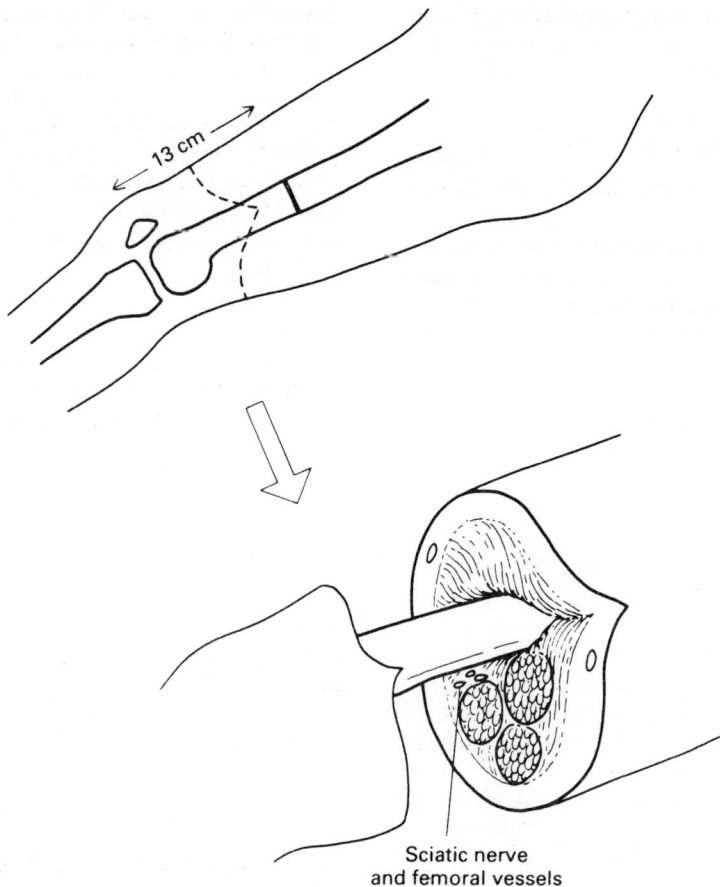

13 cm

Sciatic nerve
and femoral vessels

Fig. 68 Above-knee amputation

4. Divide the muscles shorter than the skin flaps and reflect them to the level of bone section.

5. Doubly ligate and divide the main vessels (femoral, profunda femoris). Cut the sciatic nerve higher than the bone cut end and ligate if bleeding from comitans nervi ischiadici to avoid future neuroma.

6. Reflect an area of periosteum (if possible) to cover the raw area of bone, retract soft tissue with a bone shield, divide bone with a saw, wax its bone marrow and cover it with the periosteum after filing the end.

7. Secure haemostasis.

8. Cover the bone end by suturing over it the lateral and medial then the anterior and posterior muscle groups in turn, opposing groups being sutured to each other.

9. Resuture the deep fascia and subcutaneous tissues and close the skin, providing two lateral drains (Redivacs) to drain deep and superficial spaces.

10. To prevent flexion deformity developing at the level of the hip joint, employ physiotherapy and splintage.

Long posterior flap of below-knee amputation (Fig. 69)

1. The patient is placed in the supine position under general anaesthesia.

2. Make a skin incision across the front of the leg 12 cm below the knee joint. Mark a 15 cm long posterior flap below the line of bone section which is 13 cm from the knee joint line. Deepen the incision down to the tibia.

3. Reflect the anterior tibial muscles and periosteum proximally for 1.25 cm.

4. Divide and bevel the tibia with a saw or Gigli saw. Dissect it out and divide the fibula 2.5 cm above this level.

5. Extend the ends of the skin incision vertically downwards thus forming the posterior flap. Reflect this flap upwards. Find the sural nerve and divide it clear of the site elected.

6. Deepen the posterior incision through the muscles down to the tibia and fibula, reflect them upwards and remove the leg. Locate and ligate the posterior tibial and perineal vessels and both saphenous veins.

7. Model muscles and then suture them over the site of bone division.

8. Achieve haemostasis.

9. Close muscle, fascia and skin with drainage.

Symes' amputation (Fig. 70)

1. Under general anaesthesia. A tourniquet may be applied while the foot is held at right angles over the end of the table.

2. Make an incision from the lateral malleolar tip vertically down to the sole, cross transversely and continue it over the medial aspect of the ankle terminating 12 mm below (not behind) the medial malleolar tip, to avoid damage to the calcaneal branch of the lateral plantar artery.

3. Dissect off the heel flap by keeping close to the bone. Divide the Achilles tendon. Depress the foot and incise across the dorsum through the tendons and down to the bone. Disarticulate the talo-tibiofibular joint by dividing the ligaments (the lateral ligament from within outwards).

4. Identify the vessels and ligate them.

5. Retract the soft tissues and remove both malleoli and tibial articular cartilage by sawing across the

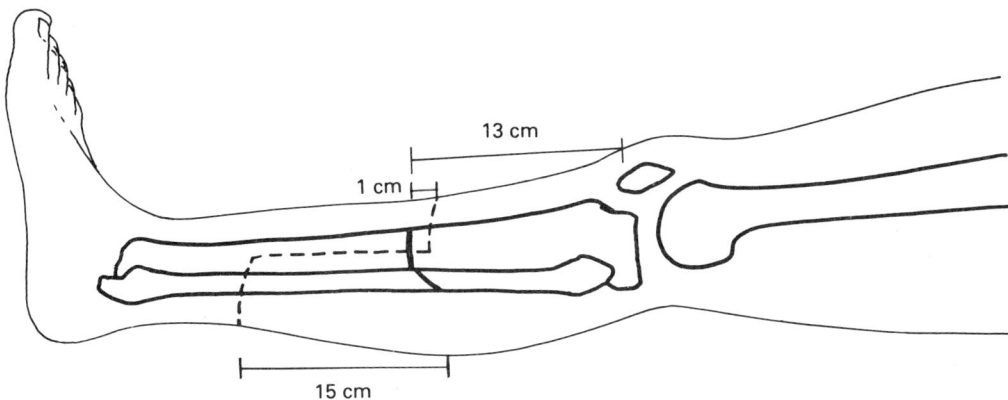

Fig. 69 Long posterior flap below-knee amputation

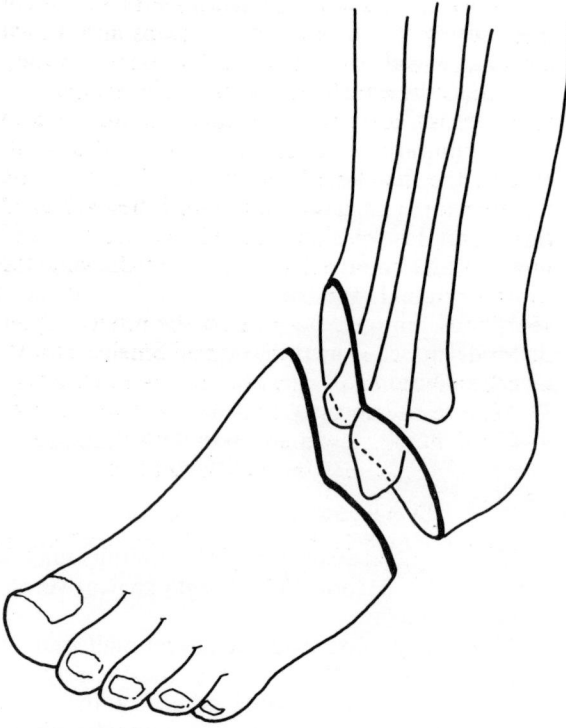

Fig. 70 Symes' amputation (lower tibial and fibular ends are cut after removal of the talocalcaneometatarsal bones of the foot)

bone as low as possible (avoid removing the epiphysis in the young).

6. Release the tourniquet, obtain haemostasis, leave in the drain and sew up the inferior skin flap anteriorly. An 'elephant boot' is used when the wound is sound.

3.26. Keller's Arthroplasty

Indicated in hallux valgus or rigidus.

Procedure (Fig. 71)

1. A tourniquet is applied under general anaesthesia and with patient in the supine position.
2. A 5 cm incision is made over the anteromedial aspect of the proximal phalanx and metatarsophal-

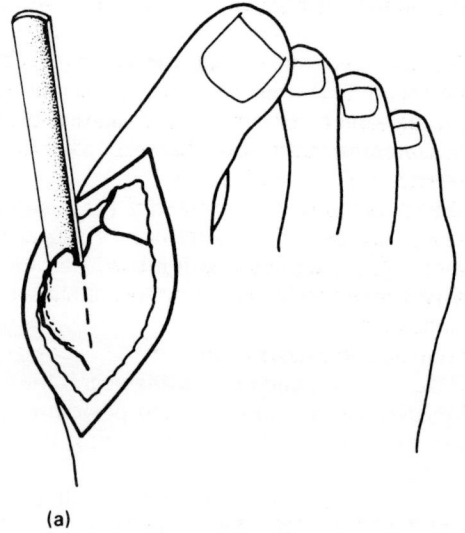

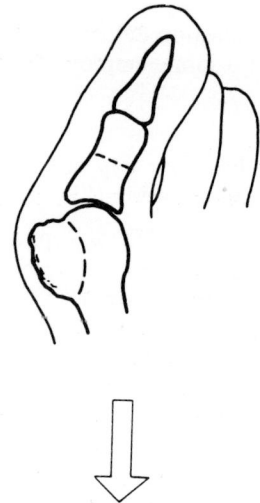

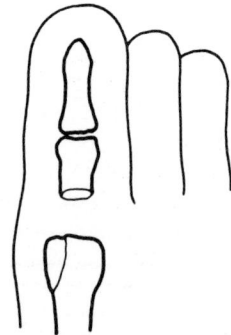

Fig. 71 Keller's operation for hallux valgus. (a) Removal of the metatarsal exostosis. (b) Removal of proximal third of the phalanx

angeal joint of the big toe—incise deep down to the bone.

3. The joint is opened medial to the extensor hallucis longus tendon.

4. The proximal third of the proximal phalanx is excised, preserving the flexor hallucis longus tendon (a Silastic implant can be used here).

5. The exostosis of the metatarsal head is excised with an osteotome. The medial collateral ligament is reconstructed, then the skin is closed.

6. A pad of gauze between the toes maintains the varus position.

7. Following the operation, early movements are initiated.

3.27. Open Medial Meniscectomy

Procedure (Fig. 72)

Preoperative quadriceps exercises and arthroscopy are required.

1. Exsanguinate with an Esmarch tourniquet and maintain exsanguination with a pneumatic tourniquet. The thigh is supported on a sandbag.

2. The skin is prepared.

3. Remove the bottom segment of the operating table while the patient is supine with knees flexed; the surgeon sits at the patient's feet with the foot of the injured side in his lap.

4. Make a 5 cm oblique incision from the lower medial corner of the patella downwards and medially to end 1 cm below the joint line (medial meniscectomy). A similar incision downwards and laterally on the outer side of the knee is used for lateral meniscectomy. Incise the capsule in the same line as the skin incision.

5. Open the synovium and inspect the joint interior, flexing and extending the knee. Look at the back of the patella.

6. The medial collateral ligament is retracted to obtain a view of the peripheral attachment of the cartilage.

7. A blunt tendon hook is applied over the free edge of the anterior horn of the meniscus which is then detached, using a scalpel horizontally between the anterior horn and tibial plateau.

8. The cartilage is firmly held in the left hand with a meniscus or Kocher's toothed forceps and drawn inwards towards the intercondylar space, dividing the peripheral attachment with a solid scalpel.

9. The posterior horn is divided, taking care to avoid injuring the posterior cruciate ligament. Rotation of the tibia laterally and flexion of the knee may help in this division. This is best achieved by keeping a Smellie's knife blade vertical to avoid injury to the collateral ligament and drawing the cartilage over it.

10. Divide the posterior rim via the intercondylar notch using a mirror-image curved Smellie's knife. Check that the entire meniscus has been removed.

11. The synovium and capsule are sutured separately. The skin is closed.

12. A crêpe pressure bandage is applied.

13. The tourniquet is removed.

Comment: Arthroscopic (closed) meniscectomy is now performed in many centres.

3.28. Internal Fixation of Femoral Neck Fractures

Procedure

1. On a special orthopaedic table with the patient in a supine position and under general anaesthesia.

2. The fracture is reduced by *traction in flexion*; this is followed by *internal rotation* and *abduction*.

3. This position is maintained and the X-ray apparatus is set up.

4. X-rays of the hip are used in two planes to ensure satisfactory reduction. An image-intensifier may be used.

5. The trochanter and the upper part of the femur are exposed through a 10 cm lateral incision.

6. Guide wires are inserted until one of them achieves the correct position, confirmed by radiograph, and the required length of nail is estimated.

7. The canalised trifid Smith–Petersen nail is then driven over the guide wire into the head after reaming the cortex. The wire is removed and the fracture is impacted. The position of the nail is

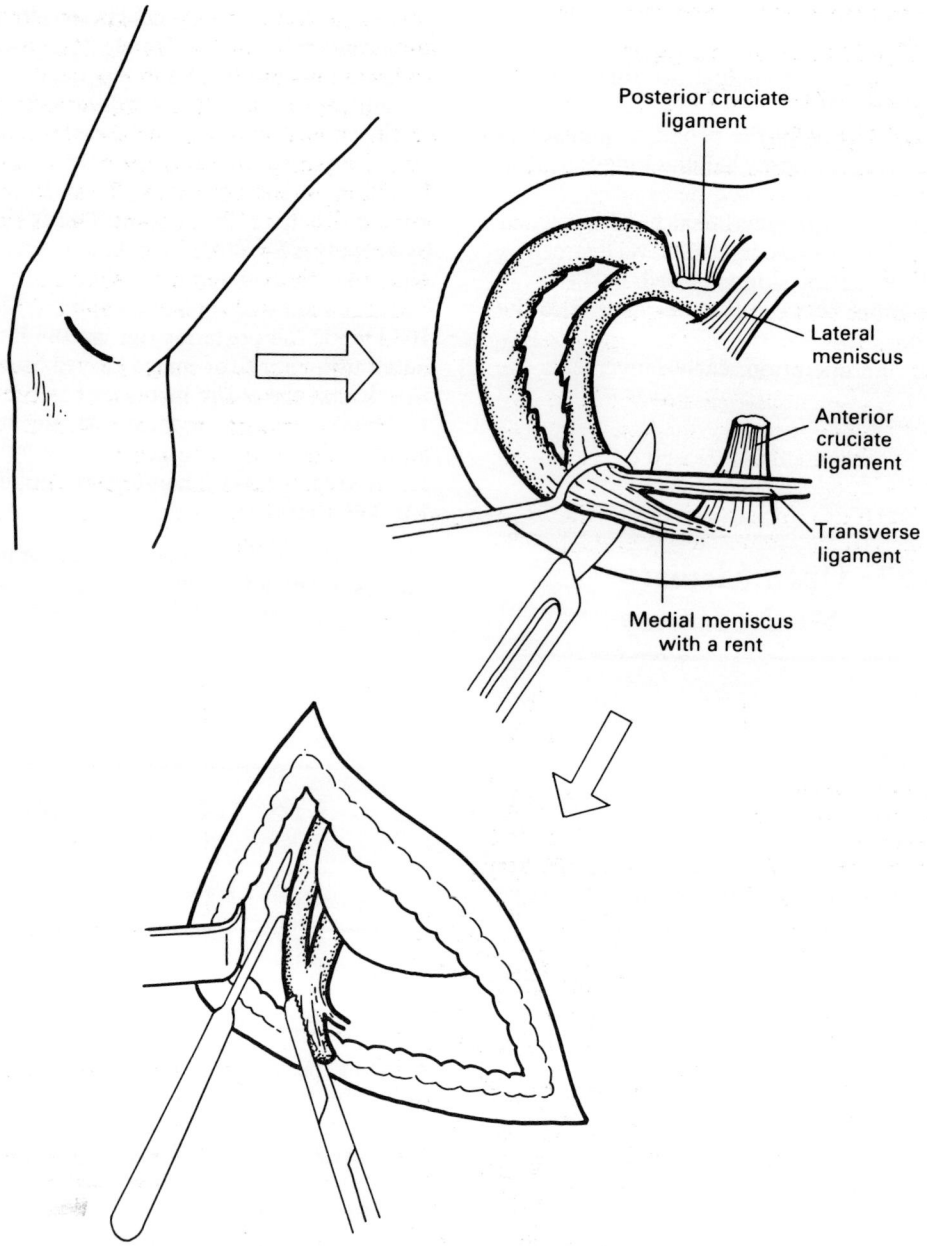

Fig. 72   Open medial meniscectomy

checked by further X-rays. In intertrochanteric or extracapsular fractures further fixation is obtained by a plate that holds the end of the nail and can be screwed down into the lateral aspect of the shaft of the femur—pin and plate or sliding (Pugh) nail.

8. The wound is closed with a Redivac drain.

9. Movements are commenced the day after the operation.

3.29. Posterior Approach and Arthroplasty of the Hip

Procedure (Fig. 73)

1. The patient lies on the unaffected side with the upper arm on a rest, and the pelvis supported by padded rests.
2. The skin is incised along the anterior border of the gluteus maximus from the posterior superior iliac spine to the greater trochanter and then downwards for approximately 15 cm.
3. The iliotibial tract is incised in line with the lower limb incision, and the gluteal bursa opened. The gluteus maximus is then separated along its fibres and retracted medially. Finally, the gluteus medius and minimus are freed and retracted.
4. The capsule is exposed by retracting the quadratus femoris and dividing the obturator internus with the gemelli marking them with stay sutures.
5. The capsule is opened in a T-shaped manner and the hip dislocated by rotating the thigh medially.
6. Arthroplasty is performed.
- Hemiarthroplasty, e.g. Thompson prosthesis may be inserted for intracapsular fractures of the femoral neck:
  - (a) The exposed femoral head is removed with a corkscrew like instrument and bone levers.
  - (b) The femoral neck is trimmed with an osteotome or power saw.
  - (c) Ream the femur. Insert the cement and prosthesis after proper anatomical orientation.

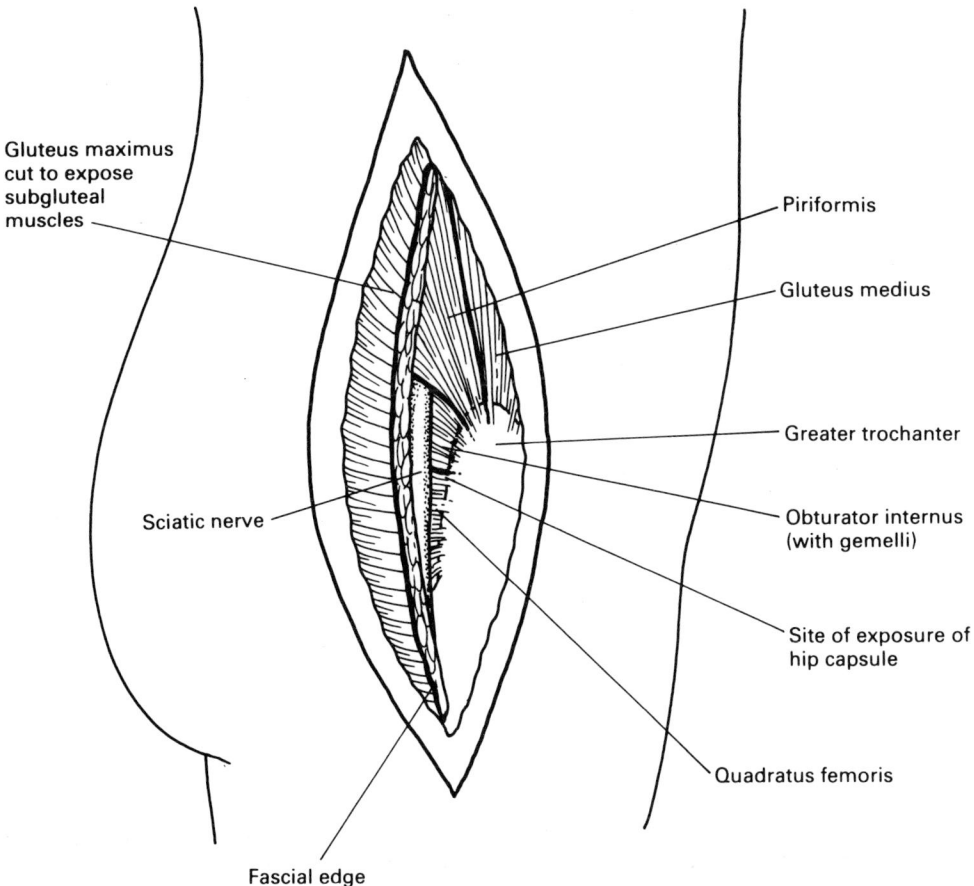

Fig. 73 Hip exposure—posterior approach

Gluteus maximus cut to expose subgluteal muscles

Piriformis

Gluteus medius

Greater trochanter

Sciatic nerve

Obturator internus (with gemelli)

Site of exposure of hip capsule

Quadratus femoris

Fascial edge

(d) Secure and reduce the prosthesis.
(e) Close the wound in layers, including a suction Redivac drain.

Comment: In hemiarthroplasty, the cementless Austin Moore prosthesis is another alternative.

- Total replacement (low friction) hip arthroplasty:
  (a) The head is dislocated and then excised using a power saw or osteotome.
  (b) The acetabulum is reamed.
  (c) The centring hole is closed by a mesh cup in the Charnley operation. The cement (antibiotic treated) is inserted followed by the acetabular component.
  (d) The femoral shaft is reamed. The cement and prosthesis are inserted after proper anatomical orientation.
  (e) The femoral prosthesis is reduced and secured.
  (f) The greater trochanter initially divided, to facilitate exposure, is replaced and fixed with wire sutures (only in Charnley's operation).
  (g) The wound is closed in layers and a suction drain is left *in situ*.

3.30. Laminectomy

Indications

- Spinal cord compression due to:
  —Intervertebral disc protrusion (prolapse), whether lateral or central.
  —Spinal stenosis, whether postdegenerative (osteoarthritis), congenital, postspondylolisthetic or unclassified (Paget's disease, tuberculosis and postoperative).
  —Vertebral trauma (due to oedema and/or fracture)—simple fenestration decompression may be adequate, but internal fixation is required in fractures or in multilevel laminectomy, using plate fixation or wiring of intact spinous processes (above and below). Posterolateral on-lay bone graft may be added for reinforcement.
  —Primary or secondary vertebral bone tumours—need fixation.
- Pain relief—chordotomy.
- Spondylolisthesis with nerve root or cauda equina compression—fusion of facet joints using screw fixation is required.

Preoperative assessment

All patients undergoing laminectomy must be assessed thoroughly.

Clinically
Persistent symptoms of sciatica (buttock and lower limb pain) with pain increased by coughing or straining; signs of slight forward tilt and lateral list (sciatic scoliosis); tenderness with limited back movement as well as limited straight leg raising may all present.

Neurologically (according to the compressed segment)
- S_1 Weak foot eversion and ankle jerk, and sensory loss along lateral border of foot.
- L_5 Weak big toe extension and knee flexion, increased knee jerk (weak antagonists) and sensory loss on the outer aspect of the leg and mediodorsal aspect of the foot.
- *Cauda equina compression* leading to urinary retention and sensory loss over the sacrum.

Radiologically
- Plain lumbar x-ray (to exclude bone diseases).
- Myelography (using metrizamide) to confirm, localise disc protrusion and exclude intrathecal tumour.
- Computerised tomography

Procedure (Fig. 74)

1. Under general anaesthesia. The patient is placed in a prone position with the spine flexed.
2. A midline incision is made. Deepen the incision to expose the spines and laminae. Reflect the erector spinae muscles with a wide raspatory and insert a self-retaining muscle retractor.
3. Remove two spines at their base and the supra- and interspinous ligaments with bone-cutting forceps and expose the dura by nibbling bone away from the laminae with bone forceps. Secure haemostasis.
4. In cases where the cord needs to be inspected clear the dura of fat and coagulate veins. Pick up the dura with stay-sutures and open it to look for intradural lesions. Later resuture it with silk. For chordotomy make a cut in the cord with a special angulated knife 3 mm deep from the denticulate ligament to the anterior nerve root on the appropriate side. (The fourth and fifth thoracic segments are opposite the second and third thoracic bodies.)
5. For removal of a prolapsed intervertebral disc, perform a hemilaminectomy: remove one spinous

Removal of
spinous
process

Lamina

Spinous
process

Angled bone
shears

Gentle retraction applied to
denticulate ligament

Posterior root

Dura opened

Rotating spinal cord to
expose the anterior surface
(in intradural lesions). One
or even two posterior roots
may be divided

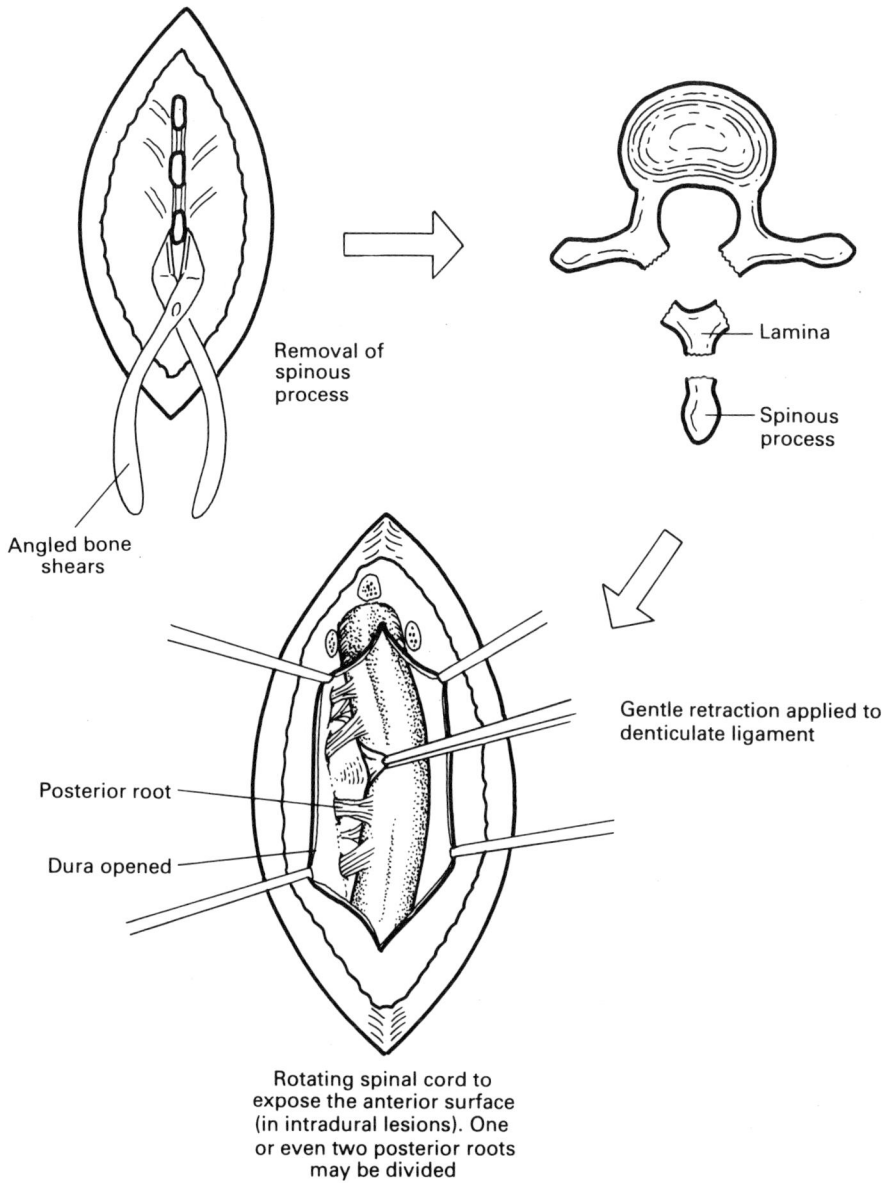

Fig. 74 Laminectomy

process and retract the cord and nerve root; divide the posterior longitudinal ligament over it, and curette it out with a rongeur.

6. Approximate the muscle and fascia with interrupted sutures and close the skin.

Note: Fenestration decompression (excising ligamentum flavum only) has now almost replaced formal laminectomy.

For more operations, see also Sections 1 and 4.

SECTION 4
Principles and Practice

Introduction

In this part, examiners test your common sense, practicality and grasp of elementary principles and are not interested in a display of encyclopaedic knowledge. Examiners want to make sure that you are familiar with your surrounding surgical atmosphere, and you are likely to be shown commonly used instruments and appliances, or confronted with clinical questions to test your clinical judgement and wisdom through discussion of X-rays. You may also be asked about controversial topics, e.g. advantages versus disadvantages of operations for breast carcinoma. It is therefore essential that you substantiate your reasoning and answer confidently. The mutual discussion may be interesting and stimulating and sometimes acts as an exchange of experience between the examiner and the candidate. If the examiner wants to tell you his practical way of management, listen to him carefully with interest. You may be questioned about the anatomical basis of surgery and may be shown bones.

This part therefore includes:

1. *General topics* already discussed in Section 1 (e.g. endoscopy, radiotherapy, chemotherapy, jaundice, shock, principles of skin grafting, postoperative pain relief, gut precancerous conditions, critical review of breast carcinoma management).
2. *Special practical questions.*
3. *Bones* (only in London College).
4. *Common instruments.*
5. *X-rays.*

4.1. Special Practical Questions

ORGANISATION OF OPERATING THEATRE
(Fig. 75)

Operating theatres should be near the intensive therapy unit (ITU), accident/emergency and X-ray departments. They should be constructed so that they are separate from the general traffic and air movement in the rest of the hospital (far from wards). A single floor reserved entirely for a suite of theatres is recommended. Alternatively a situation in a cul-de-sac rather than near a main thoroughfare is ideal. In order to reduce solar heat-gain, a position on a lower level in the hospital is favoured rather than on the top floor of a tall building. Clean and dirty streams of traffic in an operating department should be segregated practically. There should be a *transfer or changeover section* at the entry to/exit from the sterile zone. This protective zone also includes the recovery area, plaster room, changing rooms and various offices; seminar or teaching facilities may also be sited here.

The *clean zone* consists of scrub room and gowning anaesthetic room, exit lobby, rest areas and sterile store. The operating theatre and sterile preparation room form the *sterile zone*. The least clean area of the whole department is the disposal sluice or sink room and disposal corridor forming the *disposal zone*. The clean zone must include adequate storage rooms for equipment (or general supplies and sterile packets—staff base or office). An X-ray dark room, small laboratory, blood storage facilities, and rest rooms for surgeons and staff may be provided.

The processing and sterilisation of drape and instrument packets is either centralised in the hospital sterilising and disinfecting unit (operates in association with the main *central sterile supply department*) or carried out in the *theatre sterile supply unit* built adjacent to the operating department.

Personnel working within the department should be able to move from one clean area to another without having to pass through unprotected or traffic areas. Air-flow direction should be from the clean to the less clean areas. There should be no air movement between one theatre suite and another. Heating and ventilation should allow comfortable climatic conditions for the patient, surgeons, anaesthetists and staff.

The construction must be such that a high standard of cleanliness can be maintained. All surfaces should be smooth and washable and all joins between walls, ceilings and floors curved to

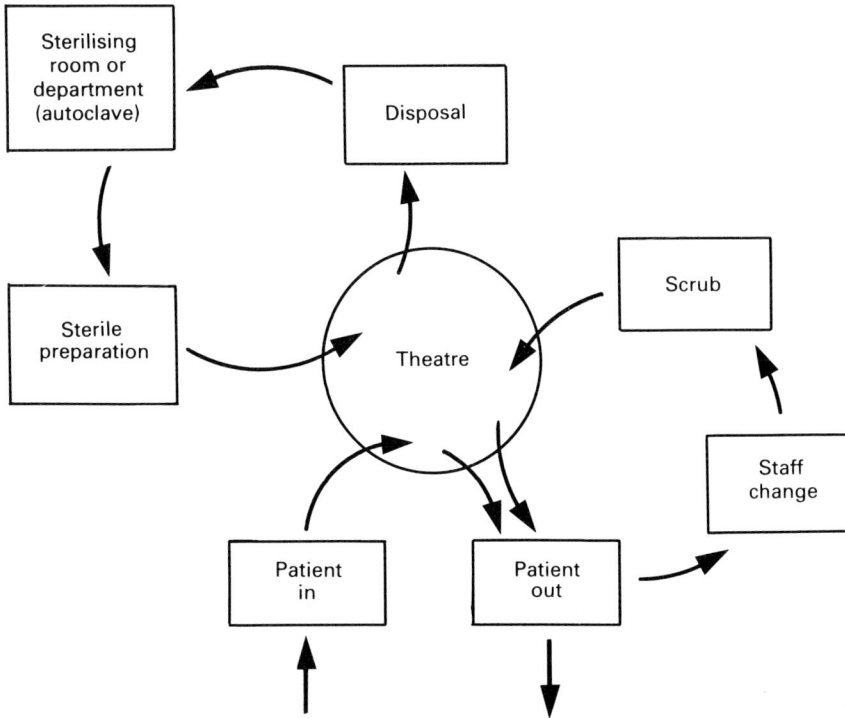

Fig. 75 Operating theatre organisation

minimise dust collection. The walls should have an impervious semi-matt surface with laminated plastic sheet finish, vinyl sheet or an epoxy resin paint (tiles are not ideal) as these finishes reflect less light. Colour is preferably pale blue, grey or green since they are less tiring to the eyes. The floor should also be impervious, made of terrazzo, rubber or vinyl with an antistatic composition to minimise the danger of an explosion due to a static spark.

There are three types of operating departments, the layout of each being dependent on the total hospital plan:
1. The single-theatre suite.
2. The two-theatre suite or twin suite.
3. Multiple-theatre departments (three or more).

Lighting and electricity

The mains voltage supplied in the UK is between 220 and 240 V, 50 Hz AC. Emergency lighting is provided either from batteries at a low voltage (12–24 V) or by a supplementary generator which provides electricity at the standard mains voltage. The artificial light makes daylight unnecessary, but the complete absence of windows is psychologically

disadvantageous to staff. If windows are fitted they should be small to minimise the solar heat gain or loss and facilitate heating and ventilation control. Provision must be made for blacking out operating areas if endoscopic operations are to be performed. This is achieved by special blinds.

The general lighting of theatres may be provided by fluorescent tubes or filament lamps (recessed in the ceiling) producing even illumination with no glare. For the actual operation (task) area, a shadowless illumination is vital and produced by directing the light from several angles to minimise shadows from the operator and his assistants.

There are three types of shadowless light fittings:
1. The *scialytic shadowless light fitting* consisting of an optical lens surrounding a single lamp of 150 W. Light rays from the lens are projected onto a circle of mirrors focusing light on the operation area with the aid of a lampholder.
2. The *metal reflector shadowless light fitting*—instead of mirrors the reflector consists of a concave, highly polished surface, either plain or made up of many facets.
3. The *multireflector shadowless light fitting*—has six to nine separate lamps instead of one lamp as in

(1) and (2) and special reflectors. Focusing is achieved by a single knob fitted to the light housing.

Surgical diathermy is a high-frequency electric current passed through the patient's body between two electrodes. As the surgeon applies the 'live' electrode to tissues, heat is generated at this point because of tissue cell electrical resistance. The effect is localised because the current from the 'live' electrode spreads out in the patient's body and travels to the 'indifferent' electrode (a large metallic sheet in contact with the patient's body). Diathermy is used for either electrocoagulation or cutting. Cutting is obtained by using higher current and a needle electrode; an arc is struck between this electrode and the underlying tissues producing a very hot arc (in excess of $1000\,^{\circ}$C) which causes tissue disintegration and has a cutting effect when moved. A surgical cautery consists of platinum wire loop or point raised to red heat by means of an electric current. This heated cautery point is then applied to tissues causing coagulation.

Static electricity, generated whenever two dissimilar materials are separated, can cause a spark especially in a dry atmosphere (with the potential danger of explosion). Static-forming materials include nylon, flannel and wool, viscose rayon, glass, cotton and linen, dry skin, wood, rubber and various plastics. Cotton, linen and viscose rayon are ideal for theatre clotting and towels, since they readily absorb moisture. Carbon black is finely dispersed through rubber resulting in an electrically conductive rubber which dissipates static electricity immediately. This black *antistatic rubber* has a distinctive yellow mark (to distinguish it from other types of rubber).

Switches and socket outlets installed on walls of operating theatres and anaesthetic rooms should be spark-free. Precautions are important to prevent an explosion from sparks or static electricity, particularly in the vicinity of anaesthetic gas leakage. Flammable gas concentrations exist only in an area extending for 25 cm from the leakage point, beyond which gases dilute to a non-flammable level.

Ventilation

This is of paramount importance:
● For the comfort of the staff.
● To remove the anaesthetic gases.
● To admit air free of pathogenic organisms.
The ventilated air passes through spinning water discs or a steam humidifier, resulting in 50–60% relative humidity. Combined with background heating (from pipes or panels within walls or ceiling) a ventilation system is a very satisfactory way of rapidly adjusting the temperature in the operating theatre and maintaining it between $18.5\,^{\circ}$C and $22\,^{\circ}$C (except during hypothermia anaesthesia). The minimum bacteriological air requirements are:
1. No detectable clostridium spores or coagulase-positive *Staphylococcus aureus*. No more than 35 bacteria-carrying particles/m³ of ventilated air is allowed (as tested on aerobic cultures).
2. During surgical operations, the concentration of bacterially contaminated airborne particles over a 5 min period should not exceed 180/m³. There are two good methods of assessing the bacterial content of the air—the *settling or sedimentation plate* (a culture plate on which bacteria in air are allowed to settle) and the *slit-sampler* (air is sucked through a narrow slit onto a rotating culture plate beneath it); the latter is a more efficient and quicker method.

Surgical sepsis has been greatly reduced as a result of installation of special ventilation systems. The following types are available:

Plenum turbulent air flow system   Positive pressure is essential to prevent contaminated air infiltrating into the theatre, and the air pressure in the theatre should be slightly greater than that outside the suite. A medium velocity system is the method of choice (at present). Air at roof level is drawn by a fan via a series of filters, humidified, cooled or warmed and forced into the theatre through high-level diffusers fitted into walls and ceiling. Filters must be changed regularly since bacteria such as Pseudomonas multiply on cooling coils and humidifier. The filter is made of disposable fabric and oiled mesh with pores of about 5 μm in diameter which are sufficient to filter airborne particles containing bacteria (not individual bacteria).

Laminar flow displacement ventilation system   Air moving at a unidirectional horizontal velocity passes through an efficient filter to remove inherent contamination. Positive pressurisation is as before but instead of turbulent air rapidly mixing with that already present in the theatre, the displaced air is introduced gently and merely displaces that in the theatre by quiet downward movement.

Others   A high impact/high exhaust enclosure was introduced by Charnley. This was improved to the Charnley–Howorth Surgicair enclosure and later to the Ex Flow Clean Zone unit (with no side walls). Another approach is a surgical plastic isolater.

ORGANISATION OF THE ACCIDENT/EMERGENCY DEPARTMENT
(Fig. 76)

An accident/emergency department is the shop window of the hospital service and is likened to Cinderella (hard working yet understaffed and not the most popular department in the hospital). Owing to the large number of injuries affecting limbs, it would be most appropriately run by an orthopaedic surgeon fully trained in the management of musculoskeletal injuries. The duties of the consultant in charge include:

● Administration and sorting of cases.
● Teaching and training.
● Resuscitation in major accidents.
● Definitive treatment of many of the less serious conditions.

Apart from the consultant in charge, registrar, senior house officers and nursing staff, there are general practitioners, ambulance service men and porters involved actively in the department's performance. It is beyond dispute that the best departments are those with consultants playing an active and full continuous role in the day-to-day work including initial treatment, continuous care and rehabilitation of injuries.

The department should include two fully equipped resuscitation rooms (for major cases), a treatment room (for potentially infected cases), a few (3–5) cubicles for examination and treatment of minor cases (dressing, suturing and foreign body removal), as well as a day ward (for observation of some cases) and a minor theatre for reduction of fractures, e.g. Colles' and dislocations. This may be combined with a plaster room (one of the resuscitation rooms may be converted into a minor theatre). Easy access by the ambulance service to

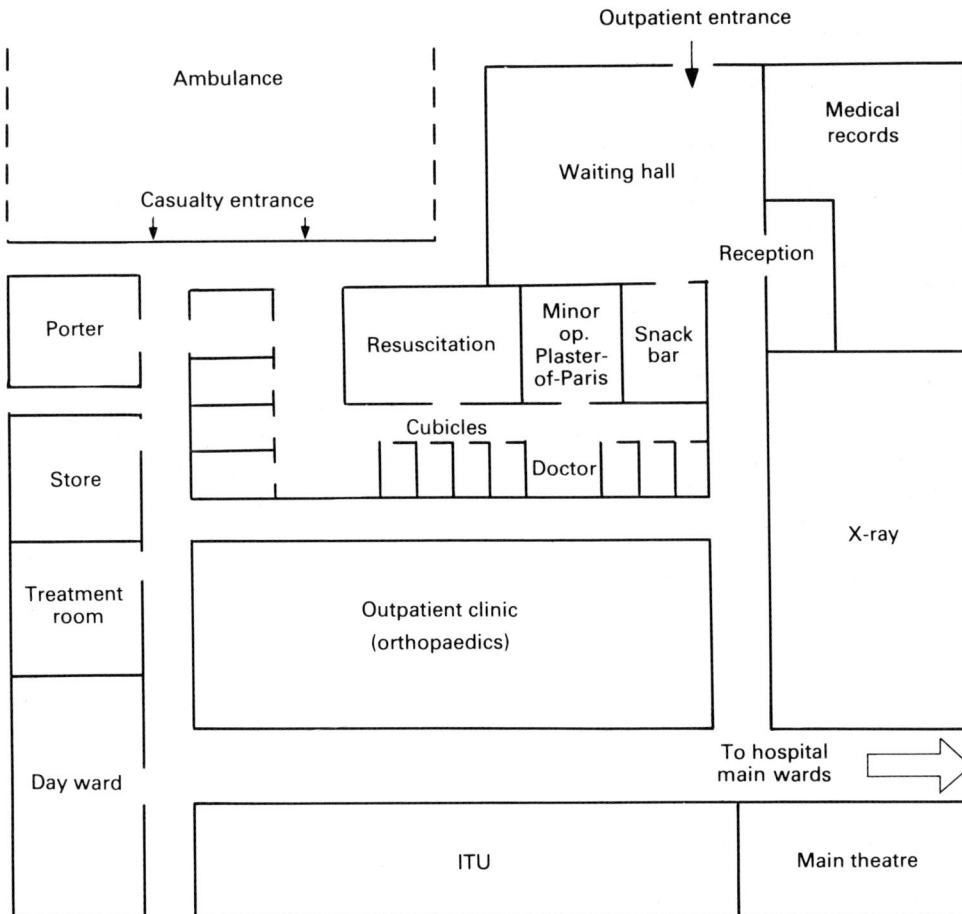

Fig. 76   Organisation of accident/emergency department

the accident/emergency department is important. Ancillary rooms include doctors' and staff rest room, porter office, reception and waiting room. The accident/emergency department should be near the X-ray department, intensive therapy unit and the main operating theatre.

The essence of a good accident/emergency service is the ability to meet sudden and particularly unforeseen needs. One of the least appealing features of such a service is that it is never off duty and it is likely to be busiest when most would prefer to be off duty and even in bed.

Major trauma cases include injuries of bones, joints, nerves and tendons which, although not likely to cause death, are serious injuries and constitute real emergencies. On the other hand, thoracic, abdominal and severe head injuries are critical and likely to be fatal. Minor cases include wounds and lacerations, as well as emotionally shocked patients. Thus in disasters (an emergency of such magnitude as to require extraordinary mobilisation of accident/emergency services) the management plan needs to be flexible and based on quick sorting of patients arriving at the hospital into three groups (triage classification):

1. Moribund and hopeless (too damaged to benefit from treatment, i.e. dying or dead).
2. Those whose lives are threatened requiring immediate attention (critically injured) and those who need attention fairly soon (seriously injured).
3. Those who can wait (minor injuries or emotional trauma).

It has been estimated that of the population examined in an accident/emergency department only 48% required the hospital services and 51% could have been treated at home. Among the 48% only 3.5% of cases were actually in danger of death (critically injured) while 44.5% were deemed real emergencies but not in danger of death. About 1% died in the accident/emergency department; and 19% of cases were admitted into hospital (11% to a surgical or specialised unit and 3% to the intensive therapy unit).

ORGANISATION OF INTENSIVE THERAPY UNIT

Ideally 1% of hospital beds should be devoted to the intensive therapy unit (ITU) (coronary care unit is excluded). The unit is under the shared responsibility of an anaesthetist as well as surgeons and/or physicians according to the nature of the case. Their duties include daily rounds (and regular follow-up), teaching, patient discharge and admission to another ward when the patient has recovered sufficiently.

Staff includes medical (anaesthetists, surgeons and/or physicians), junior medical (registrars, senior house officers and house officers), nursing (should be one nurse per patient per session or four nurses per bed per 24 h) and ancillary staff (porters, cleaners and technicians).

The ITU should be near the operating theatre, recovery area and hospital wards. Radiological and biochemical facilities should be available (especially blood gases analysis). The design, which should include dirty and clean areas (for infected and clean cases respectively), can be either: *open-plan* or *closed-plan* cubicles (to minimise infection and psychological trauma).

Whatever the design is, an ITU should be very clean, with a good air conditioning and ventilation system so that airborne cross-infection will be avoided. Such an efficient air flow pattern and air conditioning obviate the need for a special respiratory exhaust system.

Every bed should be specially equipped and provided with electrical outlets. Additional outlets for X-ray and domestic use are needed and should have separate grounding systems. Piped oxygen and suction outlets (two of each) are required for each bed. Pipeline supplies of both nitrous oxide and compressed air and a modern ventilator per bed are also required. Bedside and/or central monitoring of patients is a matter of individual choice. A monitor screen that can display signals from all beds should be sited in the staff sitting or conference room.

Rapid and frequent service, especially determination of blood gases, serum electrolytes, blood sugar and ESR, may demand the provision of a small computerised on-site laboratory with radiation protection material.

There should be sufficient storage space for drugs, linen, sterile supplies, i.v. fluids, respiratory, electric and diagnostic equipment and domestic cleaning machines. Equipment should be wall-mounted.

Accommodation for unit secretary/receptionist and visitors should be provided.

USE OF THE STETHOSCOPE IN SURGERY

Preoperative

- Checking blood pressure.
- Assessment of valvular and cardiac lesions. Murmurs necessitate prophylactic antibiotics to

prevent subacute bacterial endocarditis. Benign systolic murmurs may indicate hyperdynamic circulation as in anaemia and arteriovenous fistula and further investigations are required.

- Assessment of major vascular diseases, e.g. systolic murmur may indicate coarctation of the aorta, bruit may indicate carotid artery atherosclerosis, renal artery stenosis and aortic aneurysm.
- Assessment of chest conditions and treatment accordingly.
- Assessment of intestinal obstruction: either loud frequent sounds (borborygmi or high-pitched sounds), tingling or no sounds in silent abdomen of paralytic ileus.
- Assessment of vascular tumours, e.g. hepatoma and haemangioma of liver or eye proptosis due to arteriovenous fistula or skeletal metastases from thyroid carcinoma.

Operative

To confirm the correct placement of the endotracheal tube by listening to breath sounds on inflation of the lungs.

Postoperative

- Assessment of pulmonary complications after major abdominal or thoracic operation, e.g. atelactasis, abscesses and bronchopneumonia.
- Bases of lung should be auscultated for possible left ventricular failure decompensated after major operation. After cardiac operations a murmur may indicate leakage from an artificial valve replacement.
- In abdominal surgery, bowel sounds are checked by auscultating McBurney's point. Good bowel sounds may indicate that nasogastric suction can be removed.

DRAINAGE IN SURGERY

Drainage can be established operatively be channelling the contents of the internal organs externally (e.g. ileostomy, colostomy, urostomy, cholecystectomy) or by diverting the visceral contents internally (e.g. gastric drainage via pyloroplasty or gastroenterostomy, cholecystojejunostomy or ureterosigmoidostomy). More importantly, drainage is established by mechanical means for removal of:
1. Contents of body organs, e.g. Foley's catheterisation of urinary bladder and nasogastric tube

aspiration. There are also specialised drains for hydrocephalus or infected obstructed kidney.
2. Secretions of body cavities, e.g. peritoneal and pleural cavities.
3. Various tissue fluids, e.g. pus, blood, secretions, introduced solutions and air.

Drains are not substitutes for careful haemostasis and meticulous dissection. Drainage is discussed with items (2) and (3) in mind.

Indications for drainage

- Removal of material foreign or harmful to a particular location, e.g. potential nidus of infection.
- Obliteration of dead space.
- Monitoring and prevention of operative complications, e.g. delayed haemorrhage and anastomotic leak.
- Therapeutic value of fibrous tract after drain removal, e.g. T-tube track can be utilised for retrieval of residual biliary stone.

The value of drainage is debatable because it is inconvenient to the patient, it increases the risk of contamination (with introduction of infection), causes delay in healing (because drains are foreign bodies) and may even cause breakdown of anastomosis. Drains themselves damage delicate tissues by mechanical pressure and can irritate and induce fluid formation and collection. On balance, however, the following conditions should be drained:

- Abscess cavity with thick shaggy walls that must collapse for healing of the deepest portion, e.g. perforated appendix.
- Insecure anastomosis because of its size, tension, poor blood supply, infection or general metabolic abnormalities (like diabetes) or because the sutured organs lack peritoneal covering (extraperitoneal rectum) or are difficult to cover with omentum or nearby bowel.
- Anticipated leakage, e.g. gall bladder bed, pancreatic and splenic surgery.
- After trauma since missed foreign bodies and massive contmination lead to incomplete healing.
- Generalised peritonitis *per se* is not an indication for drainage since this would be physically and physiologically impossible. Therefore there should be other reasons for drainage, e.g. perforated viscus or a localised source of peritonitis.

Complications of drains

- Infection (exaggerated).
- Anastomotic leak and duodenal stump perfor-

ation (if in contact with suture line as a result of mechanical pressure necrosis).
- A vessel may be cut when the stab wound is made leading to haemorrhage.
- Bowel may herniate alongside a drain and become obstructed.
- Wound dehiscence and postoperative hernia formation if the drain is brought out through the primary incision.
- Loss of the drain, e.g. inside the abdomen. The drain should, therefore, be fixed to the skin for security.

Types of drain

Gauze packs and ribbon gauze wicks   Act by capillary action. They may be soaked in EUSol-paraffin to prevent adhesions to the raw healing surface.

Twisted nylon suture threads   Used sometimes after breast mass excision and minor operations.

Penrose   Very thin rubber tube of 2.5 cm diameter which can be filled with gauze and acts as a cigarette drain. Used in abscess cavities like wicks.

Sheet drains   Corrugated drain in which the fluid tracks to the surface in the gutter. Yeates drain (a sheet formed from parallel plastic tubes) in which fluid passes through tubes; once these have filled, it tends to track alongside the drain.

Tube drains   In abdominal surgery they are connected to bags, thus forming a closed system, but in pneumo- or haemothorax or post-thoracotomy they are connected to an underwater seal closed system. Multiple holes at the end are essential in case one hole becomes obstructed. A sump drain consists of two tubes. A large outer tube creates a sump in which fluid collects. A smaller tube lies freely at the bottom of this sump and is attached to a suction source (tissue can not be drawn into the holes of the smaller suction tube). A Shirley sump drain incorporates a side tube guarded by a bacterial filter so that sterile air can be drawn to the drain tip. When suction is applied, the air leak prevents tissues being sucked into the holes of the drain and blocking them.

Vacuum drains   A Redon trocar needle is used to attach the drain to the Redivac, Sterivac or Surgivac apparatus to create negative pressure with no need for a suction machine.

Drains must not be too rigid as they may damage viscera, nor too soft as they may twist or kink and become blocked. They should not be made of irritant material, e.g. rubber, but rather of silicone, Silastic or polyethylene. To serve its purpose the drain should be wide, patent and left *in situ* for an adequate period until drainage is minimal. If used prophylactically, e.g. duodenal stump or anastomotic leak, the drain should be left in place as long as the danger of perforation exists, i.e. for 10 days, until a fibrous track is formed which will act as an external fistula (with a safety-valve action).

RADIOACTIVE ISOTOPES IN SURGERY

Are used in three ways:

In vivo—**diagnostic scanning**

Diagnosis of space-occupying lesions (in bones, thyroid, brain, liver or mediastinum), assessment of function (renogram in kidney diseases, blood flow measurement and lung scanning in pulmonary infarction due to embolism). For example:
- ^{99m}Tc pertechnetate intravenously for scanning of skeletal metastases (bone isotope scan), vascular diseases and lung scan.
- ^{131}I in goitre and brain scan.
- ^{67}Ga for hepatic and mediastinal scanning (in Hodgkin's and non-Hodgkin's lymphomas).

A carrier material is needed as a radioactive marker, e.g. ^{131}I-labelled albumen is used in diagnosis of venous thrombosis and estimation of blood volume loss in shock, and ^{99m}Tc-labelled microspheres are used in lung scanning.

In vivo—**therapy**

Such radioactive isotopes are used for palliation and rarely for cure of tumours. Available as interstitial radiotherapy (e.g. radioactive gold grains, seeds and wires), as an intracavitory colloidal solution (e.g. radioactive gold solution to prevent recurrent pleural effusion in pleurodesis and to prevent malignant ascitic fluid accumulation) or as a special i.v. systemic radiotherapy (e.g. ^{32}P for polycythaemia rubra vera). Radioactive isotope therapy can also be administered using a linear accelerator, e.g. telecobalt (^{60}CO) in the radiotherapy of many solid tumours. Radioactive isotopes are used in non-malignant disease such as thyrotoxicosis and certain skin diseases, and also for pituitary and hormonal manipulation in terminal cases for pain relief.

In vitro—**radioimmunoassay in research**

- Physiology of fluid compartment measurement such as total body water, plasma volume, extracellular fluid, blood flow and cardiac output.
- Respiratory physiology using labelled O_2 and CO_2.
- Metabolism of protein, fat and carbohydrate.
- Electrolytes and membrane permeability.
- Formation and fate of lymphocytes and blood elements and RBC life-cycle and synthesis.
- Intracellular digestive enzymes.

MICROSURGERY

Telescopic spectacles or a simple operating microscope with high-intensity illumination can provide a stereoscopic magnified field of vision up to × 6 and × 40 respectively. The focal distance between the surgeon's eyepieces and his hands is 150–200 mm. The operating microscope needs to be sterilised and maintained. The instruments required are fine and delicate, e.g. ridge or beak-tipped forceps, titanium microsurgical needle holder, microscissors, suction cutter, fine needles with very fine suture materials such as 7/0, 8/0 silk and 9/0, 10/0 nylon or Prolene. Teaching is possible with a microscopic teaching aid.

Uses

Otolaryngology: in middle ear surgery fenestration, stapes operations, tympanoplasties and acoustic neuroma treatment.

Ophthalmology: in cataract surgery, keratoplasty, glaucoma and vitrectomy.

Neurosurgery: in intracranial aneurysms, thromboembolectomy and tumour surgery especially in spinal cord and bypass extracranial–intracranial anastomosis for stroke.

Plastic surgery: in micro- (below wrist) and macro- (above wrist) reimplantation surgery of the hand with anastomosis of vessels and nerves, and in transplantation of the great toe for use as a thumb. Also in vascular graft surgery.

Vascular surgery: in renal, carotid and small blood vessel anastomoses (it is technically possible to join vessels as small as 1 mm in diameter).

Gynaecology: in dissection and anastomosis of the Fallopian tubes in sterility cases.

Urology: in ureteric anastomosis and sphincteric surgery and in vasovasotomy in patients with bilateral vasectomy reversal.

Others:

- Casualty—for removal of foreign bodies and repair surgery.
- Paediatrics—for catheterisation of minute vessels in small babies.
- Dermatology—for diagnosis and treatment of skin lesions.

ASCITES

Either cirrhotic or malignant (tuberculous ascites is not discussed here). In malignant ascites there is no cure and the mechanism is unknown but there is mucous secretion and peritoneal infiltration. In cirrhosis, hypoproteinuria and portal hypertension are the main factors. Treatment of intractable ascites includes the following.

Medical treatment

With diuretics and chemotherapy, e.g. spironolactone therapy up to 450 mg/24 h (response time is 10–28 days), intracavitary chemotherapy with thiotepa or bleomycin cytotoxics.

Repeated tapping

Is uncomfortable, causes hypoalbuminaemia, marasmus and subcutaneous implantations and is expensive.

Peritoneovenous (PV) shunt

With Denver or LeVeen valves under local anaesthesia and prophylactic antibiotics. This will increase plasma volume and urine volume and improve nutrition. The valve is inserted intraperitoneally with the valve pump connected by an abdominal tube that is drained subcutaneously into an internal jugular vein.

Postoperative therapy

Includes diuretics, inhalation against resistance, probably a corset or binder, and sometimes anticoagulants.

Complications of PV shunts

- Death due to fluid overload.
- Blockage of the shunt is the major problem and is due to the recurrence of ascites, a non-compressible Denver valve or direct puncture of

venous tubing. The leak is detected by a shunto-gram and treated by regular Valsalva's man-oeuvres, and an increase in diuretics. Shuntogram may be diagnostic and therapeutic. The Denver valve may need to be pumped and the shunt may need revision.

- Failure.
- Sepsis and fever.
- Emboli, e.g. clots, tumour pieces, cholesterol or air.
- Tumour spread locally or systemically.
- Venous thrombosis.
- Catheter migration.
- PV shunt coagulopathy with bleeding (rarely).

Contraindications for PV shunts

- Short life expectancy.
- Cardiorespiratory cripple.
- Poor liver function.
- Loculated viscous or blood-stained ascites (block PV shunt quickly).

ADHESIONS

Adhesions are the commonest cause of intestinal obstruction in the Western world accounting for one-third of intestinal obstructions in general and 50% of small bowel intestinal obstructions. They are also the most likely cause of intestinal strangulation.

In developing countries where laparotomies are a rarity and where hernias go untreated until they reach an enormous size or strangulate, intestinal obstruction due to adhesions is uncommon and strangulated external hernias head the list of causes of intestinal obstruction.

Peritoneal healing and aetiology of adhesions

Clinical and experimental studies have shown that unsutured peritoneal defects heal rapidly and usually without adhesion formation. Centripetal growth from the wound margins contributes little to the healing process. The entire defect becomes endothelialised simultaneously and not gradually from the border as in epithelialisation of skin wounds. The new mesothelium is derived from subperitoneal perivascular connective tissue cells which resemble primitive mesenchymal cells. If there is ischaemic injury (e.g. if the tissues were crushed) and the peritoneum is sutured or ligated, because of a marked decrease in fibrinolytic activity,

fibrin adhesions almost invariably form and later become fibrous intra-abdominal adhesions. Many substances may contaminate the peritoneal cavity at the time of laparotomy and induce foreign body granuloma and adhesion formation, e.g. fragments of gauze, lint or cotton wool, clumps of antibiotic powder or glove dust powder such as talc (magnesium silicate), lycopodium and starch powder.

Classification of adhesions

Congenital (about 2%) e.g. Meckel's diverticulum, malrotation of the colon or congenital bands. Although they are rare, they may occasionally give rise to strangulation.

Acquired These are the most common type.
1. Postoperative (about 80%), e.g. appendicectomy and gynaecological surgery. Although much less commonly, abdominoperineal rectal excision and total colectomy are also particularly likely to be followed by obstructive adhesions.
2. Postinflammatory (about 18%), e.g. acute appendicitis, diverticulitis, pelvic infection, Crohn's disease and cholecystitis in this order of frequency.

Prevention of adhesions

Various methods have been used in an attempt to prevent adhesions. They are probably ineffective but may be harmful and may even increase the incidence of adhesions.

- The instillation of various fluids, e.g. Dextran 70, povidone-iodine, or distension with gas introduced intraperitoneally to hold the damaged surfaces apart.
- Enhancement of peristalsis in an attempt to disrupt early fibrinous adhesions.
- The covering of peritoneal surfaces with an extraordinary variety of inert membranes and lubricants or with grafts of peritoneum.
- The use of enzymes to digest adhesions, e.g. trypsin and hyaluronidase.
- The instillation of substances to inhibit deposition of fibrin, e.g. steroids, anticoagulants and fibrinolytic agents.

Treatment

- The vast majority of adhesions are completely harmless and in many instances are life-saving by promoting anastomotic healing and localising intra-abdominal inflammation.

- Conservative nasogastric suction and i.v. drip are indicated in early postoperative intestinal obstruction and where there have been previous episodes of subacute intestinal obstruction or several previous operations for division of adhesions.
- The majority of acute intestinal obstructions due to adhesions, however, require immediate surgical relief by freeing of a kinked or compressed loop of bowel; rarely resection or bypass (short circuit) may be needed.
- Recurrent adhesive small intestinal obstruction may need small bowel intubation for 7–10 days with a 300 cm long, 18 Fr Foley tube inserted via a jejunostomy. It is threaded through and splints the small bowel. Once the tube tip reaches the caecum the balloon can be inflated. The gastrointestinal tract should be sucked out and emptied prior to intubation.
- Rarely plication operations are carried out for recurrent intestinal obstruction due to adhesions, e.g. Noble's seromuscular bowel plication, Childs and Phillips mesenteric plication and Takita's operation of anchoring the greater omentum to the lesser sac and plicating bowel loops by their mesentery.

Comment

It is highly recommended that after any laparotomy, wherever possible, the omentum is brought down between the gut and the abdominal wall (after placing the small intestine in organised loops). This avoids dangerous small bowel adhesions to the posterior aspect of the midline incision; instead omental adhesions to the posterior aspect of the anterior abdominal wall are formed and are easy to detach.

SUDDEN DEATH DURING SURGICAL OPERATION

Anaesthetic error

Hypoxia May be induced by the following. Undetected respiratory obstruction, kinked or displaced endotracheal tube, vagal stimulation caused rarely by intubation, oesophagoscopy, mediastinoscopy or bronchoscopy. Wrong gas or wrong connection. Tension pneumothorax due to rupture of emphysematous bulla after positive pressure ventilation. Mendelson's syndrome or chemical pneumonitis due to hydrochloric acid aspiration during anaesthesia while gag reflex is absent and endotracheal tube is not cuffed or inflated properly. Undetected hypotension and falling blood pressure due to internal bleeding. Air embolism via undiscovered disconnected i.v. line especially the subclavian one.

Wrong drugs or misadministration Anaphylactic reaction to anaesthetic agent, to dextran or undetected incompatible blood transfusion (detected during operation only by falling blood pressure and sudden unexplained wound bleeding). Overdosage of local anaesthetic, e.g. procaine released systemically after regional i.v. anaesthesia. Accidental injection of direct or indirect depressant (vasodilator), hypotension induced by ganglion blockers, lignocaine and aminophylline. Cardioplegic action of hyperkalaemia. Arrhythmia due to cardiac irritation by chloroform or cyclopropane and adrenaline.

Patient problems

Operation after recent myocardial infarction or in a patient with a diseased myocardium or cardiogenic shock, severe dehydration and electrolyte imbalance (in intestinal obstruction), pulmonary oedema or severe chest disease can all lead to death. Other risk factors include shocked patient due to leaking aneurysm, upper gastrointestinal tract bleeding or ruptured ectopic gestation. Also amniotic fluid embolism during delivery.

Surgical error

- Hypotension induced by rough manipulation of bowel and mesenteric stretching, and rarely by sympathectomy.
- Cardiac arrhythmia induced by cardiac catheterisation, open heart surgery and wrong non-synchronised DC shock (S on T phenomenon).
- Oculocardiac reflex induced by pressure on eyeballs in ophthalmic operation (vagal stimulation).
- Accidental incision of groin aneurysm misdiagnosed as abscess with uncontrollable bleeding.

CAUSES OF SECOND DAY POSTOPERATIVE JAUNDICE

- Anaesthetic toxicity, e.g. halothane.
- Drug toxicity, e.g. chlorpromazine (Largactil).
- Operative stress superimposed upon pre-existing liver disease or viral hepatitis.

- Liver hypoxia, e.g. underperfusion and hypotension.
- Haemolysis due to excessive or incompatible blood.
- Extrahepatic biliary residual stone or cholestasis.
- Ligated or injured common bile duct.
- Leakage of bile into peritoneal cavity (with transperitoneal absorption of bile, often associated with sepsis and shock).
- Septicaemia and cholangitis (late).
- Pulmonary embolism (after 7th day).

4.2. Bones

These are only shown in the English College to open discussion on selective orthopaedic topics, e.g.

Humerus to discuss the effect of fractures on the nerves which are in contact with it (radial nerve in shaft fracture, ulnar nerve in medial epicondyle fracture and axillary nerve in shoulder dislocation).

Tibia to discuss structures attached to the tibial plateau, and the mechanism and types of meniscus injury as well as the operative procedure of meniscectomy.

Femur to discuss fractures of the neck and their management as well as hip dislocation (both traumatic and congenital) with its management.

Skull (is rarely shown) to discuss the foramina in the cranial fossae. Difficult questions on this bone may be asked purposely to fail certain candidates who performed badly in the written and/or clinical part of the examination.

4.3. Common Instruments and Appliances

The purpose of showing an instrument is to open discussion on the surgical management of a particular condition, e.g. Bakes dilator, Desjardin gall stone forceps and T-tube are shown to discuss exploration of the common bile duct for biliary stone. The following are short notes on commonly presented instruments at the examination:

1. *Bronchoscope*: made of brass with lamp carrier. The metallic tube is fenestrated with two distal holes to allow for inflation of the lung when the bronchoscope is introduced into the other lung. There is no graduation. The distal end is bevelled to lift the epiglottis during introduction. There is a proximal short small tube that serves as an anaesthetic attachment.

2. *Negus rigid oesophagoscope*: made of polished brass and differs from the bronchoscope in the following ways:
- No fenestration.
- The tube is graduated in centimetres to measure the level of scoped oesophagus.
- Has twin lamp carriers on its sides.
- The distal end is not bevelled but is guttered or fissured to allow for suction and better biopsy performance.
- No proximal anaesthetic attachment piece since oesophagoscopy is *always* performed under separate endotracheal intubation (general anaesthesia) while bronchoscopy can be performed *either* under local anaesthetic spray of the oropharynx or under general anaesthesia.

3. *T-tube*: used for biliary drainage after common bile duct exploration or as a splint for ureteric anastomosis. The size is French gauge, i.e. circumference in mm so that a T-tube size 12 Fr has a circumference of 12 mm and a diameter of 12 divided by 3 ($d = \frac{c}{\pi}$) = 4 mm. T-tubes should be of latex or rubber but never of plastic since the latter is hardened by bile, making the tube difficult to remove. Furthermore latex and rubber stimulate fibrinous adhesion leading to a safe track. There is little reaction to a plastic tube and therefore the risk of biliary peritonitis is greater. T-tube is used once only.

4. *Foley catheter*: A self-retaining balloon catheter usually used for drainage of urinary bladder retention or monitoring urine outflow. It can be used for cholecystostomy, caecostomy, peroperative large bowel irrigation and for common bile duct peroperative cholangiography. The size is by French gauge as in T-tubes. The larger the capacity of the balloon the more is the residual urine or fluid (more infection). The balloon can be pulled to sit snugly over the prostatic bed after enucleation or transurethral resection (TUR) of the prostate with the therapeutic value of haemostasis accomplished by balloon pressure over the prostatic bed. The Teflon-coated latex type of catheter with or without

Bardcomatic (already inflated balloon) is not favoured owing to its small lumen, irritant material (crystallisation and infection around catheter tip), possible balloon puncture and bubbling of its material. They are usually used for short periods in catheterising patients with acute urinary retention who are waiting for cystoscopy and/or TUR of the prostate. After TUR of a prostate or bladder tumour a three-way *Simplastic Foley catheter* is used (size 22 or 24 Fr) for continuous irrigation of the bladder for a short period (usually 7 days).

Permanent indwelling Foley catheters (changed every 3 months) of Silikon 100, e.g. Dover type, are preferred to those made of Silastic (latex outer surface with silicone elastomer coating the drainage lumen) because the former have a wider lumen and are made of very inert material that does not bubble after long use.

5. *Joll thyroid retractor* with twin sharp prongs and threaded expanding bar for retraction of upper and lower cervical skin flaps in thyroidectomy.

6. *Joll thyroid aneurysm needle* for threading the suture around thyroid vessels prior to ligation and division.

7. *Ochsner trocar* with cannula and sucker attachment; in gall bladder decompression introduced through a purse-string prior to cholecystectomy or bypass. You may also be shown *Desjardin gall stone forceps.*

8. *Hurst oesophageal bougie*: rubber filled with mercury.

9. *Mousseau barbin tube* ⎫ inserted for palliative
⎬ bypass in oesophageal
10. *Celestine tube* ⎭ carcinoma.

11. *Sengstaken Blakemore triluminal decompression tube*: used in acute bleeding from oesophageal varices in portal hypertension. It is rubber, X-ray opaque and serves for gastric suction and, with a gastric balloon and oesophageal balloon, to decompress the gastric and oesophageal varices respectively.

12. *Lane clamp* for gastroenterostomy (non-crushing occluding clamp).

13. *Payr stomach clamp* (crushing clamp for partial gastrectomy).

14. *Doyen clamp* (non-crushing occluding) traditional soft intestinal clamp.

15. *Bakes dilator* with malleable shaft for common bile duct surgery. It has an olive head to avoid trauma during pushing and pulling of the dilator through the duodenal papilla.

16(a) *Martin endarterectomy stripper.*
  (b) *Cannon endarterectomy loops.*

17. *Tibbs arterial cannula* for filling distal artery (with heparinised saline) after embolectomy.

18. *Fogarty embolectomy catheter* with a guide wire inside and a terminal latex balloon.

19. *Myers varicose vein stripper.*

20. *Dormia basket stone dislodger.*

21. *Bladder (Lister) metallic sound.*

22. *Smellie meniscectomy knife.*

23. *Brodie director* with a probe for fistula surgery. The proximal part helps in division of tongue tie.

24. *Humby skin graft knife.*

25. *Lloyd–Davies operating sigmoidoscope.*

26. *Colostomy bag*: made of disposable plastic. It is not drainable (no outlet) and comes with or without a deodorising filter.

27. *Ileostomy bag*: drainable with a special security clip. Used many times. No deodorising filter.

28. *Urostomy bag*: drainable but with a non-reflux valve which can fit wide-bore night drainage tube. No deodorising filter.

29. *Parks rectal retractor, Goligher rectal speculum* and *ordinary proctoscope* (how to assemble them and how to apply them to the rectum).

30. *Periosteal elevator, Doyen rib raspatory, rib approximator and spreader.*

4.4. Clinical Radiology: Questions on General Principles

Q1

1. (Fig. 77).
(a) What is the abnormality?
(b) How do you treat?

Answers on p. 290

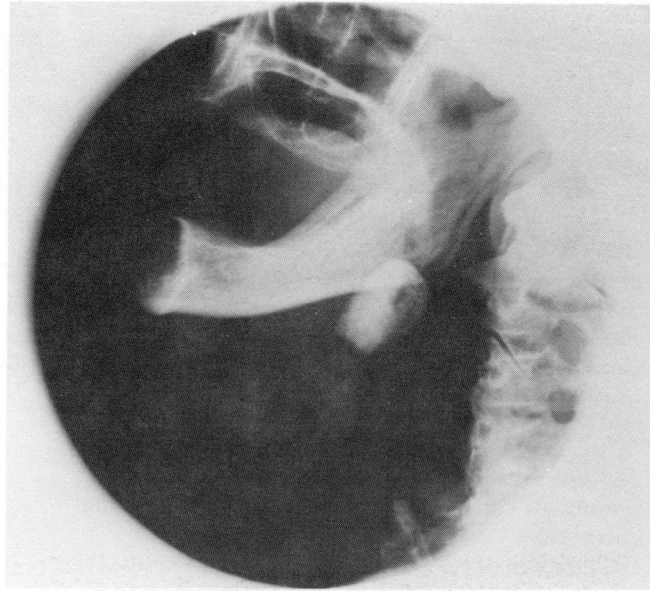

Fig. 77

Q2

2. A 40-year-old man with dysphagia (Fig. 78).
(a) What is this investigation?
(b) What is the lesion?
(c) What is your treatment?

Answers on p. 290

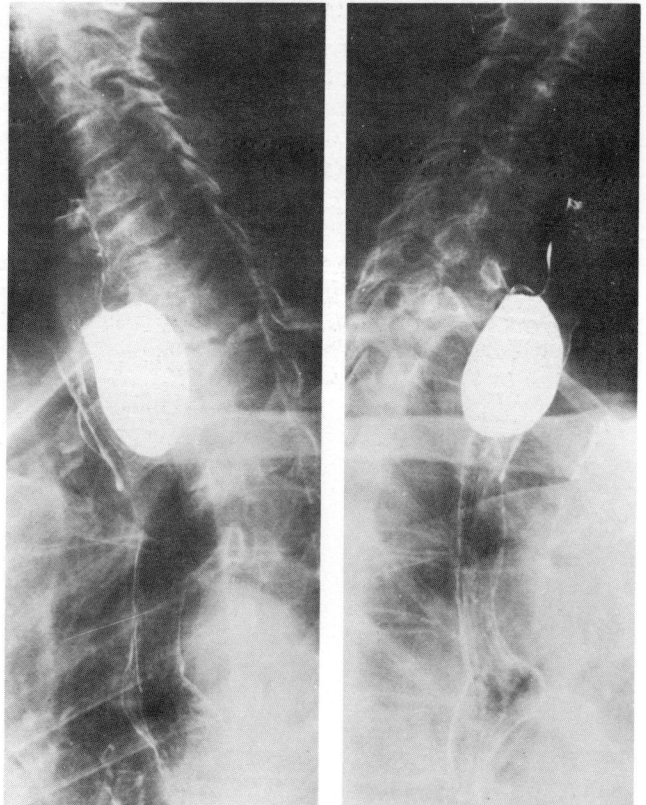

Fig. 78

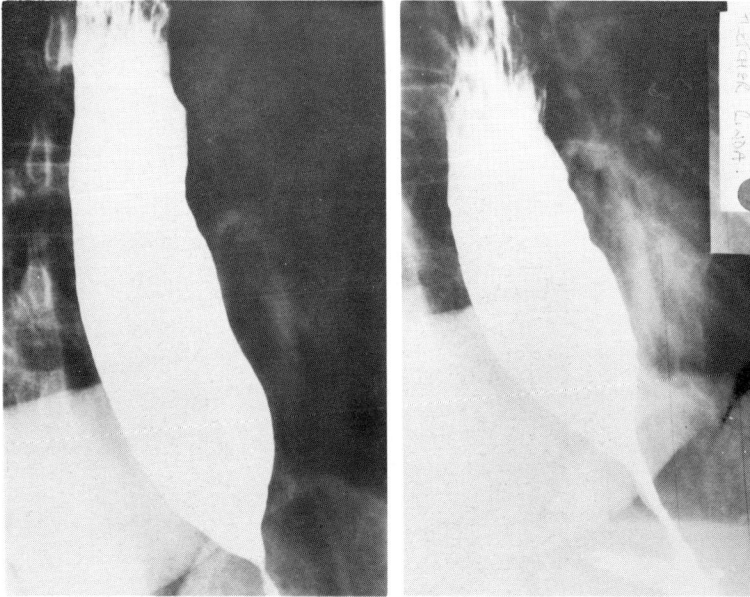

Fig. 79

Q3

3. A 40-year-old woman with dysphagia (Fig. 79).
(a) What is the abnormality?
(b) What are the complications?
(c) How do you treat?

Answers on p. 290

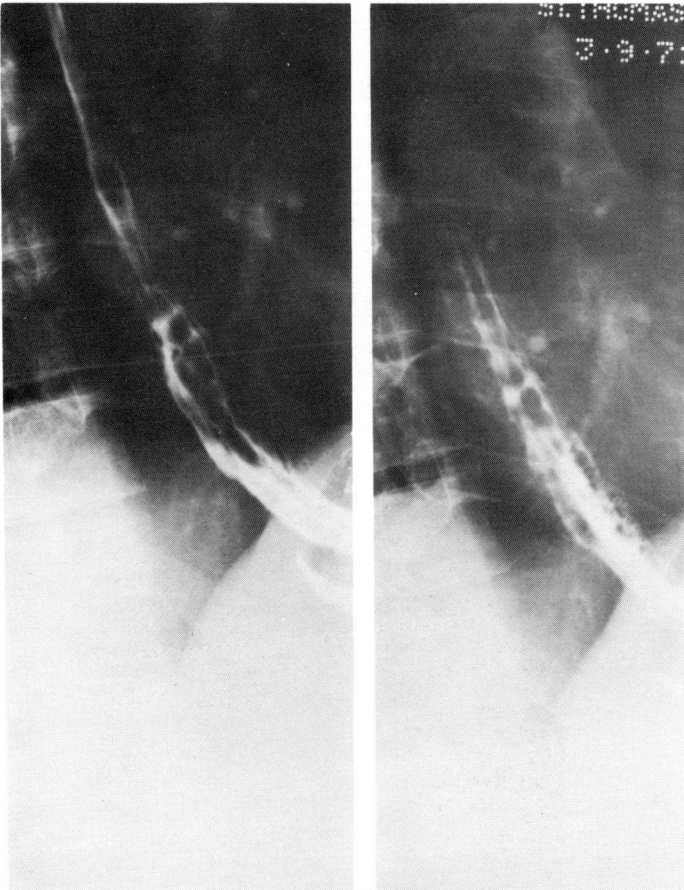

Fig. 80

Q4

4. A 45-year-old man admitted to hospital
   with splenomegaly (Fig. 80).
(a) What is the investigation and the
    abnormality?
(b) What is the diagnosis?
(c) Are there any other valuable radiolog-
    ical investigations?
(d) How do you treat now?
(e) What is the main complication and
    how do you treat it?

Answers on p. 290

Q5

5. A 45-year-old man with periodic abdominal pain and vomiting (Fig. 81).
(a) What is the investigation?
(b) What is the diagnosis?
(c) Discuss your management.
(d) What are the indications for surgery?

Answers on p. 291

Fig. 81

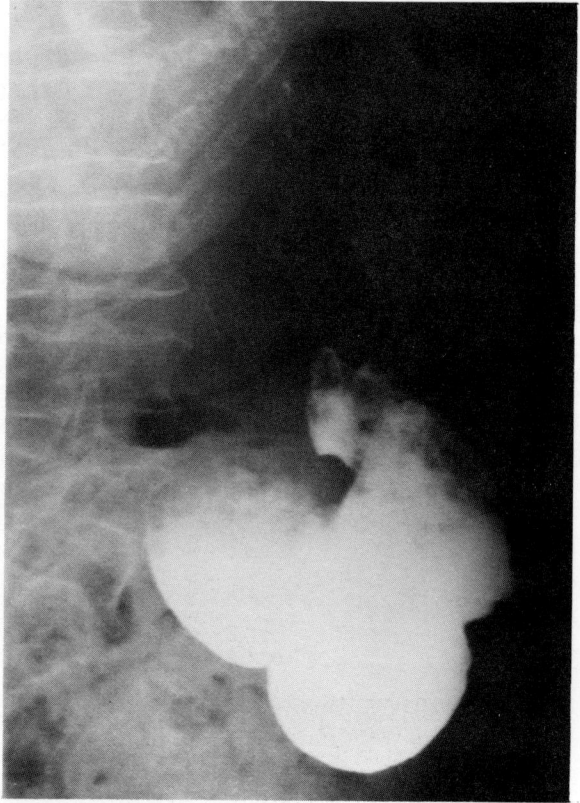

Q6

6. A 60-year-old woman with severe abdominal pain (Fig. 82).
(a) What is the abnormality?
(b) What is the most likely diagnosis?
(c) List the conditions that can produce a similar appearance.
(d) How do you treat?
(e) What advice do you give the patient postoperatively?

Answers on p. 292

Fig. 82

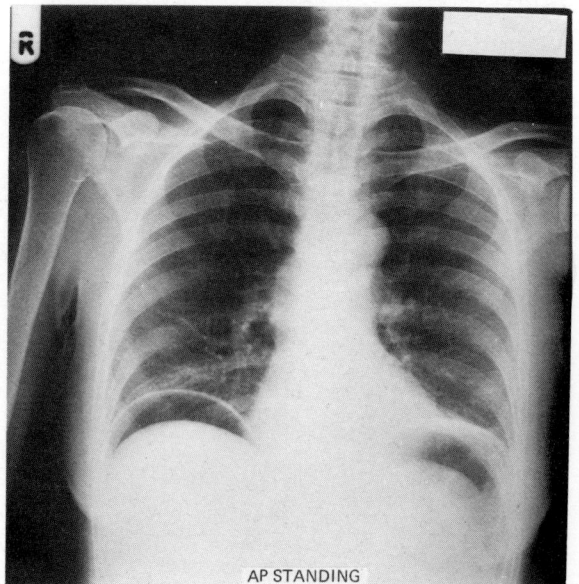

AP STANDING

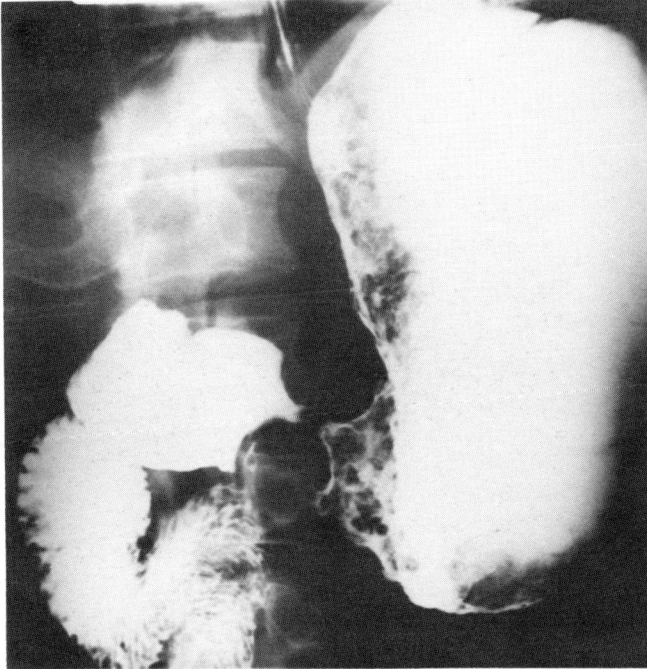

Fig. 83

Q7

7. A 50-year-old man with vague upper abdominal pain (Fig. 83).
(a) What is your diagnosis?
(b) How do you manage?

Answers on p. 293

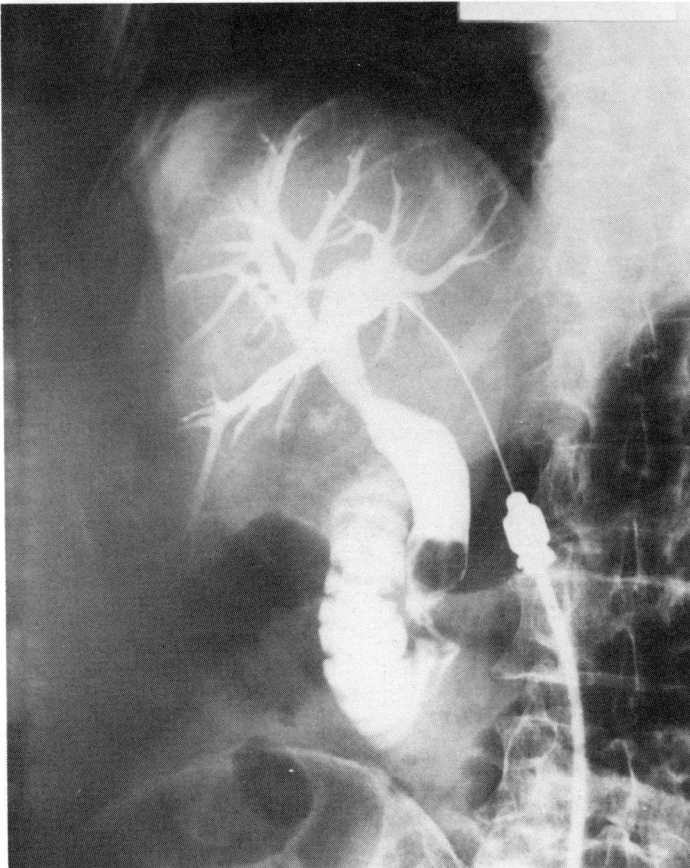

Fig. 84

Q8

8. A 60-year-old man with pain (Fig. 84).
(a) What is this investigation and what are the procedural requirements?
(b) What is the abnormality?
(c) What is the clinical presentation?
(d) How do you treat?

Answers on p. 293

Q9

9. (Fig. 85).
(a) What is this investigation and diagnosis?
(b) What are the indications for common bile duct exploration?

Answers on p. 293

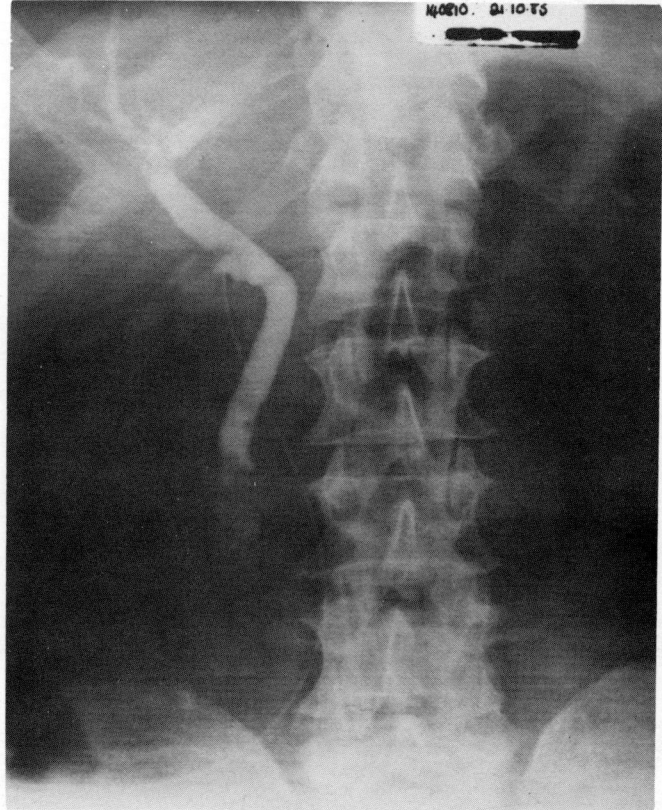

Fig. 85

Q10

10. A 50-year-old woman in her 10th post-operative day (Fig. 86).
(a) What is this investigation and diagnosis?
(b) How do you treat?

Answers on p. 294

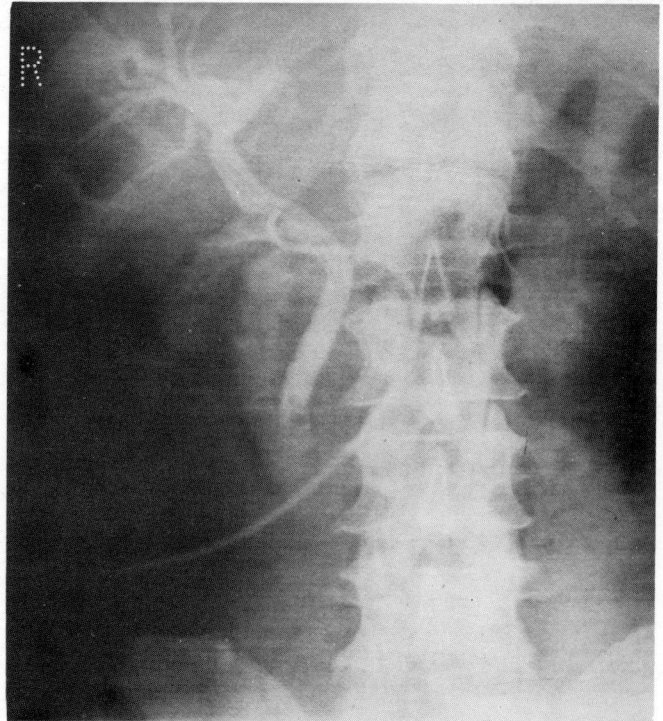

Fig. 86

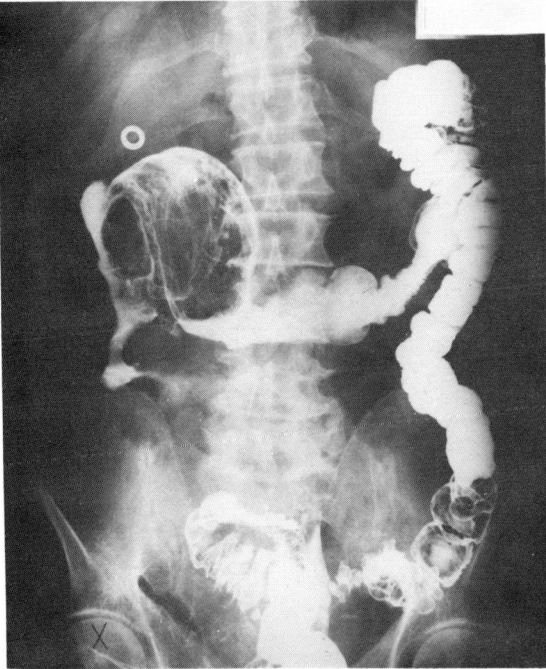

Fig. 87

Q11

11. A 55-year-old woman with vague acute abdominal pain (Fig. 87).
(a) What is the investigation and diagnosis?
(b) What one other clinical presentation is there?
(c) What is the definitive treatment?

Answers on p. 294

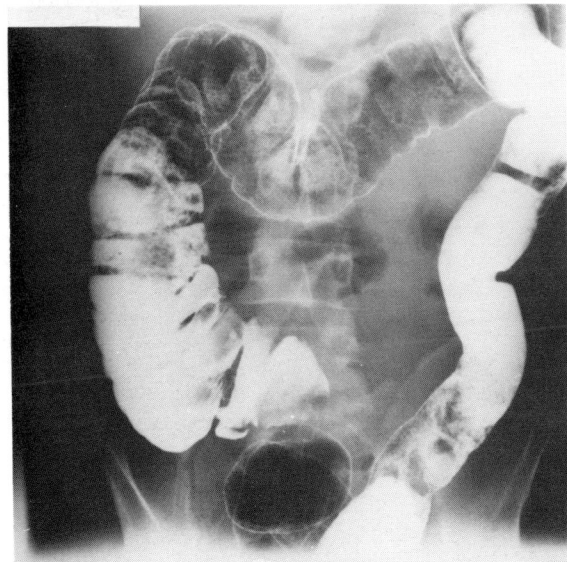

Fig. 88

Q12

12. A 27-year-old man with diarrhoea (Fig. 88).
(a) What are the radiological findings in this barium enema?
(b) What is your diagnosis?
(c) What are the indications for surgery?

Answers on p. 295

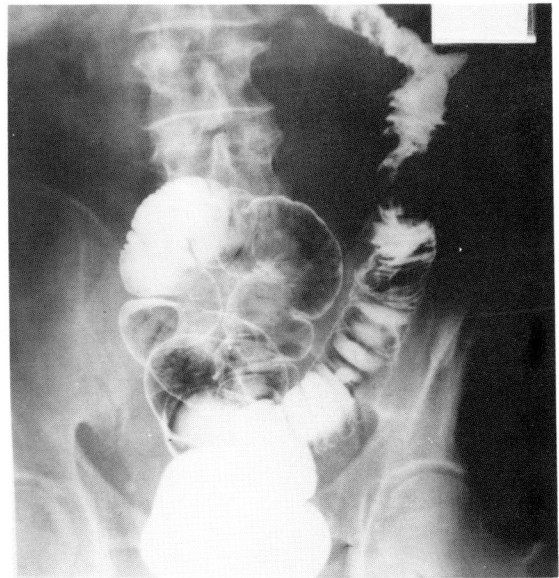

Fig. 89

Q13

13. A 57-year-old man with recent change of bowel habits (Fig. 89).
(a) What is the investigation and abnormality?
(b) What is your diagnosis?
(c) How do you treat?

Answers on p. 295

Q14

14. A 60-year-old woman with vague abdominal
    pain of 4 h duration (Fig. 90).
(a) What is the investigation and diagnosis?
(b) What are the other clinical presentations?
(c) Discuss the treatment.

Answers on p. 296

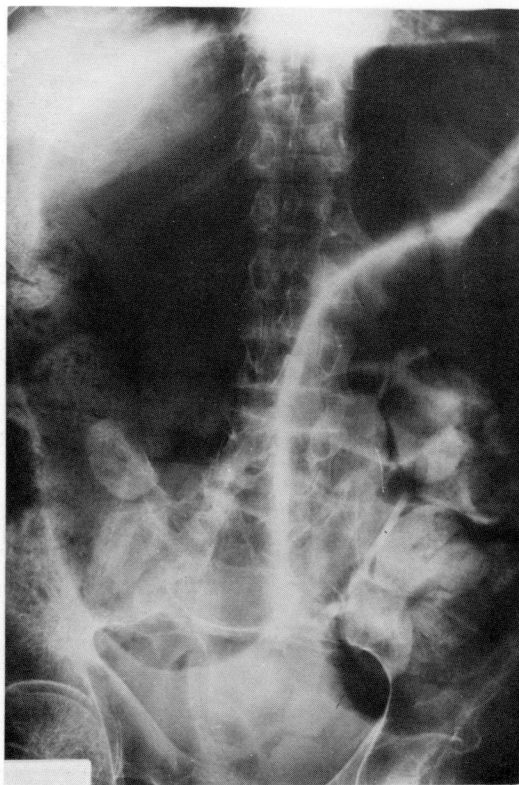

Fig. 90

Q15

15. A 50-year-old man involved in a road traffic
    accident (Fig. 91).
(a) What is the investigation?
(b) What is the diagnosis?
(c) What is the clinical presentation?
(d) How do you treat?

Answers on p. 296

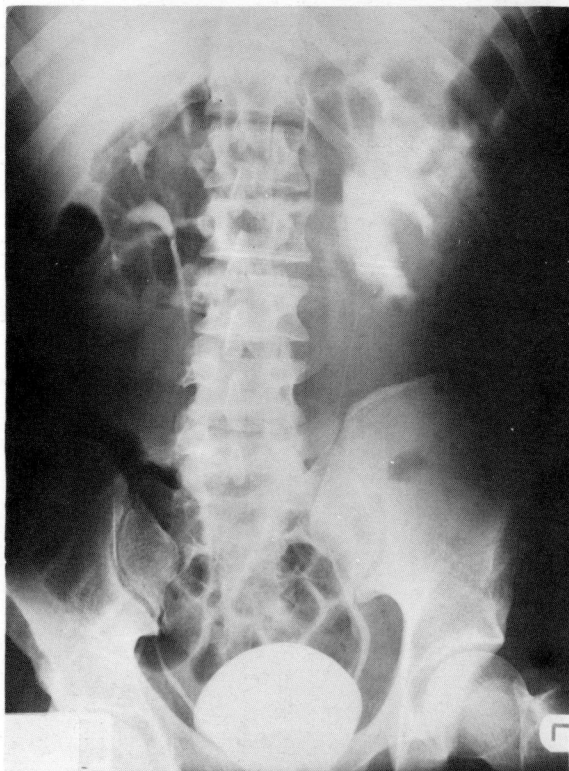

Fig. 91

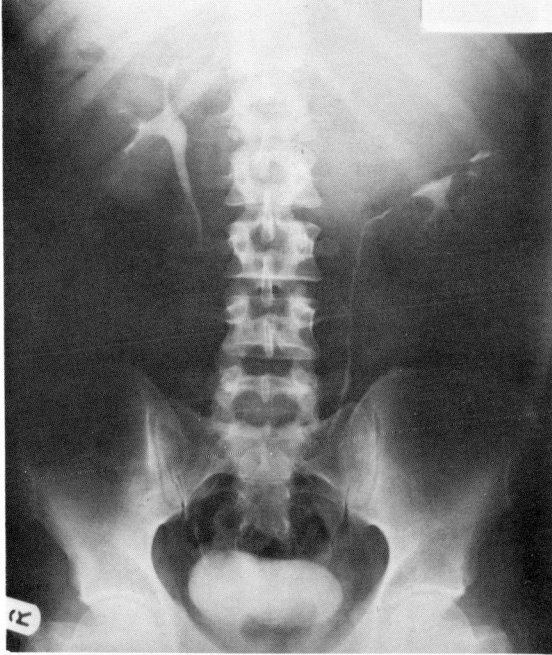

Fig. 92

Q16

16. A 35-year-old man presenting with pyrexia (Fig. 92).
(a) What is the investigation and diagnosis?
(b) What are the other presentations of this condition?
(c) What is your treatment?

Answers on p. 298

Q17

17. A 55-year-old man presenting with vague lower abdominal pain (Fig. 93).
(a) What is the investigation?
(b) Describe three abnormalities.
(c) How do you treat?

Answers on p. 299

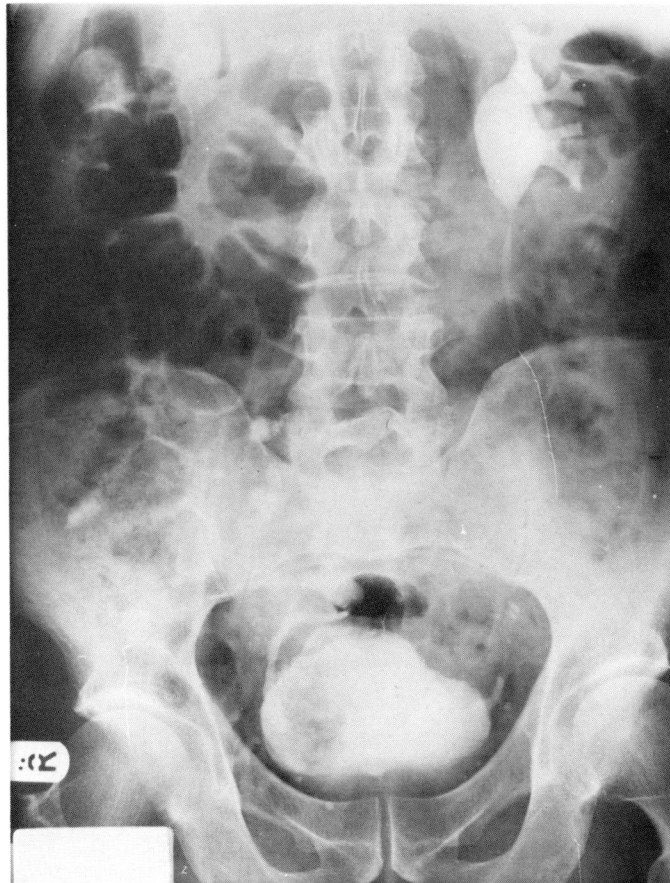

Fig. 93

Q18

18. A 65-year-old man complaining of difficult micturition (Fig. 94).
(a) Describe three abnormalities.
(b) What is the diagnosis?
(c) How do you treat?

Answers on p. 299

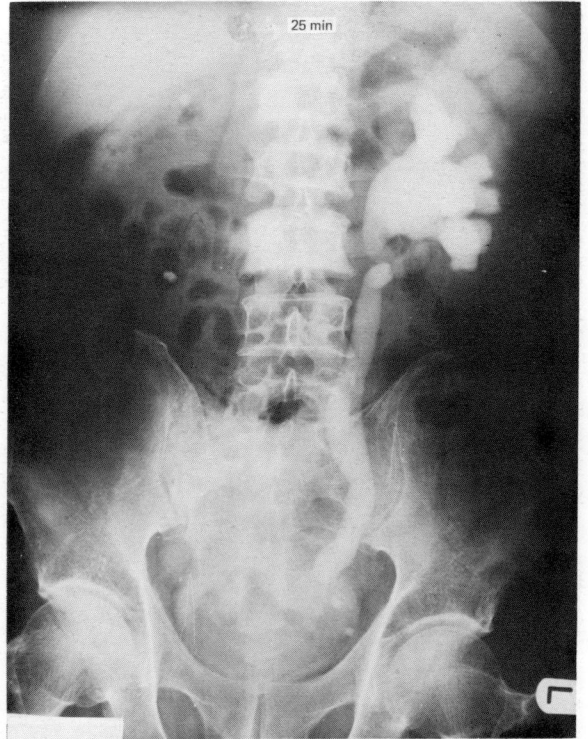

Fig. 94

Q19

19. A 60-year-old man with right abdominal pain (Fig. 95a and b).
(a) What is the investigation?
(b) Spot three abnormalities.
(c) What is the treatment?

Answers on p. 299

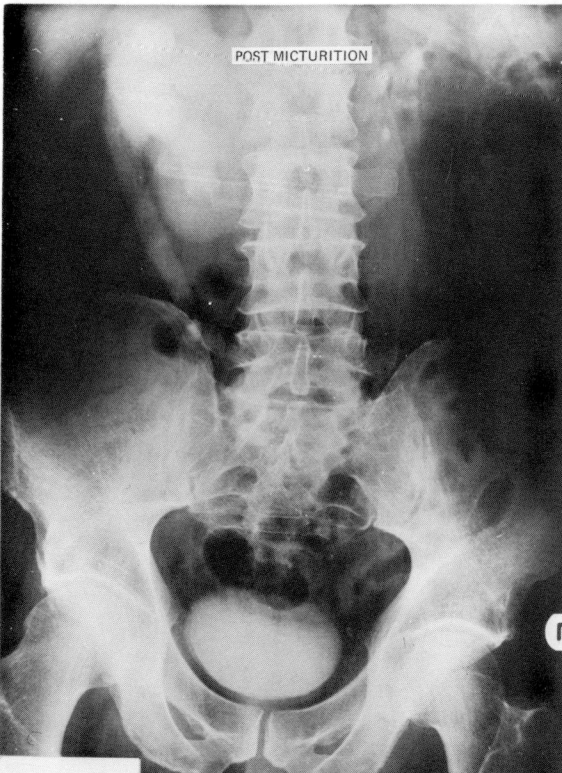

(a)

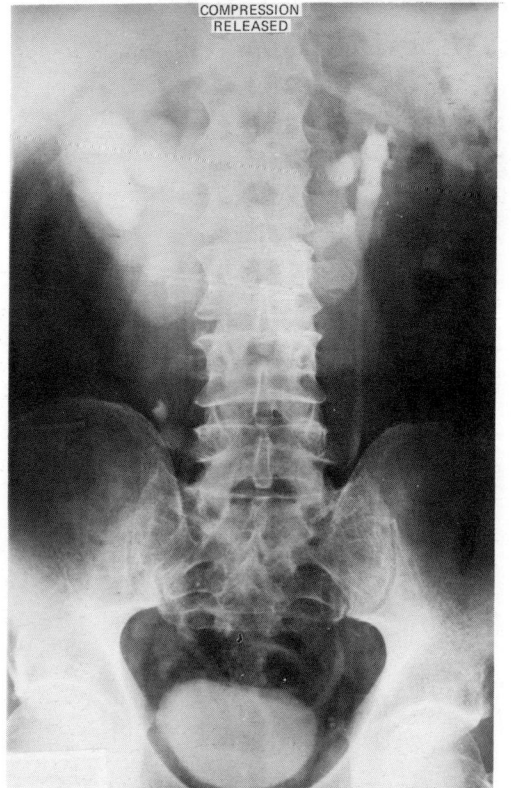

Fig. 95

(b)

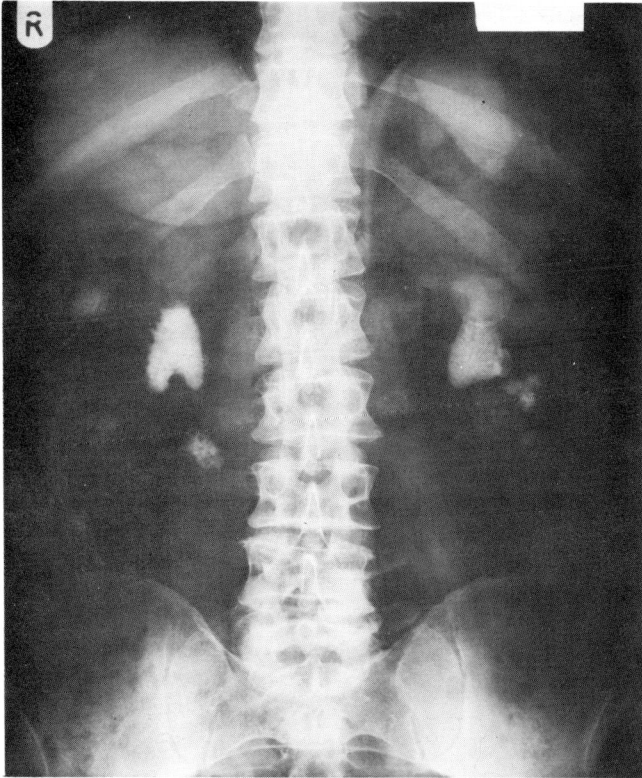

Q20

20. A 59-year-old woman presenting with recurrent problem 5 years after operation (Fig. 96a and b).
(a) What is the abnormality? and diagnosis? How do you confirm it?
(b) What is your management?

Answers on p. 301.

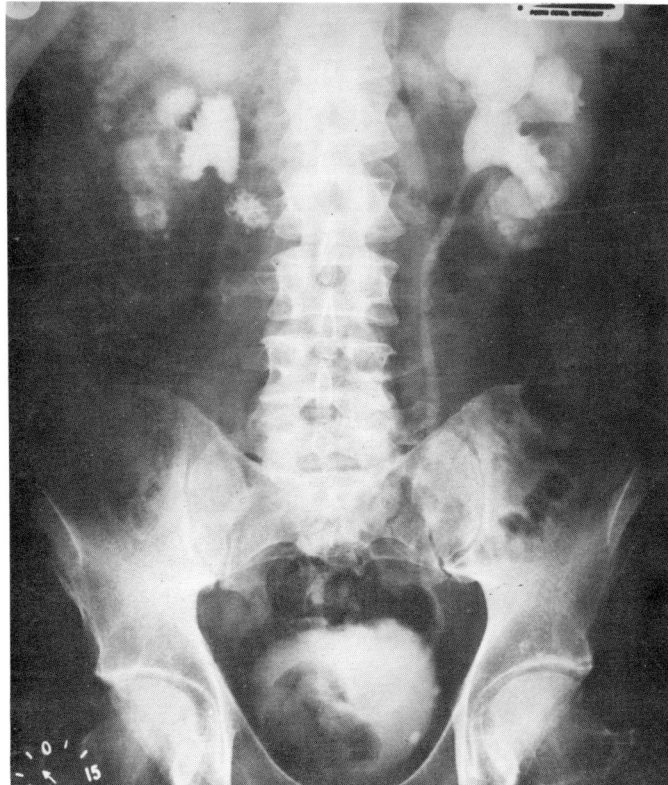

Fig. 96

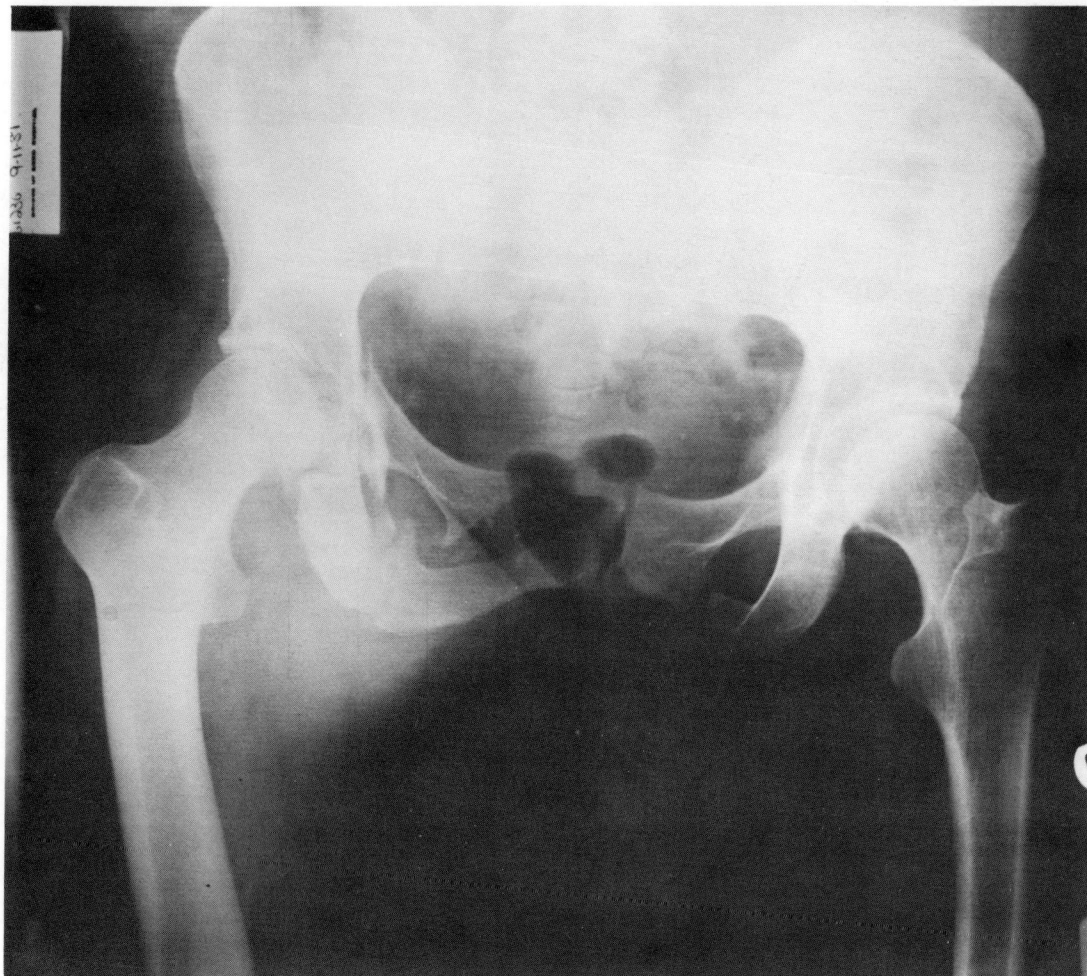

Fig. 97

Q21

21. A 50-year-old man admitted to hospital because of a road traffic accident (Fig. 97).
(a) What are the abnormalities?
(b) How do you treat?

Answers on p. 301

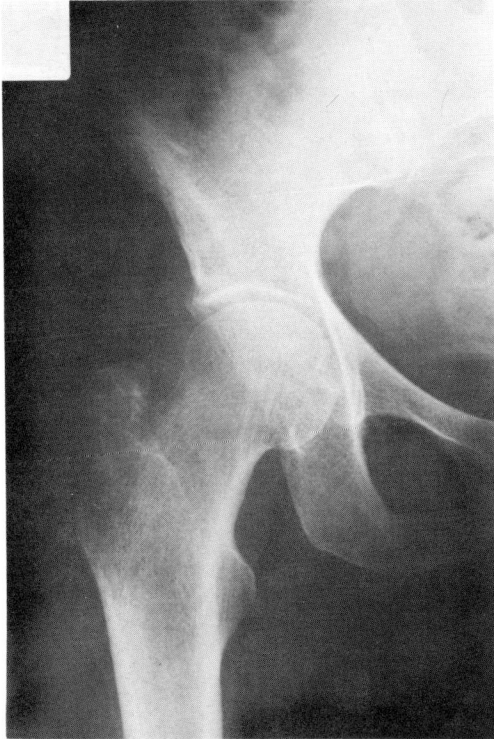

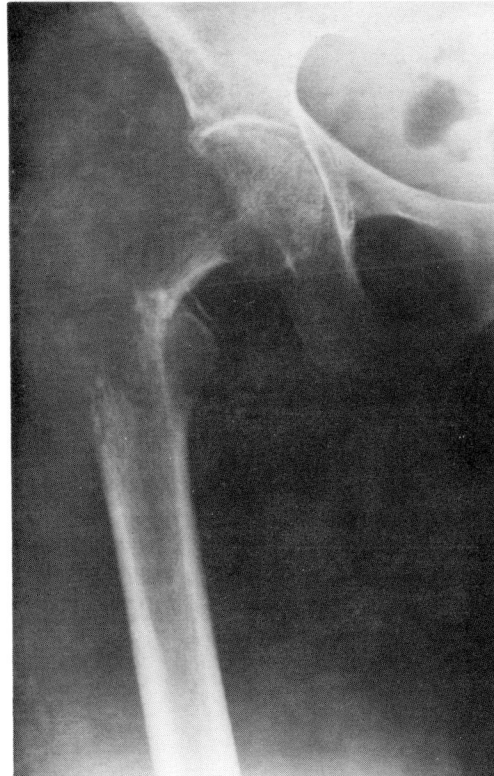

(a)

(b)

Q22

22. A 57-year-old woman with severe right hip pain and limited movement. She was never operated on (Fig. 98a and b).
(a) What is the abnormality?
(b) What are your next steps in diagnosis?
(c) Discuss the causes of such an abnormality.
(d) What is the complication and treatment?

Answers on p. 303

Fig. 98

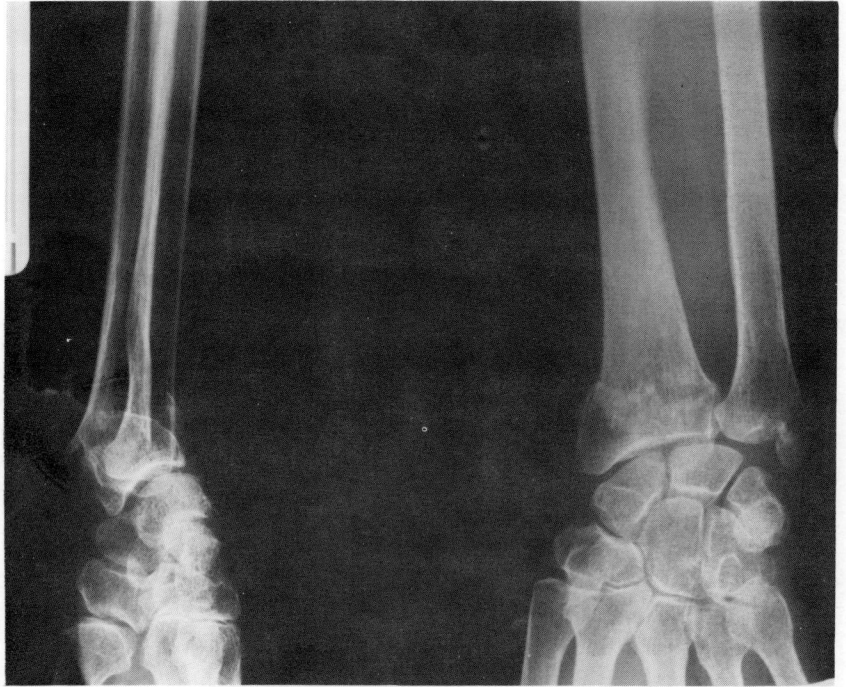

Fig. 99

Q23

23. A 55-year-old woman who fell on her right outstretched hand (Fig. 99).
(a) Spot all the radiological findings.
(b) What is the diagnosis?
(c) How do you treat?
(d) What are the complications and treatment?

Answers on p. 303

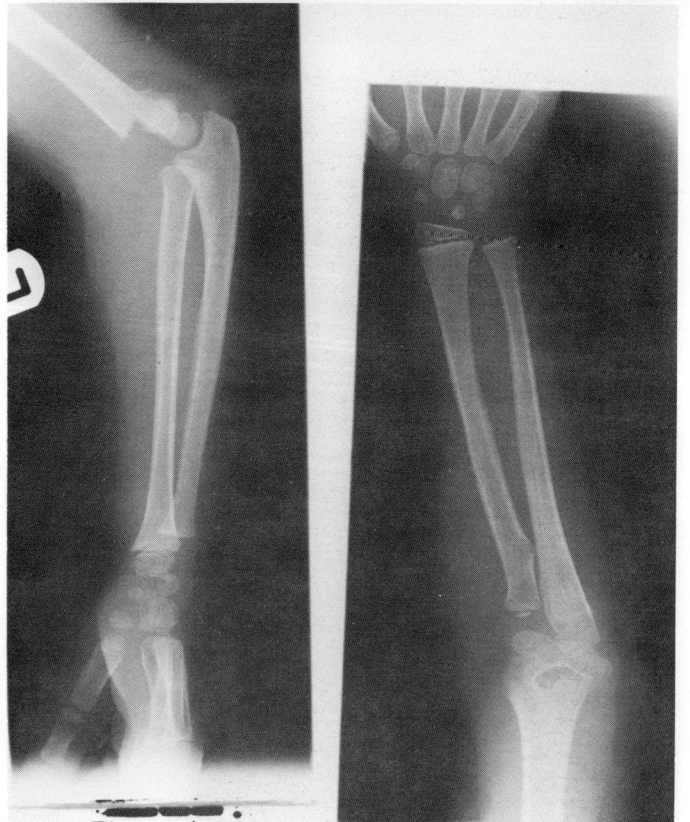

Q24

24. An 8-year-old boy who fell on his left arm (Fig. 100a and b).
(a) What are the abnormalities and diagnosis?
(b) How do you treat?
(c) Enumerate the fractures around the elbow in children.
(d) Discuss details of the most serious complications.

Answers on p. 304

Fig. 100   (a)   (b)

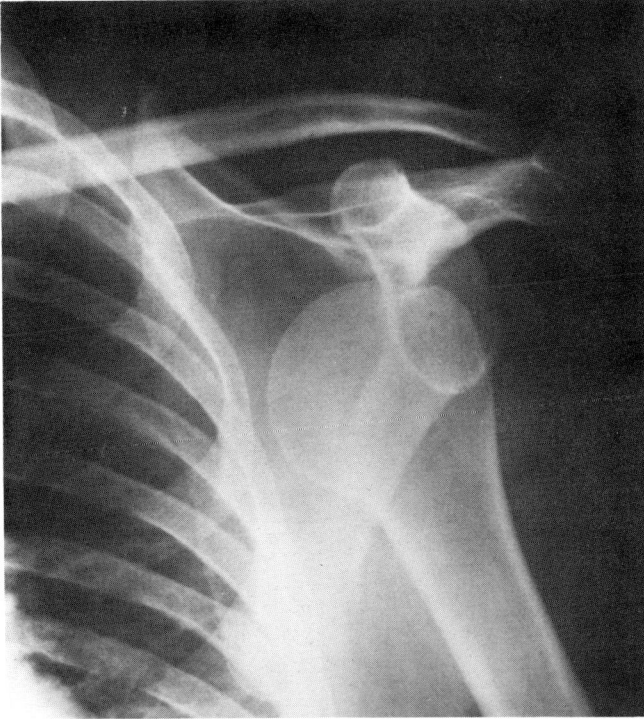

Fig. 101

Q25

25. A 28-year-old man was playing tennis and suddenly could not move his left shoulder (Fig. 101).
(a) What is the diagnosis?
(b) What are the physical signs?
(c) How do you treat?

Answers on p. 305

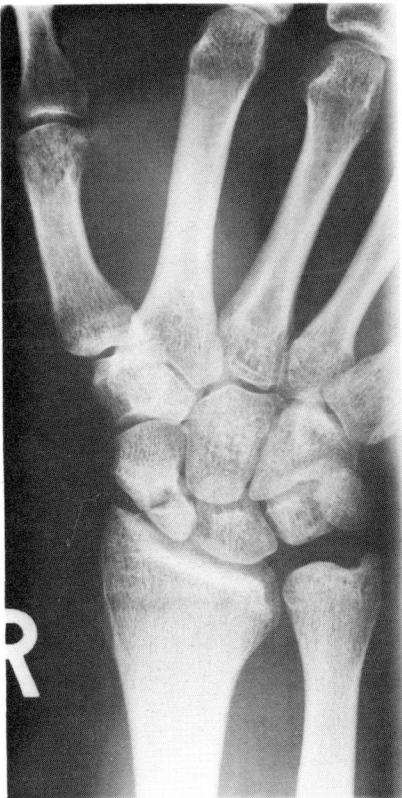

Fig. 102

Q26

26. A 30-year-old man who fell on his right outstretched hand (Fig. 102).
(a) What is the diagnosis?
(b) How do you manage this case?

Answers on p. 306

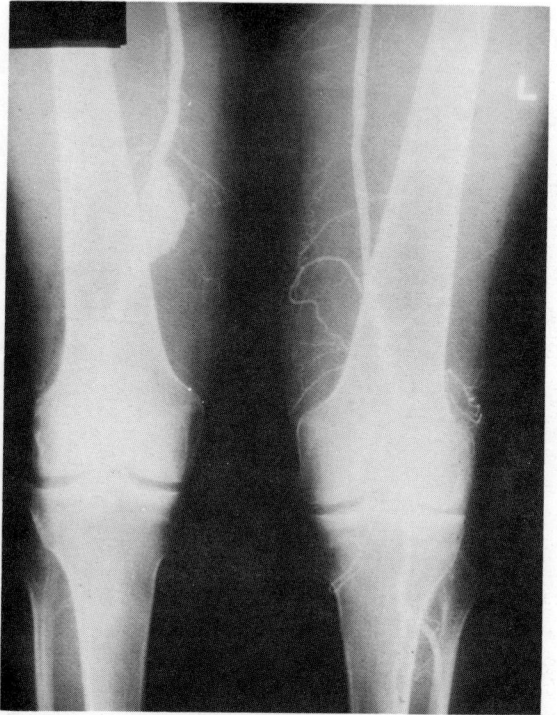

Fig. 103

Q27

27. A 50-year-old man with right thigh mass (Fig. 103).
(a) What is the investigation?
(b) What is the diagnosis?
(c) How do you treat?

Answers on p. 306

Q28

28. A 30-year-old man with a swollen painful lower limb (Fig. 104).
(a) What is the investigation and diagnosis?
(b) What is your treatment?

Answers on p. 307

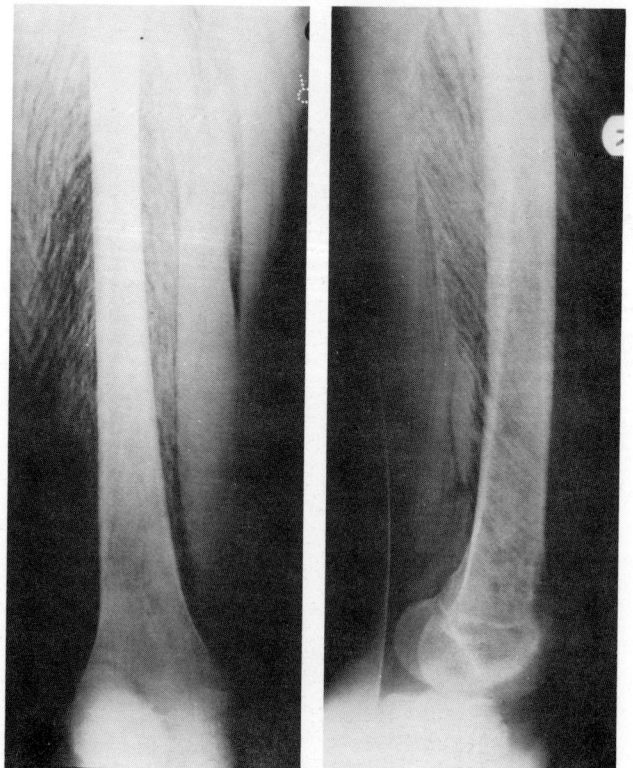

Fig. 104

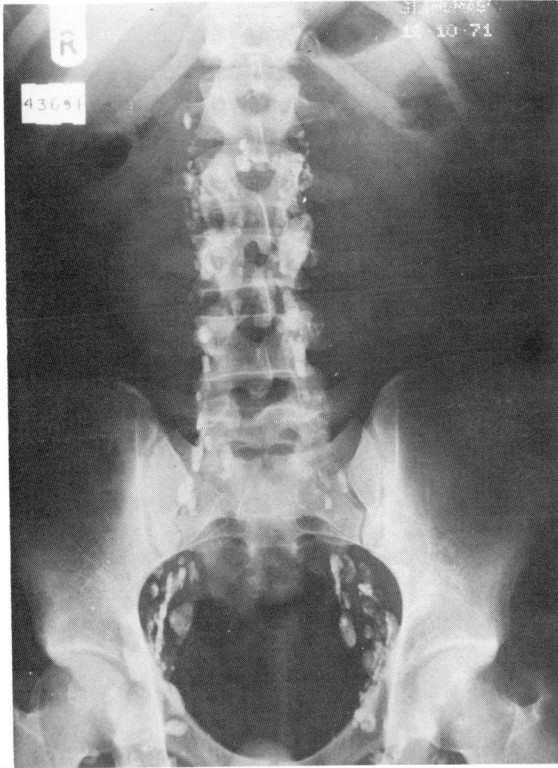

Fig. 105

Q29

29. A 30-year-old man with a large bilateral cervical rubbery lymphadcnopathy (Fig. 105).
(a) What is this investigation?
(b) What is the provisional diagnosis? What other investigations can be done to confirm it?
(c) How do you perform this procedure?

Answers on p. 308

Q30

30. A 30-year-old woman with right upper limb pain (Fig. 106).
(a) What is the diagnosis?
(b) What are the clinical findings?
(c) How do you treat?

Answers on p. 309

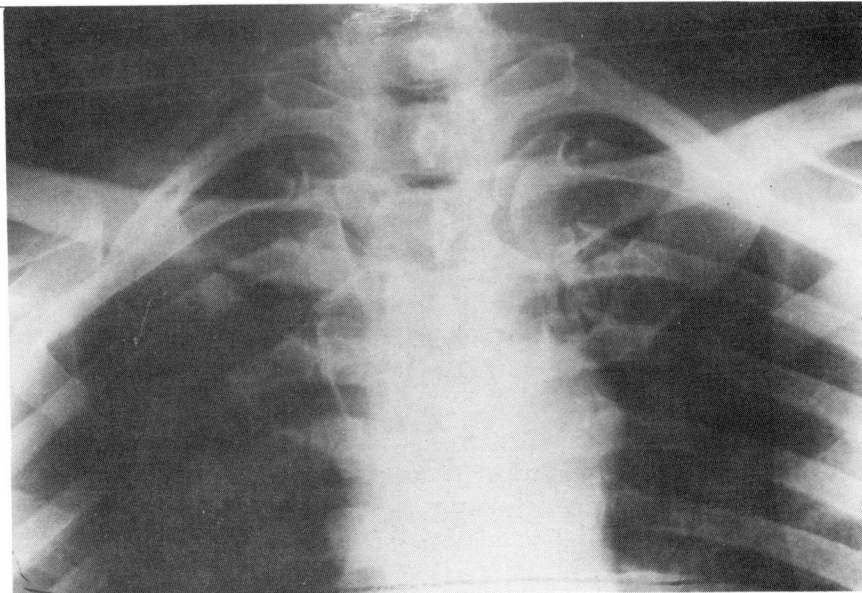

Fig. 106

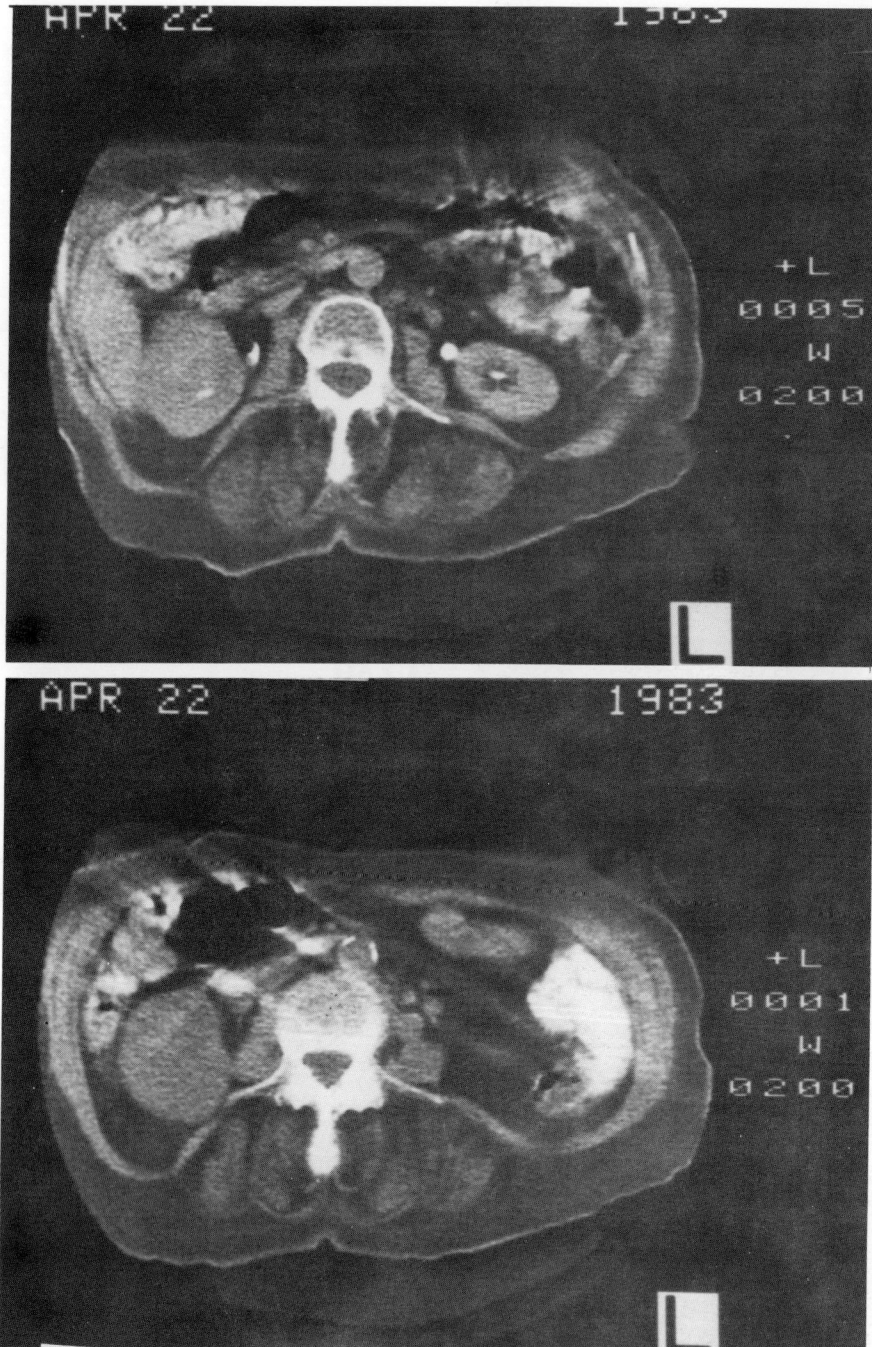

Fig. 107

Q31

31. A 45-year-old man who presented with pathological fracture of the tibia (Fig. 107).
(a) What is this investigation?
(b) What does it show?
(c) What is your treatment?

Answers on p. 309

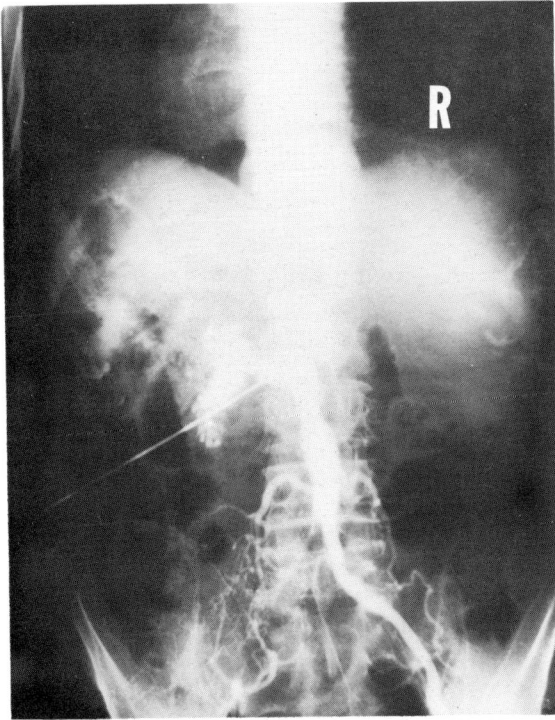

Fig. 108

Q32

32. A 59-year-old man with right buttock intermittent claudication with recent impotence (Fig. 108).
(a) What is this investigation?
(b) What are the abnormalities and diagnosis?
(c) How do you treat?

Answers on p. 309

Q33

33. A 57-year-old man with intermittent claudication of the left lower limb (Fig. 109).
(a) What is this?

Answers on p. 309

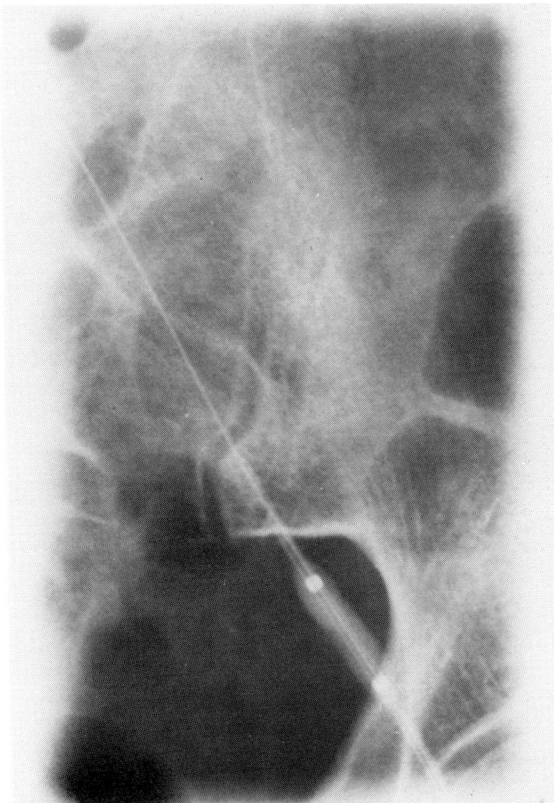

Fig. 109

Q34

34. A 60-year-old man with lower limb intermittent claudication (Fig. 110).
(a) What is the investigation?
(b) Spot all the abnormalities.
(c) How do you treat?

Answers on p. 309

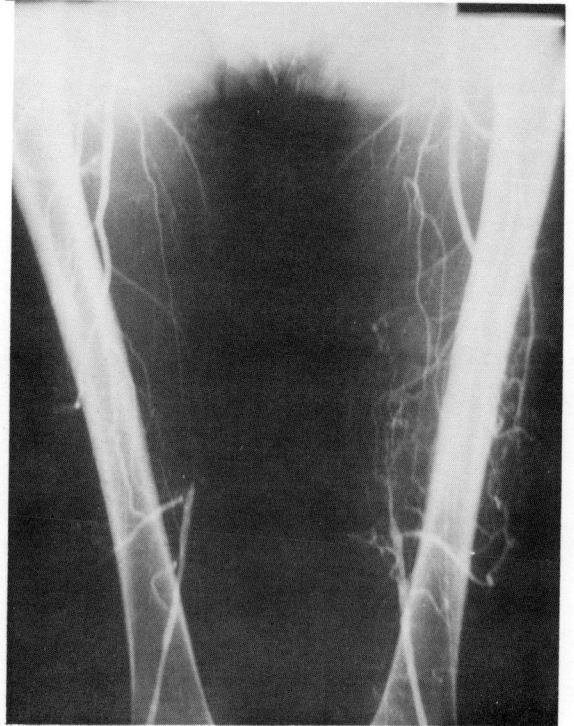

Fig. 110

Q35

35. A 63-year-old man was admitted to hospital with left renal colic (Fig. 111).
(a) What is the diagnosis?
(b) How do you treat?

Answers on p. 310

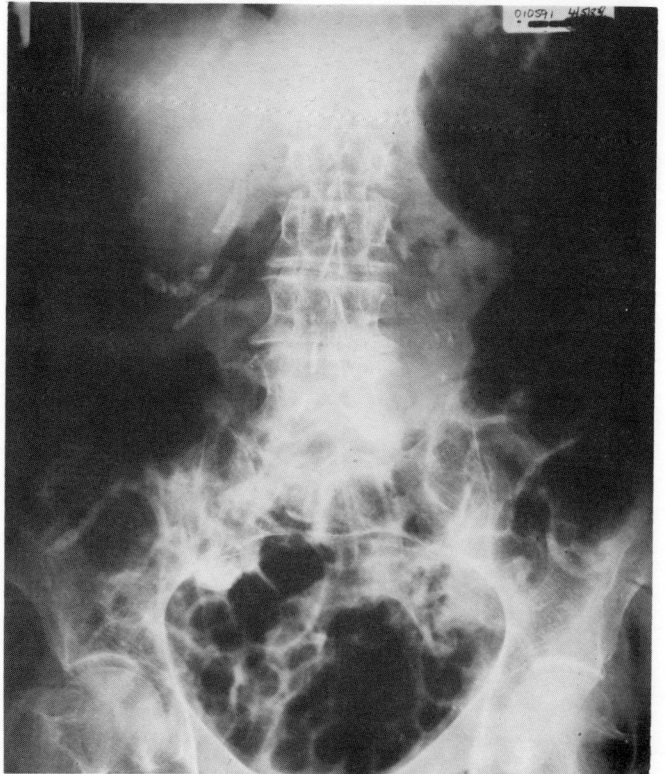

Fig. 111

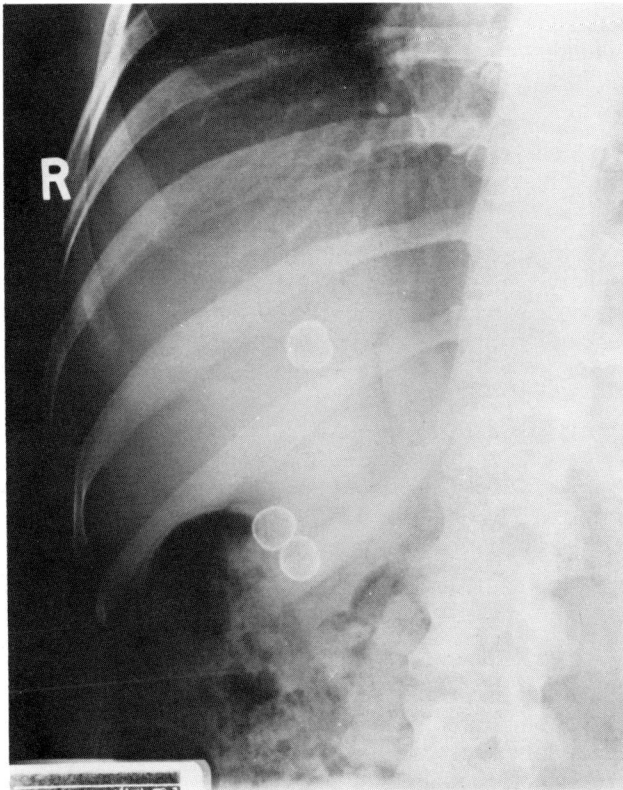

Fig. 112

Q36

36. A 53-year-old woman was admitted to hospital with severe continuous upper abdominal pain following a meal of fish and chips at night (Fig. 112).
(a) What is the abnormality(ies)?
(b) What is your diagnosis?
(c) Comment on investigations available for such a condition.
(d) Do you perform emergency or elective operation and why?

Answers on p. 310

Answers

A1

(a) Left submandibular salivary calculus shown on a plain X-ray.

(b) Excision of left submandibular salivary gland. Submandibular calculi are much more common than parotid calculi because of the antigravity course of Wharton's duct in the former. Small stones within the duct are approached intra-orally; stay sutures are applied to the incised mucosa over the duct opening and the stone is milked bimanually. If the stone is large and deep within the intraglandular part of the duct, or the gland is severely damaged by chronic infection, or suspected superimposed tumour cannot be ruled out, excision of the gland is indicated (extra-orally). In the parotid gland only the stone should be removed (whether by the intra-oral or extra-oral approach). Presents clinically as painful swellings and confirmed by bimanual palpation and plain X-ray. Sialograms are necessary to identify and locate parotid stones in Stensen's duct. Salivary stones are not systemic and have no relation to calcium metabolism. They are usually unilateral.

A2

(a) Semilateral view of thin emulsion barium swallow.

(b) Posterior pharyngeal pouch.

(c) Surgical excision. Pharyngeal pouch is caused by pressure exerted by a bolus on Killian's dehiscence (a weak area between the upper thyropharyngeus fibres and lower cricopharyngeus fibres of the inferior constrictor muscle) in the presence of cricopharyngeus spasm. Elderly men are the victims with progressive swelling and gurgling noises in the neck occurring after drinking. It starts asymptomatically and ends with dysphagia and emaciation. Oesophagoscopy or bougienage is contraindicated. The pouch is approached surgically by a left incision along the anterior border of the sternomastoid with mobilisation and forward retraction of the lateral thyroid lobe (middle and inferior thyroid arterial ligation) with carotid sheath retraction backwards. The anaesthetist passes a nasogastric tube as a guide. The pouch neck is identified and dissected and closed in two layers. The area is drained and the wound closed. Postoperatively the patient is fed through a nasogastric tube for 3 days followed by fluids for 3 days. Antibiotics are given prophylactically to prevent mediastinitis. (Preliminary temporary gastrostomy or jejunostomy may be required in extreme emaciation.)

A3

(a) Achalasia of the oesophagus or cardiospasm (smooth pencil-shaped narrowing).

(b) It predisposes to diverticula and carcinoma (precancerous) and leads to dysphagia as well as anaemia, aspiration pneumonia (usually right middle lobe) and arthritis (toxic rheumatoid arthritis). Achalasia is due to absence (or defect) of Auerbach's parasympathetic plexus.

(c) Heller's operation (oesophagocardiomyotomy) by the abdominal or thoracic approach. A longitudinal 10 cm long incision (5 cm proximal and 5 cm distal to the constricted portion) is deepened down to (and without puncturing) the mucosa which will bulge. Eighty per cent of cases have satisfactory postoperative results; 20% will continue with reflux oesophagitis.

A4

(a) Barium swallow showing soap bubble appearance.

(b) Oesophageal varices.

(c) Yes. Splenic portography (Fig. 113) to test the portal vein patency as a prerequisite to shunt.

(d) No prophylactic operation in portal hypertension (i.e. shunt) unless the patient is bleeding or has had bleeding before, because:

● It has no benefit.

● It may cause severe encephalopathy and increase mortality.

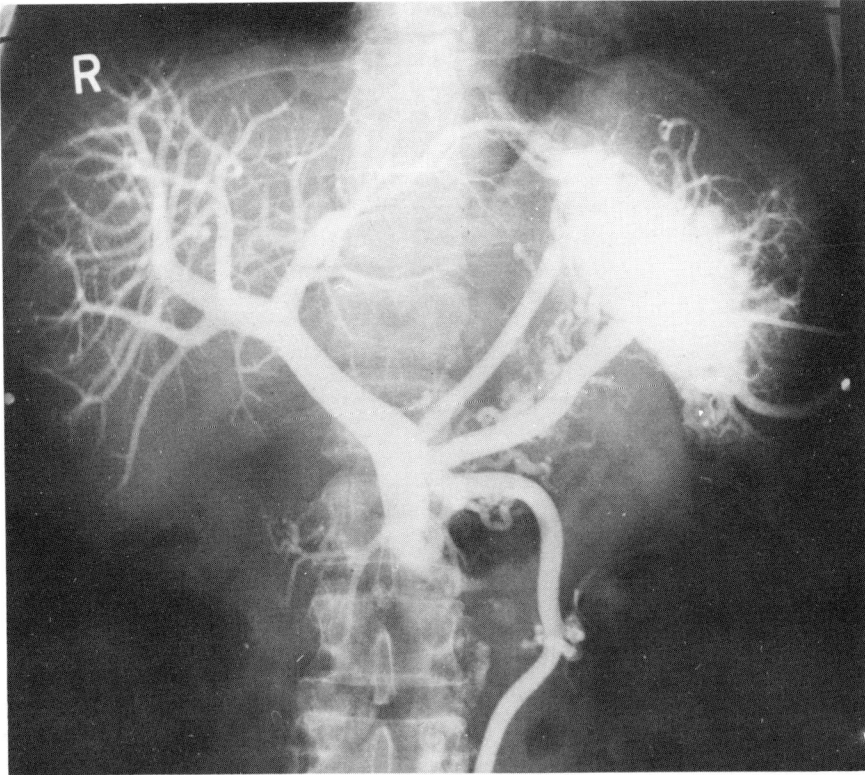

Fig. 113

(e) Massive haemorrhage treated conservatively at first (rest, sedation, fresh blood transfusion, with CVP and blood pressure monitoring. Oral magnesium sulphate and neomycin with prevention of protein intake. Pitressin 20 units/200 ml of normal saline per 20 min. Occasionally, ice water gastric lavage to reduce bleeding and remove clots). If these methods fail then try tamponade with a Sengstaken triluminal tube (should not be left in for more than 72 h as the pressure causes ulceration and oesophageal rupture. It also leads to saliva inspiration into the lungs). If bleeding recurs after removal of the Sengstaken tube then emergency operation (whether direct oesophageal or decompressing shunt) is indicated. Elective shunting is only indicated if the patient (known to have portal hypertension) has bled in the past.

Comment. Splenomegaly in upper gastrointestinal tract bleeding is not diagnostic of portal hypertension (unless varices are documented radiologically as in this case) since cirrhotics (with splenomegaly) may bleed:

- From peptic gastric or duodenal ulcer secondary to hypergastrinaemia (not metabolised by liver) in up to 20% of cases.
- From gastric erosions due to alcoholism.
- From Mallory–Weiss syndrome due to alcoholism.
- From gastric fundal varices and not oesophageal varices.

Furthermore splenomegaly alone may be due to the leukaemia causing upper gastrointestinal tract bleeding (very rarely).

A5

(a) Barium meal.

(b) Benign giant lesser curve peptic ulcer.

(c) Endoscopy and biopsy to confirm the benign radiological appearance (no everted ulcer margin, peristalsis moves through it, rugae radiate immediately from ulcer. In ulcer cancer the margin is everted and because of surrounding infiltration the peristalsis and rugae stop a distance away from it). H_2-receptor antagonist (e.g. cimetidine or ranitidine) is given over 6 weeks (duodenal ulcer requires 6 months) with endoscopic monitoring to assess healing. If still symptomatic and/or no healing then surgery is indicated (partial gastrectomy and Billroth I or II or alternatively wide excision of ulcer-bearing segment with simple closure of the defect).

(d) Indications for surgery are:

● Any ulcer complications, e.g. perforation, pyloric stenosis and bleeding (continuous or intermittent).
● Failure of medical treatment and/or economic considerations and expediency.
● Combined gastric and duodenal ulcers.
● Serious persistent hour-glass deformity.
● Suspicion of malignancy, e.g. greater curve ulcer and/or positive cytology, very long ulcer history (size is not criterion for malignancy) and ulcer in patient over 60 with short history.

A6

(a) Gas crescent under right hemidiaphragm.

(b) Perforated peptic (probably duodenal) ulcer.

(c) Pneumoperitoneum and right subphrenic gas are most commonly seen after laparotomy (as a normal finding). Perforated viscus (peptic duodenal or gastric ulcer, colonic diverticula, gall bladder empyema and rarely appendicitis) is the next most common cause. They are also seen in open (or closed) abdominal trauma. Subphrenic abscess (mainly postoperative), amoebic liver abscess and infected liver hydatid cyst cause a right subphrenic fluid level (rather than a crescent), with basal lung consolidation (Fig. 114).

(d) Emergency simple closure of the perforation with an omental tag and peritoneal toilet and drainage. Quick i.v. rehydration, nasogastric suction, prophylactic antibiotics with BP, PR and CVP monitoring are recommended. Up to 8 % of abdominal conditions subjected to urgent laparotomy are perforated peptic ulcers and it is important to remember that 10 % will have had no prior recognisable ulcer symptoms and that about 30 % of perforated ulcers show no positive radiological evidence of pneumoperitoneum. Simple closure has 7 % operative mortality which becomes even less with early diagnosis and prompt treatment since delay causes a change from a mainly chemical peritonitis in the first 6 h to 100 % demonstrable bacterial peritonitis after 12 h.

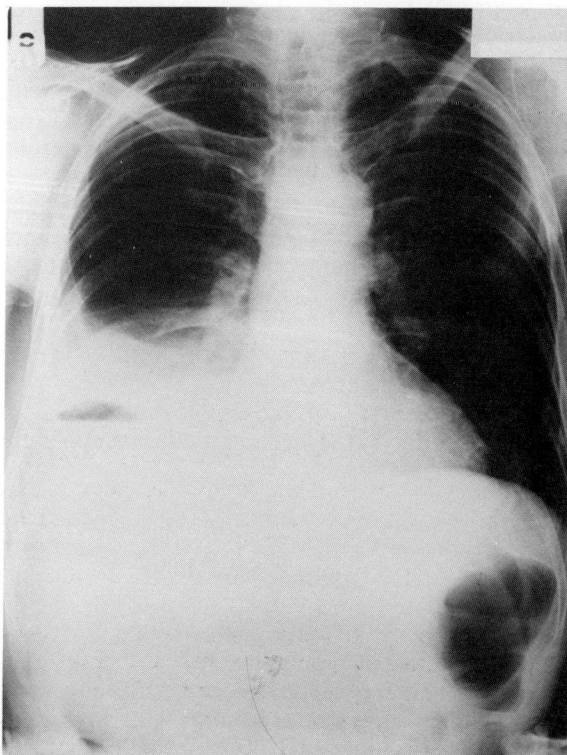

Fig. 114

(e) To have the definitive treatment of truncal vagotomy with drainage procedure (preferably gastroenterostomy) as an elective operation. Roughly one-third of closed perforations will recover permanently postoperatively, another one-third continue as a symptomatic ulcer and the last third proceed to ulcer complications, i.e. recurrent perforations, bleeding and stenosis.

A7

(a) Prepyloric non-obstructing tumour (filling defect seen in barium meal).
(b) Endoscopy and biopsy then operation. If carcinoma then do distal radical gastrectomy. If the tumour is benign, do endoscopic snaring (if pedunculated) or open local surgical excision (if sessile).

A8

(a) Percutaneous transhepatic cholangiography—PTC (using a fine Chiba needle under prophylactic antibiotic cover, e.g. cefuroxime in a patient with normal prothrombin time). Complications include intraperitoneal bleeding, biliary peritonitis and infection.
(b) Two biliary stones at the lower end of the common bile duct (CBD) with proximal biliary dilatation (due to incomplete obstruction).
(c) Charcot's triad of intermittent jaundice, biliary colic and fever with rigor (due to ascending cholangitis).
(d) Cholecystectomy, CBD supraduodenal exploration and stone removal (choledocholithotomy) with T-tube drainage. If the CBD is packed with stones or it is impossible to remove all stones then a permanent prophylactic drainage procedure such as choledochoduodenostomy is recommended.
Comment. This technique (i.e. PTC) has now been extended into external biliary drainage (decompression), transhepatic dilatation of biliary strictures and endoprosthesis insertion.

A9

(a) Peroperative pre-exploratory cholangiography showing multiple obstructing stones in the lower end of the CBD (no dye passed down to duodenum). This procedure should be performed routinely in all cholecystectomy cases (*see below*).
(b) The indications or *classical criteria* for CBD exploration are:
● Preoperative, e.g. history of jaundice or Charcot's triad, gall stone pancreatitis, oral cholecystography revealing multiple small stones with patent or dilated cystic duct.
● Peroperative, e.g. palpation of CBD stone, dilated CBD more than 10–12 mm, periductal fibrosis, cholecystectomised gall bladder showing single-faceted stone or thick wall with no stone, indurated pancreas, or biliary sludge or mud on needle aspiration of CBD. Peroperative pre-exploratory cholangiogram (revealing one of four findings: a filling defect, dilated CBD, no flow to duodenum and/or stenosis or non-visualisation of lower intramural narrow segment of duct) is far more accurate (over 95%) than the above criteria and is the best available method for this purpose.
● Postoperative T-tube cholangiography revealing residual stone.
Comment. Exploration of the CBD is associated with high mortality (3%, a fourfold increase over cholecystectomy alone) and with more morbidity (T-tube biliary intraperitoneal leakage). Since out of 60–80% of patients with one of the above criteria only 20% have CBD pathology, operative cholangiogram is used for CBD pathology detection, biliary anatomy demonstration, and identification of patients who do not need choledochotomy. It is the best available method and should be practised routinely with cholecystectomy to avoid the high risk of residual biliary stone which can reach 30% of explored cases done without operative cholangiogram.

However, this policy is not universally accepted. The argument is that for practically every 100 patients with gall stones only 20 will require choledochotomy, suggesting that 80 do not require cholangiography. However 60–80% of patients have at least one of the *criteria* for CBD exploration and it would seem reasonable to omit cholangiography in the 20–40% *who have no such criteria*. It is claimed that such a selective policy would result in less than 1% of residual stone incidence.

A10

(a) T-tube postoperative cholangiography showing two residual obstructing stones at the lower end of the CBD.

(b) Residual stone accounts for 10–20% of recurrences after choledochotomy. Re-exploration carries a mortality in excess of primary choledochotomy. The following steps in management recommended in chronological order:

A. Leave T-tube *in situ*.

1. A proportion of CBD small stones will pass into the duodenum spontaneously especially if amyl nitrite or an antispasmodic is given to relax the sphincter.

2. Gall stone dissolution by giving oral chenodeoxycholic acid (Chendol) or using T-tube lavage with various solutions, e.g. saline heparin, cholate or, more effectively, glyceryl mono-octanoate (GMO). Irrigation using 500 ml normal saline with 5000 units heparin (to prevent haemobilia) coupled with 20 mg i.v. Buscopan is a common practice. Lavage should be monitored and consequent diarrhoea (due to bowel irritation by bowel salts) controlled by cholestyramine (GMO can induce erosive duodenitis). This method is time-consuming and requires hospitalisation and repeated cholangiogram to see if the stone has passed. The success rate is 50%.

3. Monitored flushing with maximal relaxation of sphincter of Oddi (Cuschieri, 1984). Massive sterile saline infusion via a disposable manometry line through the T-tube with i.v. continuous infusion of cerulitide 2 ng/kg per min via a constant infusion pump. Cerulitide is an analogue of caerulein with a powerful cholecystokinin effect causing maximal relaxation of the sphincter of Oddi. The amount of saline infused is 1–3 litres at a rate that will maintain the biliary pressure at 25–30 cmH$_2$O. Prophylactic antibiotic (i.e. cefuroxime single dose 1 g) should be given $\frac{1}{2}$ hour prior to the procedure. T-tube cholangiography should be performed before and after the procedure. This method is simpler, more effective, less time-consuming and less invasive than the above method and is side-effect free (only watery diarrhoea).

B. Remove T-tube after 4–6 weeks.

1. Percutaneous stone extraction: do T-tube cholangiogram (to ensure that stone is still present) before T-tube removal. The stone retrieval system (Dormia basket, Fogarty balloon catheter or preferably a Burhenne steerable catheter) is passed down the T-tube track under X-ray screening by a skilled radiologist. It is for this reason that the surgeon is advised to use a size 16 Fr (or larger) T-tube in the right upper quadrant so that the track is *short, straight* and *large* enough for such manoeuvring.

2. Endoscopic sphincterotomy: followed by passage of Dormia basket or Fogarty balloon for stone retrieval. A skilled team of surgeon and radiologist is necessary to achieve the 90% success rate. It has a 1% mortality and 8% morbidity but this compares favourably with surgical re-exploration. Complications are pancreatitis, bleeding, cholangitis and rarely perforation and stone impaction.

3. Surgical re-exploration should be reserved for the few patients in whom the above methods fail or are not available and where the risk is justified.

C. In the absence of a T-tube from the start (the residual stone was diagnosed with intravenous cholangiography after clinical suspicion following cholecystectomy), gall stone dissolution should be tried with chenodeoxycholic acid or ursodeoxycholic acid (suitable stones must be radiolucent indicating a high cholesterol content and measure less than 1 cm with a patent duct to permit entry of the solvent). Dissolution generally takes 6–24 months. If this fails try endoscopic extraction and if this fails then surgical re-exploration (if the risk is justified).

A11

(a) Barium enema revealing carcinoma of caecum causing ileocolic intussusception—a rare presentation. (Appendix is shown connected to the mass and lifted to right hypochondrium.)

(b) Severe anaemia due to bleeding cauliflower tumour (gastric and caecal carcinomas are notorious for their tendency to bleed and cause anaemia), right iliac fossa mass and rarely secondary acute appendicitis.

(c) Right hemicolectomy (with primary ileocolic anastomosis).

1. Intravenous drip, nasogastric suction and indwelling urinary catheter after 2 days' bowel preparation.

2. General anaesthesia, supine position and long right paramedian incision (rectus muscle-splitting).

3. Quick exploration for tumour size and fixity, and for liver, mesenteric lymph nodes and peritoneal metastases as well as for double primary colonic carcinomas (up to 20% of cases). Pack off small intestine to the left.

4. Dissect and resect the greater omentum off the right side of the transverse colon. Mobilise the ascending colon by dividing the right paracolic peritoneum and freeing the hepatic flexure and terminal ileum by blunt dissection, taking absolute care to safeguard the duodenum, right ureter and genital vessels.

5. Ligate and divide the ileocolic and right colic arteries through artificially created windows in the mesocolon and mesentery, visualising them under a spotlight.

6. Apply a non-crushing (occluding) intestinal clamp to the antimesocolic border (just enough to occlude the lumen of the proposed site of division) as well as a crushing clamp and cut between. Ideally 15 cm of terminal ileum should be resected. However, the viability of the ileal end must be confirmed on the basis of a good extramural blood supply. Re-resection and examination may be necessary until a viable end is obtained.

7. Ileocolic anastomosis should be performed under near aseptic conditions (pack off the area and mop up the contents with an antiseptic-soaked swab). End-to-end, end-to-side, side-to-end or side-to-side anastomosis is optional. The ileal end can be enlarged by a Cheetle longitudinal antimesenteric cut. Either a double-layered (interrupted waxed seromuscular 2/0 silk and continuous mucosal 2/0 chromic catgut) or a single-layered (waxed interrupted serososubmucosal 2/0 silk) technique may be used.

8. Close the mesenteric gap and remove the packs.

9. Anal stretch to prevent increased intracolic pressure from straining the anastomosis.

10. Drain and close.

A12

(a) Narrowing of left colon with loss of haustration (pipe-stem colon) and multiple fine filling defects of pseudopolyps (due to intervening mucosal undermining secondary to ulcers).

(b) Ulcerative colitis.

(c) *Emergency surgery* in toxic megacolon (fulminating cases), severe haemorrhage and perforation.
Elective surgery in:

- Local complications, e.g. pseudopolyposis, fibrous stricture, rectovaginal fistulae, fistula *in ano*, ischiorectal abscess, haemorrhoids.
- General complications, e.g. liver cirrhosis and sclerosing cholangitis, skin lesions of pyodermia gangrenosum and erythema nodosum, arthritis, iritis, ankylosing spondylitis, stomatitis, anaemia and renal disease.
- Suspicion of neoplastic change. Ulcerative colitis is precancerous in 3.5% of cases and the risk increases with disease duration (i.e. after 20 years the risk is 12%), with whole colon involvement and in the presence of pseudopolyposis. Thus 10 years after diagnosis, regular radiological and sigmoidoscopic checks must be done even if the disease seems to be quiescent.
- Onset in children or adolescents.
- Chronic invalidism.

A13

(a) Barium enema showing irregular filling defect of left descending colon.

(b) Left colonic carcinoma.

(c) Left hemicolectomy (with primary colocolic anastomosis). This is almost a mirror-image of right hemicolectomy with similar steps: the incision will be a long left paramedian, the bowel is packed to the right side and then the left colon is mobilised (by dividing the left paracolic peritoneum up to the splenic flexure, excising part of the greater omentum, mobilising the transverse colon and finally mobilising the splenic flexure fully with enlargement of the paramedian incision or transverse extension if necessary). Safeguard the left ureter and genital vessels. The left colic and, if necessary, the middle colic vessels are divided. The area is packed off, the left colon is resected, and the transverse colon is anastomosed to the pelvic colon. The mesenteric gap is repaired, the anus stretched, area drained and abdomen closed.

A14

(a) Plain abdominal X-ray revealing massive colonic distension with gas in an inverted U sign (with its opening directed towards the right iliac fossa). The appearance is characteristic of volvulus of the sigmoid colon (it can affect the mid-gut in infants — volvulus neonatorum due to arrested rotation and/or band of Ladd; in adults it affects the small intestine or caecum in addition to the sigmoid colon).

(b) Sudden volvulus is manifested by severe abdominal pain which is followed either by quick (in 6 h) massive abdominal distension (as here) or spontaneous untwisting of the bowel followed by passage of large quantities of flatus and faeces. Absolute constipation with hiccough or retching may occur. Vomiting is late.

(c) Rectal tube deflation of the twisted bowel (via sigmoidoscopy) is the first step and the operation can be done electively after a few days of bowel preparation. If deflation is impossible, immediate laparotomy and untwisting with rectal tube deflation is carried out followed by resection. In an emergency operation and/or when the bowel is non-viable it is better to clamp the afferent and efferent limbs, exteriorise the volvulus segment and excise it on the abdominal surface immediately or after 48 h, performing Paul–Mikulicz double-barrelled colostomy, the spur of which is crushed by an enterotome after a few days. Closure of colostomy is carried out 4 weeks later when there is no oedema and the colon has established an extraperitoneal location. In elective resection, primary end-to-end colocolic anastomosis is preferred.

A15

(a) Emergency intravenous urography revealing extensive extrarenal (extraperitoneal) extravasation of contrast in the left kidney.

(b) Left traumatic renal rupture (complete) (Fig. 115).

(c) Left loin pain, tenderness (rarely superficial bruising or penetrating wound). Haematuria is the cardinal sign of a damaged kidney with possible clot colic and late clot dislodgement leading to severe delayed

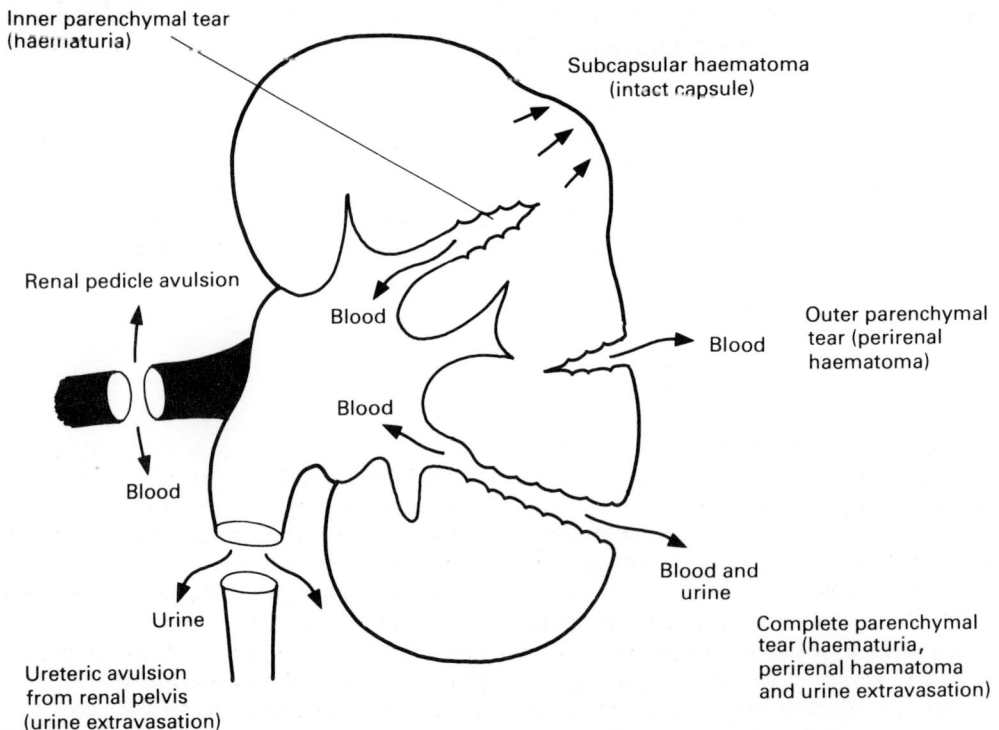

Fig. 115 Renal injuries

haematuria (from third day to third week). Palpable loin mass (perinephric haematoma) as well as abdominal distension 24–48 h later due to splanchnic nerve implication by retroperitoneal haematoma (meteorism).
(d) Conservative treatment should be stressed and is usually successful (bed rest—flat position until macroscopic haematuria becomes microscopic or absent for 1 week, analgesia for pain, antibiotics to prevent infection of haematoma, hourly monitoring of pulse rate, blood pressure and urine output. Each specimen of urine passed should be sampled, blood should be grouped and crossmatched and blood transfusion should be instituted in shock or continuous bleeding).

Surgical exploration is indicated in 20 % of patients only in:
- Progressive haemorrhage (hypotension).
- Loin swelling due to extravasated urine (since this leads to infection and is not controllable by antibiotics).
- Signs of perirenal infection of haematoma.
- Severe delayed or secondary haemorrhage.
- Early hypertension as a sequel to renal vascular injury.

It is essential to confirm the presence of a contralateral functioning kidney before operating on an injured kidney. Emergency intravenous urography or chromocystoscopy (i.v. 7 ml of 0.4 % solution of indigo-carmine watched cystoscopically as excreted by ureter within 5 min) is sufficient. The transperitoneal approach is recommended to allow full laparotomy and to deal with other injured organs. Renal vessels can be controlled before the kidney is exposed. The kidney should be exposed by opening Gerota's fascia to relieve tamponade. Drainage of haematoma or extravasated urine should be performed together with repair of the renal injury.

Surgical repair should be conservative. Small tears (in small or large subcapsular haematomas) should be sutured over Oxycel, pieces of detached muscle or mobilised omentum. Larger single rents (in cortical not medullary lacerations) are dealt with by nephrostomy through the rent and suturing the kidney on either side of a Malecot nephrostomy tube. Laceration confined to one pole of the kidney is dealt with by partial nephrectomy. Repair of a solitary damaged kidney must be attempted, but if this is not possible, the wound is packed firmly with gauze so that the bleeding is controlled and the ruptured kidney may heal.

However, in a multiple massively ruptured kidney or in avulsion of the renal pedicle (in the presence of a contralateral functioning kidney) nephrectomy must be undertaken. The standard loin extraperitoneal approach is recommended in patients presenting several days after the injury because of perirenal haematoma or urine extravasation and since associated abdominal organ injuries are unlikely by that time.

Comment on ureteric injuries

These are uncommon and usually iatrogenic following pelvic surgery (e.g. colorectal resection and hysterectomy) or Dormia basket extraction of stone. They are either unilateral or bilateral (anuria). The former are asymptomatic with silent renal atrophy, pyonephrosis with loin pain and fever, or urinary fistula which develops via an abdominal incision or following hysterectomy via the vagina. In bilateral injuries, each ureter is damaged inadvertently in one of the following ways.
- Divided.
- Crushed.
- Portion of its wall has been removed.
- Blood supply is damaged (avascular necrosis).
- Ligated.

Ureteric cut leads to retro- or intraperitoneal extravasation of urine with paralytic ileus and peritonitis. When ureteric ligation causes obstruction, the injury may be recognised at the time it is inflicted and repaired immediately or it may not be diagnosed until later (in which case do a temporary nephrostomy and repair the injury later when oedema and infection have abated after 6 weeks). Prophylactic ureteric catheterisation for easy identification and protection prior to pelvic surgery is sometimes practised.

The type of repair depends on the level of ureteric injury. For a low injury, reimplantation into the bladder is the treatment of choice (preferably with a non-refluxing anastomosis). The gap between the ureter and bladder can be bridged by a psoas hitch or Boari flap. An injury at or just above the bifurcation of the common iliac vessels is dealt with by transureteroureterostomy or replacement by an ileal segment. With more proximal (higher) abdominal ureteric injuries, direct repair (splinted spatulated anastomosis) with a Malecot nephrostomy tube is recommended. Very rarely nephrectomy (in the presence of a contralateral functioning kidney) or kidney transplantation into the iliac fossa may be attempted (Fig. 116).

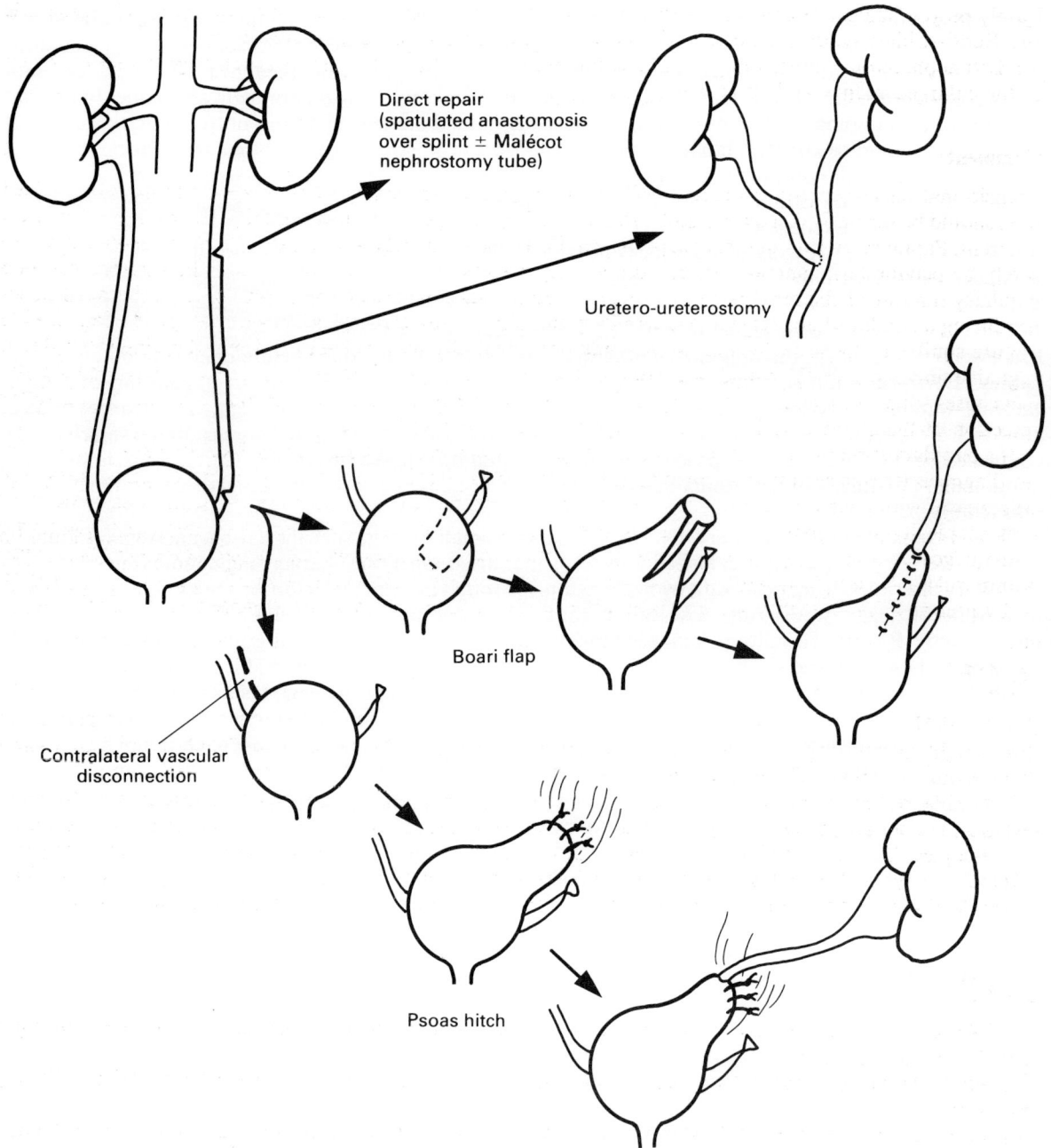

Fig. 116   Repair of various ureteric injuries

A16

(a) Intravenous urogram (IVU) revealing a huge filling defect involving the upper pole of the left kidney (hypernephroma).

(b) Painless haematuria (can be painful as a result of clot colic), palpable mass, pyrexia of unknown origin. Sometimes pathological fracture (due to skeletal metastasis) or pulmonary secondaries (with haemoptysis).

Rarely polycythaemia or anaemia. Very rarely persistent hypertension, nephrotic syndrome, left varicocele and Budd–Chiari syndrome due to infiltration of hepatic veins in *right* renal tumour.
(c) Left nephrectomy preferably via a transabdominal (rather than lumbar) approach to gain wide exposure of the enlarged kidney and its pedicle.

Comment

Transitional cell carcinoma of the renal pelvis (in the form of a papillary tumour, a solid tumour or a mixed one) should be seriously considered and differentiated from hypernephroma since the treatment is completely different. Papillary tumour of the renal pelvis manifests itself clinically by haematuria (and clot colic) and very rarely by pelviureteric junction obstruction and hydronephrosis. The characteristic filling defect seen in a papillary tumour of the renal pelvis may be misleading since hypernephroma can infiltrate the renal pelvis producing a similar filling defect while papillary tumour can infiltrate the kidney proper producing an IVU picture similar to hypernephroma. Retrograde ureterography may be used to define the diagnosis (this is arguable since a good IVU should be as good as a retrograde picture). Because of multiple ureteric and bladder metastases (due to papillary tumour spread by seeding) the treatment is a nephroureterectomy with sleeve resection of the bladder wall followed by cystoscopic follow-up for life.

If a papillary tumour of the renal pelvis was treated by nephrectomy alone, based on clinical and operative misdiagnosis (frozen section may sometimes be required to reveal the nature of the tumour), then the patient will present with haematuria probably from a ureteric metastatic or recurrent tumour which can be detected cystoscopically (if the papillary tumour is at the ureteric orifice or in the bladder), by retrograde ureterogram with image intensifier or by CT scan of the pelvis. Such cases are usually advanced and excision of the ureteric stump will not be sufficient. They are therefore treated with intravesical fulguration if the tumour is accessible or by ureteroscopic fulguration and chemotherapy if it is extensive, and are regarded as terminal cases.

A17

(a) An IVU.
(b) A right congenital pelvic kidney (due to renal ectopia), right-sided filling defect (bladder carcinoma) and left pelviureteric junction obstruction.
(c) The bladder carcinoma (threatening to obstruct the right pelvic kidney) should be assessed by cystoscopy, examined under anaesthesia and possibly treated by transurethral resection, and monitored by regular check cystoscopies. The left pelviureteric junction obstruction should be tackled thereafter by reconstructive pyeloplasty by the dismembered Anderson–Hynes operation (if obstruction is high), or Culp rotational flap, Foley Y-V plastic operation or longitudinal cut sutured transversely (if obstruction is low) (Fig. 117).

A18

(a) IVU shows left hydroureter and hydronephrosis, osteoblastic metastatic lesion of L3 vertebra and right non-functioning kidney.
(b) All the above abnormalities are due to obstructive prostatic carcinomatous uropathy (revealed indirectly by its metastasis).
(c) Transurethral resection of prostatic carcinoma to relieve the obstruction followed by hormonal therapy (stilboestrol 1 mg three times a day initially for 1 week followed by 1 mg a day for life) and/or radiotherapy for painful skeletal metastasis. Prostatic coagulopathy or stilboestrol thromboembolic complications may necessitate subcapsular orchidectomy.

A19

(a) An IVU.
(b) Congenital horse-shoe kidney (with characteristic bilateral reversed lower calyx), right obstructing ureteric stone and right hemihydronephrosis.

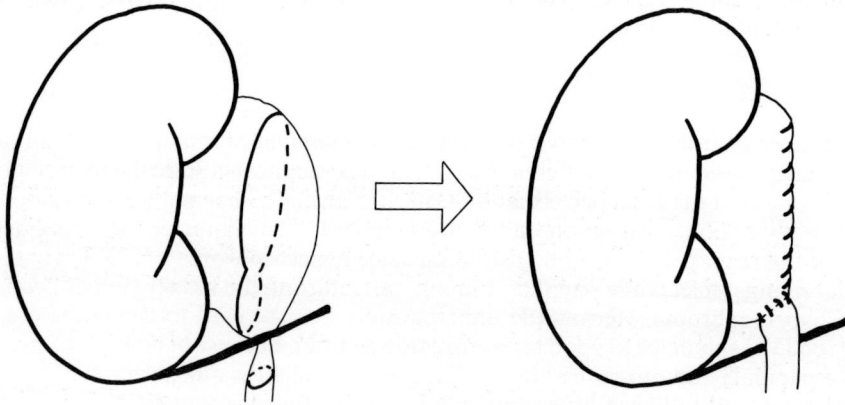

Anderson–Hynes pyeloplasty

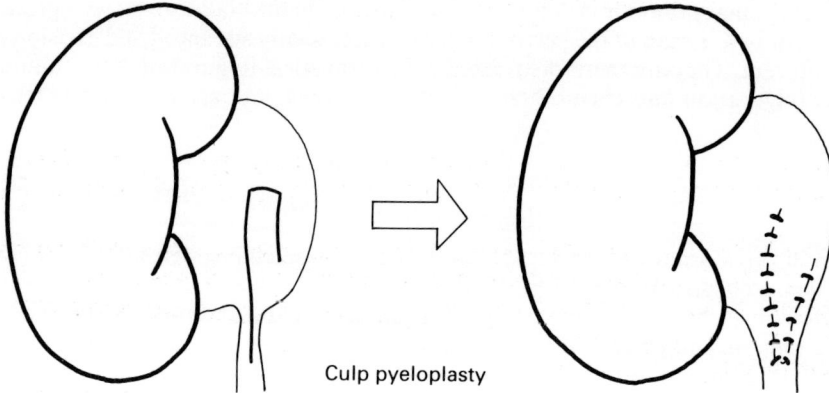

Culp pyeloplasty

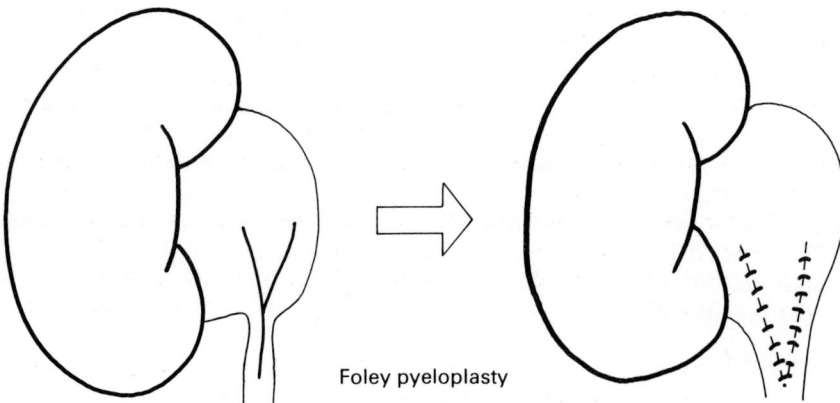

Foley pyeloplasty

Fig. 117 Types of pyeloplasty

(c) Transabdominal intraperitoneal approach to divide the median fusing isthmus and extraction of the right ureteric calculus. However, the area should be drained extraperitoneally. Conservation of renal tissue is essential, and right heminephrectomy should only be done for irreparably diseased half (e.g. huge calculus or neoplasm).

A20

(a) Recurrent bilateral renal staghorn calculi with delayed functioning right kidney. The condition is very much suggestive of primary hyperparathyroidism and should be confirmed biochemically (high serum calcium, low serum phosphorus, high urinary calcium and phosphorus with high alkaline phosphatase). In hyperparathyroidism the classic renal lesion is nephrocalcinosis which if treatment is delayed can lead to a huge stone.
(b) The primary cause of hyperparathyroidism should be treated first; then renal stones are treated when indicated by complications:
● High blood urea due to pelviureteric junction obstruction secondary to ball valve mechanism.
● Pyonephrosis due to infection and urinary stasis
● Severe pain.
   In bilateral disease the painful kidney should be operated on. However, renal isotope scan should be done to assess the best functioning kidney which should then be operated on first.

A21

(a) Multiple bilateral pubic rami fractures with disruption of the symphysis pubis. There is incomplete undisplaced basal intracapsular fracture of the left femoral neck with right central acetabular fracture without hip dislocation.
(b) Correction of shock then treatment of pelvic visceral injuries (when confirmed) followed by treatment of the fracture itself which needs external pelvic compression either by suspending it in a pelvic sling from an overhead beam, nursing the patient between sandbags (or on his side) or by applying hip spica divided in the centre and bandaged by rubber.
   The pelvic visceral injuries and treatment are:
● Intrapelvic rupture of membranous urethra (patient cannot pass urine, blood leak from urethral meatus, bladder distension before extravasation occurs and Vermooten's sign). Urethrocystography and immediate catheterisation are contraindicated since they may destroy any residual intact urethral wall. The patient should be taken to theatre, the bladder opened and the position of the prostate assessed. *If the prostate is not floating high* (indicating incomplete partial injury), the bladder is closed round a large (28 Fr) Malecot catheter (orthopaedic reduction of pelvic fracture can be attempted) and antibiotic cover given. If, 3 weeks later, urethroscopy and metallic sound are successful then the suprapubic catheter is clamped to allow the patient to micturate. *If the prostate is floating* (indicating complete total rupture), then a catheter is railroaded across the gap using two metallic bougies or the little finger and a metallic bougie. Traction on a Foley catheter is used to replace the prostate in position. The bladder is closed around the Malecot catheter with separate drainage of the prevesical space. The Foley catheter is removed after 12 days. The suprapubic drain may be clamped and removed after 2–3 weeks.
● Extraperitoneal rupture of bladder (bladder impalpable with dullness and tenderness suprapubically)— carry out laparotomy, suture the bladder with the urethral Foley catheter *in situ* and drain the prevesical space.
● Rectal injury (assessed by rectal examination) may necessitate a defunctioning loop iliac colostomy.
● Sciatic nerve injury with anaesthesia and weakness of part of the leg may be associated with vertical disruption of the pelvic ring and is treated by reduction of the pelvic fracture.
● Injury to blood vessels is rare; repair is indicated if lower limb pulses are absent or there is evidence of ischaemia.
● In a female patient, very rarely the vagina can be injured, and it should be sutured (not applicable here).

Comment

Posterior urethral injuries

Managment of posterior urethral injuries resulting from pelvic fractures in males is controversial. The conservative approach and late surgery is based on the fact that the majority of such injuries are incomplete ruptures. Because urethral catheterisation, as well as urethrography or urethroscopy, may complete the rupture, suprapubic bladder catheterisation is done initially followed by definitive repair 3 weeks later. Those who advocate such an approach suggest that complete posterior urethral ruptures will always heal with stricture formation whereas incomplete lesions may heal spontaneously without subsequent stricture. They believe many of the complications are due to the initial treatment rather than to the injury itself (Mitchell). The early operative approach (advocated here) is based on the fact that incomplete rupture of the posterior urethra often results in formation of a stricture which may be long and tortuous. In complete rupture re-apposition of the ends of the ruptured urethra will allow healing without stricture formation or will result in a short stricture which can be managed easily by urethral dilatation; thus, when posterior urethral injury is suspected clinically, attempted urethral catheterisation causes no harm and the most difficult strictures occur when early approximation of the ruptured urethral ends is not attempted. In such cases the urethral gap may be considerable and the ends will not meet as the pelvic haematoma resolves (Blandy).

Pelvic fractures

Are the shared responsibility of orthopaedic and general surgeons. They are classified as:

Isolated (not destroying pelvic ring integrity)   These are not significant and need only 3 weeks' rest with leg exercises.

Pelvic ring integrity disruption (due to ring fracture at two points)   The pelvis is no longer a stable weight-bearing structure, the separated fragments may be displaced and the fracture may be difficult or impossible to reduce. The fracture receives secondary consideration while every effort should be made to exclude or confirm and treat the fracture complications inflicted on the pelvic viscera. The fracture may be slight (bed rest), disrupted symphysis pubis (*see above*) or upward proximal displacement (skeletal traction through tibia of the affected side is essential for 2 months to prevent sciatic nerve compression).

Hip dislocation (*see also* Section 1.33)

Uncommon injuries, classified as:

Posterior dislocation   Occurs in flexed adducted and internally rotated hip position (since the femoral head becomes covered posteriorly by the capsule only and not by bone, force applied to the long axis of the femoral shaft may dislocate the head over the posterior hip of the acetabulum). Such injuries occur in front seat car passengers who are thrown forwards and strike their knees on the dash board. Also in motorcycle accidents and in roof fall accidents. The femoral head is displaced into the sciatic notch (damaging the sciatic nerve) and then into the ilium dorsum. Pain is referred along the sciatic nerve. The dislocation is reduced under general anaesthesia on the floor with the patient's iliac crests steadied by an assistant. The surgeon stands over the limb and flexes the knee and hip, then adducts with vertical lifting of the femur (sometimes with internal rotation). Reduction is maintained by skeletal traction on the tibia of the affected side for 6 weeks with no weight-bearing for 6 months (because of possible unpredicted avascular necrosis of the femoral head in 10% of cases).

Complications are:
- Sciatic nerve injury: treated by reduction of dislocation.
- Avascular necrosis of femoral head: treated by hemi- or total hip replacement arthroplasty.
- Femoral neck fracture (rarely): treated by operation and dislocation open reduction. Avascular necrosis is invariable.
- Fracture of posterior hip of acetabulum: treated by open reduction and internal fixation with a screw with open reduction of dislocated hip.
- Hip osteoarthrosis with post-traumatic ossification.

Anterior dislocation Rare. The femoral head lies in either the obturator or the pubic position with the limb flexed, abducted and externally rotated. Treated by reduction.

Central dislocation Usually accompanied by other pelvic fractures and is due to a blow on the greater trochanter driving the head through the acetabular floor resulting in comminuted acetabular fracture. Treated by reduction of the femoral head to its anatomical position; this is maintained by tibial skeletal traction with mobilisation as soon as pain allows. The result is unsatisfactory because of hip osteoarthrosis regardless of treatment. (Open reduction is difficult and one should accept the displacement and later osteoarthrosis.)

A22

(a) Progressive osteolytic lesion affecting the greater trochanter of the right femoral head.
(b) Bone biopsy (the histology in this case was consistent with a secondary rather than a primary bone tumour), skeletal survey and radioactive isotope bone scan (hot spots in the latter are not always due to tumour as prior skeletal survey may show recently fractured bone with callus formation, Paget's disease of the bone or even osteoarthrosis). A thorough clinical examination of both breasts, chest, thyroid gland and kidneys should follow including chest X-ray, mammogram, IVU and thyroid radioactive scan. The primary is treated, although a solitary metastasis could be treated as well. Multiple secondaries indicate advanced carcinomatosis beyond treatment.
(c) Rarely primary bone tumour (osteogenic sarcoma) but more commonly secondary bony metastases (more than two-thirds of cases). The primary origin tends to be breast carcinoma or (in males) prostatic carcinoma in two-thirds of all secondary bony deposits. One-sixth arise from the bronchus, kidney and thyroid (in that order). In the remaining one-sixth of cases no primary tumour can be identified. The majority of tumours are osteolytic (radiolucent) but prostatic and rarely bony breast deposits are osteoblastic (sclerotic).
Comment. Bone biopsy under general anaesthesia revealed a subclinical abdominal mass in this obese woman. Barium studies revealed displacement of the transverse colon; abdominal ultrasound and IVU excluded kidney origin. Exploratory laparotomy revealed an inoperable small bowel carcinoma (bypassed and biopsy taken). Histology was similar to bone biopsy and both showed non-Hodgkin's lymphoma or anaplastic carcinoma. Since skeletal survey and bone scan revealed only this solitary hot spot in the right hip, this rare case was reported as a solitary skeletal metastasis from small bowel carcinoma and represents one of unidentified origin. Skeletal metastases are usually multiple and very rarely solitary. When presented clinically such metastases can reveal the subclinical occult primary tumour.
(d) Pathological fracture which could be treated by hip replacement (hemiarthroplasty). Classically, pathological fractures of bone shafts (e.g. femoral shaft) are treated with internal fixation followed by radiotherapy (in malignant cases only).
Comment. Bone fracture following trivial trauma may be due to local or general causes.
- Local bony lesions: simple cyst, osteoclastoma, eosinophilic granuloma, hydatid cyst, aneurysmal bone cyst, haemangioma, fibrous dysplasia and Brodie's abscess (localised chronic osteomyelitis) and primary bone tumour.
- General causes: Paget's disease, primary osteoporosis, vitamin D deficiency (rickets in children and osteomalacia in adults), scurvy (vitamin C deficiency), endocrine disorders such as hyperparathyroidism and secondary osteoporosis (in pituitary or adrenal cortical tumour), secondary skeletal metastases and multiple myeloma.

A23

(a) Fracture of distal 2 cm of radius with dinner-fork deformity. The distal fragment is:
- Displaced dorsally.
- Angulated dorsally.
- Driven proximally, overlapping the shaft (shortening).
- Angulated laterally.
- Supinated.
There is an associated fracture of the ulnar styloid process.

(b) Colles' fracture.

(c) The fracture is reduced under general anaesthesia or Bier's block. The surgeon shakes hands with the patient's affected hand, and applies firm traction (with assistant exerting countertraction on the elbow), disimpacting the distal radial fragment by pressing it into palmar-flexion, ulnar deviation and pronation. Dorsal plaster slab is applied in this position from the elbow to the metacarpal heads. Satisfactory reduction is confirmed by X-ray. The slab is converted into Colles' plaster 24 h later (if the reduction is maintained with satisfactory circulation to the fingers) and maintained for 6 weeks.

(d) Complications (with their treatment) are malunion (osteotomy and realignment), subluxation of inferior radioulnar joint (excision of ulnar tail), stiffness of fingers or shoulder (exercises), fraying attrition rupture of extensor pollicis longus (extensor indicis transfer) and Sudeck's post-traumatic osteodystrophy (physiotherapy).

A24

(a) Fracture through the distal metaphysis of the humerus with complex distal fragment displacement consisting of three elements:
- Backward displacement.
- Backward angulation.
- Pronation (since the hand is usually pronated at the time of injury) producing internal rotation and adduction of the distal fragment.

The diagnosis is supracondylar fracture of the humerus.

(b) Examine the radial pulse of the affected arm since the brachial artery may be injured by the distal fragment, compressed by haematoma or contracted as a result of spasm. Reduction under general anaesthesia with X-ray screening is essential. The assistant grasps the upper arm and the surgeon shakes hands with the affected forearm exerting:

1. Firm steady traction in the long axis of the forearm (while in flexion) for 2 min; then
2. Traction and extension of the elbow (feel radial pulse); then
3. Supination and external rotation, which are compared with range of supination and external rotation of unaffected arm; then
4. Gradual maximal flexion (90°) of elbow with palpable radial pulse done by pressing the olecranon with the thumbs (and fingers over biceps) to move it and the distal fragment forward into flexion.
5. A light back slab is applied over padding and postreduction X-ray is checked immediately, 48 h and 1 week later. A collar and cuff may be used but never a full encircling plaster. Radial pulse should be examined when the patient is admitted to hospital and for 48 h.

(c) Fractures around the elbow in children are very important because their complications or malmanagement result in disabling problems. They are:
- Supracondylar fracture of the humerus (65% of cases).
- Lateral condyle = external condyle = capitellum fracture.
- Medial epicondylar fracture.
- Fracture separating upper radial epiphysis.
- Olecranon fracture.
- Posterior dislocation of elbow with possible fracture of coronoid process, radial head or distal humeral articular surface.
- Monteggia fracture-dislocation (ulnar fracture with dislocated superior radioulnar joint) may be included.

(d) The most serious complication of supracondylar fracture of the humerus is: *Vascular occlusion* leading to gangrene or ischaemic Volkmann's contracture (of flexor muscles and peripheral nerves). Other complications are *injury to the median nerve*; and *deformity from malunion* causing cubitus varus (treated by supracondylar osteotomy).

Comment on vascular occlusion

Diagnosis of incipient stage

Vascular occlusion is suggested by impaired circulatory signs including:

- Colour (pale).
- Temperature (cool).
- Pulses (feeble or absent).
- Capillary return (poor).
- Nerve conduction — digital sensory loss in the absence of nerve injury (motor testing is less reliable):
- Inability of patient to extend fingers fully.
- Marked pain on passive extension in the forearm.

Diagnosis of established stage

History of fracture and the characteristic flexion contraction of the wrist and fingers (flexor muscles are affected more than extensor muscles).

Treatment

Incipient Volkmann's ischaemia

1. First steps.
- Remove external splints or bandage.
- Reduce fracture (if not already reduced).
- Hot water bottles — to produce vasodilatation.
- Dextran 40 i.v. infusion.
2. Second step (if first steps fail). Explore for:
- Free brachial artery kinking and if in spasm paint it with papaveretum or apply a warm pack.
- Punctured or contused and thrombosed artery. Excise and end-to-end suture or use vein graft.

Established Volkmann's ischaemic contracture

Restoration to normal function is impossible. The following options are available:
- Overcome shortening by prolonged stretching with spring splints.
- Shorten bones.
- Muscle slide operation (detachment and distal displacement of flexor muscles).
- Excise dead muscles and transfer healthy muscle, e.g. wrist flexor or wrist extensor, to the tendon of flexor digitorum profundus and flexor pollicis longus.
- Arthrodesis of wrist.
- Grafting of median nerve damaged by the ischaemic injury.

A25

(a) Anterior subcoracoid left shoulder dislocation (of humeral head).
(b) There is a triad of physical signs:
- Outer aspect of the shoulder is flattened and the arm appears to originate from under the junction of the middle and outer thirds of the clavicle.
- Immobility of the shoulder (due to mechanical problem, spasm and pain).
- Abduction position.
(c) Reduction under general anaesthesia producing muscle relaxation. Kocher's method consists of flexing the elbow and:
1. Applying traction in the long axis of the humerus for 2 min; then
2. Rotating the humerus externally; then
3. Adducting the shoulder fully; then
4. Rotating the shoulder internally fully.
The postreduction X-ray is checked and the position is maintained for 3 weeks by a sling and bandage.

Comment

In acute shoulder dislocation, the humeral head takes one of four positions:
1. Anterior subcoracoid (the commonest).
2. Subglenoid.
3. Subclavicular.
4. Posterior or dorsal.

Recurrent shoulder dislocation is due to instability following maltreated acute dislocation and is treated only by operation.

Bankart's operation for recurrent shoulder dislocation

1. A sandbag is placed between the scapulae to allow the shoulder to fall backwards. The incision commences above the coracoid process, extends downwards one finger's breadth lateral to the deltopectoral groove for 12.5 cm, safeguarding the cephalic vein, dividing the deep fascia and splitting the deltoid in line with the incision. (If exposure is inadequate identify and divide the coracoid process; retract the tip and its attached muscles — coracobrachialis and biceps — downwards.)
2. Rotate the arm externally and divide the subscapularis and the capsule 2.5 cm from the muscle insertion.
3. Open and inspect the capsule, and retract the humeral head with Bankart's retractor. Notice the voluminous capsule, labrum glenoidale tear, humeral head defect and possibly loose bodies.
4. If the labrum is detached, raise a shaving from the front of the glenoid cavity to produce a raw area, drill holes in the anterior edge of the glenoid with an angled dental drill and suture the detached glenoidal labrum to the raw area, using wire, nylon or other suitable ligatures.
5. Repair the subscapularis (in the Putti–Platt operation the muscle and capsule are overlapped (double-breasted) for 2.5 cm).
6. Resuture the coracoid process into position (if divided) and bandage the arm to the side with the elbow held forwards for 5 weeks.

A26

(a) Fracture of the waist of the right scaphoid bone.

(b) Patient presents clinically with a painful wrist (but with no major impairment of wrist function). On examination there is tenderness in the anatomical snuff-box (over the scaphoid) with little swelling. Pinch test by pressing the thumb against the index finger of the affected side causes severe pain in the anatomical snuff-box. X-ray should include three views: anteroposterior, lateral and *two oblique*. Since there is no displacement immediately after injury the fracture may not be displayed radiologically. The case is misdiagnosed as sprained wrist and mobilisation carried out, leading to avascular necrosis, non-union and osteoarthrosis of the wrist or stiff wrist in later treatment. Therefore suspected fracture, even if not confirmed radiologically, should be treated in a scaphoid plaster (like a Colles' plaster from the elbow down to the metacarpal heads *but also set up to the interphalangeal joint of the thumb* while the hand is in a functioning position as if holding a glass of water) for 2 weeks, after which the plaster is removed and the wrist X-rayed again; by this time the original unrevealed scaphoid fracture becomes obvious radiologically. If the fracture is confirmed at this time or diagnosed from the start the scaphoid plaster should be applied for 8 weeks.

Non-union is either immobilised for a year (may result in stiff wrist), treated by bone grafting and internal fixation with a small screw followed by 8 weeks' immobilisation in plaster or accepted as it is (non-union will not always give rise to significant disability).

A27

(a) Arteriography.

(b) Right popliteal artery aneurysm with wide lumen (although the presence and extent of thrombus cannot be assessed). The left popliteal artery is healthy with good filling of its trifurcation (perineal, anterior and posterior tibial arteries).

(c) Surgery by wide exposure with proximal and distal control followed by femoropopliteal bypass (using reversed autogenous vein graft or gore graft) combined with either aneurysmal excision or exclusion. Occasionally Matas' aneurysmorrhaphic reconstruction may be performed if practically possible.

Comment on aneurysm classification

Aneurysm is an abnormal arterial dilatation and is either:
- True: dilated artery (whether fusiform, saccular or dissecting);
- False: an organised sac communicating with the artery through an opening in its wall. It is traumatic in origin; or:
- Arteriovenous fistula (congenital or acquired).

The causes of aneurysms are:
- Congenital: berry aneurysm (of cerebral circle of Willis) and dissecting aneurysm of Marfan's syndrome.
- Traumatic (false and arteriovenous aneurysm such as cirsoid aneurysm).
- Atherosclerosis as in abdominal aortic aneurysm.
- Hypertension.
- Infective: wrongly called mycotic — they are usually bacterial or syphilitic.
- Infarction: left ventricular aneurysm after myocardial infarction (containing mural thrombus).

The eventual outcome of aneurysms is either spontaneous healing (consolidation), infection, development of a slow leak or sudden rupture.

A28

(a) Plain X-ray of lower limb revealing a bipennate muscle structure (of the right thigh) due to the presence of gas in the intramuscular planes. The diagnosis is gas gangrene.

(b) The condition is extremely life-threatening and treatment should include:
1. Preparation for immediate operation with
   (i) Blood transfusion.
   (ii) Penicillin 8 mega-units (stat. i.v. injection) followed by 4 mega-units 4-hourly for 8 days together with 2 g streptomycin injection daily.
   (iii) Anti-gas gangrene serum (3 ampoules immediately and repeated 6-hourly i.v.).
   (iv) 100% oxygen or hyperbaric oxygen to reduce the amount of toxin produced by the anaerobic organisms (*Clostridium welchii*, *Cl. septicum* and *Cl. oedematiens*).
2. Operation aiming at early and meticulous excision of all dead and dying muscular tissues, either done via bilateral long incisions of the affected limb with secondary suture or (if such total clearance is impossible) amputation via hip disarticulation. Although uncommon, gas gangrene carries a high mortality in the victims of accidents and classically complicates high amputation stumps in the presence of arterial disease (since Clostridia are present in the intestine, prophylactic antibiotics are required in amputation with a fluffy bandage to prevent faecal contamination of stump). The mortality is due to rapid gangrene involving muscles initially (swollen tense limb with sickly foul odour due to gas and thin brownish foul exudate) and, when septicaemia occurs, involving the abdominal organs (e.g. foaming liver).

Comment

Gas gangrene and tetanus are the two acute specific infections that are commonly asked about in the final FRCS. Tetanus is caused by *Clostridium tetani* which produces a powerful exotoxin that:
- Interferes with ACh/Ch-esterase balance leading to sustained muscular tonic spasm due to ACh excess.
- Causes extreme hyperexcitability of motor neurons in the anterior horn cells leading to explosive muscle reflex spasm in response to minor stimuli.
- Causes concomitant sympathetic overactivity.

The time between the first symptom and the first reflex spasm is '*the period of onset*' which serves as a prognostic index (the longer it is, the better the prognosis). First symptoms are difficult swallowing, jaw stiffness, and painful neck, back and abdomen. Risus sardonicus (smile), opisthotonos and muscle rupture (psoas, rectus abdominis, pectoral) are due to reflex convulsions which occur spontaneously or in response to trivial stimuli. Cyanosis, pneumonia, respiratory failure and death are the ultimate outcome. Prophylactically active immunity can be induced by administration of tetanus toxoid followed by a booster dose every 5 years. Passive immunisation with 250 units human antitetanus globulin (ATG) should always be given with toxoid. Established tetanus is treated by isolation of the patient in a quiet dark place, wound toilet, and administration of ATG (one dose) and penicillin (heavy doses). In addition: in mild cases—sedation with i.m. promazine and amylobarbitone 6-hourly; in seriously ill patients—nasogastric tube (for feeding) and tracheostomy; and in dangerously ill patients—intermittent positive pressure ventilation with curare is indicated.

A29

(a) Lymphangiography.
(b) Probably Stage 2 Hodgkin's disease but cervical lymph node biopsy and staging laparotomy are required for accurate diagnosis.
(c) Patent blue dye is injected into the web between toes to show the lymphatics on the dorsum of both feet which thereafter are exposed, cannulated and then injected with a radiopaque solution (Lipiodol Ultra-Fluid) using a size 30 E needle and an infusion pump, so that deeper main trunks in the leg may be visualised on X-ray.

Comment

Normal radiological appearance of the lymphatic system

1. Lymph nodes—uniform in opacity (no filling defect).
2. Lymph vessels—uniform in size with beaded appearance due to the presence of valves.

Abnormal radiological appearance of lymphatic system

1. Lymph nodes (direct signs)
   (a) May be normal in size or slightly enlarged and typically with filling defect.
   (b) Foamy reticular appearance.
   (c) Discontinuity of lymph node chain.
2. Lymphatic vessels (indirect signs)
   (a) Displaced lymphatics.
   (b) Collateral lymph channels.
   (c) Lymphatic obstruction causing variation in the calibre of vessels.
   (d) Persistence of contrast medium in vessel after 24 h.
   (e) Dermal backflow (bullae in skin, papules or vesicles).

The clinical applications of lymphography

1. Preoperative for early detection of lymph involvement to facilitate clearance.
2. In radiotherapy
   (a) To plan field of irradiation.
   (b) To assess response to radiation.
3. To diagnose nature of lesion
   (a) Distinguish abdominal or pelvic from retroperitoneal masses.
   (b) Lymphoma causing pyrexia of unknown origin.
   (c) Nature of lymphoedema of extremities.
4. For endolymphatic injection of cytotoxic drugs or radioisotopes in the treatment of certain malignant disease, e.g. malignant melanoma.

A30

(a) Right cervical rib producing thoracic outlet syndrome.
(b) Locally there is a cervical bony fixed lump and supraclavicular tenderness. Forearm ischaemic pain radiating to the upper arm is brought on by use of the arm, especially in elevation, and relieved by rest. The hand is cold with colour changes (pale when held aloft and blue when dependent). The radial pulse is absent or feeble especially after abduction of the arm with possible systolic bruit on subclavian auscultation. Skin trophic changes are preceded by finger numbness, leading to ulceration, gangrene or nerve pressure symptoms (pain, paraesthesia and weakness in hand and forearm with wasting of the thenar and hypothenar muscles are attributed to cervical rib only after exclusion of cervical spondylosis and carpal tunnel syndrome).
(c) Extraperiosteal excision of cervical rib (with periosteum).

Comment

Cervical ribs are present in up to 1 % of the population. They are usually asymptomatic and commonly bilateral (in this case unilateral). Thoracic outlet syndrome is caused by:
● Bones (cervical rib, clavicle fracture, transverse process of C7).
● Muscles (scalenus anterior, pectoralis minor).
● Bands (fibromuscular band related to any of the above structures).
The syndrome is also known as costoclavicular, scalenus anterior, shoulder girdle, pectoralis minor, hyperabduction, Adson's or cervical rib syndrome. Arch arteriography is required to show subclavian stenosis and post-stenotic dilatation with local thrombus formation (which can lead to distal embolisation). Treatment in the absence of cervical rib is scalenotomy, band removal, first rib removal or even sympathectomy.

A31

(a) Computerised axial tomography (CT) scan.
(b) A renal mass in the lower pole of the right kidney, confirmed by repeating the scan after contrast injection. The left kidney is normal. The diagnosis is that of right hypernephroma.
(c) Right radical nephrectomy.

A32

(a) Lumbar aortogram.
(b) Aortogram shows an extravasation at the injection site as the aorta is very narrow (due to atheroma). The left common iliac artery is narrow but patent. The right common iliac artery is blocked at its origin. Collateral circulation is visualised through the lumbar arteries and part of the internal iliac vessels. Diagnosis: Leriche's disease (in progress, not yet occluding the origin of the left common iliac artery).
(c) Either right aortofemoral bypass using a Dacron tube graft or preferably inverted Y (trouser or bifurcated Dacron graft) aortofemoral bypass.

A33

(a) Left percutaneous transfemoral balloon angiography; balloon mounted on guide wire was passed retrogradely for dilatation of stenotic external iliac segment (angioplasty).

A34

(a) Angiography (cannot tell from this film whether it is a retrograde femoral or lumbar aortogram).
(b) Bilateral occlusion of the superficial femoral arteries with irregular narrow lumens (normally the superficial femoral arteries run parallel to the femur). Both deep femoral arteries are patent and normal. There

is good run-off on both sides with more pronounced collaterals on the left side.

(c) Surgery indicated in severe intermittent claudication, in rest pain in pregangrenous state and in distal embolisation (sudden dislodgement and showering of atheromatous plaque distally could cause, for example, gangrenous toe with silent proximal vascular disease). Operation will be bilateral femoropopliteal end-to-side bypass using reversed autogenous vein or gore graft (recommended below the inguinal ligament). Endarterectomy and profundoplasty may be added.

A35

(a) Leaking aortic aneurysm. Notice the left paramedian linear calcification surrounded by soft tissue swelling (leaking retroperitoneal haematoma which can be manifested clinically by flank ecchymosis—the Grey–Turner sign as seen in acute pancreatitis).

(b) Very urgent aortic clamping followed by aortic aneurysm repair.

A36

(a) Plain abdominal X-ray showing three radiopaque gall stones, one of them having moved to obstruct Hartmann's pouch.

(b) Acute calculous obstructed cholecystitis.

(c) Available investigations are:

Plain abdominal X-ray—may reveal radiopaque gall stones in 10–15% of cases (since 85–90% are radiolucent, this is exactly opposite to urinary stones where 85–90% are radiopaque).

Oral cholecystogram—to confirm the presence of gall stones or non-visualisation of the gall bladder (a negative sign of positive diagnostic value). In acute cholecystitis, this test is limited because of vomiting and inability to swallow tablets. It is worthwhile in patients who are not nauseous or jaundiced.

Intravenous cholangiogram (bolus)—produces relatively poor opacification of the extrahepatic biliary system and the dye fails to concentrate adequately even in a normally functioning gall bladder.

Infusion i.v. cholangiogram—probably the most reliable diagnostic procedure with accuracy of more than 90%. It requires tomographic facilities and the long infusion time may prove inconvenient.

Grey scale ultrasound—detects gall stones in both acute and chronic stages and provides information on dilated ducts. Its effectiveness is impaired by bowel gas in the gall bladder area masking the stones in approximately 30% of patients on the initial scan. Repeat scanning is important.

Isotope scanning—i.v. technetium isotope HIDA is the most successful test for diagnosis of acute cholecystitis. Failure of isotope uptake by the gall bladder is diagnostic. Delay of excretion of common bile duct dye in the duodenum is indicative of common bile duct obstruction.

(d) Traditionally most British surgeons proceed with conservative treatment (bed rest, pain relief with antispasmodic drug, e.g. hyoscine butylbromide (Buscopan) and analgesic, e.g. pethidine, antibiotics and possibly nasogastric suction and i.v. drip in persistent vomiting), so that the condition resolves and definitive investigations can take place in the recovery period; definitive elective cholecystectomy is done 6–12 weeks later. Elective cholecystectomy has the advantage of allowing confirmation of the provisional clinical diagnosis with more investigations and avoiding operation on an acutely inflamed friable gall bladder with, for example, obscure anatomy in an obese patient. It also means that a convenient time can be chosen with experienced anaesthetic and surgical staff and appropriate facilities (e.g. operative cholangiogram) available. However, its disadvantages are prolongation of the patient's symptoms (persistent pain and/or fever) in 6–33% of cases and possible complications, i.e. extrahepatic obstructive jaundice (with or without cholangitis and septicaemia), empyema of the gall bladder and perforation of the gall bladder (in 3–12% of acute cholecystitis cases), that may require the surgeon to undertake emergency operation with potentially poorer results. Many surgeons consider this too high a price to pay for the traditional approach and are now beginning to follow the policy of early surgery, i.e. *urgent* but not emergency cholecystectomy done within 1 week of admission (to allow the surgeon to carry out the necessary investigations and the acutely inflamed gall bladder to settle). The advantages of the early operative approach are as follows:

- The accuracy of clinical diagnosis supplemented by investigations (plain abdominal X-ray, ultrasound, oral cholecystogram and/or infusion, i.v. cholangiogram with HIDA scan when available) has become very close to 100%.
- The pathology of the removed gall bladder during first admission reveals that 65% have chronic cholecystitis with acute inflammation, 25% chronic cholecystitis and 10% acute cholecystitis. Long-term follow-up of such patients indicates a high incidence of recurrence and development of complications.
- The mortality of urgent surgery is exaggerated. Studies reveal that the operative mortality rate is equal to that of elective cholecystectomy. Indeed 20% of patients treated conservatively will require re-admission for a further attack before their elective operation; in addition 17% of patients are defaulters—they either refuse subsequent admission or are lost (owing to false impression of being cured) only to present later with complications. Thus the *overall* mortality of late operation is probably higher than that of early intervention. However, morbidity (i.e. wound infection) was found to be higher in urgent operation because of highly infected bile.
- Technically, urgent cholecystectomy in patients with chronic cholecystitis is as easy as elective operation. In 75% (with acute inflammation) oedema may make the operation easier by creating a plane of cleavage. However, surgery should be avoided if acute symptoms have continued for 7 days or more as the granulation tissue and adhesions are more advanced (perforation of the gall bladder is extremely rare after 7 days of continuous symptoms and these patients are best treated conservatively with surgery at a second admission).
- Acalculous cholecystitis presents with severe systemic illness and rarely responds well to conservative treatment. The gall bladder is thick-walled, grossly oedematous with leucocyte infiltration and full of pus and fibrin mixed with bile with mucosal ulcerations. Aetiology is obscure (e.g. associated with torsion of the vascular pedicle, bile stasis with prolonged fasting, clostridial organisms, trauma, burns and specific diseases such as diabetes, sarcoidosis and chronic renal failure). Surgical delay in such patients only increases the hazards of the illness.

Summary   The policy should be as follows:
- Patients unfit for operation at any time are managed conservatively.
- Patients with acute symptoms of more than 7 days receive conservative treatment with elective operation 6 weeks later.
- Patients with symptoms of less than 7 days' duration have an operation on the next list after diagnosis (urgent but not emergency operation) by a competent surgeon.
- Emergency operation for patients presenting with a perforated gall bladder (toxic signs with peritonitis) or increasing local signs.

Technical points in early operation   Handling of the perforated, gangrenous or friable gall bladder may result in rupture and dissemination of infected material. This can be minimised by aspirating some of the contents to relieve the tension and the gall bladder can then be mobilised in a retrograde manner. This allows the gall bladder to hang by the pedicle of cystic duct and artery. These can be divided close to or even across the neck of the gall bladder allowing better visualisation of the common bile duct. Prophylactic antibiotics and operative cholangiogram are mandatory. Subtotal cholecystectomy or cholecystostomy may be used only in difficult situations.

SECTION 5
Surgical Pathology

Surgical pathology is an integral part in the *viva* of the Final FRCS with the exception of the Irish Fellowship. In the London Fellowship, both microscopy (slides) and macroscopy (specimens) are important. In Edinburgh only macroscopy is included in the form of specimens, while in Glasgow the surgical pathology in the *viva* usually proceeds without specimens.

A. How to Handle a Surgical Specimen

1. Hold it in your hands and look at it from different angles.
2. Identify the organ, usually by spotting a key structure, e.g. the presence of appendix in a bowel segment means ileocaecal region, typical mucosal folds are seen in the stomach, skin identified by hair in a bowel segment indicates anorectal junction, taenia coli and/or appendices epiploicae indicate large bowel, tooth in a bone segment indicates a jaw, pyriform hollow viscus with or without a stone indicates gall bladder, nipple and areola indicates breast, globular hollow viscus with two ureters and urethra with stricture or prostatic obstruction indicates a bladder, and so on.
3. Once you have identified the organ, the lesion should be easily recognised. If in difficulty describe what you see and do not stop talking. Remember that the organ's identity will give you a clue about the pathology, e.g. anorectal junction usually indicates a rectal carcinoma excised by the abdominoperineal approach, an ileocaecal segment possibly indicates Crohn's disease, carcinoma or carcinoid and breast always indicates carcinoma.
4. Having identified the organ and the lesion, it is a bonus (but not essential) to comment on whether the specimen is surgical or postmortem. In the latter you will see a discrepancy between the size of the removed organ and the lesion, e.g. a specimen showing the whole stomach of a child with congenital pyloric stenosis, a lung with more than one metastasis, a whole urinary system (two kidneys, two ureters and bladder) showing prostatic obstruction, part of a heart or skull.

B. Examples with Discussion

The following examples of specimens with discussion between the candidate (C) and the examiner (E) should provide a better understanding of what to expect in this part of the examination.

B1. MECKEL'S DIVERTICULUM

The examiner hands the candidate a specimen of Meckel's diverticulum (Fig. 118).

E: What is this?

C: A segment of bowel with mesentery. It is a small bowel since there is no taeni coli, appendices epiploicae or haustration. There is an antimesenteric diverticulum. It is a Meckel's diverticulum.

E: What is a Meckel's diverticulum?

C: It is a remnant of the vitellointestinal duct and represents a true congenital diverticulum.

E: Are there any false diverticula?

C: Yes, sir. The acquired diverticula are false since they represent herniation of mucosa through a mesenteric blood vessel hole; they are mucososerosal pouches and do not contain all the wall layers. An example is diverticular disease of the sigmoid colon.

E: What are the complications of Meckel's diverticulum?

C: Bleeding, inflammation and possibly perforation, peritonitis, intussusception, peptic ulcer due to ectopic gastric mucosa, intestinal obstruction across the band of Meckel's diverti-

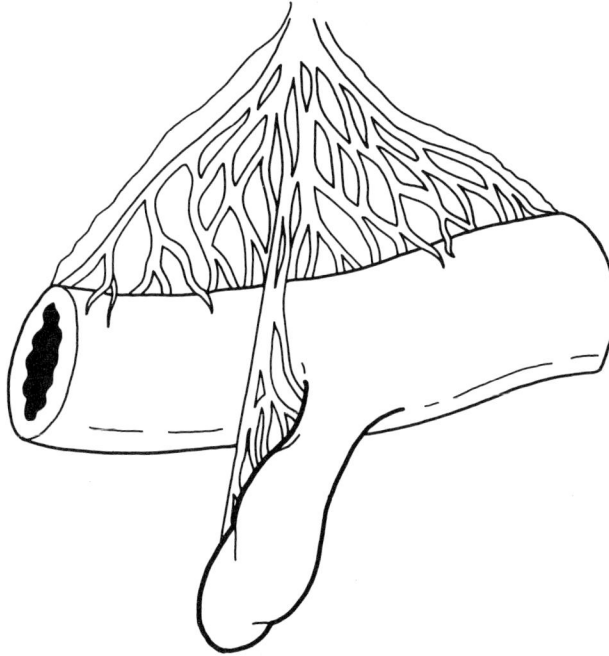

Fig. 118 Meckel's diverticulum

culum connected to the umbilicus, herniation into the inguinal or femoral canal (Littre's hernia).

E: If you find it accidentally in laparotomy, do you remove it?

C: Symptomless Meckel's diverticulum is better removed unless the patient is being explored for a vascular lesion (e.g. leaking aortic aneurysm or bypass graft operation), is undergoing emergency abdominal operation or is in a generally poor condition.

E: How do you remove it?

C: Meckel's diverticulectomy via a wedge excision of its base, but if the base is indurated it is better to do a limited resection of the diverticulum-bearing segment of the ileum and do an end-to-end anastomosis with two layers using 2/0 chromic catgut.

B2. GASTRIC OUTLET OBSTRUCTION

E: What is this (Fig. 119)?

C: A specimen of tissue with characteristic mucosal folds—it is gastric mucosa with distal pyloric obstruction.

E: What is the cause of the obstruction here?

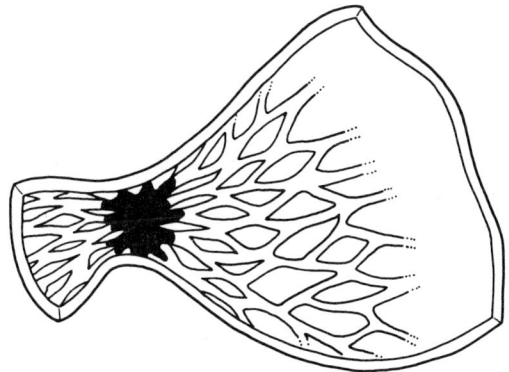

Fig. 119 Scarred duodenal ulcer

C: Most likely a scarred peptic ulcer since the absence of a mass in the pylorus and the presence of normal mucosal gastric folds near the obstruction excludes the possibility of pyloric gastric carcinoma.

E: All right. What is the cause of the obstruction here? (He hands the candidate a specimen exhibiting congenital pyloric stenosis.) (Fig. 120).

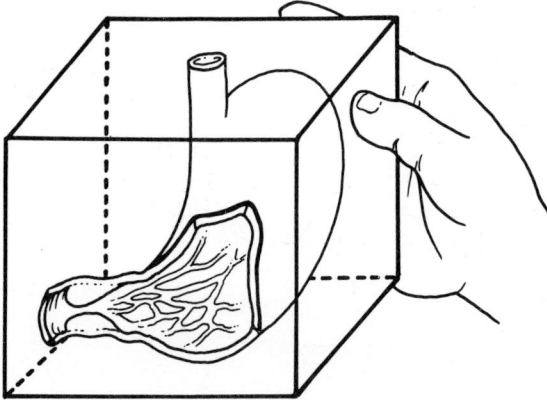

Fig. 120 Congenital pyloric stenosis

C: There is a thickened muscular layer of pyloric canal with obstruction. Since the whole stomach is shown this is a postmortem specimen of a child who died from congenital pyloric stenosis.

E: What are the physical signs of pyloric obstruction in general?

C: Visible peristalsis (from left to right), a succussion splash is heard and the outline of the enlarged stomach can sometimes be observed. Epigastric mass can be felt in carcinoma and congenital pyloric stenosis. Signs of carcinomatosis are obstructive jaundice, ascites, Krukenberg's tumour (bilateral ovarian tumours felt per rectum), palpable Virchow's left supraclavicular lymph nodes (Troisier's sign), phlebothrombosis of superficial veins of the leg (Trousseau's sign) and Sister Joseph nodule (secondary tumour in umbilicus via falciform ligament). The patient is mentally confused as a result of frequent projectile vomiting leading ultimately to metabolic alkalosis with hypokalaemia. In very advanced stages there will be paradoxical aciduria (acidic urine in the face of systemic alkalosis due to secretion of H^+ ions in the urine for Na^+ exchange because of very low K^+ stores ready for exchange).

E: What is the treatment for congenital pyloric stenosis?

C: A quick preparation including rehydration and correction of electrolyte disturbances with i.v. fluids, followed by Ramstedt's operation (pyloromyotomy), preserving mucosa only. Medical treatment with atropine-like drugs (Eumydrin) could be tried but usually fails.

E: What about the treatment of chronic duodenal or prepyloric ulcer?

C: Truncal vagotomy and gastroenterostomy.

E: Give me other alternatives.

C: Truncal vagotomy with pyloroplasty (constructed through the unhealthy scarred tissue) or proximal gastric vagotomy with Hegar or finger dilatation through a small gastrostomy window.

E: Tell me what you know about postvagotomy diarrhoea.

C: It is a misnomer since it has the following causes:
- Rapid gastrointestinal transit, i.e. dumping.
- Abnormal small bowel bacterial colonisation due to less peristalsis after vagotomy.
- Because of dumping, hypertonic meals are less well absorbed, leading to an osmotic fluidy diarrhoea as a result of withdrawal of water from the gut.
- Reabsorption of bile salts from terminal ileum is interfered with because of excessive hydrolysis of conjugated bile salts (by bacterial colonisation); thus fat is not absorbed, leading to steatorrhoea.
- Since the vagus is a secretomotor but a sphincter inhibitor, the gall bladder is distended with spasm of the sphincter of Oddi. As a result of continuous bile secretion, overflow incontinence of bile occurs and bile is poured into the bowel passively, preventing water absorption, irritating the colon and producing diarrhoea.

E: What do you do in gastric carcinoma?

C: That depends on whether it is early or late. In early carcinoma, distal radical gastrectomy should be done. In late cases with signs of carcinomatosis, a palliative *high* anterior gastrojejunostomy is my choice to protect the anastomosis from tumour invasion.

B3. ILEOCAECAL JUNCTION

E: This specimen was taken from an elderly man. What is it (Fig. 121)?

C: This is part of the bowel. The presence of mesentery indicates small bowel but the other part shows haustration, taenia and appendices epiploicae, indicating large bowel. It is an ileocaecal junction of the bowel with a large tumour about 10 cm in diameter.

E: Where is the appendix?

C: I have looked for it but cannot see it; either it is involved in the mass or the patient has had an appendicectomy.

E: What is the diagnosis?

C: Carcinoma of the caecum or appendicular mass.

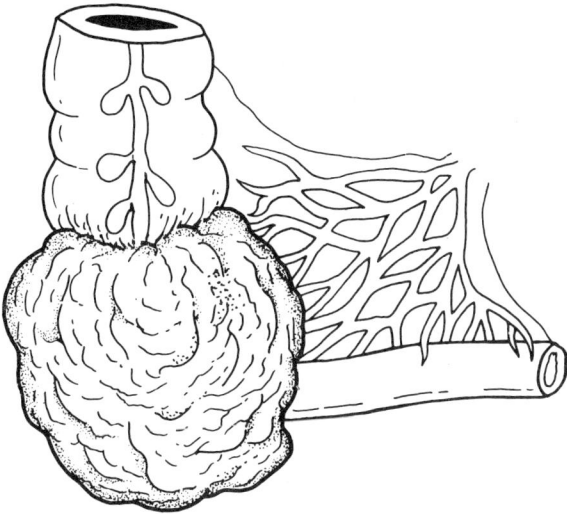

Fig. 121 Caecal carcinoma or appendicular mass

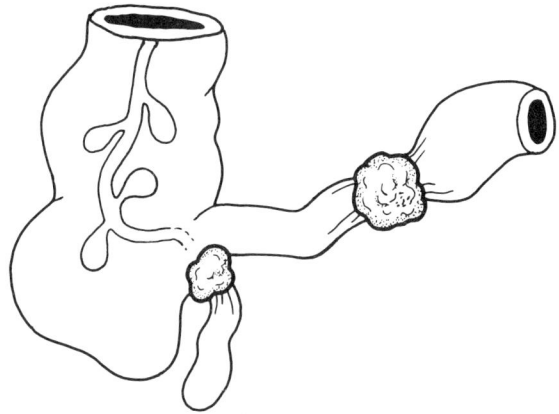

Fig. 122 Carcinoid tumours

E: Can you link the two diagnoses in one?

C: Yes. Carcinoma of the caecum can lead to secondary appendicitis (by obstructing the appendix base).

E: What are the clinical features?

C: Anaemia, right iliac fossa mass, secondary appendicitis and less commonly intussusception with abdominal pain which may be referred to the periumbilical central area.

E: What is your treatment?

C: Right hemicolectomy even for doubtful appendicular mass (which proves later by histology to be appendicitis) since leaving a mass that may prove to be carcinoma of the caecum is a fatal mistake.

Comments

Carcinoid tumour can lead to secondary appendicitis. The tumour usually affects the appendix (60 % of cases) or ileum (40 %) and is a golden yellow well-defined mass (Fig. 122). Carcinoid tumour can also present as bleeding from the gastrointestinal tract, intussusception, subacute intestinal obstruction and rarely (1 %) carcinoid syndrome—facial flushing, wheezes due to bronchial spasm, diarrhoea, borborygmi, and pulmonary stenosis and tricuspid incompetence due to chemical mediator, commonly 5-hydroxytryptophan (5-HT). Normally 5-HT is destroyed by liver but when there are hepatic secondaries from ileal carcinoid (appendicular carcinoids almost never have secondaries) the syn-

drome manifests itself. The treatment is right hemicolectomy. The presence of hepatic secondaries may require hepatic resection but the prognosis is still good. 5-Fluorouracil (5-FU) can be used locally or systemically for hepatic secondaries; methysergide, being a 5-HT antagonist is used for diarrhoea and bronchospasm; *p*-chlorophenylalanine is used for diarrhoea and to improve appetite and well-being; and α-methyldopa for flushing.

Ileocaecal tuberculosis can lead to a similar tumour. Tumour caseation and caseating mesenteric lymph nodes are present accompanied clinically by a change in bowel habits (subacute intestinal obstruction) and a history of pulmonary tuberculosis (especially in the ulcerative type) as well as anaemia, steatorrhoea, weight loss and right iliac fossa mass. Right hemicolectomy is recommended. If the patient's general condition is poor, biopsy and defunctioning ileocolostomy should be done initially, followed by chemotherapy (on histology reporting). Right hemicolectomy is undertaken later on.

Crohn's disease is similar but the bowel that is not involved in the mass may be fiery red and thickened. Again presentations are anaemia, intestinal obstruction and internal fistulae as well as anal lesions (if colon is involved). Obstruction and fistulae necessitate surgery; otherwise the disease should be treated medically. Ileocolic anastomosis is recommended for young patients. However, in elderly patients with stricture or enterocolic fistula limited resection is recommended.

B4. RECTAL TUMOUR

E: What is this (Fig. 123)?

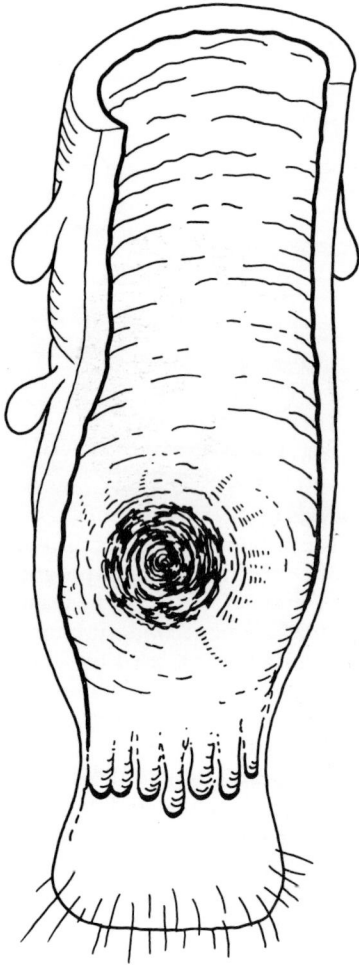

Fig. 123 Abdominoperineal specimen of rectal carcinoma

C: This is a specimen showing an ulcerative lesion 5 cm in diameter with everted edges involving part of the bowel. The presence of appendices epiploicae in the upper part and the skin with hair in the lower part indicates it is a surgical specimen from abdominoperineal resection for rectal carcinoma.

E: What are other lesions that may be excised by abdominoperineal resection?

C: Villous adenoma, rectal carcinoid tumour, ulcerative colitis and polyposis coli (proctocolectomy with terminal ileostomy in the latter two cases).

Comment

Discussion may continue on the clinical presentation of rectal carcinoma in general, on Dukes'

classification and on the pros and cons of restorative resection versus abdominoperineal resection.

B5.   BILATERAL HYDRONEPHROSIS

E: Can you tell me what this is (Fig. 124)?

C: A specimen of the whole urinary system revealing bilateral hydronephrosis, bilateral hydroureters, dilated trabeculated sacculated bladder with bladder neck obstruction by huge bulging prostatic enlargement. This is a postmortem specimen.

E: What do you think the cause of death was here?

C: Chronic renal failure due to back pressure from urinary outflow obstruction.

E: O.K. What were the clinical features before death?

C: Prostatism: difficulty in micturition, hesitancy, poor flow and possibly frequency (diurnal and nocturnal) due to detrusor instability. Acute or chronic retention, haematuria and superadded infection may also occur.

E: What are the indications for surgery?

C: Obstruction (in the form of acute or chronic retention) and bleeding. Frequency alone is not an indication for surgery.

E: What are the available methods of surgery?

C: Either open prostatectomy (suprapubic transvesical, retropubic or mixed vesicocapsular and transperineal) or closed endoscopic prostatectomy (transurethral resection of prostate—TURP).

E: What are the indications and contraindications for TURP?

C: 1. Size: large prostate—as estimated roughly by rectal examination—should be removed by the open method. Small prostate and carcinoma are ideal for TURP, but nowadays TURP can be done even if the prostate is 100 g or more.
2. With associated pathology, e.g. stone, large diverticulum, the open method is better than TURP.
3. If the patient's condition is poor or risky due to cardiothoracic status then TURP is preferable to the open method (*see also* Prostatic carcinoma, p. 136).

E: What are the other causes of *bilateral* hydronephrosis?

C: Either *congenital* (urethral matal stricture, congenital valves of the posterior urethra or congenital contracture of bladder neck) or *acquired* (bladder tumour involving both ureteric orifices; prostatic enlargement—benign or malign-

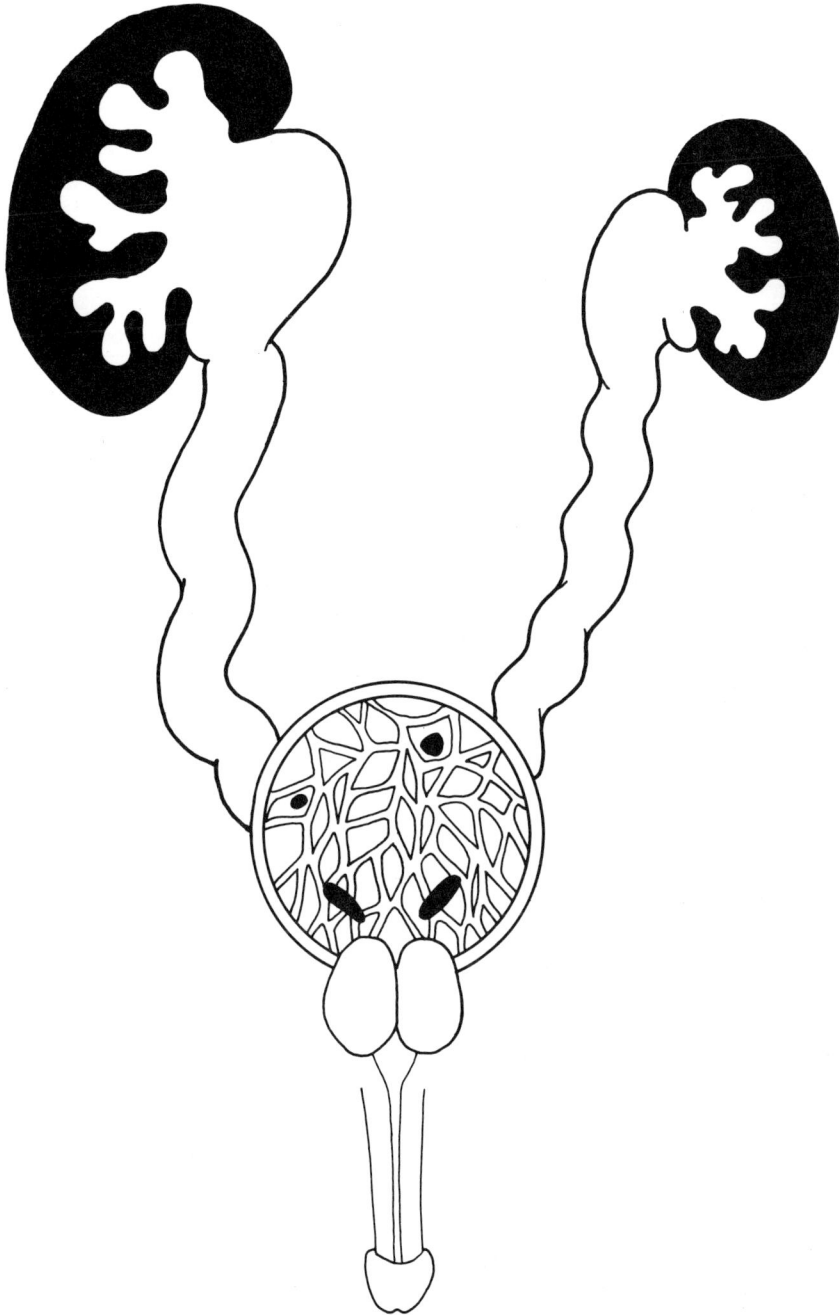

Fig. 124 Bilateral hydronephrosis

ant; carcinoma of the cervix and occasionally of the rectum involving both ureters; or inflammatory or traumatic urethral stricture or phimosis).

Comments

Hydronephrosis

Is an aseptic dilatation of the whole or part of the kidney caused by partial or intermittent obstruction to urine outflow. The causes of unilateral hydronephrosis lie in the upper urinary system (pelviureteric junction and ureter) while those of the bilateral type are in the lower urinary system (bladder and urethra). *Unilateral* hydronephrosis may be shown as a specimen. The causes are:

Extraluminal
● Congenital: e.g. aberrant blood vessel and postcaval ureter.
● Neoplastic: e.g. carcinoma of cervix, prostate, rectum, colon and caecum.
● Idiopathic retroperitoneal fibrosis (may follow administration of some drugs such as methysergide and methyldopa).

Transmural
● Congenital: e.g. stenosis, physiological narrowing or achalasia at pelviureteric junction, congenital megaureter and duplicated pelvis (more prone to hydronephrosis than normal pelvis). Ureterocele and congenital small ureteric orifice.
● Inflammatory: stricture of ureter (due to stone), tuberculosis of ureter or cicatrised tuberculosis at pelviureteric junction.
● Traumatic: after stone retrieval or stricture following ureteroureteric anastomosis or ureter trauma during pelvic operation.
● Neoplastic: tumour of the ureter or bladder involving the ureteric orifice.

Intramural
● A ureteric stone or small stone in the renal pelvis leading to intermittent hydronephrosis.

Specimen of whole urinary system in a child

This is a postmortem specimen of either the congenital valves of a prostatic urethra or Marion's disease. Suprapubic drainage of urine is life-saving. The definitive treatment is transurethral division in prostatic urethra and Y-V plasty in Marion's disease.

Bladder neck obstruction

Is a common problem resulting from intraluminal pathology, e.g. calculus or clot, but more importantly from transmural pathology:
● Congenital urethral prostatic valves or bladder neck contraction in Marion's disease (the hypertrophied interureteric bar is analogous to hypertrophic pyloric stenosis of infants).
● Neoplastic: e.g. benign adenomatous or hyperplastic prostate, carcinoma of the prostate or primary bladder cancer involving the bladder neck.
● Inflammatory: e.g. prostatic urethral stricture, post-prostatitis or fibrotic prostate; bilharziasis and tuberculosis are other causes.
● Traumatic stricture after instrumentation or ruptured membranous urethra.
● Spasm of external sphincter is quite common postoperatively and may lead to a similar effect as bladder neck obstruction.

Small capacity bladder due to contraction

The examiner may discuss this with you. The causes are:
● Tuberculosis.
● Bilharziasis.
● Interstitial cystitis or Hunner's ulcer.
● Hypertonic neuropathic bladder.
● Late contraction following radiotherapy or intravesical chemotherapy or partial cystectomy.
● Disseminated bladder tumour or papillomatosis.

B6. CHOLESTEROSIS

E: What is this (Fig. 125)?
C: A hollow viscus, pyriform in shape, opened on one side revealing tough mucosa with yellow specks. It is a surgical specimen of a gall bladder with chronic cholecystitis.
E: Which type of chronic cholecystitis?
C: Cholesterosis.
E: What is the route of precipitation of cholesterol particles here? Is it via bile or blood?
C: Via bile passed to the gall bladder for storage and concentration where the ratio of cholesterol to bile acids is already high.
E: What is the bile acids/cholesterol ratio?
C: Normally it is 25:1 when bile acids keep cholesterol soluble in bile, but when the ratio reaches the critical level of 13:1 the cholesterol crystals

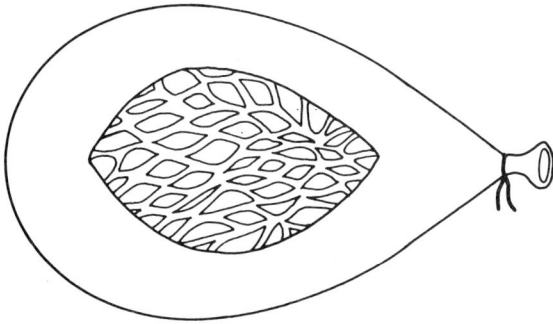

Fig. 125 Cholesterosis

(micelles) precipitate out on gall bladder mucosa. Each crystal sets off an inflammatory reaction in the wall, thus acting as a nidus for stone formation. Such bile is called 'lithogenic'.

E: O.K. What are the theories of gall stone formation?

C: These are:

1. *Metabolic factors*: include the bile acids/cholesterol ratio which I have discussed as well as bile pigment stones in excessive haemolysis, e.g. acholuric jaundice.

2. *Infection*: bacteria carried by blood or coming from the bowel via the lymphatics, infestations with Ascaris, or ingested foreign bodies, e.g. plum or tomato skin.

3. *Bile stasis*: e.g. during pregnancy; explains the increased stone incidence in multipara. Stasis may be secondary to distal obstruction or dyskinesia.

E: How do you treat chronic cholecystitis?

C: Cholecystectomy.

B7. OSTEOSARCOMA

E: What is this (Fig. 126)?

C: A specimen of long bone bisected longitudinally. It shows an expanding tumour at the upper metaphyseal end which is eroding the cortex and elevating the periosteum. It is a bone tumour.

E: What sort of bone tumour do you think it is?

C: It could be a secondary bone tumour (by far the commonest—more than 80 % of bone tumours) or it could be a primary bone tumour (less than 20 % of all bone tumours).

E: O.K. If I tell you that this is a primary one, what is your diagnosis?

C: Osteogenic sarcoma.

E: And what are the causes?

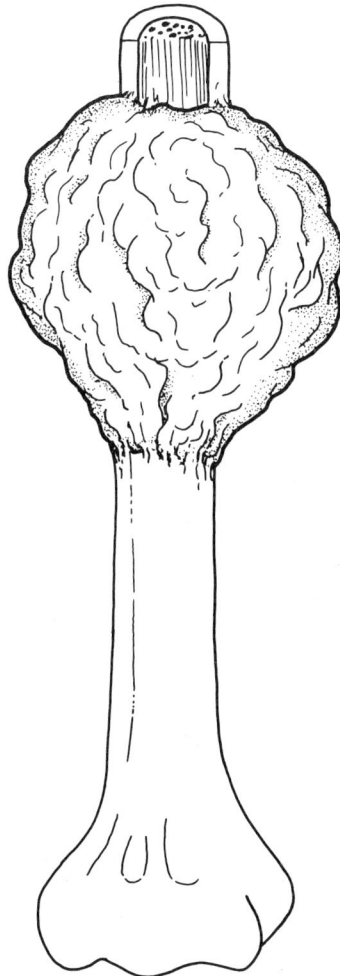

Fig. 126 Osteosarcoma

C: It develops in hitherto normal bone (second and third decades of life), in Paget's disease of bone (late in life), or following excessive irradiation.

E: What are the clinical and radiological findings?

C: Clinically, a painful swelling and/or pathological fracture. Radiologically, osteolytic destroyed bony areas with ill-defined edges, soft tissue shadow due to tumour transgressing the bone, sunray appearance (irregular spicules of bone radiating away from the shaft), Codman's triangle (elevated periosteum with new bone formation subperiosteally), pathological fracture and metastasis such as pulmonary secondaries.

E: How do you manage osteogenic sarcoma?

C: Open biopsy is a must to confirm the diagnosis, followed by preliminary radiotherapy (9000 rad) over 3 months; if this controls the tumour locally then follow-up 6 months later to detect any pulmonary metastasis. If the chest X-ray is clear then amputate, but if chest X-ray shows pulmonary secondaries amputation should not be attempted. Solitary pulmonary metastasis can be treated by lobectomy. Palliative amputation is performed if the tumour was not controlled locally after preliminary radiotherapy. Chemotherapy can be given (methotrexate, vincristine and adriamycin) for 1 year following the amputation.

E: Cade's method is time-consuming and I personally prefer immediate amputation to rid the patient of the tumour; such a prompt debulking procedure could be followed by more successful chemotherapy. Anyway, where are you going to amputate?

C: The site of election is through the bone or joint immediately proximal to the involved one, e.g. upper tibia (mid-thigh amputation), lower femur (high amputation), upper femur (hip disarticulation or hind-quarter amputation).

B8. HAND SKIN TUMOUR

E: What is this (Fig. 127)?

C: A specimen showing the right hand cut off at the wrist. There is a circular growth on the dorsum of the hand 7 cm in diameter with everted margin. It is a postmortem specimen of squamous cell carcinoma of the skin.

E: What are the causes, in general?

C: Causes can be placed in two groups:

1. *Premalignant skin conditions*: Bowen's intradermal disease (cells are similar to those found in Paget's disease of the nipple); leukoplakia, senile or solar keratosis (ultraviolet sunlight exposure is a predisposing factor, especially in the Celtic race); radiodermatitis (e.g. in radiologist or postirradiation areas of ringworms and thyrotoxicosis); chronic scars; or Marjolin's ulcer.

2. *Predisposing factors*: Exposure to long wavelengths leading to Kangri cancer of Kashmir; sleeping on oven bed leading to Kong cancer and charcoal burns. Chemicals such as tar and arsenic, and soot as in chimney-sweep's carcinoma. Infection such as chronic lupus vulgaris or tuberculosis of the skin. Postmastectomy lymphoedema may be superimposed by lymphangiosarcoma. Hereditary conditions such as

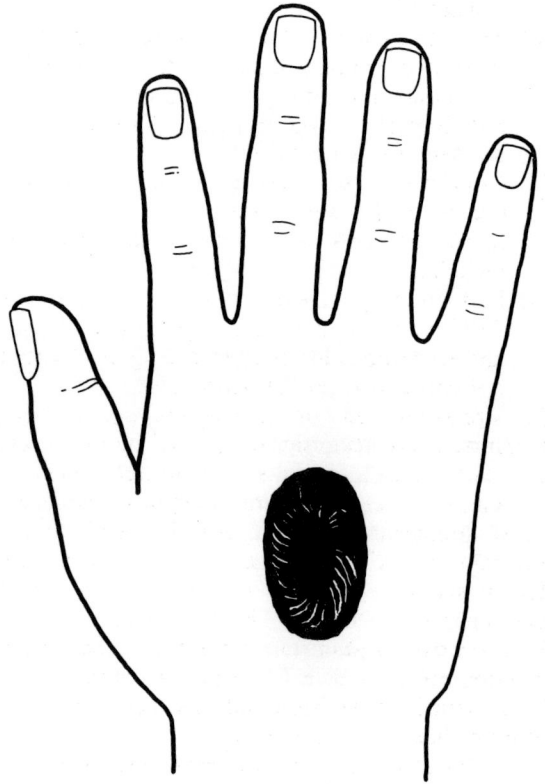

Fig. 127   Squamous cell carcinoma

xeroderma pigmentosa, albinism and Von Recklinghausen's disease.

E: How do you treat?

C: Biopsy from tumour and normal skin, followed by wide excision with closure or skin graft (if the gap is large). Enlarged lymph nodes may be treated with antibiotics initially; if they subside secondary infection is the cause but if they persist block dissection may be needed (if the lymph nodes are mobile). If draining lymph nodes are fixed, block dissection is contraindicated (regression may occur after radiotherapy). Alternatively, the skin tumour could be treated with radiotherapy alone (especially in an elderly patient with a small mobile skin tumour).

B9. PANCREATIC PATHOLOGY

This is one of the most interesting subjects to discuss even without specimens (though you may be shown a postmortem specimen of acute haemorrhagic pancreatitis with fatty necroses or carcinoma of the pancreatic head to open a wide discussion).

1. *Congenital*
(a) Annular pancreas due to failure of complete rotation of the ventral segment thus obstructing the duodenum and producing double-bubble radiological appearance. Treated by duodenojejunostomy.
(b) Congenital cystic disease and mucoviscidosis.

2. *Inflammatory* (pancreatitis)

3. *Neoplastic*: This is a very large topic and includes:
(a) Endocrine pancreatic tumours: these are APUDomas (Amine content Precursor Uptake and Decarboxylation cells) arising mostly (but not entirely) from the neural crest.

(i) Alpha-cell tumour (glucagonoma): diabetes mellitus, necrolytic migratory erythematous rash and catabolism and low serum proteins. There is associated normochromic normocytic anaemia, angular stomatitis, glossitis, infection and venous thrombosis with psychological disturbances. Diagnosis is on clinical grounds together with demonstration of a high glucagon level. Preoperative localisation with selective pancreatic arteriography and CT scan is carried out. Treatment is by excision and therapeutic embolisation of hepatic secondaries.

(ii) Beta-cell tumour (insulinoma) is usually benign and solitary. Episodic hypoglycaemia may be misdiagnosed as a psychiatric case. Whipple's triad is present (attack is brought on by fasting during which hypoglycaemia occurs and is relieved with i.v. glucose). Preoperative localisation (as in glucagonoma). Cure by excision (enucleation or partial pancreatectomy). Inoperable cases are treated with diazoxide to control hypoglycaemia and streptozotocin for liver secondaries (therapeutic embolisation is preferable in the latter).

(iii) G-cell hyperplasia of pancreas (Zollinger–Ellison syndrome); can also occur in G-cell tumours of the gastric antrum and duodenum. Concomitant with hyperparathyroidism it may indicate multiple endocrine adenopathy. There is intractable peptic ulceration (in odd sites, e.g. postbulbar duodenum or jejunum), hypergastrinaemia with massive acid hypersecretion, and diarrhoea, steatorrhoea or hypokalaemia. The protective value of cimetidine usually makes total gastrectomy unnecessary (especially if given with pirenzepine to enhance the H_2 receptor blocker). If there is no response then carry out total gastrectomy. The primary tumour of the pancreas (or gastric antrum) should be removed.

(iv) D-cell tumour (somatostatinoma) produces excessive somatostatin leading to diabetes, steatorrhoea, diarrhoea, hypochlorhydria, cholelithiasis and weight loss. Diagnosis by somatostatin assay.

(v) VIPoma.

(vi) PPoma: Pancreatic polypeptide is secreted in many of the above tumours and is also found in their metastases.

(b) Exocrine pancreatic tumours
(i) Head (70% of cases), involving:
● Head proper (two-thirds).
● Periampullary region (one-third).
(ii) Body and tail (30%).

These tumours present generally either as painless progressive obstructive jaundice or as an intractable pain without jaundice. Diagnosis is on clinical findings and radiologically by barium meal (pad sign and reversed 3 sign in head proper and periampullary carcinoma respectively) and hypotonic duodenography with pancreatic function tests. Treatment depends on site and stage of disease (to decide whether radical or palliative procedure is required).

B10. MISCELLANEOUS

You may be shown one of the following specimens:
● Piece of small bowel with marks of constricting band around part of its circumference and gangrene in the constricted part. It is Richter's hernia (strangulated partial enterocele) usually due to femoral hernia.
● Piece of bone with a cavity containing one tooth (jaw). The diagnosis is dentigerous cyst due to non-erupted permanent tooth. A dental cyst is usually attached to the root of a pulpless tooth. Treatment is by excision of the whole epithelial lining of the cyst, and the bone cavity is obliterated by a soft-tissue 'push-in' or with bone chips and wound suturing.
● Upper thoracic cage with accessory rib with discussion of symptomatology and treatment.
● Bony osteoma as a benign tumour (treatment is surgical excision).
● Saccular aneurysm of an artery with classification of aneurysm and treatment.
● Testicular tumour (seminoma or teratoma).
● Large bowel with polyposis coli with discussion of symptomatology and treatment.
● Jejunal diverticulosis.
● Postmortem specimen of carcinoma of oesophagus.
● Oesophageal stricture.

C. Histopathology Slides

There is no substitute for a histopathology atlas or actual slides borrowed from the pathology department of your hospital in order to familiarise yourself with their appearance. This part is only required in the Final FRCS (England). You will be given three slides: you must examine these under the microscope in 10 min and state the diagnosis of each disease. Each slide comes with a very useful typed card containing a short history of the patient; the name of the organ or tissue is usually shown on the slide. Dividing the time equally, write the slide number on the paper along with its abnormal microscopic findings, then write your possible diagnosis (concluded from correlation of the findings). Remember that each organ or tissue has a list of common diseases so go through them and come up with the most likely diagnosis. The examiners know very well that you are not a professional pathologist so only histopathology of the common diseases will be covered. When you finish you will be taken to meet the examiner and with the help of a slide magnifying projection screen you will discuss your three slides. The diagnosis of each one will open the discussion covering different aspects of that particular disease from aetiology to surgical management. The following are the most common slides with the most important abnormal microscopic findings seen in each.

C1. LYMPH NODE

Tuberculous lymphadenitis Caseating granuloma with central caseation (amorphous pink necrosis) surrounded by epithelioid cells, lymphocytes and, more importantly, Langhan giant cells (multinucleated cells with peripheral nuclei).

Hodgkin's disease Commonly the nodular sclerosis phase with destruction of lymph node architecture and replacement with patches of fibrosis. Cellular areas reveal lymphocytes, macrophages and, more importantly, the characteristic Reed–Sternberg cells (double nucleated cells with a mirror image arrangement of nuclei). Lymphocyte predominance, mixed cellularity and lymphocyte depletion are other phases (rarely shown).

Metastatic carcinoma Commonly adenocarcinoma from gastrointestinal tract (or elsewhere) showing patchy replacement of lymphatic structure with islands of mucoid and clear cells (clear cytoplasm with central or occasionally eccentric nucleus—signet ring appearance) indicating their primary origin.

C2. SKIN

Squamous cell carcinoma With breach of epithelial continuity and everted border. The tumour grows down deeply with undermining of epidermis. Atypical cells with polychromatic nuclei and abnormal mitotic figures can be seen particularly easily in their characteristic cell nests or as epithelial pearls with central keratin.

Basal cell carcinoma (rodent ulcer) The skin ulceration is surrounded by a beaded margin. The tumour grows down but superficially in the form of masses or columns undermining epidermis. Each column or mass is composed characteristically of polyhedral epithelial cells with a peripheral palisade formation.

Malignant melanoma With dark brown or black epidermal melanocytes not confined to the basal layer of skin, but infiltrating the whole section up and down.

Paget's disease of the nipple The section is composed of breast tissue and overlying skin (*see* 'Breast').

C3. BREAST

Hard pericanalicular fibroadenoma (the common fibroadenoma) Normal ductules within a background of dense fibrous tissue. Usually multifocal but very well encapsulated. It is benign.

Fibroadenosis The adenosis element (budding of glandular acini) is associated with epitheliosis (hyperplasia of acinar lining) or even papillomatosis (extensive epithelial hyperplasia causing overgrowth within ducts). The other element is fibrosis with dense fibrous trabeculae replacing fat and elastic tissues and compressing ducts leading to cyst formation. The interstitial tissues may be infiltrated by round cells (lymphocytes). Its possible premalignancy status is debatable.

Intraduct papilloma and carcinoma The papilloma shows epithelial proliferation in one of the larger lactiferous ducts (usually one duct and occasionally two or more). It is premalignant. The carcinoma is similar but the cells are atypical with various sizes of nuclei and pigmentation (malignant).

Scirrhous carcinoma (the commonest—63% of cases) The ductal carcinomatous cells break the epithelial basement membrane, causing intense reactionary fibrosis which leads to a very hard mass with an irregular contour due to puckering of surrounding tissues to variable degrees. Notice the criteria of the malignant cells within fibrous tissue.

Paget's disease of the nipple (rare—1%) Breast tissue is seen with overlying skin. This is not a premalignant disease but an actual breast malignancy. It is an *intraduct carcinoma* that slowly grows upward infiltrating the epithelial covering of the nipple. Large rounded vacuolated cells with small deeply staining nuclei (hydropic appearance) are seen in the deeper layer of the epidermis. Some lymphocyte infiltration of the dermis occurs. Notice that in duct carcinoma, malignant cells are confined to ducts. If the cells break the basement membrane, they provoke interstitial fibrosis causing scirrhous carcinoma and if the cells creep upward to infiltrate nipple skin they cause Paget's disease of the nipple. Paget's disease is usually unilateral (with no vesicles), occurs in the menopause and does not respond to treatment (unlike eczema of lactating mothers).

C4. BONE

Osteogenic sarcoma (commonly idiopathic in children and rarely occurs in Paget's disease of the bone in adults) The normal bone structure is infiltrated by spindle cells with marked nuclear hyperchromatosis and islands of osteoid formation. Malignant giant cells and high vascularity are obvious.

C5. THYROID GLAND

Colloid goitre Owing to increased colloid storage the acini distend and the gland shows a fine honeycomb appearance. It is caused by alternating periods of iodine sufficiency and deprivation.

Thyrotoxicosis While normal thyroid gland consists of acini lined by flat cuboidal epithelium and filled with homogeneous colloid, in hyperthyroidism, hyperplastic acini are lined by high columnar epithelium with empty or vacuolated colloid follicles. There is lymphocyte infiltration with lymph

follicle formation. Following treatment the acinar lining becomes low, cuboidal and full of colloid.

Hashimoto's autoimmune thyroiditis (struma lymphomatosa) There is widespread atrophy of parenchyma, diffuse fibrosis, diffuse lymphocyte infiltration and localised collections of lymphocytes with germinal centres. Acinar cells are enlarged and rounded with granular cytoplasm (characteristic Askanazy cells). Mild initial hyperthyroidism will be followed eventually by inevitable hypothyroidism.

Papillary carcinoma (the commonest thyroid carcinoma—60%) There is papillary formation, often follicular structure and sometimes solid masses of cells. The cells are well differentiated with a characteristic appearance (large pale ground-glass nuclei and small nucleoli). There may be a breach of the thyroid capsule. This carcinoma is multifocal so total thyroidectomy is needed. Lymphatic spread may necessitate a block dissection which should be carried out one side at a time (never do simultaneous bilateral block dissection). Prognosis is good.

Follicular carcinoma (17%) The well-differentiated cells are arranged in follicles which sometimes contain colloid. Thyroid capsule is invaded and the tumour is very vascular. Lobectomy is satisfactory since it is not multifocal. Blood spread necessitates hormonal therapy with thyroxine and multiple metastases necessitate ^{131}I therapy.

Medullary carcinoma (6%) Undifferentiated round or polygonal cells in fibrous stroma with no papillary or follicular structure. The characteristic 'amyloid' in globoid masses in stroma and within some malignant cells is the most important finding. This tumour arises from parafollicular (C) cells and is associated with high levels of serum calcitonin. The tumour is familial and is associated with phaeochromocytoma, parathyroid tumour and Von Recklinghausen's disease of skin. Treatment is by total thyroidectomy.

C6. PARATHYROIDS

In hyperparathyroidism, calcium in the blood and urine is high while phosphate is low.

Adenoma Composed of interlacing compact cords or solid masses of cells of uniform type (chief cells with regular nuclei and scanty cytoplasm) in a scanty vascular stroma.

C7. PAROTID SALIVARY GLANDS

Pleomorphic adenoma (mixed parotid tumour—the commonest parotid tumour) Shows a complex structure of epithelial, glandular and mucoid material. The epithelial cells are arranged in irregular strands and masses or branching columns (sometimes with glandular acini). The myoepithelium proliferates in sheets. The varying amounts of mucoid material give a myxomatous appearance (like cartilage). Clinically it is a firm circumscribed lobulated mass on the jaw angle usually unilateral with no sex predilection.

Adenolymphoma (Warthin's tumour; less common than pleomorphic adenoma) This benign tumour has a markedly eosinophilic epithelium folded into cavities (cystic formation) with papillary appearance. The tall columnar cells are arranged in regular palisade formation or in glandular acini. There are characteristic lymphocyte follicles in the stroma. Unlike pleomorphic adenoma adenolymphoma has a monomorphic eosinophilic papillary structure with lymphoid follicles. Clinically it is a soft cystic fluctuant tumour in the lower pole of the parotid and can be bilateral, affecting middle-aged or elderly males. Unlike all other tumours, which produce a cold spot, adenolymphoma produces a 'hot' spot in a ^{99m}Tc pertechnetate scan (a firm preoperative diagnosis without biopsy). Fine needle aspiration cytology is an accepted preoperative diagnostic test.

C8. STOMACH AND DUODENUM

Peptic ulcer Mucosal continuity is breached. The excavation of the wall is deep and reaches the muscular layer, producing four layers from the mucosa towards the muscularis:
1. Exudate with pus cells.
2. Fibrinoid necrosis.
3. Granulation and capillary formation.
4. Fibrotic base due to chronicity.

Gastric carcinoma There is mucosal discontinuity but the ulcer edges are everted. Whereas benign ulcer erodes a large gap in the muscular coat, carcinoma infiltrates between muscles without destroying them. There are no dilated vessels in the base and the cells are typically malignant (various sizes of cells, cytoplasm nuclei and different pigmentation with infiltration of surrounding normal tissues). Clear cells or even signet ring cells can be seen (as a result of much of the cytoplasm displacing the nucleus to one side).

C9. SMALL AND LARGE BOWEL

Carcinoid tumour The tumour is golden yellow due to its high lipid content. The characteristic Kulschitsky cells are related to bases of crypts of Lieberkuhn and present as solid masses of small clear (lipid-containing) cells closely packed together within a fibrous stroma. The cells may show a palisade or rosette arrangement (and are capable of reducing silver salts). Classically the tumour affects the terminal ileum or appendix (but it may occur elsewhere).

Crohn's disease (granulomatous ileitis) Usually no mucosal discontinuity but transmural thickening of the wall affecting submucosa mainly with chronic non-caseating granulomatous reaction (sarcoid formation). Epithelioid cells and giant cells (Langhan's type) are seen. Macroscopically, Crohn's disease distribution is segmental, involving the ileum (may be extensive) and rectum in 50% of cases, with anal lesions in 75% and internal fistulae in 8% when colon is involved. The mucosal fissuring and cracking (with no or patchy ulceration and transmural thickening) produce a characteristic cobblestoning (a macroscopic pathological appearance rather than a radiological appearance).

Ulcerative colitis (more correctly called haemorrhagic proctocolitis) Is mainly a mucosal disease with ulceration of mucosa (discontinuity) and suppurative acute inflammation with an oedematous vascular submucosal background infiltrated by polymorphs. Focal collection of polymorphs and frank crypt abscesses are seen.

Unlike Crohn's disease, ulcerative colitis has a continuous distribution, involving the rectum in all cases, with limited or no ileal involvement. There are no internal fistulae but anal lesions occur in 25%. No cobblestoning is seen but mucososubmucosal hypertrophy produces pseudopolyps, which are unusual in Crohn's disease.

Acute appendicitis Hollow viscus with suppurative inflammation (pus cells and vascular oedematous wall).

Colonic carcinoma Whether adenocarcinoma or anaplastic depends on the degree of differentiation. Identify the signs of malignancy (atypical appearance with mitotic figures and infiltration of surrounding normal tissues). Depending on amount, clear cells or signet rings can be seen.

Ileocaecal tuberculosis   Tuberculosis may affect any part of the human body (e.g. kidney, bone, testis, skin). The tubercle is the characteristic lesion exhibiting typical central caseation (coagulative necrosis of epithelioid cells) surrounded by epithelioid cells and peripheral lymphocytes in a concentric mass around a clump of bacilli. The epithelioid (or endothelioid) cells occupy the central zone of the tuberculous follicle and are oval faintly-staining nuclei with abundant clear cytoplasm. The lymphocytes are arranged in the peripheral zone usually with giant cells of Langhan's type (horse-shoe peripheral nuclei).

C10. URINARY SYSTEM

Hypernephroma (*adenocarcinoma or clear cell carcinoma of kidney*)   Solid masses of large cells with small central nuclei and abundant clear cytoplasm (due to its rich glycogen and doubly refractile lipid content) infiltrate the kidney stroma (notice the glomeruli) with inflammatory cells in the normal part as a response to the infiltrating malignant cells.

Transitional cell carcinoma of urinary bladder   Notice the transitional cells of the bladder mucosa arranged in papillary style with mitotic figures and deep infiltration.

Prostatic enlargement   Benign adenomas or hyperplasia in the prostate are similar to those in the breast. The small rounded acini are lined by well-differentiated cuboidal or columnar epithelium set in a fibromuscular stroma. Some of the acini are dilated and contain concentric laminated bodies (called corpora amylacea). Adenocarcinomas show more irregular hyperchromatic acini arranged in solid masses with evidence of local invasion.

Testicular seminoma   There is great uniformity. The tumour is made up of solid sheets or columns of cells mostly polygonal (of uniform size) with clear cytoplasm and rounded nuclei (well-marked chromatin network and one or two nucleoli). Tumour giant cells may be seen and often there is a well-marked lymphocyte infiltration.

C11. GALL BLADDER

Chronic cholecystitis   Hollow viscus with mild inflammation. Large foamy cells in stroma (lipid material) are seen in cholesterosis.

PART II

Background

SECTION 1
The Royal Colleges (of the UK and Ireland)

All the Colleges retain the same high surgical standard and are recognised as important world centres of education and control of professional training in surgery. The Fellowship is usually gained through qualification (on an examination basis conducted according to College regulations) or rarely granted as an honorary degree to outstanding surgeons and authorities in different parts of the world. The FRCS is not a specialist degree but a visa to higher surgical training leading ultimately to a consultant post or academic career.

In spite of the technical differences in the way the examination is conducted in these Colleges, the requirements for admission to the Final FRCS are basically similar:

- Possession of the primary (Part 1) FRCS (which is now no longer reciprocal).
- Postgraduate surgical training in hospitals recognised by the College (covering at least 1 year of general surgery, 6 months in accidents and emergencies and 6 months in one of the surgical specialities) at the level of SHO or Registrar.
- Candidates should be at least 25 years old.

At the end of the examination, only successful candidates will be admitted to the College hall to meet the President and court of examiners for congratulation. Those failed will be notified by post usually with details of performance (available only to unsuccessful candidates).

Each College will be discussed briefly here to familiarise the candidate with the differences in regulations, examination techniques and parts relevant to the Final FRCS in general surgery. The differences between the Colleges (though probably minor) merit stress since they may influence the candidate's preparation in sitting the final FRCS of that particular College.

ROYAL COLLEGE OF SURGEONS OF ENGLAND

The Guild of Surgeons was formed in about 1300. The first mention of the surgeons in the city of London records was in 1354. In 1540 came the incorporation of the Barbers Company and the Guild of Surgeons as the Company of Barbers and Surgeons. However, in 1745 London Surgeons broke away from the barbers and formed the Company of Surgeons (John Ranby was the first Master) largely through the initiative of William Cheselden of St Thomas' Hospital. By 1800, the Company of Surgeons was chartered by George III and it became the Royal College of Surgeons in London (first Master of the College was Charles Hawkins). In 1822 the title of Master changed to President (last Master and first President was Sir Everard Home). In 1843, a new charter was granted by Queen Victoria and the title of the College changed to The Royal College of Surgeons of England. Initially, 300 distinguished members were elected to become Fellows of the College. The council of the College retained the right to confer fellowship by election. However, regulations for fellowship by examination were instituted and in December 1844 the first examination (FRCS) was conducted; 24 candidates successfully passed and were admitted as Fellows. Ever since, London has retained its importance as a world centre of surgery and it attained world supremacy during the middle years of the 19th century (1830–1870) (see Part II, Section 6).

The College conducts two examinations per year exclusively in London (no overseas examination).

Requirements

For sitting the final FRCS (Eng) the requirements are:

1. A candidate of 25 years or over with a good character.

2. Primary FRCS from the Royal College of Surgeons of England only. (No reciprocity since 1st July 1980; however, possession of the primary FRCS from any of the Royal Colleges before 1980 is still acceptable).

3. Original testimonials of postgraduate training which should include at least *18 months general surgery*, 6 months accidents and emergencies and 6 months in a surgical speciality. These posts should be at least at the level of SHO — full-time residential

jobs in hospitals recognised by the college. This training *should include 1 year (obligatory) in the UK or Ireland in a recognised hospital.*

4. Filled application form with the examination fee.

The full regulations are obtained by writing to:

The Registrar,
Royal College of Surgeons of England,
Lincoln's Inn Fields,
London WC2A 3PN,
UK.

Examination procedure

Takes 2 days per candidate to finish all the different parts:

1. *Written Part:* takes 1 day (morning and afternoon sessions; each two questions with 2 hours' time).

2. *Clinical Part:* conducted in special examination hall (not in hospitals). The long case and short cases are therefore transportable — not acutely ill and commonly repeated in the examinations. Both the long case and the short cases will be discussed in the examination hall with two examiners.

3. *Oral Part:* conducted on two tables (each has two examiners) in the college pathology museum (sometimes partly conducted in the examination hall):

(a) Surgical topic — operative surgery and surgical anatomy *viva*, with discussion on instruments, human models and bones.

(b) Surgical pathology *viva*: involves examination of three histopathological slides (microscopy), later discussed with one examiner using microprojection, followed by examination of gross pathology specimens (in pots).

The clinical and oral parts take 1 day (morning and afternoon sessions respectively). There is no separate principles and practice table, but the surgical principles and practice are discussed implicitly within the oral parts. The College scoring system (of nines) makes it impossible for the candidate to pass without passing clearly the written and clinical parts individually. A borderline score in the oral parts could be compensated for after discussion and agreement by the College court of examiners.

The College announces and displays the successful candidates by number (not by names — the results are confidential).

ROYAL COLLEGE OF SURGEONS OF EDINBURGH

The Surgeons–Barbers Association, the forerunner of the College, was founded in 1505 making it the oldest surgical college. Edinburgh rose to the highest surgical standard at the end of the 18th century and maintained its world supremacy for almost half a century (*see* Part II, Section 6). The Edinburgh school was derived from that in Leiden in Holland. The Monro dynasty of anatomists (grandfather, father and son — all named Alexander Monro) made the Edinburgh teaching of anatomy famous to the extent that in 1828, the classes of its spectacular teacher (and founder of the College museum), Robert Knox, regularly attracted 504 students per lecture in the dissecting room which does not accommodate more than 200. The museum now has one of the largest collections of surgical pathology in the UK. Many of the specimens are of unique historical interest and there is a series of oil paintings of war wounds executed by Sir Charles Bell, a capable artist as well as surgeon, after the Battle of Waterloo. The College officially finished its association with barbers in 1722 and received the 'Royal' status from George III in 1778.

The first FRCS examination was conducted in 1884 as a one-part examination which later became bipartite as in England and Dublin. The College currently conducts three examinations per year in Edinburgh. It also conducts the final FRCS examination overseas in Hong Kong and Kuala Lumpur.

Requirements

For sitting the final FRCS (Ed) the requirements are:

1. A candidate of 25 years or above with a good character.

2. Primary FRCS from any of the Royal Colleges (reciprocal).

3. Original testimonials of postgraduate training which should include at least 12 months general surgery, 6 months accidents and emergencies and 6 months in a surgical speciality (e.g. cardiothoracic, urology, orthopaedic surgery). These posts should be at least at the level of SHO — full-time jobs in recognised hospitals, *anywhere in the world* (no obligatory 1 year in hospitals in the UK or Ireland).

4. Filled application form with the examination fee.

The full regulations are obtained by writing to:

The Registrar,
Royal College of Surgeons of Edinburgh,
18 Nicolson Street,
Edinburgh EH8 9DW,
UK.

Examination procedure

Takes 4 days per candidate to complete all the different parts:

1. *Written Part*: takes 2 days (3 hours on first day for operative surgery/surgical pathology and 3 hours on second day for principles/practice). The written part attracts double marking (7 + 7). This will usually be followed by a weekend.

2. *Clinical Part*: conducted in Edinburgh hospitals and other Scottish hospitals. Candidates will be taken by coach to hospitals outside Edinburgh. Both the long case and the short cases will be discussed in the wards with two examiners. The clinical part attracts double marking (7 for the long case and 7 for the short cases). Recently the long case has been replaced with short cases.

3. *Oral Part*: conducted on three tables (each has two examiners) in the college museum and halls.
  (a) Surgical pathology: surgical and postmortem specimens in pots (no microscopy slides). However, clinical and gross pathological slides may be shown.
  (b) Operative surgery (no bones).
  (c) Principles and practice.

  The candidates (according to a recent regulation) are allowed to have their written and oral parts first; those who are successful or borderline are allowed to proceed to their clinical part (which even if they pass is no guarantee that they pass the whole examination since their score in other parts may be borderline). Those who fail the written and/or oral parts are not allowed to proceed with their clinical part (without examination fee forfeited). Thus it is essential to pass clearly in *both* written and clinical parts. Of course candidates have to pass the oral part but borderline marks here can be compensated for by good marks in other parts.

ROYAL COLLEGE OF PHYSICIANS AND SURGEONS OF GLASGOW

This was founded in 1599 under the charter of James VI of Scotland, granted in response to the plea of Maister Peter Lowe (the founder of the Brethren of Chirurgerie, the forerunner of the College). For over 200 years it was known as the Faculty of Physicians and Surgeons. Authority to add the prefix 'Royal' was granted by Edward VII in 1909. The change to Royal College of Physicians and Surgeons of Glasgow was made by Act of Parliament on 6th December 1962.

The College conducts three examinations per year exclusively in Glasgow (no overseas examination).

Requirements

For sitting the final FRCS (Glas) the requirements are:

1. A candidate of 25 years or over with a good character.

2. Primary FRCS from any of the Royal Colleges (reciprocal).

3. Original testimonials of postgraduate training which should include at least 12 months general surgery, 6 months accidents and emergencies and 6 months in any surgical speciality (e.g. gynaecology, orthopaedic surgery, urology, cardiothoracic surgery). These posts should be at least at the level of SHO — full-time jobs in recognised hospitals. This training *should include 1 year (obligatory) in the UK or Ireland in a recognised hospital*.

4. Filled application form with the examination fee.

  The full regulations are obtained by writing to:

The Registrar,
Royal College of Physicians and Surgeons,
234 – 242 St Vincent Street,
Glasgow G2 5RJ,
UK.

Examination procedure

Takes 2 days per candidate to complete all the different parts:

1. *Written Part*: takes 1 day (morning and afternoon sessions for operative surgery/surgical pathology and principles/practice—3 hours each).

2. *Clinical Part*: conducted in various Glasgow hospitals. Both the long case and the short cases will be discussed in the wards with two examiners.

3. *Oral Part*: conducted on three tables (each has two examiners) in the College halls:
  (a) Surgical pathology: proceeds without specimens (pots) or histology (slides).
  (b) Operative surgery (no bones).
  (c) Principles and practice.

  The clinical and oral parts take 1 day (morning and afternoon sessions respectively).

Both Edinburgh and Glasgow Colleges announce the successful candidates by name and *display their names and numbers on the board.* (No confidentiality with successful candidates.)

ROYAL COLLEGE OF SURGEONS IN IRELAND

In Dublin the barbers and surgeons were members of the Guild of St Mary Magdalene, established by Henry VI in 1446, an association which persisted well into the 18th century to the disadvantage of the surgeons. The Dublin College of Surgeons was founded in 1780 by an Irishman, Sylvester O'Halloran, who studied surgery, ophthalmology and midwifery and worked in London, Leiden and Paris. The College received its Royal charter on 11th February, 1784. Dublin is well known for many international figures (e.g. Colles', Smith's and Bennett's fractures, Fegan's injection-compression technique of varicose veins, anal valves of Houston, and Cheyne–Stokes' breathing in head injury).

The College conducts three examinations per year in Dublin and Belfast (no overseas examination).

Requirements

For sitting the final FRCSI the requirements are:
1. A candidate of 25 years or over with a good character.
2. Primary FRCS from any of the Royal Colleges (reciprocal).
3. Original testimonials of postgraduate training which should include at least 12 months general surgery, 6 months accidents and emergencies and 6 months in a surgical speciality. These posts should be at the level of Registrar or equivalent status — full-time job in hospitals recognised by the College.

This training *should include 1 year (obligatory) in general surgery in the UK or Ireland in a recognised hospital.*
4. Filled application form with the examination fee.

The full regulations are obtained by writing to:

The Registrar,
Royal College of Surgeons in Ireland,
123 St Stephens Green,
Dublin 2,
Republic of Ireland.

Examination procedure

Takes 2 days per candidate to complete all the different parts:
1. *Written Part:* takes 1 day (morning and afternoon sessions for Paper A and Paper B — 3 hours each).
2. *Clinical Part:* conducted in various Dublin hospitals. The long case and short cases will be discussed in the wards with two examiners each. (The only College with four different examiners per clinical part taken by each candidate.)
3. *Oral Part:* conducted on two tables (each has two examiners) in the College hall.
(a) Operative surgery: with instruments and X-rays (no bones).
(b) Principles and practice: with extensive discussion of X-rays.

The clinical and oral parts take 1 day (morning and afternoon sessions respectively). There is no surgical pathology table (so no surgical specimens or slides). X-rays feature extensively in the oral parts. To be successful, each candidate *has to score a total of 360 marks and should score 120 in the clinical part.* (The marks are divided equally between the three parts and 60 is the pass mark.) The results are confidential. The College will announce and display successful candidates by number only.

SECTION 2

Samples of the Written Examination from the Four Colleges for the Past 5–10 Years

Examination papers are the copyright of each College. Permission was given only by the Royal College of Surgeons of England and the Royal College of Surgeons of Edinburgh to publish them here in the exact style; examination papers from the other two Colleges, therefore, appear in a similar but not the exact style. Although there is no limit to the number of different styles of questions asked, we believe that the carefully selected questions presented here comprehensively cover the material. When reviewed and worked on by the candidate, they will no doubt form an excellent basis for the theory of surgery. Many of the questions are based on special clinical situations and necessitate mature clinical judgement and a reasonable therapeutic approach.

It is very unusual for candidates who fail the written part and/or the clinical part to pass the final FRCS and therefore tremendous effort has gone into choosing these examination questions carefully. Some of them are shared between many Colleges (e.g. management of chronic pain, systemic bleeding in surgery, parenteral nutrition, endocrine therapy and chemotherapy of advanced cancer) and produced in different styles. Candidates who would like to review a particular College's examination papers for the last 5 years prior to their attempt, may obtain these direct from the Royal Colleges of Glasgow and Ireland. Examination papers of the Royal College of Surgeons of England are obtained from Adrian Press Limited, Ilford, Essex and those of the Royal College of Surgeons of Edinburgh from Donald Ferrier Limited, 5 Teviot Place, Edinburgh EH1 2RB. We have collected a broad spectrum of questions and consider that quick scanning is far more fruitful than a mere review of the last 5 years' questions. The first written part of each College will be provided with the exact examination details. The written part is finished in 1 day in all Colleges except in Edinburgh where it takes 2 days.

ROYAL COLLEGE OF SURGEONS OF ENGLAND

DIPLOMA OF FELLOW

FINAL EXAMINATION-I

PATHOLOGY, THERAPEUTICS AND SURGERY

10 A. M. *to* 12 NOON

BOTH *questions must be answered*

FINAL EXAMINATION-II

PATHOLOGY, THERAPEUTICS AND SURGERY

1.30 P. M. *to* 3.30 P. M.

BOTH *questions must be answered*

I *Paper I*
1. Discuss the problem of diabetes mellitus in surgical practice.
2. A young soldier has been admitted because of a high-velocity gunshot wound of the upper third of his right leg causing comminuted fractures of tibia and fibula. Describe procedure, complications and their management.

Paper II
3. Discuss the management of a patient, aged 65 years, admitted with a diagnosis of large bowel obstruction.
4. Describe the causes of hydronephrosis in a child (under 15 years of age). How should this be investigated and treated?

II *Paper I*
1. A woman, aged 30, has just discovered a lump in her breast, lateral to the nipple. Discuss the management of this patient.
2. Discuss immediate and subsequent management of a patient who has sustained a deep laceration of the front of the wrist.

Paper II
3. Discuss the causes and management of cardiac arrest during surgical procedures.
4. On cystoscopy a woman of 50 is found to have a neoplasm of the bladder. Discuss the pathology and management.

III *Paper I*
1. A youth of 18 years is admitted to hospital after having been thrown from his motorcycle. His right upper limb is found to be completely paralysed. This is his only disability and there has been no loss of consciousness. Discuss diagnosis, management and prognosis.
2. Discuss management in the first 48 hours of a patient with tetraplegia following fracture of the neck, and indicate principles governing his long-term care.

Paper II

3. Discuss the management of a man aged 50 admitted to hospital with severe haematemesis.
4. Discuss aetiology and management of intestinal obstruction in the first month of life.

IV *Paper I*

1. A young motorcyclist is admitted to hospital after a road accident. He is found to be restless and confused and to have multiple fractures of the ribs. Describe how you would manage this case during the first 48 hours after admission.
2. Discuss the management of uncomplicated duodenal ulceration. Describe the possible sequelae of procedures you mention.

Paper II

3. A woman aged 30 has passed a calculus per urethram following an attack of right renal colic. Intravenous pyelogram shows a further shadow (0.5 cm in diameter) in the lower pole of the right kidney. Discuss the management of this patient.
4. Describe management of disseminated breast cancer in a woman of 50 years. Indicate the basic scientific principles underlying the treatment that you recommend.

V *Paper I*

1. Discuss the management of a 55-year-old man extensively burned from the waist down.
2. A woman of 45 complains of food sticking behind the lower sternum. Discuss the diagnosis, pathology and management of the patient.

Paper II

3. A man of 65 presents with recent oedema of the left ankle, and mild obstructive urinary symptoms of 1 year's duration. Rectal examination reveals a hard left lobe of the prostate gland. How would you establish the diagnosis? Describe your management of the case.
4. Discuss clinical presentation of lumbar intervertebral disc disease and the place of surgery in its management.

VI *Paper I*

1. Discuss the place of surgery in the treatment of chronic inflammatory disease of the large bowel.
2. An adult presents with a suspected retroperitoneal swelling. Discuss the diagnosis and investigations.

Paper II

3. Discuss the management of a stab wound in the groin.
4. Discuss the causes, prevention and management of stricture of the male urethra.

VII *Paper I*

1. Discuss the management of a patient with a persistent external abdominal fistula.
2. Discuss the surgical management of osteoarthritis of the hip.

Paper II

3. Discuss causes, diagnosis and management of pulmonary complications that may follow major abdominal operations.
4. A 25-year-old woman with a goitre presents with a suggested diagnosis of thyrotoxicosis. How would you investigate this case? Discuss indications for operation.

VIII *Paper I*

1. A man aged 35 injured in a road accident is found to have blood coming from his urethra. On examination a swelling is found rising from the pelvis midway to the umbilicus. Describe your management of this patient, confining your answers to urogenital tract injuries. Discuss critically other accepted methods of treatment of this patient, giving reasons for your own choice of procedure.
2. Give an account of surgical disorders of the salivary glands and their management.

Paper II
3. Give an account of treatment of fractures in the region of the elbow in an 8-year-old child. What complications may arise and how are they managed?
4. Discuss diagnosis and treatment of a limp in a child of 10 years of age.

IX *Paper I*
1. Discuss causes of collapse of a vertebral body. Describe your investigations.
2. Discuss management of vascular complications of closed fractures of the long bones of the lower limb.

Paper II
3. Discuss differential diagnosis, treatment and investigation of a patient with unilateral proptosis.
4. Discuss pathology, diagnosis and treatment of acquired intestinovesical fistulae.

X *Paper I*
1. A man of 45 years presents with a recent epileptic attack affecting the right side of the body. Discuss the investigation and management of this patient.
2. Discuss the methods used for the investigation and treatment of obstructive jaundice.

Paper II
3. A 20-year-old man, following an injury at football, develops a gross swelling of the knee-joint. Discuss the management.
4. Discuss the clinical importance of vomiting.

XI *Paper I*
1. Describe the methods of urinary diversion and evaluate their place in treatment.
2. A 25-year-old man is admitted to Casualty after having been shot in the left lower chest. An X-ray shows the bullet is lodged on the left side of the 4th lumbar vertebra. Discuss the management.

Paper II
3. Discuss the investigation of a woman of 45 years with an early carcinoma of the breast. Describe the management of such a case treated by mastectomy and radiotherapy.
4. Discuss the management of an elderly patient presenting as an emergency with severe rectal haemorrhage.

XII *Paper I*
1. Discuss the diagnosis and management of renal cell carcinoma (hypernephroma).
2. Discuss the prevention, diagnosis and treatment of deep venous thrombosis.

Paper II
3. Discuss the management of a closed chest wound.
4. Discuss the uses of ultrasound in surgery.

XIII *Paper I*
1. Discuss the management of upper gastrointestinal tract bleeding in a patient with hepatosplenomegaly.
2. Discuss the management of an incised wound of the flexor aspect of the wrist.

Paper II
3. A man of 50 develops epigastric pain 3 years after a vagotomy and pyloroplasty done for duodenal ulcer. Discuss the diagnosis and management of such a patient.
4. Discuss the place of surgery in the treatment of rheumatoid arthritis.

XIV *Paper I*
1. Discuss the diagnosis and management of obstruction of the lower third of the oesophagus.
2. Discuss the management of a woman of 70 years who sustains a fracture of the femoral neck. What are the aetiological factors?

Paper II
3. Describe the management of a patient who fails to pass urine after an operation.
4. Discuss clinical presentations and management of aortic aneurysm.

XV *Paper I*
1. A healthy man aged 76 presents with a 6-month history of deterioration of urinary flow with frequency and urgency. Three years previously he underwent a transurethral resection for benign prostatic hypertrophy. Discuss your investigations and treatment.
2. Discuss the management of fracture-dislocation of the hip. What are the possible long-term consequences?

Paper II
3. Discuss the investigation and treatment of a patient who, on clinical examination, has an enlargement of one lobe of the thyroid gland.
4. Discuss the management of a severe penetrating wound of the axilla.

ROYAL COLLEGE OF SURGEONS OF EDINBURGH

FELLOWSHIP EXAMINATION

PART II

I *DAY 1 (OPERATIVE SURGERY AND SURGICAL PATHOLOGY)*   *(09.30–12.30)*
1. Discuss the investigations of a patient presenting with a unilateral swelling in the anterior triangle of the neck.
2. Describe investigation and management of a 60-year-old man with severe continuing melaena of 48 hours' duration.
3. Discuss the use of chemotherapeutic agents in the management of a solid malignant tumour.

DAY 2 (THE PRINCIPLES AND PRACTICE OF SURGERY)   *(09.30–12.30)*
1. Discuss the surgical implications of the use of the oral contraceptive pill.
2. Discuss the causes and treatment of postoperative ileus.
3. Describe methods by which an airway can be provided in a patient with laryngeal obstruction. Describe the indications for tracheostomy and a technique for operation. What postoperative complications may occur?

II *DAY 1*
1. Discuss the surgical significance of variations in total serum calcium concentration. Indicate how you would make a diagnosis of hyperparathyroidism.
2. Discuss the use of blood and blood products in surgical practice.
3. Discuss the value of population screening procedures for the detection of presymptomatic malignant disease.

DAY 2
1. Discuss the causes and management of superior mesenteric artery occlusion.
2. Give an account of the pathology of calculous disease of the biliary tract and describe in detail the management of obstructive jaundice due to gall stones.
3. Discuss the management of a patient brought to hospital unconscious and suspected of having internal injuries of chest and abdomen.

III *DAY 1*
1. Discuss factors that influence the choice of incision in surgery of the abdominal contents.
2. Discuss pathology of solitary thyroid nodule and give an account of management of the patient.
3. Discuss systemic causes of excessive bleeding at operation and their management.

DAY 2
1. What are the indications for surgical intervention in a middle-aged man with atherosclerotic occlusion of the left superficial femoral artery? Discuss the advantages and disadvantages of surgical procedures available.
2. Discuss the factors on which the success of an intestinal anastomosis depends.
3. Discuss indications, method of administration and complications of parenteral nutrition in surgery.

IV *DAY 1*
1. Discuss the management of a patient with rectal bleeding and a mucosal lesion just within reach of the examining finger.
2. Discuss the diagnosis and treatment of cancer of the prostate.
3. Give an account of techniques used to monitor a critically ill surgical patient.

DAY 2

1. Outline pathological changes in diverticular disease of the distal colon and discuss operative treatment of its complications.
2. Describe causes of arteriovenous fistula. Discuss the effects of this condition and methods of treatment.
3. Describe the pathology of osteoarthritis of the hip joint and discuss surgical management.

V *DAY 1*

1. Discuss the management of a 50-year-old man with inoperable bronchogenic carcinoma.
2. Discuss uses of radioisotopes in surgical practice.
3. Define the term 'shock'. Compare and contrast pathogenesis, clinical features and treatment of haemorrhagic and septic shock.

DAY 2

1. Describe the pathological changes that may follow the development of a renal calculus. Discuss surgical procedures that may be employed for removal of a stone obstructing the lower third of the ureter.
2. Discuss diagnosis, complications and treatment of traumatic dislocation of the hip.
3. Discuss aetiology, pathological sequelae and clinical features of gastro-oesophageal reflux. Describe an operation for relief of this condition.

VI *DAY 1*

1. Discuss local and general management of a patient who develops an external small bowel fistula.
2. Outline various methods used in the treatment of cancer and refer to the limitations of each method.
3. Discuss methods of assessing the adequacy of the arterial supply to a limb.

DAY 2

1. Describe the aetiology and pathology of degenerative osteoarthrosis of the hip and discuss surgical methods of treatment.
2. Describe the pathology of coronary arterial disease and its cardiac complications. Outline the surgical techniques available for treatment of this condition.
3. Describe how you would treat a patient with jaundice caused by multiple stones in the common bile duct.

VII *DAY 1*

1. Discuss the pathological and clinical features of thoracic outlet compression syndrome. Describe the surgical management of this condition.
2. Describe the pathological changes in acute pancreatitis and discuss aetiology. Discuss the management of the early stages of pancreatitis and describe the operative treatment of an established pancreatic pseudocyst.
3. Discuss the aetiology, pathology and treatment of maldescent of the testis.

DAY 2

1. Discuss the prevention and control of infection in a surgical ward.
2. Discuss the advantages and disadvantages of different types of suture material.
3. Discuss the management of closed head injury.

VIII *DAY 1*

1. Discuss conditions included in the term 'nerve entrapment syndrome'. Describe the operation of anterior transposition of the ulnar nerve at the elbow.
2. Discuss the operative treatment of portal hypertension complicated by oesophageal varices.
3. Discuss the operative procedures in management of carcinoma of the rectum. Indicate the relative roles of various techniques which you can employ.

DAY 2

1. Describe the investigation of a patient presenting with acute bleeding from the alimentary tract. What are the relative values of endoscopy and radiology in such emergencies.

2. What do you consider to be the essential requirements of a modern accident and emergency service? Give your reasons.
3. Discuss the merits and demerits of regional lymph gland excision as an adjunct to the surgical removal of a primary malignancy, illustrating your argument by reference to particular types and locations of tumours.

IX DAY 1

1. Discuss the diagnosis, management and procedure of tumours of the testis.
2. Discuss the aetiology of right subphrenic abscess and its possible sequelae. Describe how you would drain it.
3. Describe various primary tumours which may arise in the small bowel.

DAY 2

1. Discuss the role of surgery in relief of pain due to advanced malignant disease.
2. Discuss the management of acute head injury from time of occurrence to end of first week in hospital.
3. Discuss the differential diagnosis of low back pain with sciatica and its management.

X DAY 1

1. Give a critical assessment of the operations currently used for the treatment of duodenal ulcer.
2. Describe the pathological changes which follow the lodgement of an embolus in the common femoral artery. Discuss the management of this condition.
3. Give an account of the causes of swelling of the parotid gland. Describe the operation of superficial parotidectomy.

DAY 2

1. Discuss the problems of infection in an intensive care unit.
2. Give an account of those types of systemic hypertension that may be amenable to surgical procedures.
3. Discuss the aetiology of renal stone formation.

XI DAY 1

1. Discuss the place of lymph node dissection in cancer. Give an account of an operation for radical removal of lymph nodes in the neck.
2. Discuss the management of a residual biliary stone.
3. Discuss the management of peritonitis due to a perforated abdominal viscus. Describe in detail a transverse loop colostomy.

DAY 2

1. Discuss the role of frozen section histopathology as an aid to surgical management.
2. What factors predispose to infection in surgical wounds? How may these be combatted?
3. Discuss the aetiology and management of acute renal failure in surgical practice.

XII DAY 1

1. A 25-year-old man is admitted with a stab wound of the left supraclavicular fossa. Discuss the management.
2. A 55-year-old man is found to have hypercalcaemia. Discuss the diagnosis and management.
3. Discuss the surgery of portal hypertension.

DAY 2

1. What are the indications for total parenteral nutrition? Discuss the daily requirements, methods of delivery and complications.
2. Discuss the management of chronic severe pain.
3. Discuss the methods of prevention and treatment of bowel and urinary continence.

ROYAL COLLEGE OF PHYSICIANS AND SURGEONS OF GLASGOW

FINAL EXAMINATION FOR THE FELLOWSHIP *QUA* SURGEON
PAPER 1 PRACTICE SURGERY

9.30 A.M. *to* 12.30 P.M.

PAPER 2 SURGICAL PATHOLOGY AND OPERATIVE SURGERY

2.00 P.M. *to* 5.00 P.M.

I *Paper 1*
1. Discuss the mechanism of rupture of the medial meniscus of the knee joint. Describe types of rupture and their surgical treatment.
2. Describe various types of maldescent of the testis and discuss management of the condition.
3. Make a comparison of various intravenous fluids used to treat hypovolaemic shock.

Paper 2
1. Discuss the pathological conditions which affect the endocrine pancreatic gland. Describe the surgical treatment of one of them.
2. Discuss the pathology associated with prolapsed intervertebral disc. Describe the surgical procedure of a lumbar disc protrusion.
3. Describe a surgical operation to treat gross obesity. Discuss postoperative complications and problems.

II *Paper 1*
1. What are the causes of bilateral hydronephrosis? Describe the management of this condition.
2. Discuss the role of X-ray in the diagnosis and of ultrasonography in the investigation of the acute abdomen.
3. What are the symptoms and signs of tuberculosis of the spine? Describe investigation and management of this condition.

Paper 2
1. Discuss the causes and complications of postcholecystectomy jaundice. Describe management of retained stones in the common bile duct following cholecystectomy.
2. Discuss the pathology and complications of arthritis in the hand. Describe surgical treatment of rheumatoid arthritis of the hand.
3. Discuss the pathology of swelling of lymph glands of the neck. Describe the operation of block dissection of cervical lymph glands.

III *Paper 1*
1. Discuss the investigations of obstructive jaundice. Indicate surgical procedures for its relief.
2. Discuss the aetiology, investigation and treatment of transient ischaemic attacks (drop attacks).
3. Discuss the role of percutaneous vascular access in the investigation and treatment of disease. Outline complications that may arise from the various procedures involved.

Paper 2
1. Discuss the pathology of tumours of the oral cavity and tongue. Describe the treatment of a malignant ulcer at the lateral margin of the tongue.
2. Discuss the pathology of ulcerative colitis and describe in detail the fashioning of an ileostomy.
3. Discuss the pathology and bacteriology of gas gangrene. Describe the operation of below-knee amputation for diabetic gangrene of the foot.

IV *Paper 1*
1. Describe the symptoms of fracture of the middle cranial fossa and possible complications. Outline management of such a patient.
2. Discuss the aetiology of rectal prolapse occurring in the adult. Describe the treatment.
3. Describe the investigation and aetiology of unilateral swelling of the parotid gland. Give a brief account of management and prognosis.

Paper 2
1. Discuss the systemic changes associated with a parathyroid adenoma. Describe an operation for removal of parathyroid adenoma.
2. Discuss the aetiology and pathological effects of arteriovenous fistula. Describe the surgical treatment of traumatic arteriovenous fistula of the common femoral vessels.
3. Discuss the nature and complications of abdominal stab wounds. Describe the surgical treatment for a stab wound in the left upper abdomen.

V *Paper 1*
1. Discuss important causes of renal failure in surgical practice. What are the indications for renal transplantation?
2. What are the causes of vomiting and regurgitation in the neonate? Discuss the investigation and management of the condition.
3. Discuss indications for surgery in acute and non-acute ulcerative colitis and state briefly the operative procedures you would perform.

Paper 2
1. Discuss the pathology of mesenteric vascular occlusion. Describe the surgical treatment of acute intestinal ischaemia due to occlusion of the superior mesenteric artery.
2. Discuss the complications associated with fractures and dislocations of the elbow. Describe the surgical treatment of a comminuted fracture of head of radius.
3. Discuss the aetiology and pathology of branchial cysts. Describe in detail the surgical removal of a branchial cyst.

VI *Paper 1*
1. What particular problems are associated with supracondylar fracture of the femur? Describe their management.
2. Discuss the surgical aspects of hypertension and give a brief account of relevant surgical treatment.
3. What tumours occur in the pancreas? Describe their clinical presentation and investigation.

Paper 2
1. Discuss surgical conditions where skin grafting is necessary. Describe methods of skin grafting and their advantages and disadvantages.
2. Discuss pathology of tumours of the testis. Describe the technique of lymphangiography and the operation of orchidectomy for a malignant tumour of the testis.
3. Discuss causes of diaphragmatic hernias. Describe the surgical treatment of a traumatic rupture of the diaphragm.

VII *Paper 1*
1. What factors are responsible for endotoxic shock? Discuss management of this condition.
2. What are the more common sites of injury to the urinary system? Explain the mechanism. Describe briefly the management of a case of rupture of membranous urethra.
3. Discuss the role of endoscopy in the investigation and management of upper alimentary disease.

Paper 2
1. Discuss factors that are important in wound healing. What are the aetiological problems associated with wound dehiscence? Describe surgical treatment for right paramedian incisional hernia.

2. Discuss the pathology of premalignant disease of the gastrointestinal tract. Describe the surgical treatment for familial polyposis coli.
3. Discuss the pathology and complications of oesophageal strictures. Describe a transthoracic repair of a simple stricture of the lower third of the oesophagus.

VIII *Paper 1*

1. Outline the risks of surgery under general anaesthesia. What measures may be taken to prevent their occurrence?
2. Describe various ways in which urogenital tuberculosis may present. How would you investigate the condition?
3. Describe the treatment of compound fractures of the tibia. Discuss particular problems and complications of the condition.

Paper 2

1. Discuss the pathology of cancer of the thyroid gland. Describe the operation of subtotal thyroidectomy.
2. Discuss briefly the pathological conditions for which splenectomy is indicated. Describe the operation of splenectomy.
3. Discuss the pathology of chronic gastric ulcer and its complications. Describe an operation for this condition.

IX *Paper 1*

1. Describe the investigation of a patient who presents with ischaemia of a lower limb. What factors influence the treatment of such a case?
2. Discuss the clinical manifestations and investigation of subphrenic abscess. Give a brief account of management.
3. What is meant by paralytic ileus? Discuss aetiology and management.

Paper 2

1. Discuss the pathology of malignant melanoma. Describe the surgical treatment of malignant melanoma of the lower leg.
2. Discuss the pathology of transient cerebral ischaemia. Describe the surgical treatment of carotid artery stenosis.
3. Discuss the pathology of midline swellings of the neck. Describe operation for excision of thyroglossal cyst.

X *Paper 1*

1. What complications might arise from fractures of the pelvis. Outline emergency treatment required in such circumstances.
2. Give an account of diagnosis, treatment and prognosis of testicular tumours.
3. A 75-year-old man who had a Polya gastrectomy 15 years previously presents with weight loss, tingling in fingers and toes and backache. Discuss the management and outline factors which are responsible for causing these symptoms after gastrectomy.

Paper 2

1. Discuss the pathology of carcinoid tumour of the intestine. Describe surgical treatment of carcinoid tumour of the ileum.
2. Discuss the pathology of hiatal hernia. Describe surgical treatment.
3. Discuss the place of drains in surgery.

ROYAL COLLEGE OF SURGEONS IN IRELAND
FINAL EXAMINATION FOR THE FELLOWSHIP OF THE COLLEGE
PAPER A

(TIME: 3 HOURS)

SURGICAL PATHOLOGY AND OPERATIVE SURGERY

PAPER B

(TIME: 3 HOURS)

PRINCIPLES AND PRACTICE OF SURGERY

I *PAPER A*
Write short notes (less than one page each) on the following questions: (All questions to be answered)
1. *THORACIC:*
a. Tracheo-oesophageal fistula.
b. Tracheal collapse.
c. Thymoma.
d. Mediastinoscopy.
e. Widened superior mediastinum after severe trauma.

2. *ORTHOPAEDICS:*
a. Pes cavus.
b. March fracture.
c. Spondylolisthesis.
d. Bamboo spine (radiological appearance).
e. Charcot joint.

3. *VASCULAR:*
a. Indications for A-V fistula.
b. Complications of A-V fistula in non-uraemic patients.
c. Raynaud's phenomenon.
d. Disseminated intravenous coagulation.
e. Berry's aneurysm.

4. *GENITOURINARY TRACT:*
a. Ureterocele.
b. Superficial extravasation of urine.
c. Enuresis in children.
d. Ectopia vesicae.
e. Gut neoplasia after ureterostomy.

5. *HEPATOBILIARY:*
a. Multiple biliary cysts (Caroli's disease).
b. Contraindications of intravenous cholangiography.
c. Gall stone ileus.
d. Sclerosing cholangitis.
e. Residual biliary stone.

6. *GASTROINTESTINAL TRACT:*
a. Lateral duodenal fistula.
b. Meleney's ulcer.
c. Giant benign rectal ulcer.
d. Richter's hernia.
e. Spontaneous intraperitoneal bleeding.

7. *ONCOLOGY:*
a. Cell cycle.
b. Alkylating agents.
c. Antimetabolites.
d. Nitrosamine compounds.
e. Large bowel epithelial dysplasia.

8. *MISCELLANEOUS:*
a. Pleural mesothelioma.
b. Monoclonal antibodies.
c. Metoclopramide.
d. Ocular plethysmography.
e. G-cell hyperplasia.

PAPER B
Candidates must attempt Question No. 1 and THREE of the remaining FOUR questions.
1. Discuss the management of acute pancreatitis. What are the aetiological factors, the most important investigations and the factors that influence the prognosis?

2. Write an essay on successful colorectal anastomosis.
3. Discuss the management of a 25-year-old man admitted with a gunshot wound just below the right nipple.
4. Describe the aetiology and management of male urethral stricture.
5. Discuss the postoperative analgesia in a surgical patient.

II *PAPER A*
1. *GASTROINTESTINAL TRACT:*
a. Radiation enteritis.
b. Peptic ulcerations of the small gut.
c. Gastrojejunocolic fistula.
d. Angiodysplasia of the gut.
e. Volvulus of the colon.

2. *HEPATOBILIARY:*
a. Fulminating acute cholangitis.
b. Emphysematous cholycystitis.
c. Biliary ductal anatomical anomalies.
d. Lithogenic bile.
e. Retained stone in common bile duct.

3. *GYNAECOLOGY AND UROLOGY:*
a. Bartholin's abscess.
b. Urethral caruncle.
c. Endometriosis.
d. Ureteric reflux.
e. Tubo-ovarian abscess.

4. *VASCULAR:*
a. Transluminal angioplasty.
b. Vena cava injury.
c. Side-effects of heparin.
d. Profundoplasty.
e. Alternatives to the saphenous vein in coronary bypass.

5. *LOCOMOTOR SYSTEM:*
a. Monteggia's fracture.
b. Cubitus valgus.
c. Patellar tap.
d. Rupture of supraspinatus.
e. Rupture of quadriceps expansion.

6. *THORACIC:*
a. Cervical rib.
b. Insertion of chest tube in pneumothorax.
c. Therapeutic bronchoscopy.
d. Dysphagia lusoria.
e. Bronchobiliary fistula.

7. *VASCULAR:*
a. Measurement of ankle blood pressure.
b. Hepatic artery occlusion.
c. Blood viscosity implications in surgery.
d. Arterial injury in knee joint trauma.

8. *MISCELLANEOUS:*
a. Significance of intra-abdominal X-ray calcification.
b. High-output renal failure.
c. Malignant life cycle.
d. Anti-smooth muscle antibodies.
e. Fractured head of radius.

PAPER B
1. Write an essay on thyroiditis. Include in your answer a *detailed* description of the macroscopic and microscopic appearances in each condition and indications for surgical intervention.

2. Classify small intestinal tumours, and describe their modes of presentation, investigation and management.
3. Write an essay on fistula-in-ano.
4. Discuss the management of an unconscious patient with multiple trauma. What factors are important in prognosis?
5. Discuss the place of surgery in the management of chronic pancreatitis.

III *PAPER A*
1. *THORACIC:*
a. Shock lung.
b. IPPV
c. EEPV
d. Slipped ribs.
e. Flail chest.

2. *HEPATOBILIARY:*
a. Solitary giant cyst of liver.
b. Calot's triangle.
c. Choledochus cyst.
d. Contact cholangiography.
e. Primary biliary stone.

3. *GASTROINTESTINAL:*
a. Mucoviscidosis.
b. Spider naevi.
c. Vipoma.
d. Therapeutic ERCP.
e. Sengstaken–Blakemore tube.

4. *ORTHOPAEDICS:*
a. Low back pain.
b. Köhler's disease.
c. Myositis ossificans.
d. Codeman's triangle.
e. Scaphoid fracture.

5. *VASCULAR:*
a. Neoplastic lymphoedema.
b. Seldinger catheter.
c. Swanz–Ganz catheter.
d. Lymphoedema tarda and praecox.
e. Therapeutic uses of the intravenous route.

6. *GENITOURINARY TRACT:*
a. Priapism.
b. Autonephrectomy.
c. Deep extravasation of urine.
d. Peyronie's disease.
e. Indications and contraindications for circumcision.

7. *ONCOLOGY:*
a. Lentigo maligna.
b. Oestrogen receptors.
c. Anti-oestrogens.
d. Premalignant colonic lesion.
e. Interferon.

8. *MISCELLANEOUS:*
a. Hirtz–Halter valve.
b. Traumatic injury of the diaphragm.
c. Intrathymic parathyroid adenoma.
d. Paradoxical breathing.
e. Fat embolism.

PAPER B
1. Describe the salient features of the usual malignant tumours of bone. In each condition, write a brief account of the gross and microscopic pathological appearances.

2. Describe the aetiology, diagnostic features and management of extradural intracranial haemorrhage.
3. Discuss the indications for and complications of intravenous feeding.
4. Discuss the management of a 45-year-old male bank clerk who presents with pain in his calf on walking.
5. Write an essay on the selection of antibiotics in abdominal surgery. Briefly comment on the following statement: 'The timing of antibiotic administration is of great importance in the overall reduction of postoperative wound sepsis.'

SECTION 3
Causes of Failure

The candidate has to pass the written and clinical parts individually and clearly with no borderline marks. Borderline marks in other parts of the examination can be discussed and compensated for. Failed candidates should investigate the causes of their failure in order to avoid them in future attempts and should not be too disappointed since many of the best surgeons fail their first attempt. It has even been said 'It is a shame to pass the final FRCS at the first attempt.' We outline here the main causes of failure of the final FRCS.

Inadequate preparation Self-explanatory. Do not attempt the final FRCS (and do not waste your money and time) before you feel that you are fully prepared theoretically and have fully mastered your operations and clinical methods practically.

Inability to express oneself Particularly applies to overseas doctors with poor command of English. You may know the operations and know what to do in emergency situations but you are either unable to express yourself and your ideas in English or are unable to discuss your operations technically and systematically. It is advisable therefore to know the key English phrases in each disease and operation and know the principles in outline since discussion and substantiation of each approach is the essence of the final FRCS examination, especially the oral parts.

Lack of common sense Always think in terms of priorities and remember that common diseases are common and rare diseases are rare. This is particularly important in the discussions when you are requested to speak in order of frequency. In the written part, however, you can discuss the diseases according to the well-known plan of congenital, traumatic, neoplastic, etc. Do not show your encyclopaedic knowledge in the clinical and oral parts but be practical and precise. Mention common lesions first and outline your management according to priorities, mentioning the most important measures first.

Your management should always be comprehensive, treating the primary cause and its effects and not just symptoms. When asked about investigations, remember always to mention the simplest relevant and cheapest investigation first since there is no place for routine blind investigation in the final FRCS. Those who mention ERCP before urine examination in jaundice investigations and barium enema before rectal examination and sigmoidoscopy with biopsy in rectal carcinoma, those who embark on palpation of the groin before asking the patient to cough in hernia examination, and those who forget to examine the mouth or ask the patient to swallow in neck swelling examination deserve to fail. Try not to be clever, but be careful.

Bad candidate – patient relationship Examiners expect you to be perfect not only in your knowledge and judgement but also in your ethics and approach. Do not fail yourself by appearing excessively hirsute or eccentrically dressed. Be polite to patients. Introduce yourself and ask permission to examine them. Thank them at the end, help them with their night clothes and tuck in the sheets and blankets. This will at least show that you are a courteous and considerate doctor. Never ever examine patients as if you are manipulating animals. Look at their faces for pain expression. Examiners may press you to discuss the causes of the patient's swelling or ascites. Do not mention the word 'malignancy' or 'tumour' in front of the patient.

Lack of confidence Talk to your examiner as you would address a distinguished senior colleague. Give the impression that you are a confident safe surgeon who knows exactly what to do. Examiners sometimes try to shake your confidence by adopting the opposite approach. If you think you are right, substantiate your approach. If you are asked, 'How do you do this operation?', do not answer by saying 'Some do it this way and others prefer that way.' You have to adopt your own practical and personal safe way, so say, 'I will do this operation this way . . . ', without mentioning other views. Remember though that overconfidence in controversial topics should be resisted.

Bad examiner – examinee relationship Never ever argue with the examiner and never ask the examiner to repeat the question. Listen carefully to his question and if he says, 'Tell me about gastric carcinoma', do not reply 'What would you like me to talk about?' but say, 'I should like to talk about its pathology because I find this particularly interesting.' If you are asked about thyroiditis, never ask the examiner, 'What do you mean?' It implies that he is not making himself clearly understood or that he is phrasing his question badly and you have not listened carefully to him. Do not smile too much and do not be a joker. Do not try to be over-confident or too humble with the examiner but smile a little bit, and answer his question politely and efficiently. If he tries to explain his own approach listen to him with interest and show him that you are quite impressed (but never argue). Keep the examiner happy and keep the discussion easygoing, comfortable and mutually interesting. Also be exact and precise and answer his question *to the point*, unless you want to lead him to a topic you know better.

Luck　There is no doubt that luck is involved. It is usual for examiners to examine in pairs so that if one is unkind or aggressive (the hawk) he will be buffered or compensated for by the other, more dove-like examiner. It is bad luck to be examined by too many hawks asking impossible questions about cardiac transplantation or hepatic resection. Examiners who remain expressionless no matter what you say (if not looking unhappy) and pedantic examiners who keep asking you the same question because you are not answering the exact point in their minds are difficult to cope with. We are sure that each Royal College always tries to maintain its high standard through careful selection of fair examiners.

We strongly advise candidates not to over-react, even when they are confronted with the most difficult examiners, because this may affect their attitude and performance in subsequent parts of the examination. It should be remembered that many apparently difficult examiners may be very helpful in the comprehensive analysis of your scores.

SECTION 4
What to Read

It is a grave mistake to think that the books read for the final MB, ChB are useless for the postgraduate diploma since these books provide the solid basis for the theory and a practical guide for the clinical part. It is more convenient to go through a book you have read before than to explore a new one for the first time. Most surgical facts are not going to change radically and only a fraction of facts will emerge and need to be added every 3–5 years. Therefore, choose as your basic text or 'skeleton of surgery' a comprehensive surgical book with which you are familiar and augment this with a few other books. Try to widen and supplement your views by accumulating information on the uncovered topics from the regular journals. (The best plan is to summarise these topics in a special file which can be reviewed in conjunction with your surgical textbook before examination.) The following useful books are listed without recommendation as to the best since this depends entirely on your personal preference. However, our personal experience with books will be mentioned in the next section. *Only one book* should be selected from each group below to cover one of the examination parts. Notice that in some books the date (or edition number) is omitted deliberately so that you can order the last published edition. It is not how much you read that is important but how well you digest the facts (quality rather than quantity of reading).

General

Comprehensive textbooks

Harding Rains A. J., Ritchie H. D. (eds). *Bailey and Love's Short Practice of Surgery*. London: H. K. Lewis.

Sabiston D. C. (ed). *Davis–Christopher Textbook of Surgery*. Philadelphia: W. B. Saunders.

Taylor S., Chisholm G. D., O'Higgins N., Shields R. (1984). *Surgical Management*. London: William Heinemann. Medical Books.

Cushieri A., Giles G. R., Moosa A. R. (eds) (1982). *Essential Surgical Practice*. Bristol: John Wright.

Schwartz S. I., Lillehei R. C., Shires G. H. *et al* (eds). *Principles of Surgery*. New York: McGraw Hill (A Blakiston Publication). (in volumes)

Hardy J. D. (1983). *Hardy Textbook of Surgery*. New York: Lippincott Company.

Dunphy J. E., Way L. (eds). *Current Surgical Diagnosis and Treatment*. Los Altos, California: Lange.

McCredie J. A. (ed). *Basic Surgery*. London: Macmillan.

Forrest A. P. M., Carter D. C., Macleod I. B. (1985). *Principles and Practice of Surgery*. Edinburgh: Churchill Livingstone.

Review books (for quick revision)

Hadfield J., Hobsley M. (eds). *Current Surgical Practice*, Vols 1, 2 and 3. London: Edward Arnold.

Smiddy F. G. *Tutorials in Surgery*, Nos. 1, 2 and 3. Tunbridge Wells: Pitman Medical.

Thomas J. M., Belstead J. S. *Aids to Postgraduate Surgery*. Edinburgh: Churchill Livingstone.

Ellis H., Calne R. Y. *Lecture Notes on General Surgery*. Oxford: Blackwell Scientific Publications.

Speciality books (to widen your views)

Abdomen

Shackelford R. T. *Surgery of the Alimentary Tract*. Philadelphia: W. B. Saunders. (in volumes)

Maingot R. (ed) (1980). *Maingot's Abdominal Operations*, Vols 1 and 2. New York: Appleton-Century-Crofts.

Golligher J. C., Duthie H. L., Nixon H. H. (eds). *Golligher's Surgery of the Anus, Rectum and Colon*. London: Baillière Tindall.

Heberer G., Denecke H. (eds) (1982). *Colo-rectal Surgery*. Berlin: Springer-Verlag.

Keith R. G., Keynes W. M. (eds) (1981). *The Pancreas*. London: William Heinemann Medical Books.

Smith, Lord R., Sherlock, Dame S., (eds) (1981). *Surgery of the Gallbladder and Bile Ducts*. London: Butterworths.

Kune G. A., Sali A. *The Practice of Biliary Surgery*. Oxford: Blackwell Scientific Publications.

Blumgart L. H. *The Biliary Tract – Clinical Surgery International*, Vol. 5. Edinburgh: Churchill Livingstone.

Dudley H. A. F. (ed). *Bailey's Emergency Surgery*. Bristol: John Wright & Sons.

Thorax

Cardiothoracic section in *Davis–Christopher Textbook of Surgery*. Philadelphia: W. B. Saunders.

D'Abreu A. L., Collis J. L., Clarke D. B. *A Practice of Thoracic Surgery*. London: Edward Arnold.

Orthopaedics

Apley A. G., Solomon L. (eds). *Apley's System of Orthopaedics and Fractures*. London: Butterworths.

Adams C. *Outline of Orthopaedics* and *Outline of Fracture including Joint Injuries*. Edinburgh: Churchill Livingstone.

Crenshaw A. G. (ed). *Campbell's Operative Orthopaedics* (2 vols). St Louis: Mosby Co.

Wilson J. N. (ed). *Watson–Jones' Fractures and Joint Injuries* (2 vols). Edinburgh: Churchill Livingstone.

Urology

Glenn J. G. (ed) (1983). *Urologic Surgery*, 3rd edn. Philadelphia: J. G. Lippincott.

Blandy J. *Urology*, Vols 1 and 2. Oxford: Blackwell Scientific Publications.

Chisholm G. D. *Urology*. London: William Heinemann Medical Books.

Vascular

Cooley D. A., Wukasch D. C. *Techniques in Vascular Surgery*. Philadelphia: W. B. Saunders.

Jamieson C. *Surgical Management of Vascular Disease*. London: William Heinemann Medical Books.

Dodd H., Cockett F. B. *The Pathology and Surgery of the Veins of the Lower Limb*. Edinburgh: Churchill Livingstone.

Kinmonth J. B. (1982). *The Lymphatics*. London: Edward Arnold.

Reid W., Pollock J. G. (1978). *The Surgeon's Management of Gangrene*. London: Pitman.

Head and neck

Stell P. M., Maran A. G. *Head and Neck Surgery*. London: William Heinemann Medical Books.

Neurosurgery

Jennett B., Galbraith S. *An Introduction to Neurosurgery*. London: William Heinemann Medical Books.

Paediatric surgery

Nixon H. H., O'Donnell B. *The Essentials of Paediatric Surgery*. London: William Heinemann Medical Books.

Nixon H. H. *Surgical Conditions in Paediatrics*. London: Butterworths.

Plastic surgery

McGregor I. A. *Fundamental Techniques of Plastic Surgery*. Edinburgh: Churchill Livingstone.

Grabb W. C., Smith J. W. *Plastic Surgery*. Boston: Little, Brown & Co.

Skoog T. *Plastic Surgery*. Philadelphia: W. B. Saunders.

Clinical surgery

Bailey H. In *Demonstration of Physical Signs in Clinical Surgery* (Clain A., ed). Bristol: John Wright.

Scott P. R. *An Aid to Clinical Surgery*. Revised by Dudley H. A. F. Edinburgh: Churchill Livingstone.

Surgical pathology

Illingworth Sir Charles, Dick B. M. *A Textbook of Surgical Pathology*. Edinburgh: Churchill Livingstone.

Guthrie W., Fawkes R. *A Colour Atlas of Surgical Pathology*. London: Wolfe Medical Publications.

Curran R. C., Jones E. L. *Gross Pathology. A Colour Atlas*. London: H. M. & M. Publishers.

Royal College of Surgeons of Edinburgh. *A Colour Atlas of Demonstrations in Surgical Pathology* (1—Alimentary System; 2—Genitourinary System; 3—Cardiovascular System; 4—Orthopaedic Lesions). Contact the College for purchases.

Smiddy F. G., Cowen P. N. *Tutorials in Surgery*. No. 4 & 5. Tunbridge Wells: Pitman Medical.

Operative surgery

Rintoul R. F. (ed). *Farquarson's Textbook of Operative Surgery*. Edinburgh: Churchill Livingstone.

Keen G. (ed). *Operative Surgery and Management*. Bristol: John Wright.

Dudley H. A. F., Carter D. (eds). *Rob & Smith's Operative Surgery* (various volumes). London: Butterworths.

Rob C., Smith R. (eds). *Atlas of General Surgery*. Compiled by Dudley H. London: Butterworths.

Shipman J. J. (1977). *Operative Surgery Revision*. London: H. K. Lewis.

Smiddy F. G. *Tutorials in Surgery*, No. 3. Tunbridge Wells: Pitman Medical.

Marston A. (ed) (1979). *Contemporary Operative Surgery*. London: Northwood Publications.

Kirk R. M. *General Surgical Operations*. Edinburgh: Churchill Livingstone.

Surgical principles and practice

Lumley J. S. P., Craven J. L. (eds) *Surgical Review*, Nos 1, 2 and 3. Tunbridge Wells: Pitman Medical.

Recent Advances in Surgery, Nos 8, 9 and 10 (edited by Taylor S.) and No. 11 (edited by Russell R. C. G.). Edinburgh: Churchill Livingstone.

N.B. The above two series are excellent and candidates are encouraged to read both of them (if not own them).

Smiddy F. G. *The Investigation of the Surgical Patient*. London: Edward Arnold.

Surgical instruments

Any comprehensive general surgical catalogue, e.g. Thackray's Manufacturer's Catalogue.

Stanek J. *Surgical Diagnostic and Therapeutic Instruments*. Oxford: Blackwell Scientific Publications.

Brigden R. J. (1980). *Operating Theatre Technique*. Edinburgh: Churchill Livingstone.

Brooks S. M. (1982). *Instrumentation for the Operating Room*. St. Louis: C. V. Mosby.

Journals

Review of the following journals of the last year is recommended to keep you up to date. (Examiners often read these journals just before the examination or on the train while travelling to the college to examine you.) However, this is not an examination necessity especially if you have mastered other fields of surgery.

The leading useful journals are:

British Journal of Surgery.

The Journal of the Royal College of Surgeons of Edinburgh.

Annals of the Royal College of Surgeons of England.

Surgery edited by J. Lumley & J. Craven (review articles).

Annual Review of General Surgery, in *Postgraduate Medical Journal* (June or July issue usually). This review is extremely useful and time saving.

British Journal of Hospital Medicine and *Hospital Update* provide excellent review articles for the final FRCS.

Surgery

Annals of Surgery

Surgery Gynecology and Obstetrics

Some of the leading articles in the *Lancet* and *British Medical Journal*.

Others

Shipman J. J. (1978). *Mnemonics and Tactics in Surgery and Medicine*. London: Lloyd-Luke.

Lourie J. (1982). *Medical Eponyms: Who Was Coudé?* London: Pitman.

Jablonski S. *Illustrated Dictionary of Eponymic Syndromes and Diseases and their Synonyms*. Philadelphia: W. B. Saunders.

Some Wolfe colour atlases (of surgical interest).

Butterworth International Medical Reviews (in surgery) including different volumes on *trauma, endocrine surgery, gastroenterological surgery, vascular surgery*.

Albin R. J. (1981). *Handbook of Cryosurgery*. New York, Basel: Mariel Dekker.

Brooks D. K., Harold A. J. (1983). Modern Emergency Department Practice. London: Edward Arnold.

Tape-slide lecture programmes provided by Audiovisual Medical Libraries, e.g. Graves, and films from the Royal Society of Medicine (operative surgery).

SECTION 5
What to Do

Be Precise and Exact Get down to the nitty gritty of the surgical facts and principles since you are bound to be asked 'Why?'. Listen carefully and answer the exact question straight to the point. It is probably wiser to fractionate the answer, leaving the examiner a chance to interrupt you and re-ask you; e.g. if the examiner asks, 'What are the causes of obstructive jaundice?' answer by mentioning the individual causes according to the order of frequency, i.e. common bile duct stone then discuss carcinoma of head of pancreas, then metastatic deposits in the porta hepatis and so on. A wise candidate will talk clearly and slowly. Do not speak unless you are spoken to. Too much talk usually leads to mistakes.

Do Not Be Clever, Be Careful Examination is not show business, it is a mutual discussion about basic surgical principles, logical approach and clinical judgement. Answer the basic simple questions with a basic simple answer. Answer to the point and try to steer the discussion into an area you feel confident about. If you are asked an unfair question, e.g. about hemihepatectomy, try to tackle it by saying 'I have never done the operation and I have never seen it done but the principles are as follows . . . ' It is not shameful to admit you do not know but it is to tell lies which will easily expose your limited experience.

Keep In Touch With Surgery Through Discussions Discussion is the best means of preparation for the final FRCS:

- If there is a friend sitting his examination with you, join him in discussions of various subjects, operations and examination of patients.
- Attend all postgraduate meetings in your hospital and nearby hospitals if possible.
- Do not miss the surgical journal club of the hospital.
- Discuss every vague point about operations with your consultant.
- Attend teaching ward rounds.
- Participate in 'mock' examinations.
- Get the best of knowledge from the paramedical staff, such as physiotherapists (e.g. ask about therapeutic ultrasounds), theatre sisters (e.g. ask about surgical instruments), bacteriologists (e.g. ask about the timing and frequency of antibiotic blood assay such as gentamicin, infections and sepsis).

Filing System of Collected Data For reference purposes, you can classify the review articles and various collected literature in a filing cabinet drawer with the required number of files according to the system you propose to use. However, you should keep summaries of the common major subjects in one file for easily manageable quick revision. This book is meant to fill this gap . . . you can add to it if you think necessary.

Read Less, Digest More and Learn Surgery by Illustrations The less you read theoretically and the more you digest of your little reading, the better. There is no place for encyclopaedic knowledge since this is for reference only and not for practical surgery. Remember key phrases. Read and re-read the same book again and again rather than getting into the habit of exploring new books. There is probably no need for journals although we do recommend reading the review articles, for instance those in the *British Journal of Hospital Medicine* and *Surgery* since it is a quick method of scanning all articles of past years (*see* Section 4). Learn surgery by drawing and diagrams since it is time-saving and an easy way to revise. Also learn surgery by mnemonics (*see* Section 4).

Put Yourself in the Examiner's Chair When you see patients in the outpatient department or in the ward try to think in terms of interesting cases that could be presented in the examination. Examine the patients as if you are performing the short cases of the FRCS examination and improve your methods so that your methodical approach becomes routine, comprehensive and reflexly performed. Examine your friends and remember their mistakes and apply what you have learned when you are under the stress of the examination.

Never Be Preoccupied By What Failed Candidates Say You will hear the full spectrum of rumours of racial discrimination, nationality discrimination, sex discrimination and hospital discrimination. Do not let them disturb your balance. Give them a deaf ear. They probably failed because they deserved to.

Examiner–Examinee and Examinee–Patient Relationship (*see* Part I, Section 4)   We stress the importance of gentle examination (never manipulate patients as if they are experimental animals). Do not be argumentative or overconfident. Be straightforward and practical (think of priorities and common things before rare ones). Keep discussions simple.

Hope for the Best and Prepare for the Worst   Make every effort to prepare, but do not be too disappointed if you fail; there is always tomorrow and you can attempt the examination in other Colleges or wait for the next session in the same College.

Comment on Courses   Advanced courses are only valuable when all the basic training is complete. They are meant for orientation and guidance and quick revision of fully prepared candidates. Candidates, particularly those coming to the United Kingdom from overseas, are strongly urged to ascertain whether or not they are *eligible* to sit the examination before embarking upon academic courses of study or clinical training.

FINAL ADVICE

There is no doubt that the final FRCS is a formidable but fair examination. The difference between success and failure is marginal. The scoring system does not often pass more than 20% of attempting candidates. If you think you are going to fail after the written part, do not withdraw but finish all of the examination parts (since you have paid for it) and get the benefit of discussions, so that you can avoid any mistakes at a future attempt. It is our belief that following the above guidelines coupled with thorough preparation is the ideal way of approaching the examination for the final FRCS diploma. We do not advise too much reading. Keep a comprehensive surgical textbook (for reference) supplemented by a file of revision (e.g. this book), a clinical book (e.g. *Bailey's Demonstration of Physical Signs in Clinical Surgery*), an operative book you are used to and a book on surgical pathology—these are more than sufficient when coupled with good clinical and operative experience. You should read a sufficient number of journals to render you *au fait* with modern advances and current surgical practice.

SECTION 6
Historical Background

It has been said that 'those who cannot remember the past are condemned to repeat it'. We include this section on the historical origin and development of modern surgical science since it is essential that candidates sitting their examination for the higher postgraduate surgical diploma are familiar with the outstanding achievements of those leaders in surgery who have made the current operations easy, safe and daily routine procedures.

Examiners become annoyed when you mention a physical sign, law or operation named after a surgeon you do not know, and it is a great bonus for you if you are conversant with the historical background or at least know the nationality of the surgeon. The magnitude of the achievement of these men in any case warrants discussion of their work.

The history and pioneers of *surgical specialities* will not be considered here but only the history of *general surgery* and those historical figures who described physical signs and operations relevant to the final FRCS. As some surgical procedures could not be attributed mainly to one surgeon, we have described these separately after the 'Names' section. The two sections have been cross-referenced where there is overlap.

THE DEVELOPMENT OF SURGERY

The history of disease is at least as old as the history of mankind. In ancient Egypt, papyri have been found dealing with medicine, surgery, obstetrics and gynaecology. The Edwin Smith papyrus written in about 1600 BC is one of the oldest and is of great interest to surgeons.

In the Babylonian code of Hammurabi there were severe penalties for the surgeon whose operations were unsuccessful (e.g. cutting off his right hand). In India, Susruta described more than 100 surgical instruments in the book *Susruta Samhita* written in Sanskrit around the eighth century BC. The Indian surgeons are best known for their skill in plastic surgery. In Greece, Hippocrates (the father of Medicine) wrote 70 books around 400 BC. His book *On the Surgery* was mainly concerned with bandaging of various types of injuries (including fractures and dislocation).

The Roman encyclopaedist of the early first century AD, Aulus Cornelius Celsus, described four characteristics of inflammation: 'Rubor (redness), Tumor (swelling), Calor (heat) and Dolor (pain)' (to which one only can add loss of function for a perfect definition). Galen of the second century AD elaborated the Hippocratic principles and differentiated between surgery and medicine. In the later Middle Ages, the Moslems took the leading role (especially in the tenth century). It was Albucasis (AD 936–1013), the Moorish physician and surgeon of Andalusia ('a remarkable man, both prolific and courageous'), who described hundreds of surgical instruments and many operations in his famous book *Al-Tasrif*. He was the first to introduce the use of catgut and cotton sutures, he accomplished successful small intestinal anastomoses and was the first to operate on blood vessels. He performed the first successful thyroidectomy operation in literature, introduced the first delivery forceps and described many operations in orthopaedics, ophthalmology and gynaecology. He therefore deserves to be called 'the father of operative surgery'. Avicenna (AD 980–1037) was another remarkable physician in that period.

From the year 1300 onward surgery was looked down upon and avoided by physicians who had received their education in the universities, where, along with theology and law, medicine was usually one of the basic faculties. Surgeons, on the other hand, were of the lower class, and were scorned in clerical circles (*Ecclesia abhorret a sanguine* = the Church abhors blood). Surgeons were taught the ways of their craft by apprenticeship and their work was combined with that of barbers.

In 1543, Andrew Vesalius published his outstanding anatomy book based on cadaveric dissection: *De humani corporis fabrica*. The Scottish surgeon Peter Lowe (1550–1613) published the first real surgical textbook written in English *A Discourse of the Whole Art of Chirurgerie* in 1597 and arranged his book under five headings: (1) to take away; (2) to help and add; (3) to put in place that which is out; (4) to separate; and (5) to join what is separated. He founded the Brethren of Chirurgerie (the forerunner of the Royal College of Physicians and Surgeons of Glasgow). He also asked for separation of surgeons from barbers.

In Paris, Ambroise Paré (1510–1590) the military surgeon stressed the importance of anatomy in surgery and made remarkable contributions to wound healing and cauterisation. Alexis Littre (the father of colostomy), François De la Peyronie and others contributed tremendously to the fame of Paris in surgery. In 1743 the association with encumbering barbers was ended by Parisian surgeons (and was followed by London surgeons in 1745). Thus during nearly the whole of the eighteenth century Paris held pride of place as the centre of medical teaching and practice. The ambitious British or American doctor regarded a visit to Paris as an essential part of his training. The French world predominance continued until 1789.

Before the fame of Paris had started to wane, Edinburgh was already rising to the high place which it held until 1830. The Edinburgh school depended for its excellence upon a far higher standard of teaching than was to be found in any other centre. The Monro dynasty of anatomists and the outstanding anatomy teacher Robert Knox contributed to its name and fame. However in 1829 the series of murders committed by Burke and Hare of Edinburgh and the tracing of at least one body to Knox's anatomy rooms created a sensation which ruined Knox and tarnished Edinburgh's good name. After a similar murder in London, the Anatomy Act of 1832 was passed which permitted authorised medical schools to acquire bodies for the purpose of dissection.

London had already started to rise before Edinburgh was passing into eclipse. The greatest of London teachers were Scots by birth or education. John Hunter left Glasgow in 1748 to study in London under William Cheselden of St Thomas' and Percival Pott of St Bartholomew's. He was later appointed to St George's Hospital. Hunter founded a school of anatomy and surgery in Leicester Square and became the leader of experimental surgery. In 1804 Charles Bell a young surgeon decided to leave Edinburgh for London (because of his poor income—£25 per year while Astley Cooper of England earned £15 000 per year). He established himself as a teacher and was appointed to the Middlesex Hospital after serving at the Battle of Waterloo. In 1835 Robert Liston, a famous surgeon of his time, left Edinburgh for University College Hospital, London. In 1839 William Fergusson left Edinburgh for King's College Hospital, thereby making that small institution behind Lincoln's Inn Fields the surgical centre of the world for a short time. As these men moved South, the centre of gravity moved with them from Edinburgh to London with an inevitable outcome: the rise of London's influence at the expense of that of Edinburgh.

The major Scottish invasion of surgical London came about as the result of the foundation of new London hospitals. For over 500 years the two medieval hospitals of St Bartholomew's and St Thomas' were the only institutions which could possibly be given the name of teaching centres, but during the eighteenth century the rapid expansion of London made the provision of free treatment for the sick poor an urgent necessity. Thus came into being, often as out-patient dispensaries in origin, the Westminster (1715), Guy's (founded as a kind of annexe for the chronically sick patients of St Thomas' in 1721), St George's (1733), the London (1740), and the Middlesex (1745). In all cases the medical schools attached to these hospitals are of a later date, the earliest being that of the Middlesex, where an organised course of lectures commenced in 1785. The year 1821 saw the foundation of the first 'teaching hospital', when Dr Benjamin Golding opened Charing Cross 'to supply the want of a university, so far as medical education is concerned'. University College Hospital, first known as the North London, and King's College Hospital were founded in 1834 and 1839 respectively, for the express purpose of providing clinical instruction for the students of University College in Gower Street and King's College in the Strand.

London maintained world supremacy from 1830 until shortly after the Franco-Prussian war of 1870 when initiative passed to the victorious Germanic nations. Germany, alone among nations, accepted Lister's antisepsis wholeheartedly (in 1875 Lister made a tour of the larger centres in Germany). Outstanding surgeons like Volkmann, Esmarch, Thiersch, Langenbeck, Mikulicz, Billroth, Kocher and others contributed to the high surgical standards of Germany which dominated the world from 1870 until the end of the nineteenth century when the USA began to move up to the leading place owing to the remarkable efforts of American surgeons like Halsted of Johns Hopkins Hospital (Baltimore), the Mayo brothers of Rochester, Murphy and Oschner of Chicago, McBurney of New York and many others. The USA maintained its supremacy until the Second World War, and since then, the American and British schools have emerged as the main leaders in the field of surgery.

NAMES TO BE REMEMBERED

The following list of names is far from complete; however it is more than sufficient for the purposes of the final FRCS.

Addison, Thomas (1793–1860) Physician, Guy's Hospital, London, UK. He described Addison's disease—adrenal medullary hypofunctioning leading to hypogyloaemia, hypotension and pigmentation with hyperkalaemia and hyponatraemia.

Adson, Alfred W. (1887–1951) Neurosurgeon, The Mayo Clinic, Rochester, Minnesota, USA. He described the Adson deep-breathing test in which the radial pulse is diminished if the patient turns his head to the side of the cervical rib and inspires deeply (because of pressure of the scalenus anterior accessory respiratory muscle).

Alcock, Benjamin (b. 1801) Professor of Anatomy, Cork, Republic of Ireland. He described Alcock's canal in ischiorectal fossa (contains pudendal nerve which is easily blocked with local anaesthetic).

Amyand, Claudius Surgeon, St George's Hospital, London, UK. Performed the first appendicectomy in 1736 (*see* 'Evolution of appendicectomy).

Apley, Alan G. Contemporary orthopaedic surgeon, St Thomas' Hospital, London, UK. He introduced Apley's test in medial meniscus injury (patient lies prone and examiner stands on the affected side and grasps that foot with both hands flexing the knee to a right angle; lateral rotation produces pain in medial ligament injury while lateral rotation with compression (grinding test) produces pain in medial meniscus injury. To test medial structures rotation should be medial).

Argyll Robertson (1837–1909) Ophthalmic surgeon, Edinburgh Royal Infirmary, UK. Argyll Robertson pupils are small irregular pupils in tabes dorsalis (accommodation reflex present and light reflex absent).

Arnold, Julius (1835–1915) Professor of Pathological Anatomy, Heidelberg, Germany. With **Chiari, Hans** (1851–1916), Professor of Pathological Anatomy, Strasburg, Germany, described Arnold–Chiari malformation (displacement of the hind brain and herniation into the spinal canal of the cerebellar tonsils obstructing the free circulation of cerebrospinal fluid leading to hydrocephalus).

Atkins, Sir Hedley Contemporary Emeritus Professor of Surgery, Guy's Hospital, London, UK. He described the extended tyelectomy treatment in breast carcinoma and introduced the macrodochectomy in intraduct papilloma.

Babiniski, Joseph F. F. (1857–1932) Head of the Neurological Clinic, Hôspital Pitie, Paris, France. He described Babiniski sign in the contralateral brain upper motor neurone lesion.

Baker, William (1838–1896) Surgeon, St Bartholomew's Hospital, London, UK. He described Baker's cyst (a popliteal swelling, often bilateral, occurring in patients over 40 years of age. It is a pressure diverticulum of the synovial membrane through a hiatus in the capsule of the knee joint. It stands out when the knee is fully extended).

Barlow, Thomas G. (1915–1975) Surgeon, Hope Hospital, Manchester, UK. Together with **Ortolani, Marino** (Contemporary Director, Centre for Congenital Subluxation of the Hip, Italy) described Barlow–Ortolani test (during abduction of the flexed hips and knees, the examiner's middle fingers on the greater trochanters can reduce the already dislocated hip with a palpable jerk. Removal of the hands leads to another jerk due to dislocation which can also be shown by pressing the thumbs on the thigh from the inside).

Bartholin, Casper (1655–1738) Professor of Medicine, Anatomy and Physics, Copenhagen, Denmark. He described Bartholin's gland in labium majus infection which leads to Bartholin's abscess.

Bassini, Edoardo (1844–1924) Senator of Italy (Paria) and pioneer of (Bassini) repair of inguinal hernia (interrupted closure of conjoined tendon to inguinal ligament) which has stood the test of time. He is also credited with the first attempt to bypass a stone impacted in the bile duct by joining the gall bladder to the duodenum (1882) and he was one of the earliest surgeons to perform a gastroenterostomy.

Battle, William H. (1855–1936) Surgeon, St Thomas' Hospital, London, UK. He advised the use of a special incision for appendicectomy. Battle's sign is the bruising over the mastoid process appearing a day or two after head injury—confirms a diagnosis of middle cranial fossa fracture.

Bell, Sir Charles (1774–1842) Scottish surgeon at Middlesex Hospital, London, UK. Later Professor of Surgery, Edinburgh, UK. He described Bell's (facial nerve) palsy as well as the nerve of Bell (nerve of latissimus dorsi which needs to be preserved in mastectomy).

Bennett, Edward H. (1837–1907) Professor of Surgery, Trinity College, Dublin, Republic of Ireland. He described Bennett's fracture (fracture-dislocation of first metacarpophalangeal joint).

Billroth, Theodor (1829–1894) German surgeon, born on the Island of Rugen in 1829 and graduated from Berlin University in 1852. He became Langenbeck's assistant at Berlin and Professor of Surgery at Zurich in 1860 and moved to Vienna 7 years later where he founded the famous Viennese School of Surgery. In 1872 he resected the oesophagus and in 1873 he performed the first total excision of the larynx for cancer. In January 1881 he performed the first successful partial gastrectomy for pyloric cancer in a 43-year-old woman. He made an incision through the abdominal wall about 8 cm long transversely over the tumour, which he found to be of large size, involving more than one-third of the lower portion of the stomach. He brought the tumour to the surface (with some difficulty because of the small incision), made openings into the stomach and duodenum above and below the tumour, then cut it away. Next he stitched up the major part of the hole in the stomach so that it exactly fitted the hole in the duodenum and sewed the two together with about 50 sutures of carbolised silk. The portion of stomach removed measured 14 cm along its greatest length. 'The operation lasted, including the slowly induced anaesthesia, about $1\frac{1}{2}$ hours', wrote Billroth. 'No weakness, no vomiting, no pain after the operation. Within the first 24 hours only ice by mouth, then peptone enema with wine. The following day, first every hour, then every half hour, one tablespoon of sour milk. Patient, a very understanding woman, feels well, lies extremely quiet, sleeps most of the night with the help of small injection of morphia. No pain in the operative area, subfebrile reaction. The dressing has not been changed.'

Billroth was an exceptional man. He turned his attention later on to rectal carcinoma and is credited with being first surgeon to remove a cancer of the rectum in 1868; by 1876 he had performed 33 such operations. Between 1878 and 1892 he became interested in intestinal resection and in what was then called 'enterorrhaphies' (short-circuiting of one part of the bowel to another).

The special method of stitching the bowel, the inverting seromuscular suture, which had been invented in 1826 by the French surgeon Antoine Lembert, did not come into more than limited use until Billroth started his series of operations. It is of some interest that, at a meeting in 1879, Howard Marsh of St Bartholomew's Hospital reported twoses in which Billroth had divided the bowel and united the cut ends by Lembert sutures. 'Such suture of the divided bowel', said Marsh, 'promises good results.' Here is a clear indication of Billroth's influence during his lifetime. Halsted later demonstrated that the tough submucosa had to be secured for reliable single-layer anastomosis.

The early surgeons often put in as many as 200 sutures when performing an ordinary gastroenterostomy to avoid peritonitis but this not infrequently defeated its own purpose by weakening the walls of the gut. In 1888 Nicholas Senn of Rush Medical College, USA, introduced perforated plates of bone, which could be inserted into the lumen of the two cut ends of the bowel. These were largely replaced by the American J. B. Murphy's 'buttons' in 1892 and the 'bobbins' devised by Mayo Robson of Leeds in 1893. The principle was the same: the divided discs or buttons were inserted into the lumen of the two cut bowel ends, anchored by a purse—string suture, clamped together and oversewn, a simple innovation which restored continuity of the bowel without multitudinous stitches.

Bowen, John T. (1857–1941) Professor of Dermatology, Harvard Medical School, Massachusetts, USA. He described premalignant Bowen's skin disease (brown induration with a well-defined edge; microscopy reveals large clear cells. It needs wide excision).

Brodie, Sir Benjamin Collins (1783–1862) Surgeon, St George's Hospital, London, UK. He was chosen to be the first President of the General Medical Council. He described Brodie's abscess of bones and serocystic disease of Brodie (sarcoma). With Trendelenburg he described the test of saphinofemoral incompetence in varicose veins.

Brown-Séquard, Charles E. (1818–1894) Professor of Medicine at Harvard, Massachusetts, USA and Paris, France. He described the Brown-Sequard syndrome in spinal cord hemisection or laterally protruded disc leading to distal loss of motor power on the side of the lesion and loss of pain on the contralateral side.

Browne, Sir Denis (1892–1967) Surgeon, Hospital for Sick Children, Great Ormond Street, London, UK. He described the Denis Browne splint for clubfoot and the Denis Browne operation for hypospadias.

Buerger, Leo (1879–1943) Professor of Urology, Polyclinic Medical School, New York, USA. He described Buerger's disease (presenile atherosclerosis or thromboangitis obliterans in males). Buerger's postural test (both legs are elevated straight for 2 min supported by the examiner; after ankle flexion and extension by the patient the sole of the foot assumes a cadaveric pallor and when legs are lowered the colour changes to a ruddy, cyanotic hue) signifies a major lower limb arterial occlusion. Buerger's position is elevation of the bed head to relieve rest pain in lower limb vascular insufficiency.

Burkitt, Denis P. Contemporary surgeon, Member of External Scientific Staff, Medical Research Council, London, UK. He described Burkitt's lymphoma in tropical parts of Africa which affects children of equal sexes manifested in 80% of cases by jaw tumour which responds dramatically to chemotherapy. The viral aetiology was supported by mosquito vector and he found that above certain heights (mosquito-free area) there were no cases of Burkitt lymphoma.

Burns, Allan (1781–1813) Lecturer in Anatomy and Surgery, Glasgow, UK. He described Burns' space, a suprasternal space, swelling of which may be dermoid, enlarged lymph node (or cold tuberculous abscess), lipoma, aneurysm of the innominate artery or, rarely, a low thyroglossal cyst.

Camper, Peter (1722–1789) Professor of Medicine, Anatomy, Surgery and Botany, Gröningen, Holland. He described Camper's fascia in the anterior abdominal wall.

Chagas, Carlos (1879–1934) Brazilian physician. He described South American trypanosomiasis which affects the oesophagus producing achalasia.

Charcot, Jean-Martin (1825–1893) Physician, Hôpital Salpetriere, Paris, France. Described Charcot's triad in ascending cholangitis due to common bile duct stone (pain, jaundice and rigors due to septicaemia). He also described the painless flail joint with effusion due to neuropathy, i.e. Charcot's joint (in tabes dorsalis) as well as Charcot's hysterical blue oedema (the dependent limb becomes cyanosed and swollen from lack of use). In the upper limbs disuse atrophy leads to bone decalcification similar to post-traumatic painful bone atrophy (described by **Sudeck Paul**, 1866–1945, Professor of Surgery in Hamburg).

Cheyne, John (1777–1836) Physician, Meath Hospital, Dublin, Republic of Ireland. With **Stokes, William** (1804–1878), Regius Professor of Physics, University of Dublin, Republic of Ireland, described Cheyne–Stokes (periodic) respiration in brain stem injury, and a variety of conditions (e.g. respiratory failure, carbon dioxide narcosis and drug poisoning).

Chvostek, František (1835–1884) Physician, Vienna, Austria. He described Chvostek sign—gentle tapping of the facial nerve in front of the external auditory meatus with a percussion hammer, producing a brisk twitch on that facial side in tetany.

Cloquet, Jules G. (1790–1883) Surgeon, Hospital St Louis, Paris, France. He described 'lymph node of Cloquet', enlargement of which simulates an irreducible femoral hernia (*see* Gimbernat).

Cock, Edward (1805–1892) Surgeon, Guy's Hospital, London, UK. He described 'Cock's Peculiar Tumour' a suppurating and ulcerating sebaceous cyst of the scalp simulating a squamous cell carcinoma.

Cockett, Frank B. Contemporary surgeon, St. Thomas' Hospital, London, UK. He described the venous 'blow-out' at sites of perforators due to reverse high-pressure reflux. He recommended subfascial ligation of perforators.

Codman, Ernest A. (1869–1940) Surgeon, Massachusetts General Hospital, Boston, USA. He described Codman's triangle—a radiological appearance seen in osteogenic sarcoma. He also described Codman's method of shoulder joint examination.

Colles, Abraham (1773–1843) Professor of Anatomy and Surgery, Dublin, Republic of Ireland. He described Colles' fascia which is fused with the triangular ligament preventing urine extravasation (backwards beyond the middle perineal point); it is continuous with Scarpa's fascia permitting superficial urine extravasation beneath the latter fascia. He also described Colles' fracture of the distal end of the radius (dinner-fork deformity).

Courvoisier, Ludwig (1843–1918) Professor of Surgery in Basle, Switzerland. He described Courvoisier's law.

Cullen, Thomas S. (1868–1953) Professor of Gynecology, Johns Hopkins University, Baltimore, Maryland, USA. He described Cullen's sign (discoloured umbilicus or black-eye sign) in ruptured ectopic pregnancy and acute pancreatitis.

Curling, T. B. (1811–1888) In 1842 described stress

ulceration in burned patients (first described by Swan in 1823).

Cushing, Harvey (1869–1939) Professor of Surgery, Harvard University, Massachusetts, USA. He described stress ulcer accompanying lesions of the CNS and following neurosurgical operations. (Billroth in 1860 noted stress ulcers after operation and sepsis.) He also described 'Cushing's syndrome' which is due to hyper-adrenocorticism; hyperadrenocorticism secondary to pituitary tumour is termed 'Cushing's disease'.

De Morgan, Campbell (1811–1876) Surgeon, Middlesex Hospital, London, UK. He described de Morgan's spots, raspberry-red tiny capillary angiomas which do not show the sign of emptying (they do not blanche when compressed). They are of no clinical significance.

Denonvilliers, Charles P. (1808–1872) Surgeon, Paris, France. He described Denonvilliers' fascia between the rectum and bladder (and prostate).

De Quervain, Fritz (1868–1940) Professor of Surgery, Berne, Switzerland. He described sub-acute 'de Quervain's thyroiditis' with viral aetiology and possible spontaneous recovery. He also described de Quervain's disease (or stenosing tenosynovitis) which affects the common tendon sheath (of abductor pollicis longus and extensor pollicis brevis) in adult females.

Dercum, Francis K. (1865–1931) Professor of Neurology, Jefferson Medical College, Philadelphia, USA. He described Dercum's disease or adiposis dolorosa—multiple subcutaneous lipomas, one of which is painful or at least tender.

Doppler, Christian J. (1803–1853) Austrian physicist who invented Doppler ultrasonic blood velocity detector.

Dormia, Enrico Contemporary Assistant Professor of Urology, Milan, Italy. He invented the Dormia basket for fishing and removal of lower ureteric stones through a cystoscope (stone should be in lower 5 cm of ureter and not more than 0.5 cm in diameter). Its uses have been extended to residual biliary stone retrieval and bronchial foreign body removal.

Dukes, Cuthbert, E. (1890–1977) Pathologist, St Mark's Hospital, London, UK. He described Dukes' staging in rectal cancer. The staging is sometimes applied to colonic and urinary bladder cancer:

Stage A: The growth is limited to the rectal wall in 15% (5 year survival is 80–90%).

Stage B: The growth is extended to extrarectal tissues (excluding lymph nodes) in 35% (5 year survival is 70–80%).

Stage C: Lymph node involvement (50%) which can be either local distal para-rectal (C_1) or proximal lymph nodes accompanying the supplying blood vessels (C_2) (5 year survival is 30–50%).

Broder's Grading (Broders, Albert C. 1885–1964, Pathologist to the Mayo Clinic, Rochester, USA) is related not to the stage of spread but to the microscopic degree of differentiation:

Grade I: Least malignant with less than 25% cellular undifferentiation.

Grade II: 25–50% undifferentiation.

Grade III: 50–75% undifferentiation.

Grade IV: Over 75% undifferentiation—anaplastic.

The classification adopted by the International Union against cancer is the TNM. Tumour size: T1 < 2 cm, T2 < 5 cm, T3 < 10 cm. Node (lymph): N0 nil, N1 unilateral mobile, N2 unilateral fixed and N3 contralateral or another regional node enlargement. Metastasis: M0 nil or M1 with metastasis. This classification is applied to many cancers especially breast cancer (but not colorectal cancer).

Dupuytren, Baron Guillaune (1777–1835) Surgeon, Paris, France. He described Dupuytren's contracture (contracted thickened palmar fascia adherent to skin puckering ring finger mainly and little finger latterly; usually affects males). It should be differentiated from bilateral congenital soft tissue contracture of the little finger (ring finger is rarely affected). He also described Dupuytren's fracture (sustained by falling on to the feet—the talus is driven upwards with the ligaments supporting it, producing inferior tibiofibular diastasis).

Esmarch, Friedrich Von (1823–1908) German military surgeon of Kiel. Wrote treatises on first aid and in 1861 organised a scheme for the proper siting of field hospitals and bandaging stations in relation to the battle line. Esmarch's bandage or tourniquet, a long rubber strip to produce a bloodless limb by compression ($1-1\frac{1}{2}$ h for upper limbs and $1\frac{1}{2}-2$ h for lower limbs) was introduced in 1873.

Ewing, James (1866–1943) Professor of Oncology, Cornell University Medical College, New York, USA. He described Ewing's sarcoma of the long bones in males with rapid response to radiotherapy.

Fegan, George Contemporary Emeritus Professor of Surgery, Trinity College, Dublin, Republic of Ireland. He introduced Fegan's 'injection-compression technique' for varicose veins. Fegan's method of seeking the sites of perforators for injection is done by marking as follows. First, with the patient in a standing position, the varicosities are marked with a skin pen. The patient then lies down, raising the affected limb and resting the heel against the examiner's chest. The marked line is palpated for gaps in the deep fascia through which perforators pass, and these are marked with an X.

Fogarty, Thomas Contemporary surgeon, University of Oregon Medical School, Portland, USA. He invented Fogarty's catheter for embolectomy. It is also used for biliary stone removal.

Foley, Frederic E. B. (1891–1966) Urologist, Miller and Ancker Hospitals, USA. He invented Foley's self-retaining urinary catheter which can be used not only for drainage of urine in urinary retention or incontinence but for its balloon pressure therapeutic effect after prostatectomy (for haemostasis). Also used in cholecystostomy, gastrostomy, jejunostomy and caecostomy. Malecot (French) is another self-retaining catheter.

Fournier (*see* Meleney).

Frey, Lucja (1889–1944) Physician, Neurological Clinic, Warsaw, Poland. She described Frey's syndrome in postparotidectomy or after incision for suppurative parotitis (e.g. in typhoid fever and typhus) manifested by unilateral facial flushing, sweating, pain and hyperaesthesia in the area supplied by the auriculotemporal nerve following eating, especially spicy or sour food (also called the gustatory sweating syndrome). Frey was killed during the German occupation of Poland.

Fröhlich, Alfred (1871–1953) Professor of Pharmacology and Toxicology, Vienna, Austria. He described Fröhlich's syndrome (hypogonadism in children with obesity due to craniopharyngioma or fractured base of the skull).

Galeazzi, Riccardo (1866–1952) Director of the Orthopaedic Clinic, Milan, Italy. He described Galeazzi fracture-dislocation (fracture of the radius with dislocation of lower radioulnar joint).

Gimbernat, Don Antonio De (1734–1816) Professor of Anatomy, Barcelona, Spain. He described Gimbernat's (lacunar) ligament as a medial concave sharp border of the femoral canal ring. The posterior border comprises Cooper's (iliopectineal) ligament and fascia covering the pectineus muscle (Sir Astley Cooper, 1768–1841, Surgeon to Guy's Hospital, London, UK. He also described ligaments of Cooper in the breast along which cancer cells creep, infiltrating and puckering the overlying skin). Anteriorly the Poupart (inguinal) ligament is found (after Francois Poupart 1661–1708, Surgeon, Hotel Dieu, Paris, France). Laterally the femoral canal is bounded by the femoral vein. The femoral canal contains lymphatic vessels and the lymph node of Cloquet.

Goodsall, David H. (1843–1906) Surgeon, St Mark's Hospital, London, UK. He described Goodsall's rule (fistulae with an external opening within the anterior half of the anus are direct while those within the posterior half of the anus are indirect, uniting first then opening into the midline posteriorly after a horseshoe course).

Graves, Robert J. (1796–1853) Physician, Meath Hospital, Dublin, Republic of Ireland. He described Graves' disease or primary thyrotoxicosis manifested by diffuse symmetrical goitre, with tremor and anxiety (CNS), eye signs and pretibial myxoedema and treated medically (different from secondary thyrotoxicosis occurring in a multinodular goitre with ectopics, arrhythmias (CVS), no eye signs or pretibial myxoedema and treated surgically).

Grawitz, Paul A. (1850–1932) Professor of Pathology, Greifswald, Germany. He described renal cell adenocarcinoma (Grawitz's tumour in adults).

Halsted, William Stewart (1852–1922) Surgeon, Johns Hopkins Hospital, USA. Introduced the use of rubber gloves for the first time (used initially for protection of his theatre nurse, Caroline Hampton, who had contact rash with antiseptics; Halsted later married her). He taught the modern doctrine that surgical safety lies in avoidance of blood loss, meticulous care and gentle handling of the tissues. He was the pioneer of radical mastectomy and Halsted's repair of hernia (closure of external oblique posterior to the cord). He invented the Halsted needle holder and fine mosquito artery forceps. Kraske (Freiburg, Germany), Wertheim and Billroth (Vienna, Austria), Miles (London, UK) and

Halsted (Baltimore, USA) were the originators of the concept of the complete operation for all malignant diseases. Halsted discovered the local anaesthetic properties of cocaine and was the first to use regional anaesthesia. However, he became an addict of narcotic drugs until he died.

Harrison, Edwin (1779–1847) Physician, St Marylebone Infirmary, London, UK. He described Harrison's sulcus or groove at the costochondral junctions in the rachitic chest.

Hashimoto, Hakaru (1881–1934) Director of the Hashimoto Hospital, Miyo, Japan. He described Hashimoto's thyroiditis (or struma lymphomatosa) with hypothyroidism.

Hasselbach, Franz K. (1759–1816) Professor of Surgery, Würzburg, Germany. He described Hasselbach's inguinal triangle through which direct inguinal hernia passes (bounded by inguinal ligament, lateral border of the rectus sheath and inferior epigastric vessels).

Hirschsprung, Harald (1830–1916) Physician, Queen Louise Hospital for Children, Copenhagen, Denmark. He described Hirschsprung's disease of congenital aganglionic (parasympathetic) megacolon manifested within 3 days of birth. Secondary acquired megacolon is also described in older children with anal fissure and also in Chagas' disease.

Hodgkin, Thomas (1798–1866) Curator of the Museum of Guy's Hospital, London, UK (after his failure to obtain the post of Physician). He described Hodgkin's lymphoma.

Homans, John (1877–1954) Professor of Clinical Surgery, Harvard University, Boston, USA. He described Homans' sign (passive dorsiflexion of the foot causes calf pain in deep venous thrombosis). Such a sign may be dangerous to elicit as it may detach the thrombus, causing embolism; furthermore, if negative, it does not exclude the diagnosis of thrombosis.

Horner, Johann F. (1831–1886) Professor of Ophthalmology, Zurich, Switzerland. He described Horner's syndrome (myosis, ptosis, enophthalmus and anhidrosis) in injury of the cervical sympathetic chain.

Houston, John (1802–1845) Physician, City of Dublin Hospital, Republic of Ireland. He described anal valves of Houston.

Hunter, John (1728–1793) The first English-speaking exponent of scientific medical research. Although a stumbling, tongue-tied lecturer he successfully demonstrated the importance of the cause of disease in relation to surgery. Born at Long Calderwood (near Glasgow) he set out for London at the age of 20 to study under William Cheseldon of St Thomas' and Percival Pott of St Bartholomew's. He was appointed to the surgical staff of St George's Hospital. His outlook can best be summed up in his quoted dictum (contained in a letter to Edward Jenner, the pioneer of vaccination) 'Why think? Why not try the experiment?'. He placed surgery on a scientific basis by correlating practice with comparative anatomy and physiological experiments. He founded a school of anatomy and surgery in Leicester Square and advocated arterial ligation to cure aneurysm. He described the Hunterian chancre (or primary syphilitic sore) but he thought that syphilis and gonorrhoea were manifestations of the same infection; to test his hypothesis he inoculated himself with a scalpel and died of an aortic aneurysm later on!

Hutchinson, Sir Jonathan (1828–1913) Surgeon, London Hospital, UK. He described Hutchinson's teeth in congenital syphilis.

Kaposi, Moricz (1837–1902) Professor and Director of the Dermatological Clinic, Vienna, Austria. He described Kaposi's sarcoma among Jews from Poland (initially) affecting middle-aged males as multiple symptomless, plum-coloured nodules usually situated on the lower limbs.

Kehr, Hans (1862–1916) Professor of Surgery, Halberstadt, Germany. He described Kehr's sign (referred shoulder pain due to irritated diaphragm when patient lies flat on the back; occurs in intra-abdominal injury of the spleen or liver or in ruptured ectopic pregnancy).

Kocher, Theodor (1841–1917) Professor of Clinical Surgery, University of Berne, Switzerland. A pupil of Langenbeck and Billroth. He developed the surgical technique of thyroidectomy and described Kocher's collar incision and subcostal incision for biliary operation. In 1878 he drained a gall bladder abscess for the first time. He performed over 2000 thyroidectomies with a mortality of 4.5% (goitre is a particularly severe disease in his native Switzerland). He also described Kocher's manoeuvre in mobilisation of the second part of the duodenum. Positive Kocher's test is stridor induced by slight compression on the lateral lobes (in goitre) and indicates that the patient has an obstructed trachea. He received the Nobel Prize in 1909 (the first time it was awarded to a surgeon).

Krukenberg, Friedrich (1871–1946) Ophthalmologist, Halle, Germany. He wrote his thesis on malignant tumours of the ovary at 24 years of age. He described bilateral Krukenberg's ovarian tumours due to transcoelomic implantation of cancer cells in gut malignancies.

Latarget, André (1876–1947) Professor of Anatomy, Lyons, France. He described nerves of Latarget in the stomach.

Leriche, René (1879–1956) Professor of Medicine at the College de France, Paris (the highest professional honour in France). He described Leriche's syndrome (thrombosis or atherosclerosis of the aortic bifurcation with intermittent claudication in the thighs or buttocks associated with impotence in men).

Lister, Joseph (1827–1912) Professor of Surgery, Glasgow, Edinburgh and King's College Hospital, London, UK. He is the leader of modern aseptic surgery, applying discoveries of Pasteur to surgery. He developed antiseptics that reduced postoperative wound infection and made possible the widespread use of sterile suture materials. He discovered bacteria in the suture strand and treated ligatures with carbolic acid.

Littré, Alexis (1658–1725) Surgeon and anatomist, Paris, France. He described the penile paraurethral Littré's glands. Littré's hernia is Meckel's diverticulum in a hernial sac. He also contributed to the development of colostomy (*see* 'Evolution of colostomy').

Lockwood, Charles B. (1856–1914) Surgeon, St Bartholomew's Hospital, London, UK. He described the low approach in femoral hernia.

Louis, Antoine (1723–1792) French surgeon. He described the angle of Louis.

Ludwig, Wilhelm Von (1790–1865) German Professor of Surgery and Midwifery. He described Ludwig's angina, a cellulitis occurring beneath the deep cervical fascia with threatening respiratory obstruction (the mouth floor becomes oedematous).

Malgaigne, Joseph F. (1806–1865) Professor of Surgery, Paris, France. He described Malgaigne's groin bulgings normally seen in thin individuals.

Marion, Jean (1869–1960) Professor of Urology, Paris, France. He described Marion's disease: bladder neck enlargement in young boys. Marion's sign relates to non-visualisation of ureteric orifices due to enlarged bladder neck.

Marjolin (1780–1850) Surgeon, Paris, France. He described Marjolin's carcinomatous ulcer in burn scar. Later the term was applied to carcinoma secondary to a venous ulcer and chronic osteomyelitis ulcer.

Mayo, Charles Horace (1865–1939) **and William James** (1861–1939) (brothers) the latter described prepyloric vein (of Mayo) as well as Mayo's operation for para-umbilical hernias (can be used for all midline hernias).

Evolution of the Mayo Clinic In 1845 William Mayo, a native of Eccles, Scotland, who had read chemistry at Owens College, Manchester, emigrated to the USA where he became a doctor. William Worrall Mayo, had two sons, William James who was born at Le Sueur, Minnesota on 29 June 1861, and Charles Horace, born on 9th July 1865 at Rochester where William Worrall had set up his practice. Both sons studied medicine; William qualified in 1883 from the University of Michigan, Charles from North Western University in 1888.

In 1883 a devastating storm swept Rochester, causing much damage and loss of life. W. W. Mayo, with his two sons and the Sisters of the Order of Saint Francis, did valiant work among the injured. The Mother Superior of the Order decided to commemorate their work by building and endowing a small hospital of 50 beds in Rochester. The hospital of St Mary opened in 1889 with 15 patients, attended by five nursing Sisters, Sister Mary Joseph as surgical assistant, and Mother Alfred as Sister-in-Charge. The Mayo family formed the entire medical staff. This hospital was not a charitable institution. From the start, every patient had to pay according to his means. But patients from charitable organisations were accepted without charge, and the patient's own word was regarded as sufficient guarantee of the scale upon which he would be required to pay.

Rochester, even today, is only a small town; in 1889 it was a village, served by no important road and not on a main railway line. For 10 years the Mayos worked quietly in something that was no more than a Cottage Hospital. Then, about the year 1900, William sent a paper to the American Annals of Surgery. His paper contained particulars of so many cases of successful treatment of gallstones that the incredulous editor came to see for himself. He was the first of many thousands of visitors to Rochester. The efficiency of the Staff Nurses could be easily concluded from the clinical observations imparted to William (about secondary cancer at the umbilicus) by Sister Joseph. This secondary deposit from the gastrointestinal tract cancer is called Sister Joseph nodule.

The brothers had kept well abreast of all the advances that had so recently been made; they were perhaps the first to understand that these advances were not only of great importance but had added to the complexity of medicine. They realised that if these 'ancillary departments' were to be fully used, they must be housed under one roof. They found that exact diagnosis demanded complete investigation. This became their basic principle: a painstaking, complete investigation of the patient by highly trained experts in a single clinic. At first the Mayos had to make themselves the experts; as their fame increased they trained others in their method until they had a team. Neither brother was any kind of a specialist at the start. It was not until after 1900 that they devoted their whole time to surgery; as the years passed 'Will' became the more expert in surgery of the abdomen, 'Charlie' in surgery of the head and neck. They made a perfect combination, bound together by a most unusual brotherly love and confidence, which manifested itself in the use of a joint wallet on which each urged the other to draw more heavily. Will was the better administrator, somewhat withdrawn, with a tendency to descend from on high to put all things in order; Charlie was the more original in thought, with a witty, friendly temperament that made for a happy and cooperative staff. Both brothers showed themselves remarkably shrewd in choosing their colleagues. It says much for the Mayos that they were so successful in building up and in keeping together their large staff, for Rochester was no cultural or social centre; the clinic and the work of the clinic had to be all-sufficing.

This work rapidly increased as their fame spread. By 1906 Will had performed 150 resections of the stomach for cancer with a 10% mortality and a 3 year survival in nearly 30% of cases; in one year (1906) he did 36 of these operations with only 1 death (Cheyne did his first in 1905). As the clinic grew in size the medical staff rose in number until there were more than 150 full-time members and twice that number of young graduates under instruction. The original small hospital expanded until the beds numbered between 1500 and 2000; in 1938 just over 1000 patients registered in a single day. The Mayos firmly believed in international exchange of knowledge and ideas. They and their staff travelled widely and they encouraged visitors to make use of their experience at Rochester. The brothers

introduced a standard case-taking form, at a time when medical recording was still haphazard, on which all details of each patient were entered. The records were open to every member of the staff for consultation and discussion; from these discussions resulted the *Proceedings of the Staff Meetings of the Mayo Clinic*, in which many new advances and discoveries have been described.

As patients paid fees, often large fees, to the Clinic, a surplus of cash rapidly accumulated. In 1913 the brothers offered a sum of a million and a half dollars to the University of Minnesota for the purposes of medical education and research. Incredible though it may seem, the State Legislature made difficulties and it needed an impassioned address by Will before the scheme got under way. The Mayo Foundation, which does so much for research and postgraduate instruction, opened in 1915.

The two brothers, who had worked closely and successfully together, were not long separated by death. Charlie died on 26th May 1939, and Will 2 months later on 28th July. Their Clinic and their methods became the model for similar ventures in the USA. As we have seen, that great country could boast some excellent surgeons during the nineteenth century; it is largely through the efforts of the Mayo brothers that the USA has made such great strides in surgery during the past 60 years.

Meckel, Johann F. (1781–1833) Professor of Anatomy and Surgery, Halle, Germany. He described Meckel's diverticulum more clearly as a congenital antimesenteric full-layered diverticulum 5 cm in length and 60 cm from the ilio-caecal junction occurring in 2% of patients. The diverticulum was first recognised by Littré and he called it an ileal appendix when he found it imprisoned in the hernial sac (Littré hernia).

Meleney, Frank L. (1889–1963) Professor of Clinical Surgery, Columbia University, New York, USA. In 1924 he described a spreading gangrene in superficial tissues following surgery, trauma or sepsis. The name necrotising fasciitis was introduced by B. Wilson (USA, 1952) to indicate non-specific redness, swelling and oedema around a primary wound which if untreated leads to acute rapid skin gangrene. The patient is usually suffering from toxaemia, dehydration and mental apathy. It is differentiated from gas gangrene by:
- Absence of crepitus.
- Absence of muscle involvement.
- Failure to isolate clostridia from tissues.

Instead streptococci and *Staphylococcus aureus* synergestics or coliforms with enterococci and streptococci are isolated.

The progressive bacterial skin gangrene may affect the scrotum and is called Fournier's gangrene (described in 1884 by **Fournier, Jean A.,** 1832–1914, a French venereologist and dermatologist).

Mikulicz–Radecki, Johannes Von (1850–1905) Professor of Surgery, Königsburg and Breslau, Germany. He devised many new operations particularly on the oesophagus and on exteriorisation of the large bowel carcinoma so that it could be removed later on (Mikulicz colostomy). He is the first surgeon to cover his hands with cotton gloves in 1885; modern rubber gloves were introduced but not invented by W. S. Halsted of Baltimore in 1894. Gauze face masks were first worn by either Mikulicz or the French surgeon Paul Berger in 1896–7, while the operating gown in its present form was originated in Italy. (Although Lord Berkeley Moynihan, Professor of Surgery, Leeds 1865–1936 claimed to have been the first surgeon to wear a gown; as well as the first British surgeon to wear gloves.)

Mikulicz was the first to attempt suture of perforated gastric ulcer in 1880 (patient died). In 1884 he was the first to recommend emergency appendecotomy even if appendix was not perforated. In 1881 he used the first direct vision instrument for the oesophagus and stomach, the forerunner of the present oesophagoscope and bronchoscope. He also described the symmetrical progressive enlargement of lachrimal and salivary glands (Mikulicz's disease), the precursor of Sjögren's syndrome in which dry eyes and rheumatoid arthritis also occur (Sjögren Tage, 1859–1939, Swedish Physician).

Milroy, William F. (1855–1942) Professor of Clinical Medicine, University of Nebraska, USA. He described Milroy's disease (primary lymphoedema due to congenital as well as familial lymphatic aplasia).

Mondor, Henri (1885–1962) Professor of Clinical Surgery, Paris, France. He described Mondor's disease (self-limiting thrombophlebitis of veins over the upper chest wall and towards the axilla leading to subcutaneous cords; if on the breast, usually mistaken for carcinoma).

Monteggia, Giovanni B. (1762–1815) Professor of Surgery, Ospedale Maggiore, Milan, Italy. He described Monteggia fracture-dislocation (fracture of ulna with dislocation of upper radioulnar joint).

Montgomery, William (1797–1859) Professor of Midwifery, Dublin, Republic of Ireland. He described Montgomery glands (nodules) of areola of the breast.

Morgagni, Giovanni B. (1682–1771) Professor of Medicine and Anatomy for 56 years, Padua, Italy. He described hydatid of Morgagni (appendix of testis), torsion of which sometimes stimulates testicular torsion. He also described Morgagni follicles (one pair) opening just behind the lips of the external urethral meatus of the penis (the follicles may become infected).

Murphy, John B. (1857–1916) Surgeon to Mercy Hospital, Chicago, USA. He described Murphy's sign: pressing on the right hypochondrium during inspiration produces a catch of breath (in inflamed gall bladder). He also described the renal angle test (Murphy's kidney punch): sharp jabbing movements with the thumb under the 12th rib lateral to the sacrospinalis muscle may reveal deep-seated tenderness.

Nuck, Anton (1650–1692) Anatomist in Leiden, the Netherlands. He described 'canal of Nuck' hydrocele which causes difficulty in diagnosis of irreducible inguinal hernia in females.

Paget, Sir James (1814–1899) Surgeon, St Bartholomew's Hospital, London, UK. He described three diseases: Paget's disease of bone (premalignant), Paget's disease of the penis (premalignant) and Paget's disease of the nipple (unilateral dry eczematous ulceration of the nipple is a malignant—not premalignant—disease due to underlying intraduct carcinoma invading the skin).

Pancoast, Henry K. (1875–1939) Professor of Roentgenology, University of Pennsylvania, Philadelphia, USA. He described Pancoast's syndrome due to apical pulmonary cancer: swollen congested face due to pressure on the superior vena cava, Horner's syndrome (pressure on the sympathetic chain) and shooting pains down the arm (pressure on brachial plexus). The first rib is eroded as seen in the X-ray.

Pasteur, Louis (1822–1895) French scientist. He described 'the germ theory of disease' and showed that fermentation and putrefaction were caused by living multiplying matter. He reasoned that pus formation, wound infection and some fevers must also be caused by minute organisms from the environment.

Paterson, Donald R. (1863–1939) Ear, Nose and Throat Surgeon, Royal Infirmary, Cardiff, UK.

Together with **Kelly, Adam B.** (1865–1941) Ear, Nose and Throat Surgeon, Victoria Infirmary, Glasgow, UK, described Paterson–Kelly syndrome in 1919 which is a sideropaenic dysphagia in middle-aged women manifested by pallor (iron deficiency anaemia), stomatitis, cheilosis, smooth tongue, koilonychia, achlorhydria and mild splenomegaly; the condition is precancerous (postcricoid carcinoma). It is sometimes called the Plummer–Vinson syndrome (**Plummer, Henry S.** 1874–1937, Physician to Mayo Clinic, Rochester, USA and **Vinson, Porter R.** 1890–1959, Physician to Medical College, Virginia USA).

Péan, Jules (1830–1898) A French surgeon and one of the first surgeons to attempt vaginal hysterectomy. He introduced small instruments for securing blood vessels. He performed the first (unsuccessful) gastric resection for cancer.

Perthes, George (1869–1927) Professor of Surgery, Tubingen, Germany. He described Perthes' disease (juvenile osteochondritis with collapsed femoral head due to mushrooming secondary to aseptic vascular necrosis). He also described Perthes' test (walking with a tourniquet placed below the saphenous opening to diagnose deep venous thrombosis in cases of pain and venous congestion of the leg).

Peutz, John I. A. (1886–1957) Head of Internal Medicine, St John's Hospital, The Hague, the Netherlands. Together with **Jeghers, Harald** (1894–1968), Professor of Medicine, Tufts University School of Medicine, Boston, USA, described Peutz–Jeghers syndrome (familial gastrointestinal hamartomatous polyposis with pigmentation around the lips and anus. It is manifested by bleeding and subacute obstruction and rarely becomes malignant).

Peyronie, François de La (1678–1747) Surgeon to Louis XV and founder of the Royal Academy of Surgery, Paris, France. Mainly due to him, Paris became a great surgical centre in the eighteenth century. He described Peyronie's disease of the penis (localised painless induration of one or both corpora cavernosa leading to lateral curvature of the erect penis).

Pott, Percival (1714–1788) Surgeon, St Bartholomew's Hospital, London, UK. He described Pott's disease of the spine due to tuberculous fracture, and 'Pott's Puffy Tumour' a localised oedema over osteomyelitis of the skull. Pott trephined the skull in fractures in the eighteenth century with instruments hardly distinguishable from those of the ancient Greek and Roman

surgeons; he considered that any fracture of the skull warranted operation. Astley Cooper, however, advised against trephining unless the skull fracture is compound.

Queyrat, Louis (1856–1933) Physician, Hôpital Cochin, Paris, France. He described erythroplasia of Queyrat (bright red, shiny lesion velvety to touch with exudate on sulcus corona usually with no induration. It is a precancerous condition of the penis).

Ramstedt, Wilhelm C. (1867–1963) German surgeon. He described the pyloromyotomy as the operation of choice in congenital pyloric stenosis (1912).

Raynaud, Maurice (1834–1881) Physician, Hôpital Lariboisière, Paris, France. He described Raynaud's disease in females in which arterial spasm occurs in cold weather with colour changes from white to blue to red. Raynaud's phenomenon in males usually occurs in vibrating-tool users.

Rhazes (AD 860–932) Arab surgeon. First to stitch abdominal wounds with harp strings made of spun strands cut from animal intestine or from tendons (usually Achilles tendon).

Richter, August G. (1742–1812) Surgeon, Gottingen, Germany. He described Richter's hernia in 1777 (strangulation of a portion of the circumference of the intestine).

Riedel, Bernhard M. C. (1846–1916) Professor of Surgery, Jena, Germany. He described Riedel's thyroiditis, a stony hard goitre (like cancer) with tracheal obstruction.

Roentgen, Wilhelm C. Von (1845–1923) Professor of Physics successively at Strasburg, Giessen, Wurzburg and Munich, Germany. He discovered X-rays in 1895.

Rosenmüller, Johann C. (1771–1820) Professor of Anatomy and Surgery, Leipzig, Germany. He described the fossa of Rosenmüller, a pharyngeal recess into which the congenital branchial fistula opens.

Scarpa, Antonio (1747–1832) Professor of Surgery, Modena, and Professor of Anatomy, Pavia, Italy. He described Scarpa's fascia in anterior abdominal wall.

Sims, James Marion (1813–1883) Founder and surgeon, State Hospital for Women, New York, USA. He described Sims' left lateral position for examination and Sims' speculum.

Smellie, Ian S. Contemporary Emeritus Professor of Orthopaedic Surgery, University of Dundee, Scotland. He described Smellie's knife for meniscectomy.

Smith, Robert W. (1807–1873) Professor of Surgery, Trinity College, Dublin, Republic of Ireland. He described Smith's fracture (reversed Colles' fracture).

Spiegel, Adriaan Van Der (1578–1625) Professor of Anatomy, Padua, Italy. He described Spiegelian hernia (hernia through linea semilunaris above inguinal ligament).

Stensen, Niels (1638–1686) Danish anatomist. He described Stensen's duct of the parotid gland.

Sudeck (*see* Charcot)

Tait, Robert Lawson (1845–1899) Surgeon, Birmingham, UK (*see* 'Cholecystectomy').

Takayasu, Mikito (1860–1938) Professor of Ophthalmology, Medical College, Kanazawa, Japan. He described Takayasu disease (pulseless disease or aortic arch syndrome in which no pulse is felt in one or both arms due to progressive atherosclerosis or arteritis leading to fainting, headache and optic nerve atrophy without papilloedema as a result of occlusion of the carotid arteries).

Thiersch, Karl (1822–1895) German surgeon of Erlanger and Leipzig. Introduced the Thiersch graft (a partial thickness (split) skin graft) in 1874. However the commonly used knife is named after T. G. Humby, plastic surgeon in Barbados, W. Indies.

Tietze, Alexander (1864–1927) Chief Surgeon in Allerheiligen Hospital, Breslau, Germany. He described Tietze disease (non-specific costochondritis affecting mainly women causing a painful lump often confirmed to be a breast mass).

Trendelenburg, Friedrich (1844–1924) Professor of Surgery, Leipzig, Germany. He described Trendelenburg's position (head down and legs up); Trendelenburg's test (for saphenofemoral incompetence); Trendelenburg's operation (midthigh high ligation of great saphenous vein—now modified to saphenofemoral junction flush ligation and disconnection); and Trendelenburg's sign (when an adult patient with a dislocated hip stands with his weight on the normal side, the opposite buttock rises and when he stands on the affected side, the opposite buttock sinks). Trendelenburg's gait occurs in bilateral congenital dislocation of the hips.

Troisier, Charles (1844–1919) Professor of Pathology, Paris, France. He described 'Troisier's sign' related to supraclavicular lymph node enlargement in carcinoma of the stomach.

Trousseau, Armand (1801–1867) French physician. He described Trousseau's test: application of sphygmomanometer cuff around the arm with pressure up to 200 mmHg produces contractions of the hand in tetany. Trousseau's sign denotes thrombophlebitis migrans in visceral cancer (e.g. pancreas or stomach).

Vater, Abraham (1684–1751) Professor of Anatomy and Botany, Wittenberg, Germany. He described ampulla of Vater.

Vermooten, Vincent (1897–1969) Professor of Urology, University of Texas, Southwestern Medical School, Dallas, USA. He described Vermooten's sign (if rectal examination reveals an upward displaced prostate then the diagnosis is that of a complete intrapelvic urethral rupture in pelvic fractures but if the prostate cannot be felt and in its position there is an indefinite doughy swelling—extravasated urine or blood—it is a case of extraperitoneal bladder rupture).

Virchow, Rudolf (1821–1902) An outstanding German physiologist and anatomist of Wurzburg and Berlin. He is the founder of the science of cellular pathology. Virchow was a versatile man, who designed the sewage system of Berlin, organised the Prussian ambulance corps in 1870 and served as a member of the German Reichstag. Born in 1821, he graduated from Berlin in 1843 and founded *Virchow's Archives* (medical journal) in 1847. In his *Cellular Pathologie* published in 1858 he defined the body as a 'cell-state in which every cell is a citizen'. He is well known for Virchow's triad of thrombosis (endothelial injury, viscosity change and platelet aggregation), and for Virchow's supraclavicular lymph nodes, enlargement of which produces 'Troisier's sign' in advanced gastric cancer (as well as in intra-abdominal, testicular and bronchial cancers).

Volkmann, Richard Von (1830–1889) Professor of Surgery at Halle and Leipzig, Germany. Mainly interested in the surgery of bones and joints but also claimed to be the first man to excise the rectum for cancer in 1878. He described Volkmann's ischaemic contracture following brachial artery trauma in supracondylar fractures.

Von Recklinghausen, Friedrich D. (1833–1910) Professor of Pathology, Strasburg, Germany. He was the first to point to the blood-borne skeletal metastases in cancer. He described the diffuse neurofibromatosis with cutaneous pigmentation and multiple tumours (von Recklinghausen's disease of nerve). He also described bone cyst formation in hyperparathyroidism (osteitis fibrosa or von Recklinghausen's disease of bone).

Wallace, Alexander B. (1906–1974) Plastic surgeon, Royal Hospital for Sick Children, Edinburgh, UK. He introduced the Rule of Nines in burns.

Warthin, Aldred S. (1866–1931) Professor of Pathology, University of Michigan, USA. He described Warthin's tumour (or adenolymphoma) of the salivary glands, a soft (sometimes fluctuant) tumour in males over age 40 years.

Wharton, Thomas (1614–1673) Physician to St Thomas' Hospital, London, UK. He described Wharton' submandibular salivary gland duct.

Willis, Thomas (1621–1675) Physician, Oxford, UK. He described circle of Willis at the base of brain, first noticed the sweet taste of diabetic urine and described myasthenia gravis.

Wilms, Max (1867–1918) Professor of Surgery, Heidelberg, Germany. He described nephroblastoma (Wilms' tumour) of the kidney in children.

Evolution of some important surgical procedures

Appendicectomy

The first appendicectomy was performed in 1736 by Claudius Amyand, Surgeon to St George's Hospital, London, UK. In a boy 12 years of age, Amyand removed the appendix, a pin that it contained, and surrounding omentum from a scrotal hernia that was complicated by a faecal fistula. Surgical treatment of appendicitis was described in France (Mestivier, 1759; Lamotte, 1766; Jadelot, 1808) and in London (Parkinson, 1812). Melier, in 1827, advised drainage of appendiceal abscesses. He also envisaged the possibility of early removal of the acute inflamed appendix. Unfortunately, Dupuytren (1835), the most influential surgeon of his day, opposed Melier's views and warmly supported the conservative treatment of what was then called 'typhlitis and perityphlitis' that had been inaugurated by Goldbeck and Puchelt (1832). Volz in 1843 described opium treatment, declaring that rest for the inflamed bowel was as important as a splint for a broken leg. Grisolle (1839) in France, Hancock (1848) in the UK, and Willard Parker (1867) in the USA recommended incision and drainage before fluctuation

appeared in inflammatory conditions of the right iliac fossa. Parker (1867), taught that there were three stages of appendicitis: gangrene, perforation and abscess. Fitz (1886) was the first surgeon to use the term appendicitis. Morton (1887), of Philadelphia, successfully diagnosed and excised an acutely inflamed appendix, and Treves (1887) advocated appendicectomy in the quiescent period. About this time McBurney described a technique for removal of the appendix that is widely used even today.

Much credit is due to the pioneers in this field (Parker, Fitz, Morton, Treves, McBurney and J. B. Murphy) who advanced the claims of surgical treatment in acute appendicitis. J. B. Murphy of Chicago wrote a classic description of the signs and symptoms of appendicitis; in the same year (1889), Charles McBurney of the Roosevelt Hospital, New York, published the results of a large investigation into the disease. In the course of his paper he enunciated one of the best-known 'signs' in surgery, still called 'McBurney's point'. This is the point of maximum tenderness when the abdominal wall is pressed with one finger and is a good localising sign in appendicitis. McBurney also described an operative technique in 1894, but the so-called McBurney or grid-iron incision was, in fact, devised by L. L. McArthur of Chicago. Another commonly used incision or approach for the appendicectomy operation was introduced by W. H. Battle of St Thomas' Hospital in 1895.

Noteworthy as these various dates are, it is doubtful whether any of them are as important in the history of the appendix operation as 24th June 1902. The coronation of King Edward VII had been arranged to take place on 26th June, but the king fell ill with abdominal pain and fever only a few days before. At a consultation of some of the most distinguished surgeons in the land, including Lord Lister, it was decided that the only chance to save his life lay in urgent operation. Frederick Treves, who had performed his first successful appendicectomy in 1887, opened the abdomen and drained an appendix abscess on 24th June; he did not, as is sometimes stated, remove the appendix. The king made a good recovery and the operation was entirely successful, a success that becomes more remarkable when one considers the advanced age (for those days) and not altogether ascetic habits of the patient. After the postponed coronation on 9th August, Treves received a knighthood and Lister was made a Privy Councillor and one of the 12 original members of the Order of Merit. When welcoming Lister to his Council, the king is supposed to have said, 'I know that if it had not been for you and your work, I would not have been here today.'

Cholecystectomy

In 1869 Lawson Tait (who did his first ovariotomy at the age of 23 when still a House Surgeon) was consulted by a patient about a discharging sinus in her abdominal wall; he followed up the track of the sinus and removed a few small stones, which must have ulcerated through from the gall bladder. In 1878 Marion Sims, the famous American 'gynaecologist', attempted to remove gall stones by opening the abdomen and slitting up the gall bladder, the operation of cholecystotomy, but his patient died; in the same year Theodor Kocher of Berne drained an abscess of the gall bladder. The first successful removal of stones from the gall bladder was by Lawson Tait in 1879. Another interesting cholecystotomy was that performed by Joseph Lister in 1883, for it is often stated wrongly that Lister never opened the abdomen. Unfortunately the patient died in April 1884.

Lawson Tait is sometimes credited with the first cholecystectomy, removal of the gall bladder itself, but he never did this operation. Cholecystectomy was first performed in 1882 by the German C. J. A. Langenbuch, who is often confused with the more famous Langenbeck. This was an isolated case, but in 1896 Hans Kehr, another German, started to do the operation as a routine procedure for removal of stones and had performed over a thousand cholecystectomies by the time of his death in 1916. Berkeley Moynihan in England and Mayo in the USA were well known for their success in cholecystectomy. After 1921 it became the operation of choice and has now entirely replaced cholecystotomy.

Colostomy

Alexis Littré of Paris may be called the father of colostomy. In 1710 he was consulted about an infant who suffered from congenital malformation of the rectum, probably an imperforate anus. The child died on the sixth day after birth; at autopsy Littré took the opportunity of investigating possible means of dealing with similar defects in life. Having practised on the infant's body, he declared it possible to 'make an incision in the belly, and open the two ends of the closed bowel and stitch them together, or at least to bring the upper part of the bowel to the surface of the belly wall where it would never close but perform the function of an anus'. This was ventral or abdominal colostomy, performed through the abdominal wall; it became known as Littré's operation.

In 1776 H. Pillore, a surgeon from Rouen, performed caecostomy which is much the same as colostomy, except that the large bowel is entered at a higher point. The operation was performed for an obstruction due to cancer of the rectum (and perhaps made worse by the two pounds of mercury which had been given by mouth in an endeavour to cure the obstruction) but the patient died 28 days later. In 1793 C. Duret of Brest, performed the first successful colostomy on a 3-day-old child suffering from imperforate anus. He made an incision in the left groin and brought the large bowel to the abdominal surface; he then cut into the bowel and allowed it to act as an artificial anus. The patient lived until the age of 45 years. An interesting little note on this operation reminds us that 1793 was the year of Terror. 'Citizen Massac, Chief of the Administration, and Citizen Coulon, Physician in Chief, were charged to provide necessary dressings.'

P. J. Desault of Paris also performed Littré's operation for imperforate anus in 1794, but the child died 4 days later. In 1797 C. L. Dumas of Montpellier, the leading French surgeon of his time, advised that colostomy should be used for the relief of intestinal obstruction and claimed to have devised the operation. In fact, Dumas never did a colostomy in his life, but his weighty approval served to arouse interest. Three years later, Professor Fine of Geneva performed colostomy in a woman aged 63 years suffering from cancer of the rectum, giving credit to Dumas for the original idea. Fine's patient survived for 3 months. Freer of Birmingham was the first to attempt Littré's operation for imperforate anus in the UK (1815), but his patient died. The first successful case in the UK was that of Daniel Pring, a surgeon from Bath, in 1817.

In about 1839, J. Z. Amussat of Paris attended his colleague, Professor Broussais, who was dying from intestinal obstruction due to cancer of the rectum. Amussat declared that he would never again stand idly by while a patient of his died so terrible a death. He collected particulars of all known colostomies since Pillore had first performed the operation on a living subject in 1776. Of 29 cases, 21 of whom were infants suffering from imperforate anus, 20 had died within a matter of hours or days. Only 4 of the infants had survived, and it is curious that all 4 were treated at Brest, where Duret had first succeeded with the operation, but that Duret had attended none of the other 3 cases. Of 8 adult patients, 5 had survived.

Amussat concluded that 20 deaths were all due to peritonitis, as we should call it today, and that Littré's abdominal approach through the peritoneum must be held to blame. After experimenting in the postmortem room, he advised opening the large bowel by an incision in the back, close to the spine, an approach which had already been practised on a dead body by Duret and by Callisen of Copenhagen in 1800. This is the lumbar colostomy or Amussat's operation, a great advance because it did not entail approaching the bowel via the peritoneal cavity and so tended to avoid peritonitis. Amussat himself performed his operation 9 times successfully between 1839 and 1856; the number of his failures is unknown.

Lumbar colostomy became the operation of choice, and retained its popularity for over 30 years. In the UK it was first performed by W. J. Clement of Shrewsbury for a stricture of the colon in 1841; Clement's patient lived for 3 years. John Erichsen of University College Hospital, who had been a pupil of Amussat and present at his first operation, became the leading exponent of this method. Another surgeon who regularly practised the Amussat technique was Caesar Hawkins of St George's; in 1852 he collected all known cases of colostomy, performed for 'stricture of the colon' but not for imperforate anus in infants, and found that in 48 patients the mortality was exactly 50%. He advised that there was little difference in the result whether Amussat's or Littré's approach was used.

In 1850 three surgeons at the London Hospital returned to the abdominal method of Littré. The London Hospital became noted for successful operations; in 1865 one of their surgeons, Nathaniel Ward, made the very important pronouncement that when a cancer of the rectum is diagnosed, colostomy should always be performed without waiting for signs of obstruction; this made the operation safer because the patients were in better general health. With the introduction of antisepsis, operations on the abdomen could be performed with less risk of peritonitis, and from 1880 onwards there was an increasing tendency to give up the Amussat method, although we occasionally find mention of lumbar colostomy in case notes during the 1890s.

A colostomy is not curative operation; it will relieve obstruction of the bowel but, if that obstruction is caused by a cancer, the cancer remains to imperil the patient's life. One of the objections put forward by the London Hospital surgeons to the lumbar colostomy was that the abdominal cavity cannot be explored through the incision; a doubtful diagnosis must remain in doubt.

In 1887, C. B. Ball of Dublin recommended abdominal colostomy with exploration of the abdomen (laparotomy) in all cases. A few years later W. Ernest Miles started to explore the abdomen through a midline incision and to make the colostomy through a separate opening. This is the method generally used today. Attempts to hack a way through a rectal growth had often been made, but it was not until 1868 that Billroth removed a cancer of the rectum for the first time; by 1876 he had done 33 cases. Billroth's operation was improved by the Swiss surgeon Theodor Kocher and by the German Paul Kraske. Kraske's operation remained the method of choice from 1885 until 1908; in that year W. E. Miles introduced the abdominoperineal approach, which is still used in suitable cases. In all previous methods the operation had been done only from below; the Miles operation is commonly performed by two surgeons working together, one from below (the perineal approach) and one from above, through the abdomen.

Femoral hernia repair

Lockwood (1889, UK) and Marcy (1892, USA) described the low femoral approach while Lotheissen (1898, Vienna, Austria) described the inguinal approach. McEvedy (1950, Manchester, UK) introduced the lateral rectus approach. Nyhus in 1955 (USA), after meticulous study of the anatomy of the groin, described the 'preperitoneal approach'. Henry (1936) described the 'midline abdominal approach' as providing good exposure of the femoral rings (discovered accidentally while exposing the lower end of the ureter).

In strangulated hernia, the first objective is to save the patient's life: wound and repair considerations become secondary. The 'pararectus' approach, whether within the rectus sheath (McEvedy) or both within and without (Nyhus), gives direct access to the neck of the sac from above. For the elderly or poor-risk patient, the 'low' approach not involving an abdominal incision has much in its favour. The midline approach has the advantages of simplicity, ample exposure and immediate control of the involved loop of intestine from within the peritoneal cavity. It is the best incision for bilateral femoral hernias. By and large the Nyhus approach is probably the best. The Lotheissen approach should be condemned since it weakens the inguinal area and predisposes to inguinal hernia.

Evolution of gastric resection and Billroth's operation

Avicenna (980–1037) gave the first account of cancer of the stomach. The first detailed memoir on malignant lesions of the stomach was written by Morgagni in 1761.

In 1810 Merrem successfully performed excision of the pylorus in dogs and suggested the possible application of pylorectomy followed by end-to-end gastroduodenostomy in humans. Pean (1879) performed the first gastric resection for cancer. The patient died 4 days later. Billroth (1881) carried out the first successful pyloric resection in the human for carcinoma of the pylorus 71 years after Merrem's work (*see also* Names section). The patient died 4 months later. In the same year, Billroth's assistant Anton Wolfer successfully made the first gastroenterostomy, bypassing the stomach without removal of pyloric growth. This became the method of choice particularly after Courvoisier of Basle (well known for his law in jaundice) introduced the posterior gastroenterostomy in 1883. Connor (1884) attempted the first total gastrectomy on cancer of the stomach. The patient died on the operating table.

Billroth, on 15th January, 1885, performed the first gastric resection with closure of the cut end of the stomach and anterior gastrojejunostomy. As his patient was emaciated and a poor surgical risk owing to the presence of a pyloric cancer, Billroth originally planned to perform a two-stage operation. He envisaged that the first stage would be an anterior gastrojejunostomy and that after a short interval the second stage would be an antrectomy with closure of the open ends of the stomach and duodenum. As the patient withstood the short-circuiting procedures satisfactorily, he proceeded with the gastric resection and with closure of the ends of the stomach and duodenum.

Krönlein, on 24th May, 1888, carried out a one-stage partial gastrectomy with an antecolic anastomosis. Antecolic anastomoses predominated in the early Billroth II variations, but were later replaced by the retrocolic type of anastomosis. Von Fiselsberg (1889) was the first to close the upper end of the gastric pouch to reduce the size of the orifice and then perform an anterior anastomosis between the greater curvature portion of the stomach and a loop of proximal jejunum. Braun and Jaboulay (1892) added an enteroanastomosis between the afferent and efferent limbs of the jejunum.

The retrocolic anastomoses were first used by Hofmeister (1896). Reichel (1908) and Polya (1911) performed partial gastrectomy with retrocolic gastroenterostomy in which the entire open end of the stomach was anastomosed to the side of the proximal loop of jejunum. Here the afferent limb was affixed to the lesser curvature. Eugene Polya of Budapest was one of the first to write about the technical details of partial gastrectomy with retrocolic end-to-side gastrojejunostomy. Polya stated 'The great majority of surgeons, however, did not know of the method at all until I called it to the attention of the surgical world and especially to the attention of William Mayo who saw in it the operation of the future and whose endorsement helped to make it the one most widely adopted'.

Hofmeister (1908) and Finsterer (1914) slightly modified the original Hofmeister procedure. They performed a retrocolic anastomosis, uniting the proximal jejunum to the lower half of the open end of the stomach after closing the top half of the stomach. The short afferent limb of jejunum was buttressed to the closed upper half of the stomach, thus producing a valve effect. This operation is often referred to as the Hofmeister-Polya operation.

Balfour (1917) reported his modification of the Krönlein operation by the performance of a side-to-side enteroanastomosis to overcome the possibility of any vicious-circle vomiting.

Moynihan (1923) reversed the position of the jejunal loop, bringing the loop from the left to the right with the afferent limb to the greater curvature. In Moynihan's original account the anastomosis was antecolic, the proximal jejunal loop was short, certainly not more than 12.7 cm from the ligament of Treitz to the greater curvature.

A few years after the publication of Moynihan's operation it became customary to reduce the size of the gastric stoma by closing the upper third or upper half of the mouth of the gastric remnant towards the lesser curvature, the lower portion of the open end of the stomach towards the greater curvature being used for the gastrojejunal anastomosis. In the Polya modification the cut end of the duodenum is closed, and a loop of jejunum is brought up through an opening in the mesocolon to form an end-to-side anastomosis with the cut end of the stomach.

Coller and associates (1941) concluded that in many cases the associated gastric nodes are inadequately excised because the lesion is extensive and only a palliative operation is done, either because the nodes are not palpable or because the surgeon is not making a conscientious attempt at complete removal of the carcinoma. They also concluded that contiguous lymph nodes need not be involved in order for distant lymphatic involvement to exist.

In 1951, McNeer and associates reviewed necropsy specimens after partial gastrectomy for carcinoma and found recurrence in the gastric remnant in half the cases. They recommended that a more radical operation be attempted, and suggested radical total gastrectomy, partial pancreatectomy (tail) and splenectomy.

In a study reported from the Mayo Clinic in 1953, great attention was paid to lymph node involvement from carcinoma of the stomach. The distance of the involved lymph nodes from the nearest edge of the lesion was found to be of great prognostic significance, as was involvement or non-involvement of the subpyloric lymph nodes.

In 1893 Roentgen discovered X-rays and in 1897 Schiatter performed the first successful total gastrectomy. The patient lived for 14 months. Cuneo (1906) and Jamieson and Dobson, following many dissections, gave the first detailed descriptions (with numerous illustrations) of the lymphatic drainage of the stomach, and these influenced the extent of gastric resections for carcinoma. During 1911–1912 Holzknecht and Hendrick-Forsell (Sweden), Cole (USA), Barclay (UK), and Carman (USA) demonstrated the potential of fluoroscopy and barium meal X-ray examination for diagnosis of cancer of the stomach.

During the early years of this century W. J. Mayo, C. H. Mayo, and Moynihan were extending the scope of partial gastrectomy for malignant lesions of the stomach. Much credit is due to them for their teachings and for their demonstration that the postoperative mortality for gastric resections can be lowered by skill and judgement.

The Wolf-Schindler flexible gastroscope was introduced in 1932. Papanicolaou (1946) introduced the method of diagnosis of malignant growths from exfoliated cells from cancerous lesions. Schoemaker devised a special clamp for closing the lesser curvature portion of the stomach so that the remaining circumference could be approximated to the cut end of the duodenum, as in the Billroth I procedure. C. H. Mayo and W. J. Mayo obtained the same result by using two curved clamps across the lower half of the stomach; the second clamp was placed almost at right angles to the first to take out a portion of the lesser curvature.

Inguinal repair

The modern technique of operations for inguinal hernia started with Bassini (1888) and Halsted (1893). Bassini's operation, which consisted of high excision of the sac and posterior repair of the inguinal canal, was a development of Marcy's operation (1887). Marcy, in *The Anatomy and Surgical Treatment of Hernia* (1892), reported results with his operation that were far superior to anything that had preceded them. Halsted at first divided the internal oblique and transversus abdominis lateral to the internal ring in order to transplant the cord laterally, repairing all the layers behind the cord to Poupart's ligament and leaving the cord subcutaneous. The cutting of the muscles, the so-called lateral cut, which was subsequently revived by Brandon (1945) in the UK and in a different form by Pratt (1948) and by Weiss (1948) in the USA gave poor results, and Halsted accordingly condemned it.

To allow the conjoined tendon and internal oblique to be approximated to Poupart's ligament without tension, a 'relaxation cut' in the anterior rectus sheath may be needed. This 'rectus-relaxing incision of the rectus sheath' or 'slide' received special emphasis from Scott (1905), Fallis (1938), McVay (1939), Reinhoff (1940) and Tanner (1942, UK). In Bloodgood's operation (1919, USA), a flap of anterior rectus sheath and a portion of the rectus muscle itself were brought downwards to cover the 'weak gap' of the inguinal canal and were anchored to the inguinal ligament with interrupted sutures of fine silk. Halsted proved that ligation and exicision of veins from a bulky cord were followed in 20 % of cases by the development of a hydrocele and in some cases by atrophy of the testis. The Wyllys Andrews operation (1895) produced a neat posterior repair, leaving the cord in a newly formed canal between the two flaps of the external oblique aponeurosis.

In 1921 Gallie and Le Mesurier (1921, Canada) described their method of repair with strips of fascia taken from the thigh. However, the recurrence rate was high: 8–10 %. Again, the needle employed for the lattice repair was large and cumbersome and traumatised the fissile inguinal ligament and also the muscular layers through which it had to be passed; doubts were cast as to whether the fascia actually 'lived' in the repair; infection was by no means infrequent, and the long scar in the thigh or the gap in the iliotibial band produced by the fasciotome in some cases gave trouble. Nevertheless, the influence of Gallie's work was profound, and although other methods of radical 'cure' were in use — including excision of the sac only (Hull, 1913), the silver filigree operation of McGavin (1909), the darn-and-stay-lace method of Handley (1918), Seelig and Tuholske's fascia-to-fascia closure (1914) and Wangensteen's pedicled flap of fascia lata reflected from the thigh up to the weak area in the inguinal canal.

In 1937 Ogilvie recognised three types of inguinal hernia:

- Those in which the only abnormality is the presence of a sac.
- Those in which there is, in addition, some stretching of the internal ring, but the muscles of the inguinal sphincter are sound.
- Large indirect and direct hernias in which the sphincter mechanism has obviously failed.

Ogilvie advised the following procedures for the three types noted above:

1. Removal of the sac alone.
2. Excision of the sac with plastic repair of the internal ring.
3. Strong lattice replacement of the inguinal mechanism.

His lattice operation was based on Gallie's operation, using silk in place of fascia. For the same purpose, Maingot (1941) introduced floss silk consisting of the individual fibrils of natural silk, which offered a perfectly pliable framework for subsequent growth of fibroblasts.

In 1973 Glassow introduced the Shouldice Hospital technique of inguinal hernia repair (continous four lines of overlapping sutures).

Pancreatic surgery

Hopes of radical treatment for carcinoma of the pancreas were first raised when Halsted (1899) resected a segment of the second part of the duodenum and a portion of the pancreas for an ampullary carcinoma. He implanted the pancreatic duct and the bile duct in line with the suture of the repair of the posterior wall duodenal defect. His patient died 6 months later from recurrence of the growth. W. J. Mayo (1900), Mayo-Robson (1900), and Koerte (1904) reported limited excisions which were unsuccessful. Successful cases of limited resection of a portion of the duodenum and of the head of the pancreas for cancer were reported by Kausch (1912), Hirschel (1914), and Tenani (1922). In 1935, Whipple, Parsons and Mullins, following a systematic study of the subject and considerable experimental work, published the first report of their successful two-stage procedure for radical en bloc

resection of the duodenum and head of the pancreas for a growth of the ampulla of Vater.

Brunschwig (1937 and 1942) was the first surgeon to perform successfully an extensive radical pancreatoduodenectomy for carcinoma of the head of the pancreas, including the head and the neck of the gland together with 90% of the duodenum. In March 1940 Whipple performed the first recorded one-stage removal of the head of the pancreas and all of the duodenum with occlusion of the pancreatic stump.

Rectal excision

It was J. P. Lockhart-Mummery, in 1907 and 1920, who was responsible for developing perineal excision (a very inadequate method) into a worthwhile cancer operation. He employed loop iliac colostomy, the opportunity being taken at this stage to perform an exploratory laparotomy to assess the operability of the growth from the abdominal aspect and to determine the presence of hepatic or peritoneal deposits. The perineal operation was performed 2 weeks or so later; during the interval the distal bowel was washed out daily from colostomy to anus. For the excision the patient was placed on the left side with the knees drawn up and a wide elliptical incision was made round the anus and extended backwards to the coccyx which was excised.

Sacral excision had been employed by Kocher in 1875, but its introduction into surgical practice was due to Kraske in 1885, and it has been associated with his name ever since. With the patient lying on the left or right side an incision was made from behind the anus over the lower sacrum, usually inclining to one or other side of the midline. By removal of the coccyx and the lowermost two pieces of the sacrum good access was obtained to the back of the rectum above the levator muscles. Inferiorly the dissection was carried as far as necessary, the operation being completed either by excising the entire rectum and anal canal and establishing a sacral anus at the posterior end of the wound — so-called amputation of the rectum — or by removing a sleeve of bowel containing the growth and restoring continuity by end-to-end anastomosis — so-called resection of the rectum. Sacral excision rapidly became the most popular method in Germany and Austria and various modifications of Kraske's original technique were introduced by Billroth and others.

A combined operation involving abdominal and perineal phases for excision of the rectum was first performed by Czerny (1883) not as a premeditated plan but as a means of finishing a sacral excision which he had found himself unable to complete from below. Undoubtedly the work of Ernest Miles (1908) established the abdominoperineal operation in the UK and USA. Following his researches into the mode of spread of rectal cancer, he concluded that a radical excision for this condition, wherever situated in the rectum, ought to embrace the following structures: the entire rectum including the anal canal and sphincters, considerable parts of the levator ani muscles and ischiorectal fat, practically all the sigmoid colon and mesocolon including the superior haemorrhoidal and inferior mesenteric vessels and glands lying in its base, and a portion of the pelvic peritoneum adjacent to the rectum. The great drawback of this operation when first introduced was that it was an extremely shocking procedure with a high initial mortality. Grey Turner in 1920 thought that if the operation were divided into two stages it might be better borne by the patient. The first stage consisted of the establishment of a colostomy alone. However, the method of two-stage combined excision has been abandoned in favour of the one-stage operation.

Gabriel (1934) subsequently developed perineoabdominal excision as a single-stage procedure and became its chief advocate. He considered it to be a less shocking operation than abdominoperineal excision and, for a surgeon familiar with perineal dissections, much simpler to perform than the Miles operation, while achieving a greater removal of bowel and using a terminal colostomy rather than a loop colostomy. With the patient in the left lateral position the rectum is freed from below exactly as in a perineal excision but, instead of dividing the superior haemorrhoidal vessels and bowel in the perineal wound, the mobilised segment is pushed up into the abdominal cavity through the cut in the pelvic peritoneum.

Bloodgood (1906) and Clogg (1923) both suggested that with a suitable arrangement of the patient the abdominal and perineal phases of a combined excision might be performed simultaneously, and both of them described such operations. But it was Kirschner of Heidelberg (1934) who demonstrated conclusively that this was a practicable procedure. Devine (1937) introduced the method afresh to the English-speaking world, and Lloyd-Davies (1939), by devising special adjustable leg rests to support the patient in the lithotomy-Trendelenburg position necessary for a synchronous approach to abdomen and perineum, and elaborating various other refinements of technique, greatly assisted the development of the operation. The advantages claimed for this method are that it saves a considerable amount of operating time, that it makes the removal of very advanced fixed growths easier because their dissection can proceed from above and below simultaneously, and that it greatly facilitates suture of the pelvic peritoneum because this takes place over an empty pelvis and not on top of the divided sigmoid colon, mesocolon and rectum, waiting to be removed from below.

Extended combined excision

Attempts have been made to increase the scope of combined excision still further.

One possibility is higher ligation of the inferior mesenteric vessels with or without extended left colectomy. Miles (1926) recommended that the main ligature should be placed opposite the bifurcation of the abdominal aorta (this tie usually lies just below the origin of the left colic or first sigmoid artery), while Moynihan (1908) and others have recommended tying the inferior mesenteric artery at its origin from the abdominal aorta to avoid leaving this remnant of artery and associated lymphatics.

Multivisceral resections, complete pelvic clearance (total cystoprostatectomy en bloc with rectal excision and urinary diversion) and translumbar amputation have also been tried.

Sphincter-saving resections

Following the work of Dukes (1930, 1940) and others, which showed that the lymphatic spread of rectal cancer is mainly in an upward direction, there was a resurgence of interest in the UK and USA in the possibility of sphincter preservation in the radical excision of carcinomas of the upper rectum and rectosigmoid, and various forms of sphincter-saving resections were revived or developed:

1. Sacral resection.
2. Abdominosacral resection (Pannett, 1935).
● Abdominotranssphincteric (York Mason, 1976).
● Abdominoanal pull-through resection by various methods.
● Abdominotransanal resection with sutured colo-anal sleeve anastomosis (Sir Alan Park, 1972).
● Abdominal or anterior resection.
  —Without anastomosis—Hartmann's operation (1923). The upper end of the rectal stump is closed and a terminal iliac colostomy established.

—With anastomosis—either as *anterior resection with restoration of continuity by telescopic or tube technique* OR *modern anterior resection with sutured anastomosis (hand)*. This procedure has nothing whatever to do with the tube technique and is completed entirely by suture. It could be termed the 'Mayo Clinic operation' (1943, 1945).

High anterior resection, which is applicable to growths of the extreme upper end of the rectum or of the rectosigmoid, can be conducted without disturbing the pelvic peritoneum or mobilising the rectum from the concavity of the sacrum. This type of operation is usually thought to be followed by uneventful healing of the suture line in the bowel and rectal function afterwards is nearly always perfect. Low anterior resection involves opening the pelvic peritoneum, dividing the lateral ligaments and freeing the rectum from its sacral bed often right down to the anorectal ring. The anastomosis is then between the colon and a rectal stump devoid of peritoneal covering. There is a considerable risk of partial breakdown of the suture line, particularly with very low anastomosis. There may be faecal incontinence (at least temporary).

Anastomosis by means of mechanical devices (with metal stapler) has been recently introduced (1965, 1975).

● *Local Removal or Destruction of the Primary Growth*: includes electrocoagulation, endocavitary contact irradiation and local excision.

The currently used operation of choice is either the combined excision or restorative rectal resection (sphincter-saving).

Splenectomy

In the USA, successful splenectomy was first reported by O'Brien (1816) for splenic prolapse following a knife wound. Karl Quittenbaum of Rostock (Germany) performed the first elective splenectomy for primary splenic disease in 1826, but his patient survived only a few hours after the operation. Zaccarelli of Naples (in 1849) is reported to have carried out splenectomy for splenomegaly in a woman aged 24 years. She was discharged from hospital 24 days after the operation. In 1866 Thomas Spencer Wells of London gave an account of the first successful splenectomy in England (1866). It has been reported that Spencer Wells' preoperative diagnosis was 'query ovarian cyst' and that during laparotomy he was surprised to find a 'floating spleen' in the left iliac fossa. He did not hesitate to ligate the long pedicle, divide it with scissors, and remove the congested enlarged 'wandering' organ. J. W. Mayo, in 1928, reported 500 splenectomies carried out by him and his colleagues at the Mayo Clinic, and special attention was devoted to the results and mortality rates.

Vagotomy and antrectomy

Distal gastric resection

At the turn of the century Billroth I began to be employed with increasing frequency for benign ulceration of the distal stomach and duodenum.

Ludwig Rydygier, in November 1881, performed the first pylorectomy with gastroduodenostomy for a benign stenotic chronic pyloric ulcer and the patient lived. Kocher (1893) implanted the end of the duodenum into the posterior wall of the stomach (after the open mouth of the stomach had been closed) in order to avoid the 'angle of sorrow', or Jammerecke. Von Haberer (1922) and Finney (1924) sutured the entire open end of the stomach to the side of the second portion of the duodenum after the duodenal stump had been securely closed and inverted. Schoemaker (1911) was among the first surgeons to extend gastric resection for both malignant and benign lesions of the stomach (as well as for duodenal ulcer) and to excise practically the whole of the lesser curvature prior to the performance of end-to-end gastroduodenostomy. He had no trouble from leakage at the Jammerecke, and his immediate and late results were most gratifying. Von Haberer (1933) performed his reefing and narrowing of the mouth of the gastric stump after partial gastrectomy.

In perforated gastric ulcers suture of the perforation was first suggested by Bernhard Von Langenbeck; he never performed the operation which was first attempted by Mikulicz-Radecki in 1880, but his patient died. Rydygier attempted some form of stomach resection in 1880, but his patient died. The first man certainly to have sutured a perforation with survival of the patient is Ludwig Heusner of Germany in 1892; this operation is sometimes attributed to another German surgeon, Kriege, who reported it. The first attempt in the UK was by Hastings Gilford of Reading in 1893, but his patient died. In the following year T. H. Morse of Norwich succeeded. In 1897 a surgeon named Braun suggested that suture of the perforation ought always to be accompanied by gastroenterostomy. His advice received little or no attention at the time, but in 1929 was resurrected as an original idea by Moynihan in the UK and by Deaver in the USA.

Another method of treating the perforation was by excising the ulcer area and then suturing the incision; first performed by J. W. Dowden in 1909, it was suggested as a routine method by H. Von Haberer of Vienna in 1919. Excision of the ulcer led naturally to excision of a larger portion of the stomach combined with gastroenterostomy, (in other words partial gastrectomy). First suggested by A. Odelberg of Stockholm in 1927, the 'emergency gastrectomy for perforation' was popularised by Doberauer of Carlsbad and Sergei Yudin of Moscow. In 1900 Mayo-Robson of Leeds declared that all peptic ulcers that did not respond to a medical regimen within a reasonable time should be treated surgically. Five years later over 500 gastroenterostomies for peptic ulcer had been performed at the Mayo Clinic alone. In 1905 Berkeley Moynihan published his important book on gastric ulcer, which had a great influence upon methods of treatment. By 1925 doubt was beginning to creep in and there were a few surgeons who had started to speak of gastroenterostomy as a 'surgically produced disease'. Results were sometimes good, but all too often the operation only gave temporary relief because a new ulcer formed at the point of anastomosis of the stomach with the small bowel. Braun first described the 'anastomotic ulcer' in 1899; Mayo-Robson wrote a paper on the subject in 1905, but he still regarded it as a rare complication.

Such outstanding surgeons as Rydygier, Jedlicka, Von Haberer, Clairmont, and Finsterer made valuable contributions and pioneered distal gastric resection for surgical treatment of duodenal ulcer.

Vagotomy

Claude Bernard, in 1858, noted arrest of gastric contractions and absence of gastric secretion following vagal denervation. Pavlov, in 1894, described the absence of hydrochloric acid in fasting gastric secretions following vagotomy, but he was able to produce an acid response with subsequent feedings. He later showed that the vagus nerves supply secretory fibres to the gastric glands and constitute the pathway for stimuli that excite the cephalic phase of gastric secretion.

In 1914, Exner and Schwarzamann were the first to perform vagotomy in a human being via the abdominal route. The operation was done mainly for tabetic crisis and functional gastrointestinal disorders. Gastric atony was clearly recognised as a significant postoperative complication, and would be controlled by passing a tube through the pylorus via a gastrostomy route. Later these investigators added gastroenterostomy. Latarjet, in 1922, advocated vagotomy for benign gastric outlet obstruction and was the first to combine vagotomy with limited pylorectomy. Schiassi, in 1925, added drainage procedures to vagotomy in cases with obstruction. The operation received severe criticism, for in many instances it was performed for various functional disorders with poor results. In addition, during the 1920's there was a rise in popularity of simple gastroenterostomy championed by Berkeley Moynihan of Leeds and William J. Mayo of Rochester. In 1943 Lester Dragstedt produced a challenge to members of the surgical world when he and Owens published an account of two patients with duodenal ulcer treated by transthoracic vagotomy, which resulted in prompt ulcer healing and marked diminution in gastric acid secretion, with a rise in intragastric pH. Similar findings were reported by subsequent investigators.

Combined operation

In 1946, Farmer and Smithwick and their associates in Boston treated 18 patients with duodenal ulcer by vagotomy and removal of approximately 50% of the distal stomach (hemigastrectomy). This combined procedure resulted in marked reductions in the quantity of free acid and hydrogen ion concentration. In January 1947, Leonard Edwards of Nashville, unaware of Smithwick's combined operation performed 3 months earlier, followed the same line of reasoning and carried out truncal vagotomy with approximately 40% resection for a complication of duodenal ulcer. He termed the resection an antrectomy and constructed a retrocolic Billroth II.

Credit should also be given to the outstanding British surgeon, H. Dantree Johnson of London, who in 1947, unaware of the operations performed by Smithwick and Edwards, carried out vagotomy and antrectomy using a Hofmeister type of reconstruction.

To complete the history of the combined operation attention should be directed to the work of Colp and associates, who in 1948 reported satisfactory results with truncal vagotomy and gastrectomy, but the resection entailed removal of approximately 75% of the distal stomach.

Appendix: Normal Values

Blood

Red cell count	$4.8 \pm 1 \times 10^{12}/l$
Haemoglobin	14 ± 2.5 g/dl
Packed cell volume (PCV or haematocrit)	0.38–0.54 (l/l)
Mean corpuscular haemoglobin concentration (MCHC)	33 ± 2 g/dl
Mean corpuscular volume (MCV)	85 ± 8 fl
Mean corpuscular haemoglobin (MCH)	30 ± 2 pg
Reticulocytes	0.2–2%
Leucocytes	$7.5 \pm 3.5 \ 10^9/l$
Prothrombin time	11–15 s
Bleeding time	Up to 11 min

Liver function tests

Bilirubin	2–17 μmol/l
Alkaline phosphatase	25–130 i.u./l
Glutamic oxalo-acetic transaminase (GOT)	10–40 i.u./l
Glutamic pyruvic transaminase (GPT)	<40 i.u./l
α-Hydroxybutyrate dehydrogenase (Hbd)	40–125 i.u./l
Proteins (total)	62–80 g/l
Albumin	35–55 g/l

Thyroid function tests

T_4	58–174 nmol/l
Free thyroxine index (FTI)	58–174
T_3	1.0–2.8 nmol/l
Thyroid-stimulating hormone (TSH)	0.4–3.5 mU/l

Blood gases

Base excess	± 2 mmol/l
Bicarbonate	24–32 mmol/l
Carbon dioxide (P_{CO_2})	4.5–6.1 kPa
Oxygen (P_{O_2})	12–15 kPa
pH	7.36–7.44

Electrolytes and plasma profile

Calcium	2.2–2.67 mmol/l
Phosphate	0.75–1.4 mmol/l
Albumin	34–48 g/l
Glucose (fasting)	4.5–5.8 mmol/l
Urea	1.6–6.7 mmol/l
Creatinine	50–100 μmol/l
Uric acid	0.12–0.42 mmol/l
Chloride	95–105 mmol/l
Potassium	3.5–5.0 mmol/l
Sodium	135–146 mmol/l
Magnesium	0.7–1.1 mmol/l
Zinc	11–18 μmol/l
Iron	14–28 μmol/l

Enzymes, hormones and other plasma parameters

Amylase	<300 s.u./dl
Acid phosphatase	0.8–2.7 i.u./l
Triglycerides	0.84–1.94 mmol/l
Cholesterol	3.6–7.8 mmol/l
Cortisol (09:00)	170–720 nmol/l
(midnight)	55–220 nmol/l
α-Fetoprotein	<10 μg/ml
β-Human chorionic gonadotrophin (HCG)	<15 μg/l
Carcinoembryonic antigen (CEA)	<10 μg/l
γ-Glutamyl transferase (γ-GT)	<50 i.u./l
Parathormone	1–6 i.u./l
Follicle-stimulating hormone (FSH)	0.5–5 u/l
Luteinising hormone (LH)	3–12 u/l
Prolactin	<360 mU/l
Renin activity (lying)	1.14–2.65 pmol/ml per h
(standing)	2.89–4.49 pmol/ml per h
Testosterone (males)	10–34 nmol/l
Osmolality	280–300 mmol/kg

Cerebrospinal fluid (CSF)

Protein	0.1–0.4 g/l
Glucose	2.8–4.5 mmol/l

Faeces

Fat	<18 mmol/24 h

Urine

Calcium	<8 mmol/24 h
Catecholamines (free) (as noradrenaline)	0.69 μmol/24 h

Creatinine	9–18 mmol/24 h	Potassium	35–90 mmol/24 h
Creatinine clearance	70–140 ml/min	Protein	<0.1 g/24 h
5-Hydroxyindole-acetic		Sodium	100–260 mmol/24 h
acid (5-HIAA)	< 52 μmol/24 h	Urea	200–600 mmol/24 h
Magnesium	3.5–15 mmol/24 h	Uric acid	1.5–6.3 mmol/24 h
Oxalate	0.14–0.46 mmol/24 h	Vanillylmandelic acid	
Phosphate	16–50 mmol/24 h	(VMA)	10–35 μmol/24 h

References and Further Reading

Nutrition in surgery

Jung R. (1981). Nutrition (annual review). *Hospital Update*; **7**: 883–898.

Silk D. B. A. (1978). Parenteral nutrition. *Hospital Update*; **4**: 611–622.

Silk D. B. A. (1980). Enteral nutrition. *Hospital Update*; **6**: 761–776.

Phillips V., Galbally B. P. (1984). *Guide to Parenteral Nutrition*. Ealing Health District.

Yarborough M. F., Curreri P. W. (1981). *Surgical Nutrition*. Edinburgh: Churchill Livingstone.

Critical review of peptic ulcer management

Johnston D. (1980). Treatment of peptic ulcer and its complications. In *Recent Advances in Surgery*, No. 10 (Taylor S., ed) pp 355–410. Edinburgh: Churchill Livingstone.

Critical review of breast cancer management

Baum M. (1980). Carcinoma of the breast. In *Recent Advances in Surgery*, No. 10. (Taylor S., ed) pp 241–258. Edinburgh: Churchill Livingstone.

Baum M. (1981). *Breast Cancer*. London: Update Publications.

Forrest A. P. M. (1969). Cancer of the breast. In *Recent Advances in Surgery*, No. 7 (Taylor S., ed) pp 84–125. London: J & A Churchill.

Preece P. E., Wood R. A. B., Mackie C. R., Cushieri A. (1982). Tamoxifen as initial sole treatment of localised breast cancer in elderly women: a pilot study. *British Medical Journal*; **284**: 869–870.

Rossi A, Bonadonna G., Valagussa P., Verunesi V. (1981). Multimodal treatment in operable cancer: five year results of the CMF programme. *British Medical Journal*; **282**: 1427–1431.

Steele R. J. C. (1983). The axillary lymph nodes in breast cancer. *Journal of the Royal College of Surgeons of Edinburgh*; **28**: 282–291.

Webster D. J. T. (1984). Early breast cancer. *Surgery*; **6**: 128–131.

Critical review of abdominal stoma

Alexander-Williams J., Irving Miles (1982). *Intestinal Fistulae*. Bristol: Wright PSG.

Abbott Laboratories (1983). *An Introduction to Stoma Care*. Kent: Abbott Laboratories.

Breckman, B. (1981). *Stoma Care*. Beaconsfield Publishers Ltd.

Everett W. G. (1978). Ileostomies and their problems. *Hospitl Update*; **4**: 355–363.

Spraggon E. M. (1975). *Urinary Diversion Stomas*, 2nd edn. Edinburgh: Churchill Livingstone.

Todd I. P. (1980). A critical review of stomas, stomatherapy and newer operative techniques. In *Recent Advances in Surgery*, No. 10. (Taylor S., ed) pp 281–292. Edinburgh: Churchill Livingstone.

Early gastric carcinoma

Doll R., Nolan D. J., Piris J., *et al* (1978). Cancer of the stomach. In *Topics in Gastroenterology – 6*, (Trulove S. C., Heyworth, M. F. eds) pp 117–220. Oxford: Blackwell Scientific Publications.

Clinical aspects of obstructive jaundice

Al-Fallouji M. A. R., Collins R. E. C. (1985). Surgical relief of obstructive jaundice in district general hospital. *Journal of Royal Society of Medicine*; **78**: 211–216.

Blamey S. L. *et al.* (1983). Prediction of risk in biliary surgery. *British Journal of Surgery*; **70**: 535–538.

Shock in surgery

Hanson G. C. (1978). *Management of Septic Shock*. Middlesex: Glaxo Laboratories Ltd.

Ledingham I., McArdle C. S., MacDonald R. C. (1980). Septic shock. In *Recent Advances in Surgery*, No. 10. (Taylor S., ed) pp 161–200. Edinburgh: Churchill Livingstone.

Urological topics, e.g. urinary stone, cancer of kidney, bladder, prostate, testis and urinary diversions

Bishop M. C. (1982). Surgical aspects of stone disease (1) and (2). *Hospital Update*; **8**: 503–510, 631–638.

Blandy J. P., Oliver R. T. (1984). Cancer of the testis. *British Journal of Surgery*; **71**: 962–963.

Hendry (1982). The diagnosis and treatment of renal cell carcinoma. *Hospital Update*; **8**: 785–798.

Lancet (1979). Improved management of testicular tumours (leading article). *Lancet*; **i**: 840.

Oliver R. T. D. (1984). Testis cancer. *British Journal of Hospital Medicine*; **31**: 23–35.

Riddle P. R. (1981). Urothelial tumours. *Hospital Update*; **7**: 909–922.

Malignant melanoma

Barclay T. L. (1980). Cutaneous malignant melanoma, the current position. A lecture delivered at a Surgical Meeting, Halifax, W. Yorkshire.

Davis N. C. (1985). Melanoma—issues of importance to the clinician. *British Journal of Hospital Medicine*; **33**: 166–169.

McCarthy W. H. (1982). Malignant melanoma. In *Recent Advances in Surgery*, No. 11 (Russell R., ed) pp 85–100. Edinburgh: Churchill Livingstone.

Union Internationale Contre le Cancer (UICC) (1978). *Clinical Oncology*, 2nd edn, pp 85–104. Berlin: Springer-Verlag.

Reflux oesophagitis

Cohen S., Snaper W. J. (1978). The pathophysiology and treatment of gastro-oesophageal reflux disease. *Archives of Internal Medicine*; **138**: 1398–1401.

Shackeleford R. T. (1978). Reflux oesophagitis. In *Surgery of the Alimentary Tract*, pp 280–433. Philadelphia, London: W. B. Saunders Company.

Sutures in surgery

Ethicon (1982). *Suture Use Manual*. Ethicon, Inc.

Ethicon (1982). *PDS*. Ethicon, Inc.

Holmlund D., Tera H., Wiberg Y., Zederfeldt B., Aberg C. (1978). *Sutures and Techniques for Wound Closure*. New York: Naimark & Barba Inc.

Introduction to clinical oncology

Union Internationale Contre le Cancer (UICC) (1978). *Clinical Oncology*, 2nd edn, pp 3–115. Berlin: Springer-Verlag.

Wiltshire C. R., Bleehen N. M. (1977). Clinical oncology. Introduction. *Hospital Update*; **3**: 451–460.

Radiotherapy

Union Internationale Contre le Cancer (UICC) (1978). *Clinical Oncology*, 2nd edn, pp 81–85. Berlin: Springer-Verlag.

Walter J. (1977). *Cancer and Radiotherapy*, 2nd edn. Edinburgh: Churchill Livingstone.

Chemotherapy

Priestman T. J. (1977). *Cancer Chemotherapy—An Introduction*. Barnet: Montedison Pharmaceutical Ltd.

The Royal Society of Medicine (1982). *Aminoglutethimide—An Alternative Endocrine Therapy for Breast Carcinoma*. (Elsdon-Dew R. W., Jackson I. M., Birdwood G. F. B., eds) London: Academic Press.

Rustin G. J. S. (1983). New ideas in cancer therapy—retinoids. *Hospital Update*; **9**: 1091–1098.

Sikord K., Smedley H. (1983). Interferon and cancer. *British Medical Journal*; **286**: 739–740.

Tumour markers and cancer screening in surgery

Bloom S. R. (1979). Alimentary hormones. *Medicine*; **15**: 733–736.

Buckman R. (1982). Tumour markers in clinical practice. *British Journal of Hospital Medicine*; **27**: 9–20.

Chamberlain J. (1982). Screening for cancer. *British Journal of Hospital Medicine*; **27**: 583–591.

Forrest A. P. M., Hawkins R. A. (1983). Hormone receptors and breast cancer—an occasional survey. *Scottish Medical Journal*; **28**: 228–238.

Neville A. M. *et al.* (1979). Biological markers and human neoplasia. In *Recent Advances in Histopathology*, No. 10 (Anthony P. P., Woolf N., eds) pp 23–44. Edinburgh: Churchill Livingstone.

Nerve injury and entrapment

Dickson R. A. (1978). Nerve repair. *British Journal of Hospital Medicine*; **2**: 295–305.

Emerson J. (1981). Peripheral nerve injury. *Hospital Update*; **7**: 595–606.

Abdominal wound dehiscence

Schwartz S. I. (1974). Complications. In *Principles of Surgery*, 2nd edn. (Schwartz S. I., Lillehei R. C., Shires G. H. *et al.*, eds) pp 461–490. New York: McGraw-Hill (A Blakiston Publication).

Deep vein thrombosis and pulmonary embolism

Handley A. (1981). Pulmonary embolism and infection. In *Thoracic Medicine* (Emerson P., ed.) pp 761–775. London: Butterworths.

Hirsh J. (1981). Prevention of deep venous thrombosis. *British Journal of Hospital Medicine*; **26**: 143–148.

Pulmonary complications after major abdominal operation

Schwartz S. I. (1974). Complications. In *Principles of Surgery*, 2nd edn. (Schwartz S. I., Lillehei R. C., Shires G. H. *et al.*, eds) pp 461–490. New York: McGraw-Hill (A Blakiston Publication).

Acute pancreatitis

Carter D. (1983). Gallstone pancreatitis. *Hospital Update*; **9**: 879–894.

Collins R. E. C., Frost S. J., Spittlehouse K. E. (1982). The P_3 iso-enzyme of serum amylase in the management of patients with acute pancreatitis. *British Journal of Surgery*; **69**: 373–375.

De Jode L. R. J. (1977). Acute pancreatitis. In *Recent Advances in Surgery*, No. 9 (Taylor S., ed) pp 83–112. Edinburgh: Churchill Livingstone.

McMahon M. J., Playforth M. S., Pickford I. R. (1980). A comparative study of methods for the prediction of severity of attacks of acute pancreatitis. *British Journal of Surgery*; **67**: 22–25.

Management of chronic inflammatory bowel disease

Badenoch D., Thomson J. P. S. (1983). Surgery for ulcerative colitis. *Hospital Update*; **9**: 841–851.

Keighley M. R. B., Ambrose N. S. (1982). Surgical Considerations of Crohn's Disease. In *Recent Advances in Surgery*, No. 11 (Russell R., ed) pp 197–208. Edinburgh: Churchill Livingstone.

Springall R., Thomson J. P. S. (1984). Surgery for Crohn's disease. *Hospital Update*; **10**: 501–516.

Stroke and surgery

Lumley J. (1980). Techniques of improving the blood flow to the brain. In *Recent Advances in Surgery*, No. 9 (Taylor S., ed) pp 113–134. Edinburgh: Churchill Livingstone.

Lumley J. S. P., Taylor G. W. (1977). Surgery for stroke. In *Recent Advances in Surgery*, No. 9 (Taylor S., ed), pp 395–422. Edinburgh: Churchill Livingstone.

Peripheral vascular disease

Campbell W. B. (1982). The ischaemic lower limb (1) and (2). *Hospital Update*; **8**: 473–484, 549–562.

Dunn D. C. (1981). Vascular surgery (annual review). *Hospital Update*; **7**: 563–576.

Common surgical conditions affecting the hip joint

Burchholz H. W., Elson R., Loden Kamper H. (1979). The infected joint implant. In *Recent Advances in Orthopaedics*, No. 3 (McKibbin B., ed) Edinburgh: Churchill Livingstone.

Catterall A. (1971). The natural history of Perthes disease. *Journal of Bone and Joint Surgery*; **53**: 37.

Charnley J. (1979). *Low Friction Arthroplasty of the Hip: Theory and Practice*. Berlin: Springer-Verlag.

Coleman S. S. (1983). Reconstructive procedures in congenital dislocation of the hip. In *Recent Advances in Orthopaedics*, No. 4 (McKibbin B., ed). Edinburgh: Churchill Livingstone.

Dimon J., Hughston J. (1967). Unstable intertrochanteric fractures of the hip. *Journal of Bone and Joint Surgery*; **49A**: 440–450.

Duthie R. B., Bentley G. (1983). *Mercer's Orthopaedic Surgery*, 8th edn. London: Edward Arnold.

Elson R. A. (ed:) (1981). *Revision Arthroplasty*: Proceedings of a symposium held at Sheffield University March 22–24 1979, 2nd edn. Oxford: Medical Education Services Ltd.

Freeman M. A. R. (1975). General considerations in the design of prostheses for the 'total' replacement of joints. In *Recent Advances in Orthopaedics* (McKibbin B., ed). Edinburgh: Churchill Livingstone.

Garden D. L. (1983). The nature and cause of osteoarthrosis. *British Medical Journal*; **286**: 418–424.

Garden R. S. (1961a). The structure and function of the proximal end of the femur. *Journal of Bone and Joint Surgery*; **43B**: 576–589.

Garden R. S. (1961b). Low angle fixation in fractures of the femoral neck. *Journal of Bone and Joint Surgery*; **43B**: 647–663.

McRae R. (1983). *Clinical Orthopaedic Examination*, 2nd edn. Edinburgh: Churchill Livingstone.

May J., Chacha P. B. (1968). Displacement of trochanteric fractures and their influence on reduction. *Journal of Bone and Joint Surgery*; **50B**: 318–323.

Sharrard W. J. W. (1979). *Paediatric Orthopaedics and Fractures*, 2nd edn. Oxford: Blackwell Scientific Publications.

Wilson J. N. (ed:) (1982). *Watson–Jones Fractures and Joint Injuries*, Vol. 2, 6th edn. Edinburgh: Churchill Livingstone.

Gastrointestinal precancerous and predisposing conditions

Anthony P. P., Woolf N. (1980). *Recent Advances in Histopathology*, No. 10. Edinburgh: Churchill Livingstone.

Duncan W. (1982). *Colorectal Cancer (Recent Results in Cancer Research)*. Berlin: Springer-Verlag.

Gibson J. B. (1983). Primary cancers of the liver. *Journal of the Royal College of Surgeons of Edinburgh*; **28**: 275–281.

Gordis L., Gold E. (1984). Epidemiology of pancreatic cancer. *World Journal of Surgery*; **8**: 808–821.

Clinical implications of contraceptive pill

Anthony P. P., Woolf N. (1980). *Recent Advances in Histopathology*, No. 10. pp 23–44. Edinburgh: Churchill Livingstone.

Antimicrobials in surgery

International Symposium (1983). *Serious Infections— Treatment and Prevention (A Review)*. London: Update Publications.

Tenenbaum M. J., Kaplan M. H. (1982). Antibiotic combinations. *Medical Clinics of North America*; **66**: 17–24.

Solitary thyroid nodule

Beahrs O. H. (1984). Surgical treatment for thyroid cancer. *British Journal of Surgery*; **71**: 976–979.

Illingworth Sir Charles, Dick Bruce M. (1979). *A Textbook of Surgical Pathology*, 12th edn, p. 66. Edinburgh: Churchill Livingstone.

Surgical treatment of obesity

Joffe S. N. (1979). Surgical approach to morbid obesity. *Hospital Update*; **5**: 869–884.

Multiple injuries, abdominal trauma, thoracic trauma and cerebrospinal trauma

Brewes P. C. (1983). Open and closed abdominal injuries. *British Journal of Hospital Medicine*; **29**: 402–411.

Carter D., Polk H. C. (1981). *Trauma* (Surgery 1—Butterworths International Medical Reviews). London: Butterworth.

Crackard H. A. (1982). Early management of head injuries. *British Journal of Hospital Medicine*; **27**: 635–646.

Evans D. K. (1984). Injuries of the cervical spine. *Surgery*; **1**: 76–79.

Galbraith S. L., Teasdale G. M. (1982). Head injuries. In *Recent Advances in Surgery*, No. 11 (Russell R., ed) pp 71–84. Edinburgh: Churchill Livingstone.

Lindsay K. W. (1984). Clinical assessment after brain damage. *Surgery*; **1**: 80–85.

Medical imaging and interventional radiology

Athanasoulis C. A., Pfister R. C., Greene R. E., Robertson E. H. (1982). *Interventional Radiology*. Philadelphia: W. B. Saunders

Cumberland D. (1982). *Percutaneous Transluminal Angioplasty*. Nyegaard UK Ltd.

De Lacey G. (1983). How to make the best use of your X-ray Department. *Hospital Update*; **9**: 455–468.

Dixon A. K. (1982). Computed tomography for abdominal masses. *Hospital Update*; **8**: 575–590.

Golding S. (1984). Indications for computed tomography of the chest. *Hospital Update*; **10**: 237–251.

Granowska M., Britton, K. (1981). Nuclear medicine. *Hospital Update*; **7**: 1239–1250.

Jones P. (1984). Intubation for ureteric obstruction. *Hospital Update*; **10**: 167–180.

Kreel L. (1979). *Medical Imaging: a Basic Course*. London: HM & M Publishers.

Oliver D. E. (1984). Pulsed electromagnetic energy—What is it? *Physiotherapy*; **70**: 458–459.

McPherson G. A. D., Benjamin I. S., Hodgson H. J. F., Bowley N. B., Allison D. J., Blumgart L. H. (1984). Preoperative percutaneous transhepatic biliary drainage: the results of a controlled trial. *British Journal of Surgery*; **71**: 371.

Steiner R. E. (ed) (1983). *Recent Advances in Radiology and Medical Imaging*, No. 7. Edinburgh: Churchill Livingstone.

Some important paediatric problems

Dykes P. W., Kieghly M. R. B. (1981). *Gastrointestinal Bleeding*. Bristol: John Wright.

Smiddy F. G. (1980). *The Investigation of the Surgical Patient*. London: Edward Arnold.

Pain in surgery

Hanningington-Kiff J. G. (1981). *Pain*, 2nd edn. London: Update Publications.

Schachter M. (1981). Enkephalins and endorphins. *British Journal of Hospital Medicine*; **25**: 128–236.

Paths to Pain Relief (Filmstrip) 1978. Winthrop Laboratories.

Postoperative analgesia

White D. C. (1982). The Relief of postoperative pain. In *Recent Advances in Anaesthesia and Analgesia*, No. 14 (Atkinson R. S., Langton Hewer C., eds) pp 121–140. Edinburgh: Churchill Livingstone.

Terminal care in surgery

The Drug Information Service (Leeds Health) (1980). Care of the Dying Patient, Part 1. *Drug Information Bulletin*; March 1980, **11**: 1–10.

The Drug Information Service (Leeds Health) (1980). Care of the Dying Patient, Part 2. *Drug Information Bulletin*; April 1980, **11**: 1–8.

Lyon H. (1982). *Terminal Care*. London: Update Publications.

Saunders D. C. (1982). Principles of symptom control in terminal care. *Medical Clinics of North America*; **66**: 1169–1183.

Diabetes and surgery

Gill G. V., Sherif I. H., Alberti K. G. (1981). Management of diabetes during open heart surgery. *British Journal of Surgery*; **68**: 171–172.

Podolsky S. (1982). Management of diabetes in the surgical patient. *Medical Clinics of North America*; **66**: 1361–1373.

Portal hypertension

Dawson J. L. (1977). Portal hypertension. In *Recent Advances in Surgery*, No. 9 (Taylor S., ed) pp 55–82. Edinburgh: Churchill Livingstone.

Endoscopy and clinical surgery

Grossman M. B. (1980). *Gastrointestinal Endoscopy*. CIBA Clinical Symposium Vol. 32, No. 3.

Swan C. H. J. (1982). *A Handbook of Gastrointestinal Endoscopy*. Stoke-on-Trent: The British Society of Gastroenterology.

Vallon A. G. (1982). Lasers and fibreoptic endoscopy. *British Journal of Hospital Medicine*; **26**: 175–179.

Bleeding in surgery

Cohen J. (1984). AIDS—a review. *British Journal of Hospital Medicine*; **31**: 250–260.

Dalgleish A. (1985). AIDS. *Hospital Doctor*. C5 May 16 and May 23.

Samson D. (1976). The bleeding patient. *Hospital Update*; **2**: 185–196.

Walter J. B., Israel M. S. (1974). *General Pathology*, pp 613–625. Edinburgh: Churchill Livingstone.

Surgery in ischaemic heart disease

Hakin M., Wallwork J. (1985). Surgery for ischaemic heart disease. *Hospital Update*; **11**: 57–67.

Raphael M. J., Donaldson R. M. (1985). Coronary transluminal angiography. *British Journal of Hospital Medicine*; **33**: 18–23.

Burns management and principles of skin grafting

Hackett M. E. J. (1980). Management during the first 48 hours. *Hospital Update*; **6**: 963–976.

Harrison D. H. (1980). Microvascular surgery. *Hospital Update*; **6**: 235–248.

Settle J. A. D. (1974). *Burns: the first 48 hours*. Essex: Smith & Nephew Pharmaceutical Ltd.

Restorative resection of carcinoma of the rectum

Al-Fallouji, M. A. R. (1984). The surgical anatomy of the colorectal intramural blood supply. *Vascular Surgery*; **18**: 364–371.

Al-Fallouji M. A. R., Tagart R. E. B. (1985). The surgical anatomy of colonic intramural blood supply and its influence on colorectal anastomosis. *Journal of the Royal College of Surgeons of Edinburgh*; **30**: 380–385.

British Medical Journal (1980). Prophylaxis of surgical wound sepsis (editorial). *British Medical Journal*; **280**: 1063–1064.

Chassin J. L. (1980). Colon resection. In *Operative Strategy in General Surgery*, Vol. 1 (Chassin J. L., ed) pp 274–280. New York, Berlin: Springer-Verlag.

Dudley H. A. F., Radcliffe A. G., McGeehan D. (1980). Intra-operative irrigation of the colon to permit primary anastomosis. *British Journal of Surgery*; **67**: 80–81.

Ethicon (1982). *Suture Use Manual*. Ethicon.

Everett N. G. (1975). A comparison of one layer and two layer techniques for colorectal anastomosis. *British Journal of Surgery*; **62**: 135–140.

Fielding L. P., Stewart–Brown S., Blesovsky L. *et al.* (1980). Anastomotic integrity after operation for large bowel cancer: a multi-centre study. *British Medical Journal*; **281**: 411–414.

Gilmour D. G., Aitkenhead A. R., Hothersall A. P. *et al.* (1980). The effect of hypovolaemia on colonic blood flow in the dog. *British Journal of Surgery*; **67**: 82–84.

Goligher J. C. (1979). Recent trends in the practice of sphincter-saving excision for rectal carcinoma. *Annals of the Royal College of Surgeons of England*; **61**: 169–176.

Goligher J. C., Lee P. W. G., Simpkins K. C., Lintott D. J. (1977). A controlled comparison of one-layer and two-layer techniques of suture for high and low colorectal anastomosis. *British Journal of Surgery*; **64**: 609–614.

Goligher J. C., Morris C., McAdam W. A. F. *et al.* (1970). A controlled trial of inverting versus everting intestinal suture in clinical large-bowel surgery. *British Journal of Surgery*; **57**: 817–822.

Hewitt J., Reeve J., Rigby J. *et al.* (1973). Whole-gut irrigation in preparation for large-bowel surgery. *Lancet*; **2**: 337–340.

Irvin T. T., Edwards J. P. (1973). Comparison of single-layer inverting, two-layer inverting, and everting anastomoses in the rabbit colon. *British Journal of Surgery*; **60**: 453–457.

Irvin T. T., Goligher J. C. (1973). Aetiology of disruption of intestinal anastomoses. *British Journal of Surgery*; **60**: 461–464.

Khoury G. A., Waxman B. P. (1983). Large bowel anastomosis. *British Journal of Surgery*; **70**: 61–63.

Matheson N. A., Irving A. D. (1975). Single layer anastomosis after rectosigmoid resection. *British Journal of Surgery*; **62**: 239–242.

Orr N. W. M. (1969). A single-layer intestinal anastomosis. *British Journal of Surgery*; **56**: 771–774.

Schrock T. R., Deveney C. W., Dunphy J. E. (1973). Factors contributing to leakage of colonic anastomoses. *Annals of Surgery*; **177**: 513–518.

Sharefkin J., Joff, N. *et al.* (1978). Anastomotic dehiscence after low anterior resection of rectum. *American Journal of Surgery*; **135**: 519–523.

Stewart R. (1973). Influence of malignant cells on healing of colonic anastomoses: experimental observations. *Proceedings of the Royal Society of Medicine*; **66**: 1089–1091.

Tagart R. E. B. (1981). Colorectal anastomosis: factors influencing success. *Journal of the Royal Society of Medicine*; **74**: 111–118.

Tagart R. E. B. (1982). Colorectal anastomosis: factors influencing success. In *Colo-rectal Surgery* (Heberer G., Denecke H., eds) pp 149–154. Berlin: Springer-Verlag.

Hand injuries

McGregor I. A. (1980). *Fundamental Techniques of Plastic Surgery*, 7th edn, pp 236–271. Edinburgh: Churchill Livingstone.

Hypercalcaemia and primary hyperparathyroidism

Lavelle M. A. (1984). Parathyroidectomy. *British Journal of Hospital Medicine*; **31**: 204–208.

Surgery for incontinence

Ball T. P. (1983). Male urinary incontinence. In *Urologic Surgery* (Glenn J. F., ed.) pp 1003–1018. Philadelphia: J. B. Lippincott.

Corman M. L. (1983). The management of anal incontinence. *Surgical Clinics of North America*; **83**: 177–192.

Henry M. M. (1981). Incontinence of faeces. *British Journal of Hospital Medicine*; **25**: 232–235.

Malvern J. (1981). Incontinence of urine in women. *British Journal of Hospital Medicine*; **25**: 224–231.

Park A. (1980). The rectum. In *Davis–Christopher Textbook of Surgery*, pp 989–1002. New York, Toronto: W. B. Saunders.

Rosen M. (1981). Male urinary incontinence. *British Journal of Hospital Medicine*; **25**: 215–223.

Waterhouse R. K. (1983). Vesicovaginal and vesicointestinal fistulas. In *Urologic Surgery* (Glenn J. F., ed.) pp 609–615. Philadelphia: J. B. Lippincott.

Webster G. D. (1983). Female urinary incontinence. In *Urologic Surgery* (Glenn J. F., ed.) pp 665–679. Philadelphia: J. B. Lippincott.

Operative surgery

See Part II, Section 4.

Principles and practice

See Part II, Section 4.

Clinical surgery

Clain A. (ed) (1980). *Hamilton Bailey's Demonstrations of Physical Signs in Clinical Surgery*, 16th edn. Bristol: John Wright.

Hunter D., Bomford R. R. (eds) (1980). *Hutchison's Clinical Methods*. London: Baillière Tindall.

Surgical pathology

See Part II, Section 4.

Royal Colleges of Surgeons

England

Correspondence letter from the Royal College of Surgeons of England.

Edinburgh

Bruce J. (1961). The Royal College of Surgeons of Edinburgh. *Scottish Medical Journal*; **6**: 578–587.

Glasgow

Illingworth Sir C. (1980). *Royal College of Physicians and Surgeons of Glasgow*. Glasgow: William Hodge.

Ireland

Lyons J. B., O'Flanagan H., MacGowan W. A. (1982). *The Irresistible Rise of the Royal College of Surgeons of Ireland*. Dublin: RCSI

The causes of failure, What to read and What to do

Pietroni M. (1983). Postgraduate diplomas FRCS Part II. *British Journal of Hospital Medicine*; **29**: 337–338.

Sewell I. A. (1982). A guide to final FRCS examinations. *Hospital Update*; **8**: 965–974.

Historical background

Cartwright F. F. (1967). *The Development of Modern Surgery*. London: Arthur Barker Ltd.

Ellis H. (1984). *Famous Operations*. Harwal Publishing Co. Media, Pa.

Meade R. H. (1968). *An Introduction to the History of General Surgery*. Philadelphia: W. B. Saunders.

See Part II, Section 4.

INDEX